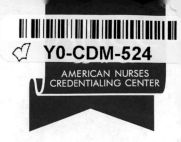

NURSING REVIEW AND RESOURCE MANUAL

Family Nurse Practitioner

Published by American Nurses Credentialing Center
Edited by Elizabeth Blunt, PhD, MSN, FNP-BC

CONTINUING EDUCATION SOURCE
NURSING CERTIFICATION REVIEW MANUAL
CLINICAL PRACTICE RESOURCE

3RD EDITION

Library of Congress Cataloging-in-Publication Data
Family nurse practitioner : review and resource manual. — 3rd ed. / edited by Elizabeth Blunt.
p. ; cm.
Includes bibliographical references and index.

1.Family nursing--Examinations, questions, etc. 2. Nurse practitioners—Examinations, questions, etc.
3. Nurses—Licenses—United States—Examinations—Study guides. I. Blunt, Elizabeth. II. American
Nurses Credentialing Center.
[DNLM: 1. Family Nursing—Examination Questions. WY 18.2 F1986 2009]

RT120.F34F3538 2009
610.73076—dc22
2008054088

ISBN 13: 978-0-9793811-5-7
ISBN 10: 0-9793811-5-0
© 2009 American Nurses Credentialing Center.
8515 Georgia Ave., Suite 400
Silver Spring, MD 20910
www.nursecredentialing.org
All rights reserved.

Family Nurse Practitioner Review and Resource Manual, 3rd Edition

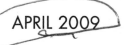

APRIL 2009

Please direct your comments and/or queries to: revmanuals@ana.org

The healthcare services delivery system is a volatile marketplace demanding superior knowledge, clinical skills, and competencies from all registered nurses. Nursing autonomy of practice and nurse career marketability and mobility in the new century hinge on affirming the profession's formative philosophy, which places a priority on a lifelong commitment to the principles of education and professional development. The knowledge base of nursing theory and practice is expanding, and while care has been taken to ensure the accuracy and timeliness of the information presented in the *Family Nurse Practitioner Review and Resource Manual, 3rd Edition*, clinicians are advised to always verify the most current national guidelines and recommendations and to practice in accordance with professional standards of care used with regard to the unique circumstances that apply in each practice situation. In addition, every effort has been made in this text to ensure accuracy and, in particular, to confirm that drug selections and dosages are in accordance with current recommendations and practice, including the ongoing research, changes to government regulations, and the developments in product information provided by pharmaceutical manufacturers. However, it is the responsibility of each nurse practitioner to verify drug product information and to practice in accordance with professional standards of care. In addition, the editors wish to note that provision of information in this text does not imply an endorsement of any particular products, procedures or services.

Therefore, the authors, editors, American Nurses Association (ANA), American Nurses Association's Publishing (ANP), American Nurses Credentialing Center (ANCC), and the Institute for Credentialing Innovation cannot accept responsibility for errors or omissions, or for any consequences or liability, injury, and/or damages to persons or property from application of the information in this manual and make no warranty, express or implied, with respect to the contents of the *Family Nurse Practitioner Review and Resource Manual, 3rd Edition*.

Published by:
The Institute for Credentialing Innovation
8515 Georgia Avenue, Suite 400
Silver Spring, MD 20910-3402
www.nursecredentialing.org

Introduction to the Continuing Education (CE) Contact Hour Application Process for *Family Nurse Practitioner Review and Resource Manual*, 3rd Edition

The Institute for Credentialing Innovation now offers the continuing education contact hours for this manual online at www.NursingWorld.org, the American Nurses Association's Web site. This process involves answering approximately 25–30 questions that test knowledge of the information contained within this manual. The continuing education contact hours can be completed at any time and a certificate can be printed from the Web site immediately upon successful completion of the test.

The *Family Nurse Practitioner Review and Resource Manual, 3rd Edition*, is designed to meet the following objectives:
1. Analyze professional issues in advanced nursing practice.
2. Compare and contrast the epidemiology, risk factors, and screening tests related to select health problems across the life span.
3. Propose patient education, health promotion, and disease prevention strategies for health problems across the life span.
4. Integrate knowledge of the pathophysiology of common acute and chronic health problems in the clinical management of clients across the life span.

5. Propose diagnostic and treatment/management approaches for select health problems across the life span.
6. Interpret and apply information from evidence-based research.

Upon completion of this manual and the online CE test, a nurse can receive a total of 61 continuing education contact hours at a price of $95. (ANA members receive a discount on CEs.) The entire process—online test and evaluation form—must be completed by December 31, 2011 in order to receive credit. **To begin the process, please e-mail revmanuals@ana.org.** Your patience with this process is greatly appreciated.

Inquiries or Comments

If you have any questions about the CE contact hours, please e-mail The Institute at revmanuals@ana.org. You may also mail any comments to Editor/Project Manager, at the address listed below.

Duplicate CE Certificates

Once you have successfully passed the CE test on NursingWorld, you may go back and re-print your certificate as often as you wish.

The Institute for Credentialing Innovation
American Nurses Credentialing Center, Attn: Editor/Project Manager
8515 Georgia Avenue, Suite 400
Silver Spring, MD 20910-3492
Fax: (301) 628-5342

The American Nurses Association is accredited as a provider of continuing nursing education by the American Nurses Credentialing Center's Commission on Accreditation.
ANA is approved by the California Board of Registered Nursing, Provider Number 6178.

Contents

Acknowledgements

The authors would like to acknowledge the editors of the previous edition of this manual for their hard work:

Marilyn W. Edmunds, PhD, ANP, GNP
Maren S. Mayhew, MS, ANP, GNP
Laurie Scudder, MS, PNP
Zoe O'Brien, MS, PNP

Family Nurse Practitioner Review and Resource Manual

3RD EDITION

Taking the Certification Examination

Elizabeth Blunt, PhD, MSN, FNP-BC

When you sign up to take a national certification exam, you will receive a packet of information from the testing agency. Review it carefully and keep it where you can frequently refer to it. It will contain information on test content and sample questions. This is critical information; review it carefully and it will give you insight into the nature of the test. The agency will also send you materials authorizing your entry into the exam. Keep these in a safe place until needed.

GENERAL SUGGESTIONS FOR PREPARING FOR THE EXAM

Step One: Control Your Anxiety
Everyone experiences anxiety when faced with the certification exam.
- Remember, your program was designed to prepare you to take this exam.
- Your instructors took a similar exam, and have probably talked to students who took exams more recently, so they know how to help you prepare.
- Taking a review course or setting up your own study plan will help you feel more confident about taking the exam.

Step Two: Do Not Listen to Gossip About the Exam

A large volume of information exists about the tests based on reports from people who have taken the exams in the past. Because information from the testing facilities is limited, it is hard not to listen to this gossip.

- Remember that gossip about the exam that you hear from others is not verifiable.
- Because this gossip is based on the imperfect memory of people in a very stressful situation, it may not be very accurate.
- People tend to remember those items that test content with which they are less comfortable; for instance, those with a limited background in women's health may say that the exam was "all women's health." In fact, the exam blueprint ensures that the exam covers multiple content areas without overemphasizing any one.

Step Three: Set Reasonable Expectations for Yourself

- Do not expect to know everything.
- Do not try to know everything in great detail.
- You do not need a perfect score to pass the exam.
- The exam is designed for a beginner level—it is testing readiness for *entry-level* practice.
- Learn the general rules, not the exceptions.
- The most likely diagnoses will be on the exam, not questions on rare diseases or atypical cases.
- Think about the most likely presentation and most common therapy.

Step Four: Prepare Mentally and Physically

- While you are getting ready to take the exam, take good physical care of yourself.
- Get plenty of sleep, exercise, and eat well while preparing for the exam.
- These things are especially important while you are studying and immediately before you take the exam.

Step Five: Access Current Knowledge

General Content

When you register to take the exam, you will be given a list of general topics that will be on the exam. In addition, examine the table of contents of this book and the test content outline, available at www.nursecredentialing.org/cert/TCOs.html.

- What content do you need to know?
- How well do you know these subjects?

Take a Review Course

- Taking a review course is an excellent method of assessing your knowledge of the content that will be included in the exam.
- If you plan to take a review course, take it well before the exam so you will have plenty of time to master any areas of weakness the course uncovers.
- If you are prepared for the exam, you will not hear anything new in the course. You will be familiar with everything that is taught.
- If some topics in the review course are new to you, concentrate on these in your studies.
- People have a tendency to study what they know; it is rewarding to study something and feel a mastery of it! Unfortunately, this will not help you master unfamiliar content. Be sure to use a review course to identify your areas of strength and weakness, then concentrate on the weaknesses.

Depth of Knowledge

How much do you need to know about a subject?

- You cannot know everything about a topic.
- Remember that the depth of knowledge required to pass the exam is for entry-level performance.
- Study the information sent to you from the testing agency, what you were taught in school, what is covered in this text, and the general guidelines given in this chapter.
- Look at practice tests designed for the exam. Practice tests for other exams will not be helpful.
- Consult your class notes or clinical diagnosis and management textbook for the major points about a disease. Additional reference books can be found online at www.nursecredentialing.org/cert/refs.html.
- For example, with regard to medications, know the drug categories and the major medications in each. Assume all drugs in a category are generally alike, and then focus on the differences among common drugs. Know the most important indications, contraindications, and side effects. Emphasize safety. The questions usually do not require you to know the exact dosage of a drug.

Step Six: Institute a Systematic Study Plan

Develop Your Study Plan

- Write a formal plan of study.
  - Include topics for study, timetable, resources, and methods of study that work for you.
  - Decide whether you want to organize a study group or work alone.
  - Schedule regular times to study.
  - Avoid cramming; it is counterproductive. Try to schedule your study periods in 1-hour increments.
- Identify resources to use for studying. To prepare for the examination, you should have the following on your shelf:
  - A good pathophysiology text
  - This review book
  - A physical assessment text
  - Your class notes
  - Other important sources, including: information from the testing facility, a clinical diagnosis textbook, favorite journal articles, notes from a review course, and practice tests
  - Know the important national standards of care for major illnesses
  - Consult the bibliography on the test blueprint. When studying less familiar material, it is helpful to study using the same references that the testing center uses.
- Study the body systems from head to toe.
- The exams emphasize health promotion, assessment, differential diagnosis, and plan of care for common problems.
- You will need to know facts and be able to interpret and analyze this information that utilizes critical thinking.

Personalize Your Study Plan

- How do you learn best? If you learn best by listening or talking, attend a review course or discuss topics with a colleague.
- Read everything the test facility sends you as soon as you receive it and several times during your preparation period. It will give you valuable information to help guide your study.

- Have a specific place with good lighting set aside for studying. Find a place with no noise or distractions. Assemble your study materials.

Implement Your Study Plan

You must have basic content knowledge. In addition, you must be able to use this information to think critically and make decisions based on facts.

- Refer to your study plan regularly.
- Stick to your schedule.
- Take breaks when you get tired.
- If you start procrastinating, get help from a friend or reorganize your study plan.
- It is not necessary to follow your plan rigidly. Adjust your focus as you learn where you need to spend more time.
- Memorize the basics of the content areas you will be required to know.

Focus on General Material

- Most of what you need to know is basic material that does not require constant updating.
- You do not need to worry about the latest information being published as you are studying for the exam. Remember, it can take 6 to 12 months for new information to be incorporated into test questions.

Pace Your Studying

- Stop studying for the examination when you are starting to feel overwhelmed and look at what is bothering you. Then make changes.
- Break overwhelming tasks into smaller tasks that you know you can do.
- Stop and take breaks while studying.

Work With Others

- Talk with classmates about your preparation for the exam.
- Keep in touch with classmates, and help each other stick to your study plans.
- If your classmates start having anxiety attacks, do not let their anxiety affect you. Walk away if you need to.
- Do not believe bad stories you hear about other people's experiences with previous exams.
- Remember, you know as much as anyone about what will be on the next exam!

Consider a Study Group

- Study groups can provide practice in analyzing cases, interpreting questions, and critical thinking.
- You can discuss a topic and take turns presenting cases for the group to analyze.
- Study groups also can provide moral support and help you continue studying.

Step Seven: Strategies Immediately Before the Exam
Final Preparation Suggestions
- Use practice exams when studying to get accustomed to the exam format and time restrictions.
  - Many books that are labeled as review books are simply a collection of examination questions.
  - If you have test anxiety, such practice tests may help alleviate the anxiety.
  - Practice tests can help you learn to judge the time you should take during an exam.
  - Practice tests are useful for gaining experience in analyzing questions.
  - Books of questions may not uncover the gaps in your knowledge that a more systematic content review text will reveal.
  - If you feel that you don't know enough about a topic, refer to a text to learn more. After you feel that you have mastered the topic, practice questions are a wonderful tool to help improve your test-taking skills.
- Know your test-taking style.
  - Do you rush through the exam without thoroughly reading the questions?
  - Do you get stuck and dwell on a question for a long time?
  - You should spend about 45 to 60 seconds per question and finish with time to review the questions you were not sure about.
  - Be sure to read the question completely, including all four answer choices. Choice "a" may be good, but "d" may be best.

The Night Before the Exam
- Be prepared to get to the exam on time.
  - Know the test site location and how long it takes to get there.
  - Take a "dry run" beforehand to make sure you know how to get to the testing site, if necessary.
  - Get a good night's sleep.
  - Eat sensibly.
  - Avoid alcohol the night before.
  - Assemble the required material—two forms of identification, admission card, pencil, and watch. Both IDs must match the name on the application, and one photo ID is preferred. Bring tissues, antacid chews, hard candy, and anything you might want to keep in your pocket.
  - Know the exam room rules.
    - You will be given scratch paper, which will be collected at the end of the exam.
    - Nothing else is allowed in the exam room.
    - You will be required to put papers, backpacks, etc., in a corner of the room or in a locker.
    - No water or food will be allowed.
    - You will be allowed to walk to a water fountain and go to the bathroom one at a time.

The Day of the Exam
- Get there early. If you are late, you may not be admitted.
- Think positively. You have studied hard and are well-prepared.
- Remember your anxiety reduction strategies.

SPECIFIC TIPS FOR DEALING WITH ANXIETY

Test anxiety is a specific type of anxiety. Symptoms include upset stomach, sweaty palms, tachycardia, trouble concentrating, and a feeling of dread. But there are ways to cope with test anxiety.
- There is no substitute for being well-prepared.
- Practice relaxation techniques.
- Avoid alcohol, excess coffee, caffeine, and any new medications that might sedate you, dull your senses, or make you feel agitated.
- Take a few deep breaths and concentrate on the task at hand.

FOCUS ON SPECIFIC TEST-TAKING SKILLS

To do well on the exam, you need good test-taking skills in addition to knowledge of the content and ability to use critical thinking.

ALL CERTIFICATION EXAMS ARE MULTIPLE CHOICE
- Multiple choice tests have specific rules for test construction.
- A multiple choice question consists of three parts: the information (or stem), the question, and the four possible answers (one correct and three distracters).
- Careful analysis of each part is necessary. Read the entire question before answering.
- Practice your test-taking skills by analyzing the practice questions in this book and on the ANCC website

ANALYZE THE INFORMATION GIVEN
- Do not assume you have more information than is given.
- Do not overanalyze.
- Remember, the writer of the question assumes this is all of the information needed to answer the question.
- If information is not given, it is not relevant and will not affect the answer.
- Do not make the question more complicated than it is.

WHAT KIND OF QUESTION IS ASKED?
- Are you supposed to recall a fact, apply facts to a situation, or understand and differentiate between options?
- Read the question thinking about what the writer is asking.
- Look for key words or phrases that lead you (see Box 1–1). These help determine what kind of answer the question requires.

Box 1-1. Examples of Key Words and Phrases

· avoid	· initial	· most
· best	· first	· significant
· except	· contributing to	· likely
· not	· appropriate	· of the following
		· most consistent with

READ ALL OF THE ANSWERS
- If you are absolutely certain that answer "a" is correct as you read it, mark it, but read the rest of the questions so you do not trick yourself into missing a better answer.
- If you are absolutely sure answer "a" is wrong, cross it off or make a note on your scratch paper and continue reading the question.
- After reading the entire question, go back, analyze the question, and select the best answer.
- Do not jump ahead.
- If the question asks you for an assessment, the best answer will be an assessment. Do not be distracted by an intervention that sounds appropriate.
- If the question asks you for an intervention, do not answer with an assessment.
- When two answer choices sound very good, the best one is usually the least expensive, least invasive way to achieve the goal. For example, if your answer choices include a physical exam maneuver or imaging, the physical exam maneuver is probably the better choice provided it will give the information needed.
- If the answers include two options that are the opposite of each other, one of the two is probably the correct answer.
- When numeric answers cover a wide range, a number in the middle is more likely to be correct.
- Watch out for distracters that are correct but do not answer the question, combine true and false information, or contain a word or phrase that is similar to the correct answer.
- Err on the side of caution.

ONLY ONE ANSWER CAN BE CORRECT
- When more than one suggested answer is correct, you must identify the one that best answers the question asked.
- If you cannot choose between two answers, you have a 50% chance of getting it right if you guess.

AVOID CHANGING ANSWERS
- Change an answer only if you have a compelling reason, such as you remembered something additional, or you understand the question better after rereading it.
- People change a choice to a wrong answer more often than to a right answer.

TIME YOURSELF TO COMPLETE THE WHOLE EXAM
- Do not spend a large amount of time on one question.
- If you cannot answer a question quickly, mark it and continue the exam.
- If time is left at the end, return to the difficult questions.
- Make educated guesses by eliminating the obviously wrong answers and choosing a likely answer even if you are not certain.
- Trust your instinct.
- Answer every question. There is no penalty for a wrong answer.
- Occasionally a question will remind you of something that helps you with a question earlier in the test. Look back at that question to see if what you are remembering affects how you would answer that question.

ABOUT THE CERTIFICATION EXAMS

The American Nurses Credentialing Center Computerized Exam

The ANCC examination is given only as a computer exam, and each exam is different. The order of the questions is scrambled for every test, so even if two people are taking the same exam, the questions will be in a different order. The exam consists of 175 multiple-choice questions.
- 150 of the 175 questions are part of the test and how you answer will count toward your score; 25 are included to refine questions and will not be scored. You will not know which ones count, so treat all questions the same.
- You will need to know how to use a mouse, scroll by either clicking arrows on the scroll bar or using the up and down arrow keys, and perform other basic computer tasks.
- The exam does not require computer expertise.
- However, if you are not comfortable with using a computer, you should practice using a mouse and computer beforehand so you do not waste time on the mechanics of using the computer.

Know what to expect during the test.
- Each ANCC test question is independent of the other questions.
  - For each case study, there is only one question. This means that a correct answer on any question does not depend on the correct answer to any other question.
  - Each question has four possible answers. There are no questions asking for combinations of correct answers (such as "a and c") or multiple-multiples.
- You can skip a question and go back to it at the end of the exam.
- You cannot mark key words in the question or right or wrong answers. If you want to do this, use the scratch paper.
- You will get your results immediately, and a grade report will be provided upon leaving the testing site.

Other Resources
- ANCC website: www.nursecredentialing.org
- ANA website: www.nursingworld.org. Catalog of ANA nursing scope and standards publications and other titles that may be listed on your test content outline can be found at www. nursebooks.org
- National Guideline Clearinghouse: www.ngc.gov

Important Factors Influencing the Nurse Practitioner Role

Elizabeth Blunt, PhD, MSN, FNP-BC

LEGAL DIMENSIONS OF THE ROLE

Legal Authority For Practice

State Nurse Practice Acts—Rules and Regulations

- Authority for nurse practitioner (NP) practice is found in state legislative statutes and in rules and regulations. The Nurse Practice Act of every state customarily authorizes the Boards of Nursing to establish statutory authority to define who may be called a nurse practitioner (title protection); what they may do (scope of practice); restrictions on their practice; the requirements an NP must meet to be credentialed within the state as an NP (education, certification, etc.); and disciplinary grounds for infraction of regulations. (See www.ncsbn.org for a listing of state nursing board requirements.) In many states, legislative acts may specifically require that an NP develop a collaborative agreement with a physician, describe what types of drugs might be prescribed, or define some form of oversight board for NP practice.
- Statutory law is implemented in regulatory language. The rules and regulations for each state may further define scope of practice, practice requirements, and/or restrictions.

- Beginning in 1999, the National Council of State Boards of Nursing (NCSBN) began implementation of an interstate compact for nursing practice to reduce state-to-state discrepancies in nursing requirements to practice. The Advanced Practice Registered Nurse (APRN) Compact addresses the need to promote consistent access to quality advanced practice nursing care within states and across state lines. The Uniform APRN Licensure/Authority to Practice Requirements, developed by NCSBN with APRN stakeholders in 2000, establishes the foundation for this APRN Compact. Similar to the existing Nurse Licensure Compact for recognition of registered nurse (RN) and licensed practical nurse (LPN) licenses, the APRN Compact offers states the mechanism for mutually recognizing APRN licenses/authority to practice. A state must be either a member of the current nurse licensure compact for RN and LPN or choose to enter into both compacts simultaneously to be eligible for the APRN Compact. To see which states participate, view the state compact map at https://www.ncsbn.org.

Nurse Practitioner Professional Practice
Licensure
- "A process by which an agency of state government grants permission to individuals accountable for the practice of a profession to engage in the practice of that profession and prohibits all others from legally doing so" (U.S. Department of Health, Education and Welfare [DHEW], 1971).
- The purpose is to protect the public by ensuring a minimum level of professional competence. "This regulatory method is used when regulated activities are complex, require specialized knowledge, skill and independent decision-making. The licensure process includes the predetermination of qualifications necessary to perform a legally defined scope of practice safely and an evaluation of licensure applications to determine that the qualifications are met. Licensure provides that a specified scope of practice may only be performed legally by licensed individuals. Licensure provides title protection for those roles. It also provides authority to take disciplinary action should the licensee violate provision of the law or rules in order to assure that the public health, safety and welfare will be reasonably well protected" (NCSBN, www.ncsbn.org/regulation/nlc_licensure_aprn.asp).

Certification
- "A process by which a non-governmental agency or association certifies that an individual licensed to practice as a professional has met certain predetermined standards specified by that profession for specialty practice" (DHEW, 1971).
- The purpose is to assure the public that an individual has mastery of a body of knowledge and has acquired the skills necessary to function in a particular specialty. Some certifications are required for entry into practice (e.g., required for licensure within a state, and thus have a regulatory function); some certifications denote professional competence and recognize excellence.

Accreditation
- "The process by which a voluntary, non-governmental agency or organization appraises and grants accreditation status to institutions and/or programs or services which meet predetermined structure, process and outcome criteria" (DHEW, 1971). The purpose is to assure that the organization has met specific standards.

Scope of Practice

- Defines a specific legal scope determined by state statues, boards of nursing, educational preparation, and common practice within a community. For example, adult nurse practitioners (ANPs) are not legally authorized to care for children. The state might require an NP to have formal educational preparation in pediatrics. Broad variation exists from state to state.
- General scope of practice is specified in many published professional documents (e.g., *Scope and Standards of Advanced Practice Registered Nursing*, ANA, 1996). In addition, many organizations have completed role delineation studies which attempt to qualify the core behaviors that all advanced practice nurses (APNs) must possess, as well as the core knowledge and behaviors required of individuals in a particular specialty. For example, core knowledge for a pediatric nurse practitioner (PNP) will be inherently different than that of a gerontological nurse practitioner (GNP). It is critical that these statements about specific scope and standards exist so that everyone—including nurses—will have access to materials to which they can refer when there are specific questions related to role. This is especially important when the traditional role of nurses is being changed or "advanced" at an uneven rate through changes in state law. As the nurse practitioner role has expanded into new practice settings, including hospice, acute care hospitals, and home care, it is important that core knowledge, as well as state law protecting NPs in these practice settings, also expand, providing the legal authorization and title protection necessary for these practice settings.
- Prescriptive authority is recognized as within the scope of practice for nurse practitioners in all 50 states, though there is significant variability from state to state. This has created inherent difficulty in collecting data related to NP prescribing practices. The *Nurse Practitioner Journal* publishes a comprehensive update of legislative requirements and recent changes in its January issue each year. Data collected by Nurse Practitioner Alternatives, Inc., since 1996 has documented stability within prescribing patterns by NPs. Data from 2004 document that the majority of NPs possess their own Drug Enforcement Administration (DEA) number (72%), write between 6 and 25 prescriptions in an average clinical day (79%), recommend between 1 and 20 over-the-counter (OTC) preparations in an average clinical day (90%), and manage between 25% and 100% of their patient encounters independently (97%; Nurse Practitioner Alternatives, Inc., 2004).

Standards of Practice

- Authoritative statements by which the quality of practice, service, or education can be judged (e.g., *Scope and Standards of Advanced Practice Registered Nursing*; ANA, 1996)
- Professional standards focus on the minimum levels of acceptable performance as a way of providing consumers with a means of measuring the quality of care they receive. They may be written at the generic level to apply to all nurses (e.g., following universal precautions), as well as to define practice by each specialty.
- The presence of accepted standards of practice may be used to legally describe the standard of care that must be met by a provider. These standards may be precise protocols that must be followed, or more recommendations for more general guidelines.

- *Healthy People 2010 Objectives* and the World Health Organization's *"Health for All"* are, respectively, national and international policy statements that describe objectives to be met to help all persons obtain a level of health that will permit them to lead socially and economically productive lives. Eventually, these objectives are expected to form the basis for international standards of practice.
- The National Organization of Nurse Practitioner Faculties (NONPF; www.nonpf.com), in partnership with the American Association of Colleges of Nursing (www.aacn.nche. edu), developed *Nurse Practitioner Primary Care Competencies in Specialty Areas: Adult, Family, Gerontological, Pediatric and Women's Health*, published by the Department of Health and Human Services' Health Resources & Services Administration, Bureau of Health Professions, Division of Nursing in 2002 (U.S. Department of Health and Human Services, 2002); *Psychiatric Mental Health Nurse Practitioner Competencies* were published in 2003; and *Acute Care Nurse Practitioner Competencies* were published in 2004. These documents outline what an NP in each of the specialty areas should be able to do (NONPF, 2008).

Patient Rights
Confidentiality

- The patient and family have a right to assume that information given to the healthcare provider will not be disclosed. This has several dimensions:
  - *Verbal information*: Healthcare providers shall not discuss any information given to them during the healthcare encounter with anyone not directly involved in providing this care without the patient's or family's permission.
  - *Written information*: Confidentiality of the healthcare encounter is protected under federal statute through the Health Insurance Portability and Accountability Act of 1996 (HIPAA). The Administrative Simplification provisions of HIPAA require the Department of Health and Human Services to establish national standards for electronic healthcare transactions and national identifiers for providers, health plans, and employers. It also addresses the security and privacy of health data. Information may be accessed at www.cms.hhs.gov/HIPAAGenInfo/07_OtherHIPAAResources.asp.
  - The individual's right to privacy is respected when requesting or responding to a request for a patient's medical record.
  - The statute requires that the provider discuss confidentiality issues with patients (parents in the case of a minor), establish consent, and clarify any questions about disclosure of information.
  - The provider is required to obtain a signed medical authorization and consent form to release medical records and information.
- Exceptions to guaranteed confidentiality occur when society determines that the need for information outweighs the principle of confidentiality. Examples might be when records are released to insurance companies; to attorneys involved in litigation; or in answering court orders, subpoenas, or summonses; in meeting state requirements for mandatory reporting of diseases or conditions; in cases of suspected child abuse; or if a patient reveals an intent to harm someone.

Informed Consent

- *Informed consent* is the right of all competent adults (age 18 or older) and emancipated minors (age 17 or younger who are married, a parent, or self-sufficient and living away from the family domicile) to accept or reject treatment by a healthcare provider. (Some states have laws concerning birth control or abortions that apply to patients younger than 18.)
- The clinician has the duty to explain relevant information to the patient so the patient can make an appropriate decision. This information usually includes diagnosis, nature and purpose of proposed treatment or procedure, risks and benefits, prognosis, alternative methods of treatment along with risks and benefits, and even the remote possibility of serious harm.
- It must be documented in the medical records that this information has been provided.
- Informed consent does not absolve the NP from allegations of malpractice should it occur.

Care of Minors

- In most jurisdictions, minors under the age of 18 cannot receive healthcare services without permission of a competent adult who is his or her parent or legal guardian.
- Exceptions to this rule may be made in some jurisdictions in the case of an emancipated minor, a pregnant minor, or in matters pertaining to sexually transmitted diseases and birth control.

Advance Directives

- When a patient is incapable of making decisions, a person's preferences may be expressed by way of a written living will or a healthcare durable power of attorney created when the patient was still competent.
    - *Living wills* are written documents prepared in advance in case of terminal illness or nonreversible loss of consciousness.
    - Their provisions go into effect when:
        - the patient has become incompetent, and
        - the patient is declared terminally ill, and
        - no further interventions will alter the patient's course to a reasonable degree of medical certainty.

Durable Power of Attorney for Health Care

- Individuals can identify in writing an agent to act on their behalf, should they become mentally incapacitated. The decisions of the designated agent are:
    - binding,
    - not limited to the circumstances of terminal illness,
    - flexible enough to carry out the patient's wishes throughout the course of an illness, and
    - often accompanied by a durable power of attorney over financial issues as well.

Ethical Decision Making
- Moral concepts such as advocacy, accountability, loyalty, caring, compassion, and human dignity are the foundations of ethical behavior.
- The ethical behavior of nurses has been defined for professional nursing in an American Nurses Association policy statement (ANA, 1988).
- Ethical behavior incorporates respect for the individual and his or her autonomy. Thus, no decision is truly ethical if the caregiver does not involve the patient in decision-making to the full extent of the patient's capacity.
- Duty to help others (beneficence), avoidance of harmful behavior (nonmaleficence), and fairness are also foundational components of ethical behavior.

Quality Assurance
- Quality assurance is a system designed to evaluate and monitor the quality of patient care and facility management.
- Formal programs provide a framework for systematic, deliberate, and continuous evaluation and monitoring of individual clinical practice. Programs promote responsibility and accountability to deliver high-quality care, assist in the evaluation and improvement of patient care, and provide for an organized means of problem solving. Thus, a good program identifies educational needs, improves the documentation of care, and reduces the clinician's overall exposure to liability.
- Programs identify components of structure, process, and outcomes of care. They also look at organizational effectiveness, efficiency, and client and provider interactions.
- May be implemented through audits, utilization review, peer review, outcome studies, and measurements of patient satisfaction.

Nurse Practitioner Legal and Financial Issues
Liability
- Sources of legal risk
  - Patients, procedures
  - Quality of medical records
- Risk reduction or management
  - Activities or systems designed to recognize and intervene to reduce the risk of injury to patients and subsequent claims against healthcare providers.
  - Malpractice insurance does not protect a clinician from charges of practicing outside their legal scope of practice. All clinicians carry their own liability insurance coverage to ensure their own legal representation by an attorney to advocate for them.
- Malpractice
  - Negligent professional acts of individuals engaged in professions requiring highly technical or professional skills
  - The plaintiff has the burden of proving the four elements of malpractice:
    - *Duty:* The clinician has the duty to exercise reasonable care when undertaking and providing treatment to the patient when a patient–clinician relationship exists.
    - *Breach of duty:* The clinician violates the applicable standard of care in treating the patient's condition.
    - *Proximate cause:* There is a causal relationship between the breach in the standard of care and the patient's injuries.
    - *Damages:* There are permanent and substantial damages to the patient as a result of the malpractice.

- National Practitioner Databank
  - The Health Care Quality Improvement Act of 1986 established a databank to scrutinize members of the healthcare profession and list those practitioners who have had a malpractice claim asserted against them.
  - Currently, very few NPs are listed in the National Practitioner Databank, but the number of NPs who have had malpractice claims filed against them is increasing as the number of NPs in practice increases.

Reimbursement

- NPs are reimbursed for their services as primary care providers under Medicare, Medicaid, Federal Employees Health Benefits Program, TRICARE (formerly known as CHAMPUS), veterans' and military programs, and federally funded school-based clinics.
- Private insurance plans may elect to reimburse for NP services even if not mandated by state law. In some states, the insurance code may be interpreted rigidly to exclude reimbursement of NPs.
- Managed care organizations (MCOs) frequently have excluded NPs from being designated as primary care providers carrying their own caseloads. Thus, in many MCOs, the only option for NPs is that of being a salaried employee. As a salaried employee, the NP contributions are often not visible and may be credited to their collaborating physicians, giving them a "ghost" provider status. Without a legitimate method to document services provided and revenue generated, the NP can find that his or her job security is often at risk. Many state NP organizations have recently focused legislative activity on enacting state laws allowing NPs to function as primary care providers in both health maintenance organizations (HMOs) and preferred provider organizations (PPOs). These efforts have led to opposition from state medical organizations.
- There is considerable flux in state and national policy on what services and procedures NPs may bill for, and whether they will be paid directly. Incorrect billing places healthcare providers at risk of fraud and abuse charges whether they knowingly violate the law or are just ignorant of the regulations.
- NPs must be aware of specific regulations and policies for patient care services. Resources include Health Care Financing Agency bulletins, among others (www.cms.hhs.gov/).

Performance Assessment

- The National Practitioner Data Bank (NPDB) and Health Integrity and Protection Data Bank (HIPDB) are maintained by the U.S. Department of Health and Human Services, Health Resources and Services Administration, Bureau of Health Professions, Division of Practitioner Data Banks. Developed as a result of the Health Care Quality and Improvement Act of 1986, the NPDB and HIPDB are flagging systems intended to facilitate a comprehensive review of healthcare practitioners' professional credentials, with a goal of improving the quality of health care. The information contained in the NPDB includes a practitioner's licensure, professional society memberships, malpractice payment history, and record of clinical privileges. NPs may perform a self-query by visiting the site at www.npdb-hipdb.com/.

- Other programs monitoring and comparing health quality include the Health Plan Employer Data and Information Set (HEDIS®) developed by the National Committee on Quality Assurance. HEDIS is a set of standardized performance measures designed to ensure that purchasers and consumers have the information they need to reliably compare the performance of managed healthcare plans (www.ncqa.org/).

Current Trends

Topics Dominating NP Discussions About the Future

Fiscal Issues

- Growing competition in the job market for NPs as numbers of NPs have increased and NPs have begun to directly compete with physicians and physician assistants.
- Reimbursement struggles with Medicare and private insurance.
- Increasing costs for malpractice insurance. Many states have launched legislative initiatives on medical tort reform in an attempt to hold down malpractice premiums.
- Effective May 2007, the Center for Medicare and Medicaid Services requires that providers obtain a National Provider Identifier (NPI). Growing concerns over reimbursement fraud and abuse issues, as well as coding issues related to overbilling and underbilling, particularly for Medicare patients, prompted the NPI initiative.
- All healthcare providers must have an NPI number. Information may be obtained at www.cms.hhs.gov/NationalProvidentStand/.

NP Education

- Recognition of the need to ensure the quality of NP education, faculty, and curricula has led to efforts by the National Organization of Nurse Practitioner Faculties (NONPF) and the American Association of Colleges of Nursing (AACN) to promulgate core competency statements. These can be viewed at www.aacn.nche.edu/education/apn.htm.
- In addition, NONPF, AACN, numerous NP professional organizations, NP accrediting bodies, and educational organizations have jointly promulgated criteria for evaluating nurse practitioner programs. In combination with accreditation standards for graduate programs and specialty areas, the criteria provide a basis for evaluating the quality of nurse practitioner programs. Documents may be viewed at www.nonpf.org/evalcriteria2002.pdf.
- AACN, working with NONPF (with input from other groups), has developed a practice doctorate in nursing. In the future, the practice doctorate is expected to be the graduate degree for advanced nursing practice preparation, including but not limited to the four current APN roles: clinical nurse specialist, nurse anesthetist, nurse midwife, and nurse practitioner.
- The Board of NONPF regards the practice doctorate of nursing as an important evolutionary step for the preparation of nurse practitioners. They anticipate that the practice doctorate degree will become the standard for entry into nurse practitioner practice; however, much like with the movement of educational preparation of NPs from the post-basic certificate to a master's degree, this evolution will be gradual. NONPF does not support any finite deadline for NP programs to be at doctoral level preparation but instead encourages NP educators to continue to sustain the highest quality programs to prepare NPs for clinical practice (NONPF, 2006).

In 2006, NONPF published a *Practice Doctorate Nurse Practitioner Entry-Level Competencies* document, viewable at www.nonpf.org/NONPF2005/PracticeDoctorateResourceCenter/ CompetencyDraftFinalApril2006.pdf.

Practice Environment

- *Health disparities:* There is growing recognition of disparities in the health services and outcomes of different populations in the United States. The National Center on Minority Health and Health Disparities at the National Institutes of Health (NIH) is a government organization with a mission to promote minority health and to lead, coordinate, support, and assess the NIH effort to reduce and ultimately eliminate health disparities. For more information, visit http://ncmhd.nih.gov/.
- *Health literacy:* Now recognized as one of the largest contributors to health outcome is the ability of a patient and family to understand and act on health information. Both the Institute of Medicine (IOM) and the Agency for Health Care Research and Quality (AHRQ) have launched efforts to quantify and offer solutions to the problems that result from inadequate health literacy. The IOM report may be viewed at www.iom.edu/report.asp?id=19723; the AHRQ study can be found at www.ahrq.gov/news/press/pr2004/litpr.htm.
- Attention is increasingly being paid to preparing registered nurses to assume emergency roles during a time of mass casualties from either natural disasters or terrorist attacks. Because other countries have had more experience with dealing with terrorism, the International Nursing Coalition for Mass Casualty Education has been established and headquartered at Vanderbilt School of Nursing to help U.S. nurses profit from others' experience and to identify the educational competencies for registered nurses responding to mass casualty incidents. The Coalition desires to improve the ability of all nurses to respond safely and effectively to mass casualty incidents through identifying existing and emerging roles of nurses, ensuring appropriateness of education for mass casualty incidents, and helping to understand response frameworks and ensure collaborative efforts. All NPs are expected to prepare themselves to play a larger role in delivery of care during a time of disaster. Information on the objectives and work that has been done towards a uniform curriculum in this area may be obtained at www.nursing.vanderbilt.edu/incmce/.
- *Direct-to-consumer advertising:* Patients frequently present to the office already having formed their diagnosis and wanting specific treatments. NPs must become knowledgeable about the newest product on the market to appropriately counsel and treat patients.
- *Complementary and alternative modalities/medicines (CAM):* There is greater recognition of the use by patients of complementary and alternative modalities and medicines. Research suggests that 40%–50% of patients are currently using a form of complementary or alternative therapy, despite the dearth of research on which to base treatment regimens. NPs as providers need to learn about common CAM treatments and particularly about how some herbal products interact with prescription drugs. The National Center for Complementary and Alternative Medicine is the federal government's lead agency for scientific research on complementary and alternative medicine (http://nccam.nih.gov).

- Since release of the Institute of Medicine's report *To Err is Human: Building A Safer Health System* (http://www.iom.edu/report.asp?id=5575), there has been increased attention on changes all healthcare providers should make to reduce medical errors. In response, The Joint Commission (formerly known as JCAHO or the Joint Commission on Accreditation of Healthcare Organizations, www.jointcommission.org/) has issued a list of abbreviations that should not be used in health care. In addition, the Institute for Safe Medication Practices has published a list of dangerous abbreviations related to medication use that it recommends should be explicitly prohibited (http://www.ismp.org/). The list of banned abbreviations includes many symbols traditionally used in patient charts and writing prescriptions.

Professional Organizations

- Participation in professional organizations is important because nurse practitioners, acting as a unified group, can influence the direction of the profession and of healthcare policy in the United States. All NPs should be involved and active in their professional organizations at the national, state, and local levels.
- State organizations work diligently to monitor and affect laws and regulations affecting NP practice and health policy. In addition, these associations provide a group of peers for discussion and continuing education. Many state NP organizations have local chapters.
- National organizations
  - The American College of Nurse Practitioners (ACNP) is focused on advocacy and keeping NPs current on legislative, regulatory, and clinical practice issues that effect NPs in the rapidly changing healthcare arena (www.acnpweb.org).
  - The mission of the American Academy of Nurse Practitioners (AANP) is to promote excellence in NP practice, education, and research; shape the future of health care through advancing health policy; serve as the source of information for NPs, the healthcare community, and consumers; and build a positive image of the NP role as a leader in the national and global healthcare community (www.aanp.org).
  - The National Organization of Nurse Practitioner Faculties (NONPF) is an organization of nurse practitioner educators who are instrumental in setting standards for nurse practitioner education. NONPF has developed core competencies describing the domains of practice with critical behaviors that should be exhibited by all entry-level NPs. Originally written in 1995, the revised edition of the core competencies became available in 2000 to reflect the current NP practice (www.nonpf.com).

THEORY AND PRINCIPLES OF FAMILY-FOCUSED CARE

The traditional family nurse practitioner (FNP) provides primary and secondary preventive care to individuals across the life span living as singles or in nuclear or extended family networks. Today's family consists of those who identify themselves as family members, not limited by walls, genetics, or legally defined relationships. Friedman (1998) defines family as "two or more persons who are joined together by bonds of sharing and emotional closeness and who identify themselves as being part of the family" (p. 9).

Family members may live either together or within close proximity in a common community, and participate in educational, social, and religious experiences. Families may form as an outgrowth of kinship bonds with others in the community or as a result of culturally specific extended family networks. Due to changes in society, family members often share multiple instrumental and expressive tasks that often overlap and are subject to communication and negotiation (Hanson, Gedaley-Duff, & Kaakinen, 2005). Family forms are varied, and the FNP will interact with nontraditional and multicultural family forms such as the gay and lesbian family, the single-parent family, the Asian- or African-American extended family, and adoptive or stepparent families, as well as traditional families.

Family-focused care is the specialized role of the family nurse practitioner. FNPs acknowledge that the family process is an interaction among family members that serves to promote mental and physical health, prevent disease, and restore health in times of illness. FNPs provide a comprehensive psychosocial approach to caring for individuals that fosters health-promoting lifestyles among family members. The FNP interacts across the interdependent roles of individual, family, and community to act as advocate, case manager, coordinator, counselor, expert provider of care, and case-finder.

The FNP assesses family structure and dynamics to help individuals maximize their health, given the realities of their personal and family health histories, psychosocial history, genetic make-up, cultural and religious values, traditions, and social and economic context. The FNP teaches family members to recognize the influences of their family health patterns and risks; to utilize family members as resources for knowledge and support during periods of health; to maintain psychosocial ties with their family of origin; and to assume functions that help optimize health in family members by utilizing resources in the community.

The FNP role is interpreted as a unique NP role. It is not, as some would suggest, an adult NP plus pediatric NP plus gerontological NP role, but requires mastery of a unique constellation of knowledge and tasks surrounding the care of an individual within a family context. The FNP is not expected to have the depth of knowledge of NPs practicing in the specialty areas but is expected to know something about many different diseases and processes affecting the individual throughout the life span. As such, the FNP will work closely with physician colleagues in the diagnosis and development of the initial treatment regimen and be prepared to refer frequently to specialists.

Family Theory: Assessment and Intervention

In general, family theory serves as a basis for assessing and coming to understand the structure, development and function of families through the process of family assessment. Authors such as Friedman (1998); Hanson, Gedaley-Duff, and Kaakinen (2005); and Wright and Leahy (2005) have developed family assessment tools. Family theory is grounded in general systems theory, including structural functional theory, family systems theory (Bowen), family development theory (Duvall, 1977), child development theory (Erickson; Havinghurst), and other social science theories, including communication, stress, and interactional theory.

Theoretical Basis For Family Theory

General Systems Theory

- General systems theory provides a framework that explains the dynamic structure and function of the family within the context of a unified whole. The family performs activities reflected by the actions of interacting parts or subsystems. The major principles of systems theory adapted from Friedman (1998); Hanson, Gedaley-Duff, and Kaakinen (2005); and Wright and Leahy (2005) include:
  - Each system has its own characteristics, and the whole is greater than the sum of the parts, rather than just the sum of the characteristics of individual parts of a system.
  - All parts of the system are dependent on one another, even though each part has its own role within the system.
  - Families are organized in such a way as to enable the interdependence and interactivity of its members.
  - Each family system has mechanisms for exchange of information within the system and between the system and the broader environment.
  - Boundaries that are open, closed, or operate at random exist within family systems.
  - Family systems change over time as both individuals and the whole respond to change in the internal and external environments. With change, families become more complex, reflecting adaptation and differentiation of its members.
  - Change occurs through feedback processes that allow for circular interaction within the family system rather than a linear cause-and-effect pattern.
  - A change affecting one part of a family manifests itself as change in the whole family system.
  - Families strive for homeostasis or a predictable steady state that reflects a balance between change and stability.
- The value of systems theory lies in understanding that families are composed of interacting parts in constant interaction with each other and the larger environment, and that change in one part of the family is reflected in change in the family as a whole. As families expand and grow and experience stress and illness, their ability to be changed and yet maintain homeostasis reflects the health and coping strategies of the family to adapt. Families with poor coping strategies may resist change or be unable to restore homeostasis after change. Stress and illness may trigger dysfunctional coping patterns or dysequilibrium. Families with closed boundaries may resist help from outside resources during periods of dysequilibrium.

Structural Functional Theory

- Families are social systems that form interdependent and independent relationships, referred to as subsystems, both within and outside of the family. Structure describes relationships within families such as the husband–wife subsystem, the parent–child subsystem, sister–brother subsystem, and so on.
- Internal family subsystems function as a microcosm of society, reflecting the larger sphere of human needs. Rank order within families is a component of structure, such as the ordering of children by birth in the family or by ages if they are adopted or stepchildren.
- Function includes the tasks that families carry out to provide members safety, reproduction, education, parenting, sexual expression, economic security, transfer of cultural traditions and inheritance, social support, play, relaxation, and health-promotion opportunities.

- Suprasystems form outside the family and reflect functional needs not met within the family. Relationships with teachers, schools, religious and civic organizations, the healthcare system, and friends are examples of suprasystems that meet needs not met by interactions within the family system. Multiple relationships are formed through suprasystems that reflect family values, beliefs, and emotional boundaries. By developing an ecomap, the FNP can visualize family members' relationship with systems outside of the family system (Wright & Leahy, 2005).
- Principles of structural functional theory adapted from Friedman (1998); Hanson, Gedaley-Duff, and Kaakinen (2005); and Wright and Leahy (2005) include:
  - Families are social systems with instrumental and expressive functions that include activities of daily living, communication, social support, role acquisition, values, beliefs, problem solving, and relationships.
  - In optimally functioning families, members take on predictable roles that meet the instrumental and expressive needs of its members.
  - Families are composed of small numbers with characteristics of small-group behavior.
  - Families are social systems that carry out functions necessary to meet the need for orderly transfer of wealth, procreation, and education of members of society.
  - Individuals adopt norms, values, and cultural traditions that are learned as part of the process of family socialization.
- Disease or ill health can interfere with the family's ability to carry out its internal functions and meet the responsibilities it has formed in relationships with systems outside the family. Families with multiple unmet needs may experience guilt, stress, dysfunction, and poor coping strategies during periods of stress and illness.

Developmental Theory

- Developmental theory explains human growth and development according to theorists such as Erikson, Piaget, and Havinghurst. The concept of development was applied further to the sociological study of families by Duvall (1977) and Duvall and Miller (1985). The model outlines the eight consecutive stages in the family life cycle that offers a predictive overview of the activities that occur in families over time and serves as a basis for anticipatory guidance when assessing and teaching families. (See Chapter 3 for more information.)
- According to Duvall (1977), families pass through eight chronological stages; as in child development theory, success in one task sets the stage for success in subsequent tasks. Failure in one task leads to frustration or delays in subsequent tasks or stages in the family life cycle. The stages supported by Duvall's model below are adapted from Friedman (1998).
  - Beginning family
  - Childbearing family (oldest child up to 30 months of age)
  - Family with preschool children (oldest child 2–5 years of age)
  - Families with schoolchildren (oldest child 6–12 years of age)
  - Family with teenagers (oldest child 13–20 years of age)
  - Launching center family (grown children leaving the home)
  - Family with middle-aged parents (empty nest, up to time of retirement)
  - Family with old age and retirement

- Underlying assumptions include
  - Families change over time due to the influence of environmental conditions.
  - Developmental tasks are the aims, though they are not completed at one time and may overlap with other developmental tasks.
  - Families demonstrate different forms of membership across developmental stages that perform age-related functions.
  - Families bring with them an experience of their past as well as current circumstances.
  - Families share common developmental processes with other families.
  - Families express developmental milestones in a variety of ways. (Adapted from Friedman, 1998; and Hanson, Gedaley-Duff, & Kaakinen, 2005)

Communication Theory

As described by Friedman (1998); Hanson, Gedaley-Duff, and Kaakinen (2005); and Wright and Leahy (2005):

- Communication theory emphasizes the interaction of individuals that includes both verbal and nonverbal communication among members of a family.
- Communication functions include emotional support, shared information, and instruction.
- The content of messages is time-bound and must be appreciated within the context of the sender.
- Communication that lacks clarity may lead to family dysfunction or poor coping strategies.
- Communication conveys values and beliefs between members and the external environment. Communication with clarity and congruence promotes positive behavior within the family.

Case Studies

Case 1. Joan graduated from a family nurse practitioner program 5 years ago and has worked part-time in a college health center since graduation. She is now accepting a job as an FNP in a family practice setting and was asked to cover the prenatal clinic 1 day a week, in addition to providing regular family practice care. The collaborating physician assures her that he will provide her with direct supervision during the first 6 to 8 weeks of her experience and that he will be present in the clinic while she is seeing patients.

1. Is Joan legally authorized to provide care to prenatal women? To children?
2. Should she accept this assignment? Why or why not?
3. What standards of care should she follow in providing care to prenatal patients?

Case 2. Lee Ann is a 14-year-old who presents in the clinic for a physical exam and immunizations. She is alone and reports that her mother is working and does not know that she has come to the clinic. Lee Ann reports that she must have the exam and immunizations for school. The school has advised you in writing that Lee Ann's immunizations are not up-to-date, and she cannot return to school until a record is provided to validate her updated immunization history.

1. What are the legal issues presented in this case?
2. What ethical principles will guide you in making a decision regarding this case?

Case 3. Alice is a 49-year-old African-American mother and grandmother. She has three children living at home and the oldest daughter, in high school, now has a baby. Alice reports that she is very angry with her teenage daughter, who does not want to help out around the house or care for her baby. Alice feels like there is chaos all the time and she complains of having frequent stress-related headaches.

1. What theoretical model will assist you in planning an intervention for Alice?
2. What additional information would you like to obtain?
3. How can you best help her today?

REFERENCES

Aldwin, C. M., Park, C. L., & Spiro, A. (2007). *Handbook of health psychology and aging*. New York: Guilford Publications.

American Nurses Association. (1988). *Ethics in nursing: Position statements and guidelines* (ANA Pub. No. G-175). Washington, DC: Author.

American Nurses Association. (1996). *Scope and standards of advanced practice registered nursing* (Pub No. ADV-10). Washington, DC: Author.

American Nurses Association. (2008). *Who pays whom for what in health care?* Retrieved February 20, 2008, from http://nursingworld.org/MainMenuCategories/ANAMarketplace/ANAPeriodicals/OJIN/TableofContents/Vol31998/Vol3No1998/References.aspx

American Nurses Credentialing Center. (2001). *ANCC certification*. Washington, DC: Author.

Ballard, K. A., Arbogast, D., & Boeckman, J. (2006). *Nursing: Scope and standards of practice*. Washington, DC: American Nurses Association.

Birren, J. E., & Schaie, K. W. (Eds). (2001). *Handbook of the psychology of aging* (5th ed.). San Diego: Academic Press.

Buppert, C. (2007). *Nurse practitioners' business practice and legal guide*. Sudbury, MA: Jones & Bartlett.

Duvall, E. M. (1977). *Marriage and family development* (5th ed.). Philadelphia: Lippencott.

Duvall, E. M., & Miller, B. C. (1985). Marriage and family development (6th ed.). Philadelphia: Lippencott.

Edmunds, M. W., & Mayhew, M. S. (2004). *Pharmacology for primary care providers* (2nd ed.). St. Louis, MO: Mosby.

Federation of State Medical Boards of the United States. (1988). *Non-physician duties and scope of practice* (Position Statement 210.003, July). Dallas: Author.

Ford, L. C. (1992). Advanced nursing practice: Future of the nurse practitioner. In L. H. Aiken & C. M. Fagin (Eds.), *Charting nursing's future: Agenda for the 1990s*. Philadelphia: JB Lippincott.

Hanson, S., Gedaley-Duff, V., & Kaakinen, J. R. (2005). *Family health care nursing: Theory, practice and research*. Philadelphia: F.A. Davis.

Harrington, C., Beverly, C. J., Maas, M. L., Buckwalter, K. C., Bennett, J. A., Young, H. M., et al. (2005). Influencing health policy for older adults. *Nursing Outlook, 54*(4), 169–256.

Institute for the Future. (2003). *Health & health care 2010: The forecast, the challenge*. Hoboken, NJ: Wiley & Sons.

Institute of Medicine. (1999). *To err is human: Building a safe healthcare system*. Retrieved February 20, 2008, from http://www.iom.edu/report.asp?id=5575

Jett, K. (2007). Alternative Medicare billing for nurse practitioners: "Incident to." *Geriatric Nursing, 28*(3), 169–170.

Josen, A. R., Winslade, W. J., & Siegler, M. (2006). *Clinical ethics: A practical approach to ethical decisions in clinical medicine*. Philadelphia: McGraw-Hill.

Mullen, F., Politzer, R. M., Lewis, C. T., Bastacky, S., Rodak, J., Jr., & Harmon, R. G. (1992). The National Practitioner Data Bank: Report from the first year. *JAMA, 268*, 73–79.

National Council of State Boards of Nursing. (1993). *Regulation of advanced nursing practice* (National Council Position Paper, 1993). Chicago: Author.

National Organization of Nurse Practitioner Faculties. (2002). *Nurse practitioner primary care competencies in specialty areas: Adult, family, gerontological, pediatric, and women's health*. Washington, DC: Author.

National Organization of Nurse Practitioner Faculties. (2006, Oct.). *Statement on the practice doctorate in nursing: Response to recommendations on clinical hours and degree title.* Retrieved September 18, 2008, from http://www.nonpf.com/NONPF2005/PracticeDoctorateResourceCenter/PDstatement1006.htm

National Organization of Nurse Practitioner Faculties. (2008). *Competencies.* Retrieved September 18, 2008, from http://www.nonpf.org/#Comp

Nurse Practitioner Alternatives, Inc. (2004). *Longitudinal nurse practitioner prescribing data—2004 cohort.* Retrieved February 20, 2008, from http://www.npedu.com/SURVEY2004.pdf

National Practitioner Data Bank. Retrieved February 28, 2008, from http://www.npdb-hipdb.hrsa.gov/

Papero, D. V., & Kerr, M. E. (1997). *Bowen family systems.* Upper Saddle River, NJ: Allyn & Bacon.

Pearson, L. J. (2008). Annual update of how each state stands on legislative issues affecting advanced nursing practice. *The Nurse Practitioner: The American Journal of Primary Health Care, 33*(1), 10–34.

Reel, S. J., & Abraham, I. L. (2006). *Business and legal essentials for nurse practitioners: From negotiating your first job through owning a practice.* Philadelphia: Elsevier Health Sciences

Sollins, H. (2006). New Medicare guidance for nurse practitioners providing services in a home care or hospice setting. *Geriatric Nursing, 27*(5), 271-272.

U.S. Department of Health, Education and Welfare. (1971). *Report on licensure and related health personnel credentials* (DHEW Pub. No. (HSM) 72-11). Washington, DC: Author.

U.S. Department of Health and Human Services, Division of Nursing. (2002). *Nurse practitioner primary care competencies in specialty areas: Adult, family, gerontological, pediatric, and women's health.* Washington, DC: U.S. Department of Health and Human Services, Health Resources and Services Administration, Bureau of Health Professions.

U.S. Office of Technology Assessment. (1986). *Nurse practitioners, physician's assistants and certified nurse midwives: A policy analysis.* Washington, DC: U.S. Government Printing Office.

Wright, L. M., & Leahy, M. (2005). *Nurses and families: A guide to family assessment and intervention.* Philadelphia: F.A. Davis.

3

Healthcare Issues

Shirlee Drayton-Brooks, PhD, FNP-BC, APRN-BC

GENERAL APPROACH

- Improving access to high-quality care to reduce health disparities is a major concern.
- There is increasing emphasis on culturally competent care and evidence-based practice.
- Medical errors and safety issues in healthcare systems remain concerns.
- 45+ million Americans are underserved because of limited access to care.
- 13% of the uninsured are children.
- High costs of insurance, fees, and medication have made health care unattainable for many poor working families.
- Causes of infant mortality have changed from primarily infectious and nutritional to noninfectious causes, such as congenital anomalies and perinatal events.

- There is increasing concern over drug-resistant organisms, bioterrorism, disaster preparedness, and pandemic flu.
- A resurgence of previously controlled infections, such as tuberculosis and syphilis, and the emergence of newer infections, such as HIV and West Nile Virus, coupled with antibiotic resistance and an increasingly global environment, make infectious disease a persistent threat to individuals at either end of the age spectrum.
- Current healthcare trends support greater emphasis on disease prevention, risk reduction, and health promotion rather than exclusive disease management.
- New emphasis on genetic research makes medical ethics a growing concern.
- Advanced practice nursing continues to expand in scope and authority.
- Managed care continues with increasing numbers of mandated restrictions.
- Healthcare technology continues to advance in general, and healthcare informatics in particular.

Red Flags

- *Health disparities:* The difference in the incidence, prevalence, mortality, and burden of disease and other adverse conditions that exist among specific population groups in the United States (National Institute on Aging, 2008)
- *Access:* The availability (or lack thereof) of healthcare services to all
- *Medically underserved community:* A setting with a shortage of personal health services
- *Vulnerability:* Open to physical, emotional, and/or socioeconomic harm
- *Disadvantaged:* Inhibited from knowledge, skills, and abilities to participate in the healthcare system as a provider and/or a receipt of health care because of economic, social, ethnic, or racial background, and/or physical or mental impairment
- *Underrepresented minorities:* Racial and ethnic populations whose representation among the health professions is lower than their proportion of the general population

EPIDEMIOLOGIC PRINCIPLES

Natural History of Disease: The course of disease development, expression, and progression in a person over time. Whether based on microbiology principles of certain organisms or large-scale research studies of causality, several stages appear to be universally descriptive:
- Stage of susceptibility (prepathological)
- Stage of presymptomatic disease (subclinical)
- Stage of clinical disease
- Stage of disability (or death)

Prevention of Disease: The goal is to intervene as early as possible to prevent disease or disability.
- Primary prevention
  - Interventions at the stage of susceptibility, directed at preventing disease from occurring
  - Ex: Education, exercise, nutrition, water fluoridation, immunizations, food-handling regulations, pollution control
- Secondary prevention
  - Interventions at the subclinical stage, directed at early detection of the illness or problem to reduce the severity of the disease
  - Ex: Genetic testing in newborns, lead screening, vision and hearing screening, smoking cessation programs, cholesterol screening, mammography, testicular self-examination

- Tertiary prevention
  - Interventions at the clinical stage of disease, directed at treatment and rehabilitation of the illness to prevent or minimize progression of the disease or its sequelae
  - Ex: Use of inhaled steroids in the management of asthma, use of penicillin prophylaxis in patients with sickle cell anemia, vitamin therapy in pregnancy

Etiology of Disease: The cause or the web of causation of a disease or problem
- Any factors (direct or indirect) that increase the likelihood of disease
- Prevalence rates describe a group at a certain point in time and the number within a group that has a particular disease or problem, like a snapshot in time.
- Incidence rates describe the rate of development of a disease in a group over a period of time, or the continuing occurrence of new cases of disease. See Table 3–2, which identifies the leading causes of death per age group.

Risk Factors
- Age, sex, social, cultural, familial, racial/ethnic, genetic occupational, and lifestyle history represent potential sources of problems and diseases that may be difficult or impossible to alter.
- Risk reduction programs may be established to decrease the vulnerability of individuals to certain problems by modifying some risks.

Communicable or Infectious Diseases: Illnesses caused by organisms that attack and invade vulnerable persons
- Involve identification of causative agents
- Rely on microbiology principles in understanding life cycle of organism
- Focus on intervention at vulnerable phases in course of disease or life cycle of organism
- Utilize selected infectious disease definitions (Table 3–1)

Table 3–1. Infectious Disease Definitions

General Definitions

Infection: Colonization and multiplication of an organism in the host, typically producing an immune response but no signs or symptoms

Disease: Stage when an infection produces signs and/or symptoms (including pathologic changes). Certain organisms (such as influenza virus) are capable of infection with or without producing disease; other organisms (such as measles virus) always produce disease in susceptible persons. Disease may vary in severity.

Colonization: The organism invades the host at a particular site, multiplies, and acts as a parasite but does not produce infection, immune response, or disease.

Carrier state: Persistence of an organism in a host; this stage may follow infection, disease, or colonization and may be infective to others.

Agent (Organism) Properties

Infectivity: Ability of an organism to invade and multiply in a susceptible host. Varicella is highly infective, rhinovirus is intermediate, and tubercle bacilli are of low infectivity.

Pathogenicity: Ability of an organism to produce disease. Rabies, rhinovirus, and varicella are highly pathogenic; adenovirus and rubella are intermediate; and tubercle bacillus is low.

Table 3-1. Infectious Disease Definitions (cont.)

Virulence: Severity of disease that an organism can produce, measured by criteria such as number of days in bed or the frequency of serious sequelae including death (fatality rate). Rabies virus is highly virulent (nearly 100% fatality rate); poliovirus is moderately virulent; varicella and rhinovirus are of low virulence (almost zero fatality rate).

Immunogenicity: Ability to produce a lasting and effective immunity. Rhinovirus, which primarily acts locally, results in a poor systemic immune response. Systemic viral infections, such as measles, produce lasting immunity.

Agent–Host Relations

Latent infection: The organism is not shedding or obtainable (likely hidden in host cells).

Patent infection: The organism is shedding and/or obtainable from such areas as feces, urine, blood, or respiratory tract. Certain infections may remain permanently patent (some cases of hepatitis B) or be intermittently patent (herpes virus), or, after being latent for a long time, reactivate and produce disease (tuberculosis and herpes zoster).

Period of communicability: The time when sufficient numbers of organisms are shed to cause transmission; usually concurrent with disease but not always

Incubation period: The time from exposure to the onset of disease

Reservoirs of infection
- Cases and carriers
- Animal carriers (lower vertebrate animals)
- Invertebrate hosts (insects)
- Inanimate objects: Some infectious agents are free-living in the environment, multiplying on inanimate objects (such as *Salmonella* in food, *Legionella* in pools of water, *Histoplasma* in oil)

Mechanisms of transmission of infection
- Direct: Through touching, kissing, sexual intercourse, childbearing, breastfeeding, transfusions
- Indirect: Through air, vector (insect, animals), vehicle (food, water, towels)

Control measures
- Measures directed against the reservoir: Isolation, quarantine, insect spraying
- Measures that interrupt the transmission of organisms: Water purification, milk pasteurization, barrier protection during sexual intercourse
- Measures that reduce host susceptibility: Immunization, appropriate use of antibiotics, improved nutrition

Concepts of epidemic vs. endemic infections
- *Generation time:* Interval between receipt of infection and the maximal communicability of the host; applied to both subclinical and clinical infections (incubation period applies only to clinical cases); used to describe and analyze the spread of infectious diseases (i.e., common vehicle, single-exposure epidemic, determined by the incubation or generation time).
- *Herd immunity:* Resistance of a group to invasion and spread of an infectious agent because a large portion of the group is immune; decreases the likelihood of an epidemic in an area.

Table 3-2. Leading Causes of Death by Age Group

Age	Cause of Death
Under 1 year	Congenital anomalies
	Short gestation
	Sudden infant death syndrome (SIDS)
	Maternal complications
	Unintentional injury
	Placenta, cord membranes
	Respiratory distress
	Bacterial sepsis
	Neonatal hemorrhage
	Circulatory system disease
1–4 years	Unintentional injuries
	Congenital anomalies
	Malignant neoplasm
	Homicide
	Influenza and pneumonia
	Septicemia
	Perinatal period
	Benign neoplasm
	Chronic low respiratory disease
	Cancer
5–14 years	Unintentional injuries
	Malignant neoplasm
	Congential anomalies
	Homicide
	Suicide
	Heart disease
	Chronic low respiratory disease
	Benign neoplasm
	Influenza and pneumonia
	Cerebrovascular disease
15–19 years	Unintentional injury
	Homicide
	Suicide
	Malignant neoplasm
	Heart disease
	Congenital anomalies
	Chronic low respiratory disease
	Influenza and pneumonia
	Anemias and benign neoplasms
20–24 years	Unintentional injury
	Homicide
	Suicide
	Malignant neoplasm
	Heart disease
	Congenital anomalies
	HIV

Table 3–2. Leading Causes of Death by Age Group (cont.)

Age	Cause of Death
	Cerebrovascular disease
	Complicated pregnancy
	Influenza and pneumonia
25–34 years	Unintentional injury
	Suicide
	Homicide
	Malignant neoplasm
	Heart disease
	HIV
	Diabetes mellitus
	Cerebrovascular disease
	Benign neoplasm
	Septicemia
35–44 years	Unintentional injury
	Malignant neoplasm
	Heart disease
	Suicide
	HIV
	Homicide
	Liver disease
	Cerebrovascular disease
	Diabetes mellitus
	Influenza and pneumonia
45–54 years	Malignant neoplasms
	Heart disease
	Unintentional injury
	Liver disease
	Suicide
	Cerebrovascular disease
	Diabetes mellitus
	HIV
	Chronic lung disease
	Septicemia
55–64 years	Malignant neoplasms
	Heart disease
	Chronic lower respiratory diseases
	Diabetes mellitus
	Cerebrovascular disease
	Unintentional injury
	Liver disease
	Suicide
	Nephritis
	Septicemia
65 years and older	Heart disease
	Malignant neoplasm

Age	Cause Of Death
	Cerebrovascular disease
	Chronic lower respiratory disease
	Unintentional injury
	Alzheimer's disease
	Diabetes mellitus
	Influenza & pneumonia
	Nephritis
	Septicemia

Table 3–2. Leading Causes of Death by Age Group (cont.)

Adapted from "Deaths: Leading Causes for 2004," by M. Heron, *National Vital Statistics Report*, 56(5). Published by U.S. Department of Health and Human Services, Centers for Disease Control and Prevention.

HUMAN DEVELOPMENT

Developmental Theory
- All development is patterned, orderly, and predictable with both a purpose and a direction.
- Development is continuous throughout life, although the degree of change in many areas decreases after adolescence.
- Development may occur simultaneously in several areas, such as physical and social, but the rate of change in each area varies.
- Development proceeds from the simple to the complex.
- The pace of development varies among individuals.
- Physical and mental stress during periods of critical developmental change, such as puberty, may make a person particularly susceptible to outside stressors.

Erikson's Stages of Psychosocial Development (Erikson, 1963)
Maintains that how well individuals accomplish developmental tasks will determine their success in accomplishing other tasks as they get older. Tasks to be mastered include:
- Trust (failure causes mistrust)
- Autonomy (failure leads to feelings of shame and doubt)
- Initiative (failure leads to feelings of guilt)
- Industry (failure leads to feelings of inferiority)
- Identity (failure leads to role confusion)
- Intimacy (failure leads to additional role confusion)
- Generativity (failure leads to stagnation)
- Ego identity (failure leads to despair)

Piaget's Cognitive Development Theory (Piaget, 1969)
Focuses on intellectual changes (ways of thinking), which occur in a sequential manner as a result of continuous interaction with the environment. The stages are:
- Sensorimotor (infancy)
- Preoperational thinking
- Concrete operations
- Formal operations (involves logic, determines possibilities, problem-solves, and makes decisions)

Bowen Family System Theory (Kerr & Bowen, 1988)

Explains current family situations in terms of past relationships and family histories.
- Connects one's past family experiences with current behaviors
- Suggests that multiple factors interacting across time influence family functioning
- Identifies the interactions among biological, genetic, psychological, and sociological factors that influence human behaviors

Sadavoy (Sadavoy, 1987)

Identified critical geriatric age-related stresses.
- Interpersonal loss, loss of social support such as loss of spouse, family, friends
- Physical disability, loss of strength
- Loss of youthful appearance and beauty
- Change in social role, such as children caring for parent
- Forced reliance on caregivers
- Change in living arrangements such as loss of house
- Confrontation with death

Infant/Child Development

- Assessment of growth is determined by routine monitoring of height, weight, head circumference (until age 2), dental development, and the appearance of secondary sex characteristics.
- Adequacy of growth is determined by comparison with normal growth parameters (Tables 3–3 through 3–6) and/or plotting the measurements of height, weight, and head circumference on a standard National Center for Health Statistics (NCHS) growth chart.
- There are two periods of rapid growth: infancy and adolescence; in between, growth is steady but slower.
- Growth of most body tissues parallels physical growth, which is most rapid in the first 2 years; lymph tissue growth is rapid in the preschool and early school-age years; growth of reproductive organs remains slow until puberty.

Patterns of development

- Sequence of development is basically the same in all children, but the rate varies.
- Attainment of developmental landmarks in one area does not always run parallel with another area of development.
- Denver Development II is a test for providers to use with children from birth to 6 years and scored based on a range of behaviors characteristic of a certain age. Children who cannot perform the activities of their age cohort then can be given special attention to identify underlying problems and strategies to overcome deficits. More information can be found at www.denverii.com.
- Development is dependent on the maturation of the nervous system.
- Generalized activity precedes specific movements (young infant kicks and waves arms with excitement, whereas the older infant reaches out and grasps).
- Development occurs in a cephalocaudal direction (head control develops before walking) and a proximal to distal direction (shoulders before fingers).
- Certain primitive reflexes must be lost before the corresponding voluntary movement is acquired (grasp reflex lost before deliberately grasping objects can occur).

Table 3-3. Normal Growth Parameters for Height and Weight

Age	Weight*	Height*
Newborn	95% of newborns weigh 5–10 lbs. Approximately 5%–10% of body weight is lost in first few days, then birthweight is regained in 7–10 days.	95% of newborns are between 18 and 22 in. long.
Birth–6 months	Weekly gain 140–200 g (5–7 ounces). Birthweight is doubled by 6 months.	Monthly gain is 2.5 cm (1 in.).
6–12 months	Weekly gain 85–140 g (3–5 ounces). Birthweight is tripled by age 1 year.	Monthly gain is 1.25 cm (0.5 in.). Birth length increases by approximately 50% by age 1 year.
Toddlers	Yearly gain 2–3 kg (4–6 lbs)	Growth is approximately 12 cm (5 in. between ages 1–2 years, 6–8 cm (2–3 inches) between ages 2–3 years. Approximately 50% of adult height is reached by age 2 years.
School age	Yearly gain approximately 2–3 kg (4–7 lbs). Growth is approximately 5–6 cm (2–3 inches) per year. Birth length doubles by age 4 years and triples by age 13 years.	
Puberty—Females (10–14 years)	Weight gain 15–55 lbs (mean 38 lbs)	Growth is approximately 5–25 cm (2–10 inches). 95% of adult height is achieved by menarche (skeletal age of 13 years).
Puberty—Males (11–16 years)	Weight gain 15–65 lbs (mean 52 lbs)	Growth is approximately 10–30 cm (4–12 inches). 95% of adult height is achieved by skeletal age of 15 years.

*These measurements are averages.

Adapted from *Whaley & Wong's nursing care of infants and children* (86th ed.) by M. J. Hockenberry, 2006, St. Louis, MO: Mosby Year Book, The National Center for Health Statistics.

Table 3–4. Normal Parameters for Heart Rate and Respiration

Age	Heart Rate* (beats/min)	Respiratory Rate (beats/min)
Newborn	70–190	30–40
12 months	80–160	20–40
2 years	80–130	25–32
4 years	80–120	23–30
6 years	75–115	21–26
12 years	Female: 70–110	18–22
	Male: 65–105	
16 years	Female: 60–100	16–20
	Male: 55–95	
Adult	60–100	10–20

*Resting measurements

Adapted from *Physical examination and health assessment* by C. Jarvis, 2007, St. Louis, MO: Elsevier Science.

Table 3–5. Blood Pressure

Category	Systolic BP (mm Hg)	Diastolic BP (mm Hg)
Normal: Child 3–5 years	116	76
Normal: Child 6–9 years	122	78
Normal: Child 10–12 years	126	82
Normal: Teen 13–15 years	136	86
Normal: Adult 20–40 years	Under 130	Under 85
Optimal: Adult	Under 120	Under 80
High Normal: Adult	130–139	85–89
Stage 1 Mild Hypertension	140–159	90–99
Stage 2 Moderate Hypertension	160–179	100–109
Stage 3 Severe Hypertension	180–209	110–119
Stage 4 Very Severe Hypertension	210 and above	120 and above

Adapted from "High blood pressure chart," by www.highbloodpressureinfo.org, in *Look after the whole family using this blood pressure reading chart*, 2006.

Table 3–6. Normal Parameters of Head Growth

Age		Size/Growth
Newborn		32–33 cm, about 2 cm larger than the chest
2 weeks–6 months		1.85 cm/month
6–12 months		0.5 cm/month
FONTANELS	Size at Birth	Closure
Posterior	0.5–1 cm	1–2 months
Anterior	2.5–4 cm	9 months–2 years

Adapted from *Physical examination and health assessment* by C. Jarvis, 2007, St. Louis, MO: Elsevier Science.

Tooth Eruption

- Deciduous teeth usually begin at 6 months of age with the central incisors and move laterally.
- All 20 deciduous teeth are in by 2–3 years of age.
- Delayed dentition is considered when no teeth have erupted by 13 months of age.
- Shedding of deciduous teeth begins at about 6 years of age and continues through age 12.
- Eruption of the first permanent teeth occurs with the first molars at about age 6 years.
- Eruption of all 32 permanent teeth may not be complete until ages 17–21 with third molars.

Developmental Landmarks/Milestones

- Development typically is assessed in 4 areas: gross motor, fine motor, language, and social skills.
- Most widely used developmental assessment tool is the Denver II (see Patterns of development, pg. 34)
- Purpose is to identify children in need of further assessment and determine if a developmental disability exists
- All states are required to have a system to identify and treat developmental disabilities in children ages 3–5 years; most states have voluntary extended this age range.

Interpreting results

- Attainment of milestones is in ranges.
- A significant finding in any developmental assessment is the loss of developmental milestones previously achieved or lack of key milestones by certain age (Table 3–7).
- Language and fine motor skills are sensitive indicators of intellectual development.
- Early attainment of gross motor skills is not a significant indicator of advanced intellectual development but does usually preclude the diagnosis of mental retardation. Developmental warning signs can be found in Table 3–8.
- No child is mentally retarded if delayed in one area but normal in all others.

Table 3-7. Developmental Milestones

Tasks	Average Age (Range)*
Gross Motor Skills	
Moves head from side to side	2 weeks
Lifts shoulders while prone	2 months
Rolls over	4 months (2–6 months)
Head control (no bobbing)	4 months
Sits alone	6 months (5–9 months)
Pulls to stand	9 months (6–10 months)
Crawls (reciprocal)	9 months (8–11 months)
Cruises	9 months (8–13 months)
Walks alone	12 months (9–15 months)
Runs, walks upstairs holding rail	18 months (14–21 months)
Throws ball overhand	19–20 months (16–24 months)
Pedals tricycle	28 months (21–36 months)
Balances on one foot	28–30 months (22–38 months)
Hops on one foot	4 years (3–4 years)
Tandem walk	5 years (3–5 years)
Skips	5 years

Table 3-7. Developmental Milestones (cont.)

Tasks	Average Age (Range)*
Fine Motor Skills	
Unfists	3–4 months
Holds objects placed in hand	3–4 months (2–5 months)
Reaches for objects	4 months (3–5 months)
Transfers objects	6 months (4–7months)
Ulnar raking	6 months (5–7 months)
Inferior pincer	9–10 months
Mature pincer	11–12 months
Deliberate throw	12–13 months
Spontaneous scribble	14–16 months (12–16 months)
Tower of 2	15 months (12–20 months)
Tower of 4	18 months (16–20 months)
Tower of 6	24 months (17–30 months)
Imitates line	24 months (19–30 months)
Tower of 10	36 months
Copies circle	36 months (2–3 years)
Uses scissors	3 years
Copies square	4 years (4–5 years)
Draws 3-part man	4 years (3–5 years)
Copies triangle	5 years
Draws 6-part man	5 years (4–6 years)
Language (Receptive and Expressive)	
Localizes sound	4–9 months
Babbling vowels	5–6 months
Babbling consonants	6–7 months
"Dada"/"mama" nonspecific	9–10 months
"Dada"/"mama" specific	10–12 months
1–3 words	11–13 months
Follows one-step command	11–15 months
10–15 words, 25% intelligible	15–18 months
Points to named pictures when asked "show me"	18–24 months
Approximately 50-word vocabulary; 2-word combinations	21–24 months
Approximately 100-word vocabulary by 2nd birthday; says "me" and "mine." (As a rule, the number of words in a sentence equals the child's age [2 by age 2, 3 by age 3].) 2- to 3-word phases	2 years
Follows 2-step commands without gesture	30 months
Few possessives ("my ball") and progressives (the –ing: I playing)	30 months
Concept of "I" questions	30 months

Table 3-7. Developmental Milestones (cont.)

Tasks	Average Age (Range)*
Knows few colors, pronouns, plurals, full name, age, approximately 250-word vocabulary, 3–4 word sentences (75% intelligible)	36 months
Counts to 4, can say a nursery rhyme, asks and answers why, how, when, knows opposite analogies, and uses past tense	4 years
Uses complex sentences, understands meaning of words, counts to 10, fluent speech, future tense	5 years

Social, Interactive, Vision

Regards face	0–1 month
Smiles responsively	1–1½ months
Hand regard	4–5 months
Smiles at mirror image	5 months
Plays peek-a-boo	5–8 months
Plays pat-a-cake	10 months
Waves bye	10 months (7–14 months)
Indicates wants	12 months (10–14 months)
Imitates housework	15 months (13–18 months)
Washes and dries hands	22 months (19 months–2 years)
Puts on clothing	22 months

*Ages will vary with different tests.

Adapted from *Nelson Essentials of Pediatrics* (5th ed.) by R. M. Kliegman, K. J. Marcdant, H. B. Jenson, & R. E. Behrman, 2006, Philadelphia: Elsevier.

Table 3-8. Developmental Warning Signs

6 weeks	Absence of auditory alertness
	Lack of visual fixation (focusing)
	Excessive head lay on pulling-to-sitting position
6 months	Persistence of hand regard
	Failure to follow 180° (for both near and far objects)
	Persistent fisting
	Preference of one hand
10 months	Absence of babble
	Absence of weight-bearing while head held
	Failure to sit without support
18 months	No spontaneous vocalizations
	No pincer grasp
	Inability to stand without support
2 years	No recognizable words
	No walking

Adolescent Pubertal Changes

Male

- Average age of onset is 10.5 to 16 years.
- Precocious puberty is the development of secondary sex characteristics prior to age 9 and is often associated with a pathological etiology in males.
- Delayed puberty is lack of changes by age 14 years.
- First change is testicular enlargement, followed by pubic hair development at the base of the penis (adrenarche); testicular size >2–2.5 cm indicates puberty has begun (see Table 3–9 for average staging)
- Penile growth occurs approximately 6–12 months after testicular enlargement; penis grows from a prepubertal size of 3.5–5.5 cm to an adult length of 12 cm (7.5–15.5 cm).
- Growth spurt begins about 1 year after the first testicular changes (average age 12.5 years), peaks after 1.5 years, and lasts 2–4 years.
- Accompanying changes, such as axillary and facial hair and deepening voice, occur later in puberty.

Female

- Average age of onset is 11 years, with a range of 8 to 13 years.
- Precocious puberty is the onset of changes prior to 8 years of age or menarche before age 10 years.
- Delayed puberty is no breast development by age 13 years or no menses by 15–16 years.
- First pubertal change is usually breast budding under the areola (the larche) and pubertal fine hair over the mons pubis (adrenarche or pubarche; see Table 3–9 for typical staging).
- Menarche occurs at an average age of 12.5 years (range 10–15).

Table 3–9. Pubertal Staging

Male Pubic Hair

Stage	Description	Average Age
1	None	Preadolescent
2	Scanty, at base of penis	12 years
3	Hair becomes darker, curlier, and coarser	13 years
4	Adult-like, but smaller amount	14 years
5	Adult-like	15 years

Female Pubic Hair

Stage	Description	Average Age
1	None	Preadolescent
2	Small amount, primarily along labia	11 years
3	Hair darkens, increases in amount, curlier	12 years
4	Adult-like, but smaller amount	12 years
5	Adult-like	14 years

Genital Development

Stage	Description	Average Age
1	None	Preadolescent
2	Testicular size increases, scrotum reddens	12 years

Breast Development

Stage	Description	Average Age
1	None	Preadolescent
2	Breast bud	11 years

Table 3-9. Pubertal Staging (cont.)

Stage	Description	Average Age	Stage	Description	Average Age
3	Penis enlarges (length)	13 years	3	Breast and areola enlargement, no contour	11 years
4	Penis enlarges (breadth and length); scrotal growth continues	14 years	4	Areola and papilla project to form second mound above breast	12 years
5	Adult-like	15 years	5	Adult-like	13 years

Adapted from *Growth of Adolescents* (2nd ed.), by J. M. Tanner, 1962, Oxford: Blackwell Scientific.

HEALTH MAINTENANCE

Current Factors Support Greater Emphasis on Health Promotion and Disease Prevention

Healthy People 2010 (U.S. Department of Health and Human Services, Office of Disease Prevention and Health Promotion, 2001; www.healthypeople.gov) is the prevention agenda for the nation as outlined by the federal government. It is a statement of national health objectives designed to identify the most significant preventable threats to health and to establish national goals to reduce these threats. It began with the 1979 Surgeon General's Report *Healthy People*, which laid the foundation for a national prevention agenda. *Healthy People 2010* national objectives emphasize disease prevention and define leading health indicators necessary to measure health over the next 10 years. As a group, these objectives reflect the major health concerns in the United States at the beginning of the 21st century. Leading health indicators were selected on the basis of their ability to motivate action, availability of data to measure progress, and importance as public health issues. They include:

- Physical activity
- Overweight and obesity
- Tobacco use
- Substance abuse
- Responsible sexual behavior
- Mental health
- Injury and violence
- Environmental quality
- Immunization
- Access to health care
- Disease prevention and health promotion emphasis has shifted away from infectious etiologies as major causes of morbidity and mortality.
- 50% of illness and disease is related to lifestyle and unhealthy decisions.
- Three groups of behaviors that would improve population health:
  - Preventative health services: Infant care, immunizations, sexually transmitted disease services

- Health protection activities: Toxic agent control, occupational safety, injury prevention, water fluoridation, infectious disease control
- Health promotion behaviors: Smoking cessation, decreased alcohol and drug use, improved exercise and fitness, stress reduction
- Changing demographics mean more people living longer with less disease and dysfunction.
- Emphasis on containing costs means prevention and early detection rather than merely treatment of illness.

MODELS AND THEORIES RELATED TO HEALTH CARE

Health Belief Model (Becker, 1972)
- Model to explain why healthy people do or do not take advantage of screening programs
- Involves variables such as perceptions of susceptibility and seriousness of a disease, benefits of treatment, perceived barriers to change, and expectations of efficacy
- Optimal interventions consider all of these factors.

Maslow's Hierarchy of Needs (Maslow, 1954)
- Some needs are more important than others and must be met before other needs can be considered. The hierarchy includes:
  - Survival needs: Water, food, sleep
  - Safety and security: Protection from hazards
  - Love and belonging: Affection, intimacy, companionship
  - Self-esteem: Sense of worth
  - Self-actualization: Achieving potential

Trans-theoretical Model of Change (Prochashka & DiClemente, 1984)
- Six predictable stages of change:
  - Pre-contemplation
  - Contemplation
  - Preparation
  - Action
  - Maintenance
  - Termination

Self-Efficacy or Social Cognitive Theory Model (Bandura, 1986)
- Self-efficacy is the perception of one's ability to perform a certain task at a certain level of accomplishment.
- Behavior change and maintenance are a function of outcome expectations and efficacy expectations.

HEALTH MAINTENANCE PRACTICE

Lifestyle/Health Behaviors

Routine counseling and chemoprophylaxis in primary prevention can prevent certain conditions (see Table 3–10).

Specific health behaviors that are amenable to intervention can be found in Table 3–11.

Table 3–10. Chemoprophylaxis for Disease Prevention

Preventing Primary Disease

Condition	Rationale	Recommendations
Neural tube defects	Neural tube defects encompass a number of disorders of the cranium, spine, and nervous system that occur when the neural tube fails to close. Folic acid supplementation has resulted in >50% reduction in these birth defects. The average North American diet includes less than half the recommended dietary intake of folic acid.	All women of childbearing years, whether pregnant or not, take 0.4 mg daily of folic acid either alone or as part of a multivitamin supplement. The dose is increased with pregnancy.
Hemorrhagic disease of the newborn	Newborn gut lacks the bacteria necessary to synthesize Vitamin K, which is used for coagulation.	Vitamin K (phytonadione), 1 mg, is administered once immediately after birth.
Ophthalmia neonatorum	Primary purpose is the prevention of gonococcal and chlamydial conjunctivitis in the neonate. Silver nitrate is not effective against chlamydia and not used as frequently.	Instilled immediately postpartum: a single application of 1% silver nitrate ophthalmic drops, 0.5% erythromycin ophthalmic ointment, or 1% tetracycline ophthalmic ointment.

Table 3–10. Chemoprophylaxis for Disease Prevention (cont.)

Condition	Rationale	Recommendations
Group B *Streptococcus* (GBS) [prevention in the newborn]	In the early 1970s, GBS was a primary cause of neonatal sepsis and meningitis. Prevention strategies began to screen women for GBS and provide antibiotic prophylaxis for those women who were positive or had specific risk factors.	Screen pregnant women for GBS in one of two ways: • Obtain vaginal and rectal cultures at 35–37 weeks gestation. • If no culture results are available, the decision for chemoprophylaxis is based on the presence of one or more risk factors: delivery at 37 weeks gestation or less, membranes ruptured for >18 hours, intrapartum fever of 38°C or higher, or if mother had a previous infant with GBS disease or had GBS bacteriuria herself. Whichever screening method is used, the treatment is the same: IV penicillin G, 5 million units, followed by 2–5 million units every 4 hours until delivery. Treatment is most effective if at least two doses of penicillin are given.
Dental caries	Reduction of dental caries can be accomplished with fluoride and sealants. Excess fluoride will cause fluoroses (mottling of the teeth).	Dose of fluoride is dependent on fluoride concentration in the water and age of the child. Sealants are plastic coverings applied by the dentist for secondary molars.

Table 3–10. Chemoprophylaxis for Disease Prevention (cont.)

Disease Prevention in High-Risk Persons

Respiratory syncytial virus (RSV)	RSV is responsible for the majority of lower respiratory tract infections in children. RSV is a paramyxovirus that produces fusion of human cells in tissue. RSV attacks the upper and lower respiratory tracts, often causing life-threatening pneumonia and bronchiolitis. Bronchiolitis may begin as a mild upper respiratory tract infection that progresses to difficulty breathing with a cough and wheeze. RSV causes potentially life-threatening airway obstruction.	Treatment is focused on symptom relief. Airway management with bronchodilators, hydration, and antivirals may be used to manage RSV.
Infective endocarditis (IE) or subacute bacterial endocarditis (SBE)	SBE prophylaxis with antibodies is recommended for persons with specific cardiac conditions who are undergoing procedures that may induce a transient bacteremia. High-risk conditions include prosthetic valves, most congenital heart malformations, rheumatic heart disease, hypertrophic cardiomyopathy, mitral valve prolapse with regurgitation and previous bacterial, endocarditis. High-risk procedures include most type of dental work (tooth extractions, cleaning, surgery) and operations within the oropharynx, gastrointestinal, and genitourinary tract. Failures may occur even with adherence to recommendations.	Recommended prophylaxis: oral amoxicillin, 50 mg/kg (maximum 2 grams) 1 hour prior to the procedure. If allergic to penicillin, use cephalexin (50 mg/kg, maximum 2 grams) or azithromycin or clarithromycin (15 mg/kg, maximum 500mg).

Table 3–10. Chemoprophylaxis for Disease Prevention (cont.)		
Disease Prevention in High-Risk Persons		
Streptococcus pneumoniae (Pneumococcal disease)	Extended (possibly lifelong) antibiotic prophylaxis is recommended for those individuals at risk for developing fulminant pneumococcal disease, particularly patients with sickle cell disease and asplenia. Pneumococcal vaccine may change these recommendations, but currently antibiotics are recommended even if vaccine is given.	Penicillin G or V <5 years of age, 125 mg bid >5 years of age, 250 mg bid Likely for life
Prevent Recurrences of Disease		
Acute rheumatic fever (ARF)	Continuous antibiotics effective against Group A *Streptococcus* are provided for individuals who have a documented history of acute rheumatic fever to prevent recurrences. Antibiotic prophylaxis should begin as soon as the diagnosis of ARF is made and continue through life.	Benzathine penicillin IM every 4 weeks or daily oral antibiotics: • Penicillin V, 125–250 mg bid, or • Erythromycin 250 mg bid, or • Sulfadiazine >60 pounds, 1 g daily <60 pounds, 0.5 g daily
Urinary tract infections (UTIs)	Children (infants to adolescents) with recurrent UTIs (>2–3 episodes) are candidates for antibiotic prophylaxis to prevent recurrences.	Daily antibiotic therapy, usually with nitrofurantoin or trimethoprim-sulfa-methoxazole, is given for various lengths of time: • Children with normal urinary tracts are usually treated until infection-free for 6–12 months • Children with vesiculoureteral reflux are treated until reflux resolves • Children with urinary tract abnormalities are often on long-term therapy

Table 3-10. Chemoprophylaxis for Disease Prevention (cont.)

Meningitis (*Neisseria meningitidis* or *Haemophilus influenzae*)	Antibiotic prophylaxis is recommended for household members and child-care contacts of infected person.	Administer rifampin within 24 hours of identifying the person at 10 mg/kg every 12 hours x 2 days (4 doses) for *Neisseria*; for *Haemophilus*, use a 4-day regimen.
Pertussis	Household contacts of infected person should receive antibiotic prophylaxis.	Administer erythromycin estolate (some experts use azithromycin) at 40–50 mg/kg/day (maximum 2 g/day) for 14 days.
Sexually transmitted diseases	Symptomatic or asymptomatic persons exposed to partners with *Chlamydia*, gonorrhea, or syphilis are treated with appropriate antibiotics.	Same treatment regimen is used for the infected and the exposed person (see Chapter 13).

Table 3-11. Specific Health Behaviors Amenable to Intervention

Factor	Strength of evidence	Benefit	Age for which recommended	Recommendation
Exercise	Good evidence	Many, including preventing cardiac disease, death	All ages; proven in men in their 90s	Individualize
Nutrition	Simple, focused intervention can be effective	Help with many chronic conditions	No upper limit	Counseling re: adequate diet
Calcium	Good evidence in high-risk patients	Reduce risk of osteoporosis	Postmenopausal women	1000–1500 mg/day for women; no recommendation for men
Cholesterol	Diet not proven to be sufficient to reduce cholesterol level; normal levels proven to protect young to middle-aged men	Reduce hyperlipidemia, atherosclerotic cardiovascular disease (ASCD)	No support for screening and treatment over age 75	Cholesterol under 200, LDL depends on risk factors
Weight Loss	Well-documented in adults up to 65	Reduce risk factor for ASCD	Not studied in elderly	Maintain ideal body weight

Table 3–11. Specific Health Behaviors Amenable to Intervention (cont.)

Factor	Strength of evidence	Benefit	Age for which recommended	Recommendation
Stop Smoking	Strongest recommendation, simple interventions can have 5%–10% quit rate	Reduce risk for cardiovascular, pulmonary, gastrointestinal diseases and malignancies	Quitting at any time improves pulmonary function and decreases risk of myocardial infarction (MI) and death	Ask about and encourage cessation at each visit
Alcohol	Cessation difficult to achieve in alcoholics	Reduce risk for falls and confusion in the elderly	No age limit to improved safety	Ask about, counsel to use in moderation
Drugs	Well-documented	Reduce many risks of polypharmacy: adverse reactions, drug interactions, death in the elderly	Never too late	Check medications at each visit; ask about over-the-counter and herbal remedies. Use only medications that are medically necessary
Safety Injury/Abuse Prevention	Little data on prevention effectiveness	Reduce risk of falls, 6th leading cause of death	Different focus in the elderly	Home safety evaluation
Aspirin	Proven in middle-aged men; few studies in elderly, look promising	Primary and secondary prevention of cardiovascular and cerebrovascular disease	Recommended for men over 40 or 50	Low dose: 80–24 mg/d for cardiovascular health
Estrogen	Well-documented; weigh risks (such as increased risk of breast cancer) versus benefits	Reduce risk of osteoporosis, coronary artery disease	Postmenopausal women with no contraindications	Progestin reduces risk of endometrial cancer, increases risk of breast cancer
Immunization				
Influenza	Well-documented	Reduce incidence, severity of influenza	65+ years	Annually
Pneumonia	60% efficacy	Prevent *Streptococcus pneumoniae* infection	65+ years	Once; may repeat in 5 years
Tetanus	Well-proven	Prevent tetanus	No age limit	Every 10 years

Exercise

- Recommendation is 30 minutes of moderate physical activity on most days of the week; does not have to be continuous
- Recommendation is as important for children as for adults

Child and Adolescent Preparticipation Sports Assessment

- Children and adolescents participating in sports should have a preparticipation evaluation (PPE). Almost all states require medical clearance prior to sports participation, although no standardization of PPEs exists and evaluations may vary. The American Academy of Pediatrics and the American Association of Sports Medicine Physicians each have developed guidelines. Suggested components can be found in Table 3–12.
- The PPE should involve parents for athletes younger than 18 years of age.
- The goal of the PPE is to identify those who may need conditioning or rehabilitation, those who need further evaluation for clearance, and those who should be excluded from participation. Particular attention of the PPE should be directed at the cardiopulmonary and musculoskeletal systems.
- Sports physicals should not replace the routine physical exam but may include preventive healthcare teaching on such topics as the use of supplemental aids and prevention of injuries.
- Results of the PPE may allow for full participation (the majority), temporary deferral (due to illness or injury), partial deferral (i.e., no contact or collision sports) and/or recommendation for an appropriate sport for certain conditions, or exclusion.

Exercise Recommendations for Adults

- Focus on fundamental fitness and not sport-specific skills
- Goal: Sustain target heart rate for 30 minutes for maximum cardiopulmonary conditioning
  - Subtract patient's age from 220
  - Multiple result by 0.8 for target heart rate
  - A 40-year-old patient's target heart rate is 144 bpm
- Before prescribing an exercise program for any patient, conduct a history and physical examination and evaluate for:
  - Fatigue, shortness of breath, chest pain
  - Risk factors for thromboembolic disease
  - Excessive bruising
  - Cardiac murmurs, clicks, hums
  - Carotid bruits
  - Other physical indicators of undiagnosed vascular disease
  - Current medications
- Decrease intensity or components of exercise program if the patient:
  - Is unable to talk while exercising
  - Is fatigued for >1 hour after finishing
  - Develops swelling or pain
- Increase intensity and/or time as patient develops tolerance

Table 3-12. Suggested Components of General Preparticipation Sports Examination

Type of Examination Activity	Observations to Make
History Family history of congenital, inherited, or early onset heart disease or sudden death Past medical history of congenital or acquired heart conditions Medication history Chronic medical condition such as asthma, sickle cell disease Seizures or recent head injuries/ concussions Obtain a history regarding drug and nutritional supplement use	General symptoms: chest pain, syncope, palpitations, dizziness, or tachycardia, especially with exercise Musculoskeletal symptoms: pain, limited movement, localized or diffuse areas of swelling Medications linked to sudden death: albuterol, imipramine, cisapride, erythromycin, antiarrhythmic drugs, pseudoephedrine, phenylpropanolamine, inhaled epinephrine, caffeine-containing products, illicit drugs—especially cocaine Enlarged organs: persons with acutely enlarged livers and spleens should not participate in any sports because of the risk of rupture. Chronic enlargements require individual assessment
Vital signs before and after 30 seconds of mild activity: stair-climbing, jumping jacks Obtain height, weight, blood pressure, pulse, and pubertal level	Increased pulse rate, irregular pulse; increased respiratory rate; perspiration Growth, including pubertal changes, is a good indicator of health Abnormalities need further evaluation
Inspection of general body stature, facing forward and backward	Look for acromioclavicular symmetry, general habitus and posture; scoliosis
Range of motion, neck	Cervical spine motion
Shoulder shrug against resistance	Trapezius strength
Abduction of shoulders against resistance	Deltoid strength
Full external rotation of arms	Shoulder motion
Flex and extend elbows	Elbow motion
Arms at sides; elbows 90° flexed; pronate and supinate wrists	Elbow and wrist motion
Spread fingers; make fist	Hand or finger motion and deformities
Contract and relax quadriceps muscles	Symmetry and knee effusion; ankle effusion
"Duck walk" 4 steps (away from examiner with buttocks on heels)	Hip, knee, and ankle motion
Knees straight, touch toes	Scoliosis, hip motion, hamstring tightness
Walk on tip-toes, heels	Calf asymmetry, leg strength

Adapted from "Cardiac evaluation of the young athlete," by C. Berul, 2000, in *Pediatric Annals*, 29(3), 163.

General Nutrition

- Goal: Maintain or achieve ideal body weight and supply all essential body nutrients to maintain or regain health.
- Normal growth requires appropriate intake of protein, fat, carbohydrates, water, vitamins, minerals, and trace elements.
- Recommended dietary allowances (RDA) are estimates of safe and adequate amounts of nutrients recommended to be consumed daily to maintain health. The RDA is the amount of nutrient needed to meet the known nutrient requirements of approximately 97% of the population.
- U.S. Department of Agriculture (USDA) food pyramid and other research suggests:
  - Bread, rice, and cereals: 6–11 servings daily
  - Fruit: 2–4 servings daily
  - Vegetables: 3–5 servings daily
  - Milk, cheese, and yogurt: 2–3 servings daily
  - Meat, fish, poultry, eggs, beans, and nuts: 2–3 servings daily
  - Use sweets, fats, and oils sparingly
  - Diets should have substantial fiber
  - Use salt and sodium in moderation
  - Limit or avoid alcohol

Infant/Childhood/Adolescent Nutrition

Diet Planning

- Energy requirements can be determined using charts or the calculations in Table 3–13.
- Adolescents who have completed their growth and desire to lose weight will need to reduce calorie intake by 500 calories per day for each pound they wish to lose each week.
- No more than 2 pounds should be lost per week.
- Weight loss is not recommended for growing children (except under special circumstances and with close supervision).
- For children older than 2 years, 55%–60% of calories should come from carbohydrates, 10%–15% from protein, and no more than 30% from fat (with saturated fat 10% or less and less than 300 mg of cholesterol per day).
- Fat and cholesterol should not be restricted in the first 2 years of life.
- Recommended fiber intake is 0.5 g/kg/day, to a maximum of 35 g/day.

Table 3–13. Determining Energy Requirements

Age	Average kcal/kg/day
0–6 months	110–120
7–12 months	90–105
1–10 years	80
Adolescence	30–55

Ex: 9-month-old infant weighing 8 kg requires approximately 800 calories/day
(8 kg x 100 kcal/kg/day = 800)

Recommended nutritional supplements
- Vitamin K, 1mg IM, given at birth to all newborns to prevent hemorrhagic disease of the newborn.
- Vitamin D, 200 units/day, recommended for all breastfed infants until they are ingesting a minimum of 500 mL/day of vitamin D-fortified formula or milk.
- Ferrous sulfate, 2–3 mg/kg/day (max 15 mg/day), recommended for breastfed preterm infants by 2 months old.
- Iron-fortified cereals should be started by 6 months of age in all infants to replace iron stores, which are depleted by the time the infant doubles birthweight at approximately 4–5 months old.
- Fluoride supplements to reduce susceptibility to dental caries.
- No fluoride supplements are recommended prior to 6 months of age and where water fluoride content is > 0.6 ppm, to avoid fluorosis (excessive mottling of the teeth; see Table 3–14).
- American Medical Association now recommends a daily vitamin for all adults.

Table 3-14. Recommended Fluoride Doses When Water Has 0.3–0.6

Age	< 0.3 ppm	0.3–0.6 ppm
6 months–3 years	0.25 mg	0
3–6 years	0.5 mg	0.25 mg
6–11 years	1.0 mg	0.5 mg

Infant Nutrition
- Breast milk and/or formulas are sufficient to meet the nutrient needs of infants up to 4–6 months of age (exceptions noted above); see Table 3–15
- Advantages of breast milk: nutritionally balanced, contains antibodies and macrophages, free of bacteria, allergic reactions are rare, savings on time and money.
- Possible disadvantages: milk supply may be insufficient, mechanical difficulties such as inverted nipples may occur, medications and infectious organisms may pass to infant, nutritional deficiencies in the mother may affect infant
- All infant formulas are 20 calories/ounce except for those specifically labeled as higher in calories (e.g., Enfamil 24).
- Evaporated milk formula should not be recommended though it may be used in extenuating circumstances (e.g., unable to breastfeed and/or cannot afford formula). It is made by mixing 1 can of evaporated milk (13 ounces) with 19 ounces of water and 3 tablespoons of corn syrup. These infants must also receive a multivitamin with iron; dosage varies with age.

Table 3-15. Infant Formulas

	Cows' Milk–Based	Soy Protein Isolate	Protein Hydrolysates
Examples	Enfamil, Similac, Good Start	Isomil, ProSobee	Nutramigen, Pregestimil, Alimentum
Composition Comments	Casein/whey ratio varies with manufacturer Lactose is usual carbohydrate (CHO) source; lactose-free formulas using corn syrup and/or fructose now widely available Available in iron-fortified and low-iron preparations; low-iron formulas never recommended	CHO—sucrose and/or glucose Methionine is added to all soy formulas to correct deficiencies All are iron-fortified	Partially hydrolyzed protein that results in peptides that do not elicit an immunologic response Most are lactose-free
Uses	Routine use in well infants	Infants with lactose intolerance Infants with cows' milk protein sensitivity (approximately 20% of infants allergic to cows' milk are also allergic to soy)	Infants with cows' milk and soy sensitivity
Contraindications	Milk protein sensitivity Lactose intolerance Galactosemia	Soy protein allergy. Preterm infants—the CHO, protein, mineral absorption of soy formulas in preterm infants is not adequately documented and American Academy of Pediatrics (2004) does not recommend their use; soy formulas specifically developed for preterm infants are available Infants with renal disease	

Food introduction
- Guidelines have been directed more by tradition than by science.
- May be introduced when infant is able to sit with support and has good neuromuscular control of head and neck, typically around 4–6 months of age.
- Tradition has held that cereals are a good place to begin; use a spoon, avoid adding to bottle.
- Start with single-ingredient foods and add one new food at a time, with up to 4–7 days between foods to identify intolerances.

Food/formula cautions
- No low-iron formula use
- No cows' milk in the first year of life
- No honey prior to age 1 year because of possible development on infantile botulism
- Avoid foods high in salt or sugar, such as canned or processed foods; RDA for sodium for infants is 17.6 mg/kg/day.
- Avoid foods that can cause choking easily such as grapes, popcorn, hot dogs, raisins, nuts, candy, and peanut butter.
- Home preparation of foods such as spinach, beets, carrots, or collard greens may have enough nitrates to cause methemoglobinemia and are therefore not recommended in infancy.
- Foods considered highly allergenic, such as eggs, wheat, seafood, and nuts, have traditionally been withheld in the first year of life to avoid a possible allergic reaction, but the validity of this practice is uncertain.

Adult Nutrition
- Calculate body mass index (BMI) to determine overweight and obesity: weight in lbs ÷ height in inches^2) x 703. BMI > 25 is considered overweight according to the National Heart, Lung, and Blood Institute (National Institute of Health, National Heart, Lung, and Blood Institute, 2001)
- An online BMI calculator can be found at www.cdc.gov/nccdphp/dnpa/bmi/adult_BMI/english_bmi_calculator/bmi_calculator.htm
  - Healthy normal weight: BMI 18.5–25
  - Overweight: BMI > 25
  - Class I Obesity: BMI 30–34.9
  - Class II Obesity: BMI 35–39.9
  - Class III Obesity: BMI > 40
- Determine ideal body weight (IBW) using charts or the formula in Table 3–16.

Table 3-16. Formula for Determining Ideal Body Weight

Build	Women	Men
Medium	Allow 100 lbs for first 5 ft. plus 5 lbs for each additional inch. Ex: If patient is 5 ft. 4 in., IBW = 120 lbs (100 + 20)	Allow 105 lbs for first 5 ft. plus 6 lbs for each additional inch. Ex: 5 ft. 10 in., IBW = 165 lbs (105 + 60)
Small	Subtract 10%	Subtract 10%
Large	Add 10%	Add 10%

Losing weight
- In establishing realistic weight goals, calculate relationship of current weight compared to ideal body weight:
  - Determine IBW using formula
  - Divide IBW by current body weight
  - Multiply by 100
  - Subtract 100
  - Result gives % over or under ideal body weight

Diet planning
- Determine caloric needs by adding basal calories (IBW x 10) and activity calories (IBW x 3) for sedentary people; or IBW x 5 for moderately active people and IBW x 10 for people involved in strenuous activity.
- Example: IBW = 120 lbs for sedentary person
  120 x 10 = 1200 basal calories; 120 x 3 = 360
  1200 + 360 = 1560 total calories needed per day
- People who wish to lose weight will need to reduce calorie intake by 500 calories per day for each pound they wish to lose each week.
- Diets should limit fat to 30% or less of total calories, carbohydrates to 55%–60% of calories, the rest of calories from protein.

Geriatric Nutrition
- Goal: Supply all essential body nutrients to maintain or regain health
- Maintain, gain, or lose weight if necessary
- Adequate calcium intake: 1,000–1,500 mg a day
- Diet moderate in fat content to keep cholesterol within normal limits
- Frail elderly at risk for malnutrition—low albumin levels.

SAFETY

Childhood Injuries
- Injuries cause approximately half of all child deaths.
- Each year about 16 million children receive care for injuries.
- More than 30,000 children become permanently disabled annually because of injuries.
- The cost of injuries to children exceeds $7.5 million yearly.
- Injury rates vary with age, gender, ethnicity, socioeconomic status, and location.
- Highest rates of injury are in adolescents, infants, males, Native Americans, African Americans, low-income areas, and rural areas.
- Injuries are preventable (see Table 3–17).

Injury Prevention in Adults/Geriatrics
- Home safety evaluation for fall prevention:
  - Bathrooms are the site of most falls
  - Throw rugs are dangerous
  - Use contrast lighting to reduce hazards
  - Sufficient lighting needed both inside and outside the home
  - Safe and appropriate assisting devices
- Driving evaluations for safety:
  - Driving essential for independence, making patients reluctant to it give up
  - Driving can be impaired due to dementia, impaired vision, slowed reflexes, musculoskeletal disorders
  - Seat belts are necessary for safety
- Smoke detectors
- Safety locks on firearms
- Tips for environmental safety can be found in Table 3–18.

Assessment for Violence and Abuse
- Clinicians should ask about and watch for signs of physical abuse during encounters with patients.
- Patients will often admit to problems, but only if they are asked.
  - Know and utilize state laws in determining requirements to report suspected abuse.
  - Learn state requirements for a rape examination.

Geriatric Abuse and Neglect
- Risk factors include age over 84; social isolation; lack of support; cognitive impairment; and physical, emotional, and financial dependency.

Table 3-17. Injury and Prevention

Type of Injury	Epidemiology	Prevention
Motor vehicle accident (MVA)	MVAs account for about half of all unintentional injury deaths; infants and adolescents usually injured as occupants while school-age children predominantly injured as pedestrians.	Use of child restraints and seat belts is the most effective way to prevent occupant injuries. There are three basic types of restraints: (1) Infant carrier for birth–22 pounds and younger than 1 year. Ride semi-inclined and backward-facing in the back seat. (2) Toddler seat for >20 pounds and >1 year. Sits forward-facing, preferably in the back seat. (3) Booster seat (outgrown a toddler seat but too small to fit properly in a seat belt). Used for 40–80 pounds, preferably in the back seat. Car seat adaptations are available for premature infants, patients in casts, on ventilators, or with special medical conditions such as spina bifida. After reaching 8 years of age and 60 pounds, a child can use the adult lap/shoulder belt if it fits properly: the shoulder strap crosses the collar bone and chest, not the neck, and the lap belt crosses the lap or hips, not the abdomen. Laws vary by state. An infant or toddler car seat fits if the child's ears are below the top of the seat's back and shoulders are below the seat strap slots. A shoulder strap should not be used if it goes across the face or throat.

Table 3-17. Injury and Prevention (cont.)

Type of Injury	Epidemiology	Prevention
Drowning	Drowning is the second leading cause of accidental death, with peak occurrences in the infant/toddler and adolescent years. Poor supervision plays a key role in drowning of young children and infants. Adolescent drowning is often associated with alcohol use. Approximately 75% of drowning occurs in bodies of water that are part of the person's home, particularly bathtubs and pools. Infants can drown in inches of water and in unusual ways such as in pails of water and toilet bowls. Approximately one third of all survivors of drowning will suffer irreversible brain injury.	Supervision is the key to prevention: (1) Leave no children unattended in or near water. (2) Keep the bathroom door closed. (3) Empty all pails of water. (4) Keep swimming pools completely fenced with a locking gate. Teach children to swim and to behave safely around water, such as using life preservers. Infant swim lessons are not recommended because of the risk of water intoxication.
Fire and burns	These injuries account for approximately 10% of all trauma deaths overall and more than 20% in children less than 5 years of age. More than one million burn injuries occur per year and as many as 30,000 persons <15 years of age are hospitalized yearly for burns. Approximately 75% of all burns are scalds that occur in the kitchen. Bathtub water if >120°F can cause burns. Skin damage rarely occurs at temperatures <110°F, but a full-thickness burn can occur in 1 second in water 160°F. Approximately 85% of all deaths from fire are due to smoke inhalation during house fires.	Keep smoke alarms on each floor of the house and check the batteries every month. (All three types—heat, photoelectric, and ionization—are effective.) Keep pot handles turned in on the stove. Keep an ABC-rated fire extinguisher in the kitchen. Do not allow children to sit in adult laps when drinking hot liquids. Teach children fire escape route and rules, and practice escapes. Keep water temperature at 120°F.

Table 3–17. Injury and Prevention (cont.)

Type of Injury	Epidemiology	Prevention
Asphyxiation and choking	This type of injury accounts for approximately 40% of all unintentional deaths in children <1 year of age. Food items commonly choked on are hot dogs, candy, nuts, grapes, raisins, and raw vegetables. Nonfood items that children choke on include balloons, undersized infant pacifiers, small toys such as balls and jacks, coins, poptops, and safety pins. Asphyxiation occurs from situations such as hanging from drapery cords or bibs tied around neck, crib strangulations (head entrapment), toy chest lids falling on a child's head and neck, or when the nose and mouth are covered in a soft pillow, beanbag, or waterbed.	Do not feed small, round, hard foods to children less than 2–3 years of age. Do not allow children to run with food. No balloons prior to age 3 years and then monitor. Keep small objects out of the reach of children; evaluate all toys for safety. Encourage parents to learn the Heimlich maneuver. Tie up all cords. Use bibs with Velcro instead of ties. Use cribs with slat spacing 2 ⅜" or less. Do not place infants on any soft or enveloping surfaces.
Poisoning	American Association of Poison Control Centers estimates that there are 1.2 million poisonings in children <6 years annually. Although the number of pediatric poisonings is high, the fatality rate is low, much less than 0.1%. Toddlers are at the greatest risk. Children 6–12 years account for a very small percent. Adolescent exposures are usually intentional (suicide or abuse) or occupational. More than half of pediatric poisonings involve nondrug products, commonly cosmetics, personal care products (deodorants), cleaning substances, and plants. Pharmaceutical preparations comprise the remainder of ingestion poisonings with vitamins (particularly iron-containing products), analgesics, cold/cough medications, and antibiotics being the most common agents.	Childproofing the home should include putting all medications and other substances out of reach and/or behind locked doors. Use child-resistant medication containers. Keep the phone number of poison control readily available. It is no longer recommended that parents keep syrup of ipecac at home.

Table 3–17. Injury and Prevention (cont.)

Type of Injury	Epidemiology	Prevention
Falls	Falls are the fifth leading cause of death in children and result in enormous morbidity. Approximately 13,000 deaths occur annually due to falls. A disproportionately large number of fall injuries are caused by falling down stairs in infant walkers and falls from bunk beds, playground equipment, skateboards, and trampolines.	Never leave infants or toddlers unattended on elevated surfaces. Keep crib rails up at all times. Avoid walker use. Gates should be placed in front of all staircases. Windowsills and bunk beds should never be used as play areas. Use window guards. Do not allow children to participate in activities beyond their physical abilities, such as skateboarding down steep hills. Discourage the use of any trampolines. Use protective gear (helmets, pads) for bike riding, skateboarding, and sports.

Adapted from *Guide to Clinical Preventive Services* AHRQ Pub. No. 07-05100), by Agency on Healthcare Research and Quality, 2007, Washington, DC: Department of Health and Human Services.

Table 3–18. Prevention of Environment-Related Health Problems

Safety Hazard	Risk	Recommendations
Secondhand smoke	Increased risk of respiratory problems and cancer	No smoking in the home, car, or around children
Carbon monoxide exposure	Range from chronic flu-like symptoms to death	Use acceptable carbon monoxide detector in home; properly use and maintain fuel-burning devices
Radon	Increased risk of cancer	Test home for radon with a home test kit; if level exceeds 4pCi/L, identify and seal basement leaks
Lead	Lead poisoning—neurological damage, anemia	Do not use lead-containing utensils for cooking or eating Renovations done with proper precautions Employment in high risk places—use precautions

Adapted from *Guide to Clinical Preventive Services* AHRQ Pub. No. 07-05100, by Agency on Healthcare Research and Quality, 2007, Washington, DC: Department of Health and Human Services.

Stress

- Stress is the emotional and physical response to an increase in the environmental demands beyond the resources of an individual to cope with those demands.
- Stress theory is based on the General Adaptation Syndrome identified by Selye (1974), who described a continuum of stress. Small amounts of stress may add excitement and variety and increase the quality of life. Large amounts of stress may be overwhelming and lead to disease.
- The goal is to find the right balance of stress in life.
- Individuals often seem to have vulnerability to stress in one system (e.g., hypertension, ulcer, mental problems).

Stress management

- Stress may be managed through various techniques:
  - Avoid unnecessary change during stressful times.
  - Manage time by keeping to predetermined goals and priorities.
  - Avoid stressful triggers (people, activities, etc.) when possible.
  - Create habits or routines to decrease stress.
  - Develop alternative activities or friendships that increase pleasure.
  - Physical exercise often decreases stress.
  - Participate in religious, motivational, or service projects that increase self-esteem or change focus to helping others.
  - Use biofeedback, tension-relaxation exercise, yoga, or imagery to control stress reactions.

Interpersonal support

- High-quality interactions with others helps individuals maintain or regain health (Pender, 1996).
  - Types of supporting behaviors (Friedman, 1998):
    - Instrumental support gives direct assistance and service.
    - Informational support uses advice, suggestions, and information in solving problem.
    - Emotional support comes when love, care, empathy, and trust are provided through relationships.
    - Appraisal support uses feedback and affirmation to help people evaluate themselves.

Stressors in the elderly

- A common myth about the elderly is that they do not tolerate change.
- The elderly do face major life changes, especially losses—death of spouse and/or friends, having to move, retiring or losing jobs, ability to do many activities, etc.; these changes cause major stress in the elderly.

Dependency

- A common personality tendency that in its extreme form causes an individual to rely on other individuals or activities, such as eating food, drinking alcohol, having sex, gambling, or other activity, to try to satisfy an emotional hunger.
- Action begun voluntarily but, through repetition, becomes involuntary.
- Dependency becomes addiction when there is loss of control (compulsivity), continuation despite adverse consequences, and obsession or preoccupation with the activity.
- Treatment may be complex and require long-term therapy.

Pharmacology in the Geriatric Population

- Polypharmacy is a common problem, causing drug interactions.
- Age-related changes increase risk of drug toxicities:
  - Absorption is slower, delayed onset
  - Distribution in tissues affected by change in fat-to-muscle ratio
  - Metabolism slowed, increasing toxicity by drugs metabolized by the P450 system
  - Excretion through the kidney is decreased due to decreased renal function
- Drug toxicities are more common and more serious in the elderly:
  - Use lower doses, titrate up slowly
  - Monitor over-the-counter drug use closely
- Noncompliance is very common.

HEALTH MAINTENANCE

Child Health Supervision

- The general health of children can be significantly improved through the effective use of healthcare supervision (e.g., disease prevention, early detection and intervention of disorders, providing anticipatory guidance).
- Health supervision should be done at regularly scheduled well visits and should include obtaining a history and physical exam, vital signs, assessment of growth and development, obtaining age-appropriate screening tests, and counseling about nutrition, safety, and other topics.
- Recommended ages for well visits are at 2 weeks; 2, 4, 6, 9, 12, 15, 18, and 24 months; yearly from ages 3–6 years; every other year from ages 6–11 years; and yearly during adolescence.
- Additional visits may be needed for children with some variations of normal, for sports physicals, and for presurgical procedures.

Pediatric Health Screening

- Purpose: early detection of treatable conditions (Table 3–19).
- Not all abnormal results are identified on screening tests and continual monitoring of patient's condition and repeat testing may be necessary.
- Use of screening tests will change as incidence of disease changes (e.g., lead testing) and as technology improves (e.g., newborn hearing tests).
- Screening tests may be recommended primarily for high-risk groups (e.g., lead, cholesterol) at certain ages; others are universal tests for all children (anemia).

Table 3–19. Pediatric Screening Recommendations

Screening Tests	Ages for Screening	Testing and Interpretation
Neonatal, metabolic, and genetic screening ("PKU Test")	All full-term infants prior to discharge and in 1–2 weeks	All states screen for phenylketonuria (PKU) and hypothyroidism; most screen for galactosemia. Other tests are determined on a state-by-state basis and may include sickle cell disease, maple syrup urine disease, homocystinuria, congenital toxoplasmosis, adrenal hyperplasia, and cystic fibrosis. All positives require immediate confirmation and/or referral.
Hearing screening	All newborns	In 1999, the American Academy of Pediatrics recommended that all newborns be screened appropriately for hearing impairment. Tools for newborns include the evoked otoacoustic emissions (EOAE); test failures with auditory brain stem response (ABR).
	3, 4, 5, 10, 12, 15, & 18 years of age	Audiometric screening: Minimal evaluation should be 20 dB HL with frequencies of 1, 2, and 4 kHz. Any unheard frequency is a failure and the child should be retested at a later date. Failure again requires a referral.
Anemia screening	Hgb and Hct are recommended once between 1 and 9 months, and once during adolescence for menstruating females	Early screening allows for detection of iron deficiency anemia and congenital anemias such as thalassemia. Complete blood count (CBC) not only identifies an anemia, but the differential (and/or smear) allows for immediate classification (e.g., microcytic) and quicker determination of etiology. Treatable anemias are followed with a repeat CBC after treatment.

Table 3–19. Pediatric Screening Recommendations (cont.)

Screening Tests	Ages for Screening	Testing and Interpretation
Lead screening	Selectively obtain blood lead levels (BLLs) at 9–12 months and possibly again at 2 years old BLLs >10 mg/dL require retesting and possible further evaluation and treatment, depending on the level	(1) Screen all children who live in communities where: 27% of housing was built before 1950 or 12% of 1–2-year-olds have BLLs >10mcg/dL. (Such information is provided by state health officials.) (2) In all other communities, screen children who live in or regularly visit homes/facilities built before 1950, or 1978 if renovated in the past 6 months, or who have siblings/playmates with elevated BLLs. (3) Screen all children on Medicaid or other forms of public assistance. (4) Screen all children where community and home information is unknown. (5) Any child may be screened if other risk factors for lead exposure exist, such as cultural practices (use of lead pottery or lead-containing folk medicines), parent occupation, or adoption from countries where lead poisoning is prevalent, or where elevated BLLs may be contributing to a problem such as developmental delays.
Cholesterol and lipid screening	Obtain cholesterol or lipid profile for at-risk children as early as 2 years (although adolescent levels more accurately reflect adult levels). Retest every 5 years if levels are acceptable Cholesterol levels >170 should be retested with lipid profile	Screen children >2 years if a *parent or grandparent* has: (1) History of premature (<55 years of age) cardiovascular disease (myocardial infarct, stroke, or peripheral vascular disease); obtain a 12-hour fasting serum lipid profile (total cholesterol, LDL and HDL cholesterol, and triglycerides), or (2) Cholesterol >240; obtain fasting lipid panel on child. Optional testing may be obtained on any child with possible risk factors such as cigarette smoking, hypertension, obesity, diabetes mellitus, and/or physical inactivity. If elevation confirmed, provide dietary recommendations.

Table 3–19. Pediatric Screening Recommendations (cont.)

Screening Tests	Ages for Screening	Testing and Interpretation
Tuberculin (TB) skin test	Annual testing, with Mantoux (PPD) skin test for children at high risk; for children with no risk factors who live in high-prevalence regions or who lack a clear history, do periodic testing at ages 1, 4–6, 11–16 years of age (suggested; can be any age)	Children at high risk include those who: (1) Have contacts with infected adults. (2) Have clinical or X-ray findings suggestive of TB. (3) Are immunosuppressed (HIV). (4) Have chronic illness (diabetes, renal disease). (5) Come from high-prevalence countries (or their parents did). (6) Have or had frequent exposure to high-risk adults: HIV-positive, homeless, drug abuser, poor health, nursing home resident, or migrant worker. Induration considered positive: >5 mm: risk factors 1–3 (see above) >10 mm: risk factors 4–6, or any child less than 4 years old >15 mm: all other persons
Vision screening	Obtain visual acuity (V/A) and binocular vision by age 4–5 years on all children and, if possible, yearly or every other year after	Test V/A with the Snellen chart standardized at 20 feet. Use a Tumbling E or Lea chart (uses symbols—apple, circle, square, and house) if letters cannot be recognized. A failed test is V/A 20/40 or greater in either eye, or if there is a two-line discrepancy between the eyes (e.g., 20/20 in one eye and 20/40 in another). All children should be tested once for color blindness. Make referrals for all failures.
Blood pressure (B/P)	Annual B/P measurements beginning at 3 years of age	If B/P is elevated, repeat. Children with persistent B/P readings >95th percentile need a thorough history, physical, labs, and possibly x-rays to determine if underlying etiology exists.

Adult/Geriatric Health Screening and Supervision

- Routine periodic health supervision visits have not been established for the adult client. The Canadian Task Force began making recommendations in 1979 for effective age-specific preventive packages designed for various risk groups rather than a standard physical examination.
- Routine screening recommendations were established by the U.S. Preventive Services Task Force in 1989 and 1996 for asymptomatic individuals, based on evidence supporting the effectiveness of preventive measures (Table 3–20).
- Various specialty groups such as the American Cancer Society, the National Cancer Institute, the American College of Obstetricians and Gynecologists (ACOG), and the American Academy of Family Physicians also make recommendations.
- As there is not always agreement among the recommending bodies, clinicians must be prepared to clearly identify and document the basis for their preventive practices.

Table 3-20. Adult/Geriatric Screening Recommendations

Problem or Issue	Generally Accepted Recommendations
Asymptomatic heart disease	Obtain baseline EKG on patients with cardiac risk factors, patients over age 40, and sedentary persons about to undergo exercise stress testing or vigorous exercise
Breast masses	Clinical breast exam and mammography every 12 months in women age 50 and over; some groups recommend age 40 and over
Cervical cancer	ACOG 2004 guidelines suggest beginning Pap smears at age 21 or within 3 years of first intercourse; women up to age 30 should have annual cervical cytology. After age 30, women who have had three negative results on annual Pap tests can be rescreened with cytology alone every 2 to 3 years; or have annual cervical cytology testing (if immunocompromised, have HIV, or were exposed to diethylstilbestrol [DES]), or have cytology with the addition of an human papillomavirus (HPV)-DNA test. If both the cervical cytology and the DNA test are negative, rescreening should occur no sooner than 3 years.
Colon cancer	Fecal occult blood tests (FOBT) annually in age 50 years and older; earlier in high-risk persons. Sigmoidoscopy every 3–5 years in those 50 years or older or colonoscopy and double-contrast barium enemas are not superior for screening purposes; positive FOBT should have colonoscopy follow-up.
Vision	Screen visual acuity of elderly with Snellen testing and refer persons at high risk for glaucoma to eye specialists.
Dental/oral	Yearly exam and counseling
Hearing	Assess hearing through physical exam and refer as needed.
Hyperlipidemia	Cholesterol and fractionated lipid profile at least every 5 years after age 35 for men, 45 for women. National Cholesterol Education Program recommends testing beginning at age 20 for both genders (2002).
Hypertension	Blood pressure screening every 2 years in normotensive patients older than 21
Menopause	Counsel all perimenopausal and postmenopausal women about potential risks and benefits of hormone replacement.
Osteoporosis	Counsel all women about the risks and benefits of hormone replacement therapy, dietary calcium, vitamin D, weight-bearing exercise, and smoking cessation. Bone density measurement should be performed in all women >65 years, earlier in women at increased risk.

Table 3-20. Adult/Geriatric Screening Recommendations (cont.)

Problem or Issue	Generally Accepted Recommendations
Prostate cancer	Digital rectal exam annually for men older than 40. No recommended routine screening for prostate cancer; digital rectal examinations, prostate-specific antigen (PSA), or transrectal ultrasound are no longer routinely recommended
Testicular cancer	Old recommendation was for clinical exam every 3 years for men ages 20 to 39 and annually for those over age 40; now, no evidence supports routine screening of asymptomatic men
Hypothyroidism	Periodic thyroid-stimulating hormone (TSH) in elderly women
Skin cancer	Periodic skin exam in older adults with sun exposure
Dementia, functional impairment	Periodic screen with standardized assessment tools in geriatric patients
Sexually transmitted diseases	Screen all sexually active women age 25 and younger, especially pregnant women, and individuals at increased risk of infection

Adapted from *Guide to Clinical Preventive Services* AHRQ Pub. No. 07-05100), by Agency on Healthcare Research and Quality, 2007, Washington, DC: Department of Health and Human Services.

GERIATRIC ASSESSMENT

Nonspecific Presentation of Illness
- A crucial aspect of geriatrics is that the elderly often present with vague complaints or deterioration in functional independence as an early subtle sign of illness.
- This generally occurs in the absence of classical (typical) symptoms and signs of disease.
- When older adults get acutely ill, they most often present with:
  - Confusion or delirium
  - Increased difficulty performing activities of daily living (ADLs)
  - Incontinence
  - Falls

Functional Assessment
- Assessment tools provide standardized data to follow trends and evaluate response to treatment.
- Cognitive and functional assessments are the keystone to providing geriatric care.
- Many assessment tools are available.

Normal Changes of Aging
- What is normal becomes less uniform as patients age.
- Normal changes usually mean less functional reserve.
- It is often difficult to differentiate normal aging, chronic disease, medication effect, and disuse.

IMMUNIZATION

- While most children are immunized by the time they enter school, many children remain unimmunized until that time, leaving them at unnecessary risk for infections.
- Many adults are inadequately immunized, either from lack of immunization as children or failure to have adequate boosters.
- Some categories of workers, such as food handlers, those working with animals, and travelers may require additional immunizations.
- The largest age group acquiring tetanus infections is the elderly, who often have not had boosters.

Immunization Guidelines
- Infants and children routinely are immunized against 11 infectious diseases (Table 3–21). In addition, influenza vaccination is encouraged for all children >6 months of age.
- Children entering school and licensed day care are required in all states to have vaccines. To check individual state laws, refer to the Immunization Action Coalition at http://immunize.org/laws/index.htm.
- Many children, particularly under 2 years of age, are not fully immunized, leaving them at risk for infections.
- When immunization is not begun in early infancy or interrupted, the immunization schedule must be modified; however, previously given vaccines do not need repeating.
- If the vaccine status is unknown, the child is considered not immunized and begun on an appropriate schedule.
- Preterm infants should be immunized with regular doses according to postnatal chronological age.
- Side effects: Common to almost all the vaccines are local injection site reactions such as pain, tenderness, and erythema that are mild and transient, and mild to moderate fevers and myalgias for 24–48 hours
- General contraindications to vaccinations include hypersensitivity reactions (urticaria, shock, wheezing) and prior encephalopathy within 7 days of pertussis vaccine, undefined illnesses where administering vaccines may confuse the diagnosis, prior severe reactions where administering the vaccine would be more harmful than withholding.
- Not contraindications: minor illnesses, family history of seizure disorders, sudden infant death syndrome or adverse reactions to vaccines, presence of a pregnant woman in the household
- There is no contraindication to simultaneous administration of the routine vaccines.
- Informed consent must be obtained prior to vaccination with information provided regarding the disease to be prevented, risks and benefits of the vaccine, and potential side effects.
- Additional vaccines may be indicated or recommended for specific illnesses and/or disorders, travel, geographical area, and/or special circumstances. Adult vaccines are listed in Table 3–22.
- Free vaccines are available through the Vaccines for Children program for uninsured and Medicaid-eligible children, children whose health insurance does not completely cover vaccines, and Native American and Alaskan Native children.

Table 3–21. Summary of Recommendations for Childhood and Adolescent Immunization

Vaccine name and route	Schedule for routine vaccination and other guidelines (any vaccine can be given with another)	Schedule for catch-up vaccination and related issues	Contraindications and precautions (mild illness is not a contraindication)
Hepatitis B *Give IM*	• Vaccinate all children age 1 through 18 yrs. • Vaccinate all newborns with monovalent vaccine prior to hospital discharge. Give dose #2 at age 1-2m and the final dose at age 6-18m (the last dose in the infant series should not be given earlier than age 24wks). After the birth dose, the series may be completed using 2 doses of single-antigen vaccine or up to 3 doses of Comvax (ages 2m, 4m, 12-15m) or Pediarix (ages 2m, 4m, 6m), which may result in giving a total of 4 doses of hepatitis B vaccine. • *If mother is HBsAg-positive:* give the newborn HBIG + dose #1 within 12hrs of birth; complete series at age 6m or, if using Comvax, at age 12-15m. • *If mother's HBsAg status is unknown:* give the newborn dose #1 within 12hrs of birth. If mother is subsequently found to be HBsAg positive, give infant HBIG within 7d of birth and follow the schedule for infants born to HBsAg-positive mothers.	• Do not restart series, no matter how long since previous dose. • 3-dose series can be started at any age. • Minimum spacing between doses: 4wks between #1 and #2, 8wks between #2 and #3, and at least 16wks between #1 and #3 (e.g., 0-, 2-, 4m; 0-, 1-, 4m). **Special Notes on Hepatitis B Vaccine (HepB)** *Dosing of HepB:* Vaccine brands are interchangeable. For persons age 0 through 19yrs, give 0.5 mL of either Engerix-B or Recombivax HB. *Alternate dosing schedule for unvaccinated adolescents age 11 through 15yrs:* Give 2 doses Recombivax HB 1.0 mL (adult formulation) spaced 4-6m apart. (Engerix-B is not licensed for a 2-dose schedule.) *For preterm infants:* Consult ACIP hepatitis B recommendations (MMWR 2005; 54 [RR-16]).	*Contraindication* Previous anaphylaxis to this vaccine or to any of its components. *Precaution* Moderate or severe acute illness.

Table 3-21. Summary of Recommendations for Childhood and Adolescent Immunization (cont.)

Vaccine name and route	Schedule for routine vaccination and other guidelines (any vaccine can be given with another)	Schedule for catch-up vaccination and related issues	Contraindications and precautions (mild illness is not a contraindication)
DTaP, DT (Diphtheria, tetanus, acellular pertussis) *Give IM*	• Give to children at ages 2m, 4m, 6m, 15-18m, 4-6yrs. • May give dose #1 as early as age 6wks. • May give #4 as early as 12m if 6m have elapsed since #3 and the child is unlikely to return at age 15-18m. • Do not give DTaP/DT to children age 7yrs and older. • If possible, use the same DTaP product for all doses.	• #2 and #3 may be given 4wks after previous dose. • #4 may be given 6m after #3. • If #4 is given before 4th birthday, wait at least 6m for #5 (age 4-6yrs). • If #4 is given after 4th birthday, #5 is not needed.	*Contraindications* • Previous anaphylaxis to this vaccine or to any of its components. • For DTaP/Tdap only: encephalopathy within 7d after DTP/DTaP. *Precautions* • Moderate or severe acute illness. • Guillain-Barré syndrome within 6wks after previous dose of tetanus toxoid-containing vaccine. • For DTaP only: Any of these occurrences following a previous dose of DTP/DTaP: 1) temperature of 105°F (40.5°C) or higher within 48hrs; 2) continuous crying for 3hrs or more within 48hrs; 3) collapse or shock-like state within 48hrs; 4) convulsion with or without fever within 3d. • For DTaP/Tdap only: Unstable neurologic disorder.
Td, Tdap (Tetanus, diphtheria, acellular pertussis) *Give IM*	• Give Tdap booster dose to adolescents age 11-12yrs if 5yrs have elapsed since last dose DTaP/DTP; boost every 10yrs with Td. • Give 1-time dose of Tdap to all adolescents who have not received previous Tdap. Special efforts should be made to give Tdap to persons age 11yrs and older who are – in contact with infants younger than age 12m. – healthcare workers with direct patient contact. • In pregnancy, when indicated, give Td or Tdap in 2nd or 3rd trimester. If not administered during pregnancy, give Tdap in immediate postpartum period.	• If never vaccinated with tetanus- and diphtheria-containing vaccine: give Td dose #1 now, dose #2 4wks later, and dose #3 6m after #2, then give booster every 10yrs. A 1-time Tdap may be substituted for any dose in the series. • Intervals of 2yrs or less between Td and Tdap may be used.	*Note:* Use of Td or Tdap is not contraindicated in pregnancy. At the provider's discretion, either vaccine may be administered during the 2nd or 3rd trimester.

Table 3-21. Summary of Recommendations for Childhood and Adolescent Immunization (cont.)

Vaccine name and route	Schedule for routine vaccination and other guidelines (any vaccine can be given with another)	Schedule for catch-up vaccination and related issues	Contraindications and precautions (mild illness is not a contraindication)
Polio (IPV) *Give SC or IM*	• Give to children at ages 2m, 4m, 6-18m, 4-6yrs. • May give #1 as early as age 6wks. • Not routinely recommended for those age 18yrs and older (except certain travelers).	• All doses should be separated by at least 4wks. • If dose #3 is given after 4th birthday, dose #4 is not needed.	*Contraindicated* Previous anaphylaxis to this vaccine or to any of its components. *Precautions* • Moderate or severe acute illness. • Pregnancy.
Human papilloma-virus (HPV) *Give IM*	• Give 3-dose series to girls at age 11-12yrs on a 0, 2, 6m schedule. (May be given as early as age 9yrs.) • Vaccinate all older girls and women (through age 26yrs) who were not previously vaccinated.	• Dose #2 may be given 4wks after dose #1. • Dose #3 may be given 12wks after dose #2.	*Contraindication* Previous anaphylaxis to this vaccine or to any of its components. *Precautions* • Moderate or severe acute illness. • Pregnancy

Table 3–21. Summary of Recommendations for Childhood and Adolescent Immunization (cont.)

Vaccine name and route	Schedule for routine vaccination and other guidelines (*any vaccine can be given with another*)	Schedule for catch-up vaccination and related issues	Contraindications and precautions (mild illness is not a contraindication)
Varicella (Var) (Chickenpox) Give SC	• Give dose #1 at age 12–15m. • Give dose #2 at age 4–6yrs. Dose #2 may be given earlier if at least 3m since dose #1. • Give a routine second dose to all older children and adolescents with history of only 1 dose. • MMRV may be used in children age 12m through 12yrs.	• If younger than age 13yrs, space dose #1 and #2 at least 3m apart. If age 13yrs or older, space at least 4wks apart. • May use as postexposure prophylaxis if given within 3-5d. • If Var and either MMR, LAIV, and/or yellow fever vaccine are not given on the same day, space them at least 28d apart.	*Contraindications* • Previous anaphylaxis to this vaccine or to any of its components. • Pregnancy or possibility of pregnancy within 4wks. • Children immunocompromised because of high doses of systemic steroids, cancer, leukemia, lymphoma, or immunodeficiency not related to HIV. *Precautions* • Moderate or severe acute illness. • If blood, plasma, and/or immune globulin (IG or VZIG) were given in past 11m, see ACIP statement General Recommendations on Immunization* regarding time to wait before vaccinating. *Note:* For patients with humoral immunodeficiency, HIV infection, or leukemia, or for patients on high doses of systemic steroids, see ACIP recommendations*.

Table 3–21. Summary of Recommendations for Childhood and Adolescent Immunization (cont.)

Vaccine name and route	Schedule for routine vaccination and other guidelines (any vaccine can be given with another)	Schedule for catch-up vaccination and related issues	Contraindications and precautions (mild illness is not a contraindication)
MMR (Measles, mumps, rubella) *Give SC*	• Give dose #1 at age 12–15m. • Give dose #2 at age 4–6yrs. Dose #2 may be given earlier if at least 4wks since dose #1. • If a dose was given before age 12m, it doesn't count as the first dose, so give #1 at age 12-15m with a minimum interval of 4wks between the invalid dose and dose #1. • MMRV may be used in children age 12m through 12yrs.	• If MMR and either Var, LAIV, and/or yellow fever vaccine are not given on the same day, space them at least 28d apart. • When using MMR (not MMRV) for both doses, minimum interval is 4wks.	*Contraindications* • Previous anaphylaxis to this vaccine or to any of its components. • Pregnancy or possibility of pregnancy within 4wks. • Severe immunodeficiency (e.g., hematologic and solid tumors; congenital immunodeficiency; long-term immunosuppressive therapy, or severely symptomatic HIV). *Precautions* • Moderate or severe acute illness. • If blood, plasma, or immune globulin given in past 11m or if on high-dose immunosuppressive therapy, see ACIP statement General Recommendations on Immunization* regarding delay time. • History of thrombocytopenia or thrombocytopenic purpura. *Note:* MMR is not contraindicated if a PPD (tuberculosis skin test) was recently applied. If PPD and MMR not given on same day, delay PPD for 4-6wks after MMR.

Table 3–21. Summary of Recommendations for Childhood and Adolescent Immunization (cont.)

Vaccine name and route	Schedule for routine vaccination and other guidelines (any vaccine can be given with another)	Schedule for catch-up vaccination and related issues	Contraindications and precautions (mild illness is not a contraindication)
Influenza Trivalent inactivated influenza vaccine (TIV) *Give IM* Live attenuated influenza vaccine (LAIV) *Give intranasally*	• Vaccinate all persons age 6m or older, including school-aged children, wanting to reduce their risk of becoming ill with influenza or of spreading it to others. • Vaccinate all children age 6-59m, as well as all siblings and household contacts of children 0-59m. • Vaccinate persons age 5yrs and older who • have a risk factor (e.g., pregnancy, heart disease, lung disease, diabetes, renal, dysfunction, hemaglobinopathy, immunosuppression, on long-term aspirin therapy, or have a condition that compromises respiratory function or the handling of respiratory secretions or that can increase the risk of aspiration) or live in a chronic-care facility. • live or work with at-risk people as listed above. • LAIV may be given to healthy, non-pregnant persons age 2–49yrs. • Give 2 doses to first-time vaccinees age 6m through 8yrs, spaced 4wks apart. • For TIV, give 0.25 mL dose to children age 6–35m and 0.5 mL dose if age 3yrs and older.		*Contraindications* • Previous anaphylaxis to this vaccine, to any of its components, or to eggs. • For LAIV only: Pregnancy, asthma, reactive airways disease, or other chronic disorder of the pulmonary or cardiovascular systems; an underlying medical condition, including metabolic diseases such as diabetes, renal dysfunction, and hemoglobinopathies; a known or suspected immune deficiency disease or receiving immunosuppressive therapy; history of Guillain-Barré syndrome. *Precautions* • Moderate or severe acute illness. • For TTV only: History of Guillain-Barré syndrome within 6wks of a previous TTV.

Table 3-21. Summary of Recommendations for Childhood and Adolescent Immunization (cont.)

Vaccine name and route	Schedule for routine vaccination and other guidelines (any vaccine can be given with another)	Schedule for catch-up vaccination and related issues	Contraindications and precautions (mild illness is not a contraindication)
Rotavirus (RV) *Give orally*	• Give a 3-dose series at age 2m, 4m, 6m. • May give dose #1 as early as age 6wks. • Give dose #3 no later than age 32wks.	• Do not begin series in infants older than age 12wks. • Dose #2 and #3 may be given 4wks after previous dose.	*Contraindication* Previous anaphylaxis to this vaccine or to any of its components, including latex for RV1. *Precautions* • Moderate or severe acute illness. • Altered immunocompetence. • Moderate to severe acute gastroenteritis or chronic gastrointestinal disease. • History of intussusception.
Hib (*Haemophilus influenzae* type b) *Give IM*	• HibTITER (HbOC) and ActHib (PRP-T): give at age 2m, 4m, 6m, 12–15m (booster dose). • PedvaxHIB or Comvax (containing PRP-OMP): give at age 2m, 4m, 12–15m. • Dose #1 of Hib vaccine may be given earlier than age 6wks. • The last dose (booster dose) is given no earlier than age 12m and a minimum of 8wks after the previous dose. • Hib vaccines are interchangeable; however, if different brands of Hib vaccines are administered, a total of 3 doses are necessary to complete the primary series in infants. • Any Hib vaccine may be used for the booster dose. • Hib is not routinely given to children age 5yrs and older.	**All Hib vaccines:** • If #1 was given at 12–14m, give booster in 8wks. • Give only 1 dose to unvaccinated children from age 15m to 5yrs. **HibTITER and ActHib:** • #2 and #3 may be given 4wks after previous dose. • If #1 was given at age 7–11m, only 3 doses are needed; #2 is given 4–8wks after #1, then boost at age 12–15m (wait at least 8wks after dose #2). **PedvaxHIB and Comvax:** • #2 may be given 4wks after dose #1.	*Contraindication* Previous anaphylaxis to this vaccine or to any of its components. *Precaution* Moderate or severe acute illness.

Table 3-21. Summary of Recommendations for Childhood and Adolescent Immunization (cont.)

Vaccine name and route	Schedule for routine vaccination and other guidelines (any vaccine can be given with another)	Schedule for catch-up vaccination and related issues	Contraindications and precautions (mild illness is not a contraindication)
Pneumo. conjugate (PCV) *Give IM*	• Give at ages 2m, 4m, 6m, 12–15m. • Dose #1 may be given as early as age 6wks. • Give 1 dose to unvaccinated healthy children age 24–59m. • Give 2 doses at least 8wks apart to high-risk** children age 24–59m. • PCV is not routinely given to children age 5yrs and older.	• For age 7–11m: If history of 0–2 doses, give additional doses 4wks apart with no more than 3 total doses by age 12m; then give booster 8wks later. • For age 12–23m: If 0–1 dose before age 12m, give 2 doses at least 8wks apart. If 2–3 doses before age 12m, give 1 dose at least 8wks after previous dose. • For age 24–59m: If patient has had no previous doses, or has a history of 1–3 doses given before age 12m but no booster dose, or has a history of only 1 dose given at age 12–23m, give 1 dose now.	*Contraindication* Previous anaphylaxis to this vaccine or to any of its components. *Precaution* Moderate or severe acute illness.
Pneumo. polysacch. (PPV) *Give IM or SC*	• Give 1 dose at least 8wks after final dose of PCV to high-risk children age 2yrs and older. • For children who are immunocompromised or have sickle cell disease or functional or anatomic asplenia, give a 2nd dose of PPV 3–5yrs after previous PPV (consult ACIP PPV recommendations [MMWR 1997;46 [RR-8] for details*).		*Contraindication* Previous anaphylaxis to this vaccine or to any of its components. *Precaution* Moderate or severe acute illness.

**High-risk: Those with sickle cell disease; anatomic/functional asplenia; chronic cardiac, pulmonary, or renal disease; diabetes; cerebrospinal fluid leaks; HIV infection; immunosuppression; or who have or will have a cochlear implant.

Table 3-21. Summary of Recommendations for Childhood and Adolescent Immunization (cont.)

Vaccine name and route	Schedule for routine vaccination and other guidelines (any vaccine can be given with another)	Schedule for catch-up vaccination and related issues	Contraindications and precautions (mild illness is not a contraindication)
Hepatitis A *Give IM*	• Give 2 doses to all children at age 1yr (12–23m) spaced 6m apart. • Vaccinate all children and adolescents age 2 years and older who • Live in a state, county, or community with a routine vaccination program already in place for children age 2yrs and older. • Travel anywhere except U.S, W. Europe, N. Zealand, Australia, Canada, or Japan. • Wish to be protected from HAV infection. • Have chronic liver disease, clotting factor disorder, or are MSM adolescents.	• Minimum interval between doses is 6m. • Consider routine vaccination of children age 2yrs and older in areas with no existing program.	*Contraindication* Previous anaphylaxis to this vaccine or to any of its components. *Precaution* Moderate or severe acute illness.
Meningococcal conjugate (MCV4) *Give IM* **polysaccharide (MPSV)** *Give SC*	• Give 1-time dose of MCV4 to adolescents age 11 through 18yrs. • Vaccinate all college freshmen living in dorms who have not been vaccinated. • Vaccinate all children age 2yrs and older who have any of the following risk factors (use MPSV if age younger than 11yrs and MCV4 if age 11yrs and older): • Anatomic or functional asplenia, or terminal complement component deficiencies. • Travel to, or reside in countries in which meningococcal disease is hyperendemic or epidemic (e.g., the "meningitis belt" of Sub-Saharan Africa).	If previously vaccinated with MPSV and risk continues, give MCV4 5yrs after MPSV. *Note:* MCV4 is not licensed for use in children younger than age 11yrs.	*Contraindication* Previous anaphylaxis to this vaccine or to any of its components, including diphtheria toxoid (for MCV4). *Precautions* • Moderate or severe acute illness. • For MCV4 only: history of Guillain-Barré syndrome (GBS).

Table 3-22. Immunization Guidelines for Adults

Type of Immunization	Recommendations for Adults
Hepatitis A	High-risk adults (see below)
Hepatitis B	All persons 12–25 years with no history of infection or previous immunization; high-risk adults
Human papillomavirus (HPV)	Females through age 26
Influenza	Pregnant women; annually for all adults 50+ years of age; others if at high risk or household contacts of those at high risk; annually for healthcare workers
Measles, mumps, and rubella (MMR)	Administer to anyone >18 years of age born after 1957 with no documented proof of immunity. Contraindicated in pregnancy, immunocompromising conditions.
Meningococcal	College freshmen living in dormitories and travelers to endemic areas with no history of prior infections; people whose spleen was damaged or removed
Pneumovax	Once at 65+; once at 50+ if at high risk and repeat if injection was more than 5 years ago
Rubella screen or immunization	Women of childbearing age
Tetanus, diphtheria, pertussis (Tdap/DTaP/Td)	Booster every 10 years; booster at 5 years for wound management
Varicella	Adults with no history of varicella or previous vaccination. Contraindicated in pregnancy and immunocompromising conditions.
Zoster	Once at 60+ for all adults with history of chicken pox infection

Vaccine Descriptions

DTaP/Tdap/Td (diphtheria, tetanus, and acellular pertussis toxoids; Td lacks acellular pertussis toxoids)

- Initial doses of DTaP at 2, 4, and 6 months of age, with the fourth dose given 6–12 months after the third (usually at 15–18 months of age) and the fifth dose at 4–6 years of age (unless the fourth dose was given after the fourth birthday, then a fifth dose is not necessary).
- If pertussis vaccine is contraindicated, an infant or child is immunized with DT up until age 7 years, Td afterward.
- Split doses of DTaP should not be used.
- Where possible, the same brand of DTaP should be used for the entire series.
- Pediatrix is a combined DTaP, Hep B recombinant, and IPV vaccine. May be used for 3-dose primary series; may not be used in infants under 6 weeks of age, nor in children >7 years.
- A Tdap booster is recommended at 11–16 years of age, and every 10 years afterwards.

Flu vaccine (influenza)

- Injected vaccines are inactivated and recommended for routine use. They are not approved for children <6 months of age. FluMist is a live, attenuated nasal vaccine that may be given to healthy children >5 years of age.

- Vaccines are developed annually based on expected strains for the coming winter.
- Immunizations are administered in the fall, before influenza season, and immunity lasts 1 year.
- Recommended annually for healthy children between 6 and 24 months of age, for household contacts and out-of-home caregivers of all children younger than 24 months of age, all adults and children with chronic illness, all adults over 50 years of age, and all healthcare workers.
- Healthy children over 24 months of age may receive vaccine if requested by parent.
- Children <9 years of age receive 2 vaccines 1 month apart the first time they are vaccinated; thereafter only one vaccine is given annually.
- Children >9 years and adults receive only one vaccine yearly, including the first year.

HAV (hepatitis A vaccine)
- Two doses given 4 weeks apart
- Indications: Anyone 2 years of age or older with increased risk of exposure to hepatitis A and no known immunity; immunity testing not required because administering vaccine to those already immune presents no risk
- Risk factors include travel to endemic areas, military personnel, homosexual or bisexual men, persons receiving plasma products, certain geographical populations (noted below).
- Routine vaccinations recommended in selected states: AZ, AK, CA, ID, NV, NM, OK, SD, UT, and WA. Considerations for: TX, CO, AR, MT, and WY.
- Specific side effects: vomiting, diarrhea, headache (rare: jaundice, erythema multiforme reactions, convulsions, syncope).

HBV (hepatitis B vaccine)
- HBV may be given at any age but is recommended to start at birth. The recommended schedule is 0, 1–2 months later, and 4–6 months after the first dose (may be shortened if necessary).
- Infants born to HBsAg-positive mothers should receive hepatitis B immune globulin (HBIg) at birth, not in the same location as HBV.
- Infants born to hepatitis B–positive mothers should have their immune status to hepatitis B checked at 9–12 months of age.
- Adults without history of vaccination should receive HBV.
- High-risk individuals: All adolescents, household contacts and sex partners of patients with hepatitis B, healthcare workers, heterosexuals with more than one sex partner in 6 months, patients recently diagnosed with other sexually transmitted disease, correctional facility inmates, certain international travelers.

Hib (Haemophilus influenzae type B vaccine)
- Three vaccines are licensed for use, with different dosing schedules. All are conjugated vaccines bound to a protein carrier. The difference in the vaccines is in the type of protein carrier used which then affects the scheduling (either a 3- or 4-dose schedule is used):
  – 4-dose schedule (Hib titer; ActHIB): 2, 4, 6 and 12–15 months of age
  – 3-dose schedule (PedvaxHIB; Comvax [Hib/Hepatitis B combination vaccine]): 2, 4, and 12–15 months of age. Any licensed product may be used for the third dose at 12–15 months of age, regardless of product used for primary series at 2–6 months.
- Because immune response to Hib vaccine increases with age, fewer doses are required at older ages. After 15 months of age, one dose of any licensed vaccine is sufficient.

- After age 5 years, Hib immunization is indicated only for children with a chronic condition associated with an increased risk of Hib disease, such as sickle cell disease, asplenia, or antibody deficiency.
- Children younger than 2 years of age with a documented Hib infection still should be vaccinated.
- Rifampin prophylaxis still should be given to immunized children exposed to Hib meningitis.

HPV vaccine (human papillomavirus vaccine)
- Gardasil protects against 4 types of HPV (6, 11, 16, 18).
- Indicated for females through ages 26 years.

IPV (inactivated polio vaccine)
- Only IPV is now used for routine vaccinations to eliminate vaccine-associated paralytic polio (VAPP).
- Given at 2, 4, 6–18 months, and 4–6 years of age
- Four doses are required for school entry unless the third dose was given after the fourth birthday (then the fourth dose is unnecessary).
- Contraindications: anaphylactic reaction to neomycin or streptomycin
- Oral polio vaccine (OPV) can be given under special circumstances, such as travel to endemic areas or during outbreaks.

Meningococcal vaccine
- Directed against Neisseria meningitidis, most common cause of bacterial meningitis in persons 2–18 years of age
- Two meningococcal vaccines are licensed for use: Menactra and Menomune.
- Menactra is recommended for all children 11–18 years of age and preferred for people aged 2–55 years in the risk groups listed below.
- Menomune is preferred for people over age 55 at risk.
- Indicated for college students (particularly freshman living in dormitories), travelers to endemic areas (sub-Saharan Africa), immunodeficiency, asplenia.

MMR (measles, mumps, rubella vaccine)
- Composed of three live, attenuated vaccines
- First dose is recommended at 12–15 months of age and the second dose at 4–6 years of age, but may be given at any time as long as 4 weeks has elapsed since the first dose.
- After exposure to measles infection, vaccination within 72 hours may be protective.
- Measles vaccine may suppress PPD reactions for 4–6 weeks; give PPD tests on the day of the vaccine or wait 6 weeks.
- Measles infection exacerbates tuberculosis (TB), but vaccination does not; TB status does not need to be known prior to vaccine administration.
- Contraindications: pregnancy; immunocompromised except by HIV (unless severely immunocompromised); anaphylactic reaction to neomycin, eggs, or gelatin
- Deferrals: Immune globulin administration within past 3–11 months or recent blood transfusion
- Not contraindications: Tuberculosis or positive PPD, persons in the household who are pregnant or immunocompromised, nonanaphylactic reactions to eggs or neomycin

- Side effects (5–12 days after vaccination): fever, rash, transient arthritis, thrombocytopenia, and (rarely) encephalopathy.

Pneumococcal vaccines
- More than 80 serotypes of pneumococci exist, and immunity to one does not protect against infection by others. Vaccines are directed against certain groups that are more responsible for causing disease than others.
- Indications: The original pneumococcal vaccine (PPV or Pneumovax) is effective against 23 serotypes but not immunogenic in children younger than 2 years of age. It is indicated for adults 65+ years of age, and for children >2 years of age with risk factors for the development of severe pneumococcal disease such as sickle cell disease, asplenia, HIV or other immunodeficiency disorders, or nephrotic syndrome.
- The newer vaccine (Prevnar), effective against 7 serotypes, is immunogenic in the under-2 age group and is now routinely administered.
- The number of vaccinations depends on the patient's age:
  - 4 shots if vaccine series begun before 7 months of age
  - 3 if 7–11 months of age
  - 2 if 12–23 months of age
  - 1 if 2 years of age or older

Respiratory syncticial virus (RSV) immune globin
- Palivizumab (Synagis) provides temporary, passive immunity for high-risk infants.
- Given at 15mg/kg IM once per month for 5 months, starting before RSV season (October or November) and continuing throughout.
- Indicated for children less than 2 years of age with chronic lung disease, and infants <32 weeks gestation.
- No alterations in routine vaccines.

Varivax (varicella zoster vaccine)
- Live attenuated vaccine
- Increasing number of states require administration prior to kindergarten entry.
- One vaccine is given usually between 12–18 months of age, but can be given anytime after 1 year of age.
- Children older than 13 years and adults with no history of chickenpox require 2 doses given at least 1 month apart.
- Give vaccine to unimmunized patients within 3–5 days after exposure to chickenpox.
- Side effects may include local injection site reaction consisting of approximately 2–3 papules (vesicles are rare with this type of reaction) and, 2 weeks postvaccine, a generalized varicella-like rash, typically on the trunk. This generalized rash carries a slight risk of infection to others through direct contact; no known cases of airborne transmission have occurred.
- Contraindications: Pregnancy, allergic reaction to neomycin, immunocompromised persons including those on high-dose steroids (exception may be asymptomatic or mildly symptomatic children with HIV), active untreated TB
- Not contraindications: Use of inhaled steroids, immunocompromised or pregnant persons in the household (these persons should avoid direct contact with a vaccine-induced generalized rash)

Other Disease Prevention Programs
Back to Sleep Program
- For the prevention of SIDS, the most common cause of death in children under 1 year of age.
- Risk factors for SIDS: Sleep position, exposure to cigarette smoke, low birthweight, and prematurity. Highest incidence in African Americans and Native Americans; lowest in Asians.
- Back to Sleep Program recommends positioning infants on their back or sides for sleeping. Incidence of SIDS has decreased dramatically with these sleeping positions.

Smoking Cessation
- More than 40% of U.S. children are exposed to environmental tobacco smoke in their own homes.
- Teenage smokers experience a decrease in physical fitness and lung function and, later, an increase in the risk of lung cancer and heart disease.
- Encourage cessation of smoking first without pharmacologic interventions; if unsuccessful, may educate regarding products available for assistance. (See Table 18–7.) They should not be used by adolescents with heart disease, especially arrhythmias, or during pregnancy (unless under supervision). Efficacy in teens has not been proven (see Treating Tobacco Use and Dependence: PHS Clinical Practice Guideline [2000].

OTHER HEALTHCARE CONSIDERATIONS

Cultural Influences
- If the healthcare provider is sensitive to issues surrounding health care and the traditional health beliefs of the patient, more comprehensive healthcare can be provided.
- Family structure and values have an impact on the health encounter.
- Ethnicity is based on the race, tribe, or nation with which a person identifies and influences the person's beliefs and behaviors.

Environmental Factors
- General circumstances such as climate, altitude, and temperature affect all people in a region and cannot be modified.
- Other factors such as air pollution, water fluoridation and contamination, crime, poverty, and transportation are examples of things that might be manipulated to have a positive effect on the community.

Evidence-Based Medicine
- To reduce the numbers of conflicting or varying recommendations for the diagnosis and treatment of common problems, the trend is to base decisions on evidence from randomized controlled research trials. These trials and meta-analyses of these trials have gained acceptance as valid foundations on which care can be provided. The availability of information about the status of research in these areas is growing through use of the Internet.

- Outcome studies will replace tradition, intuition, and preference for how different clinical problems should be handled. Nurse practitioners should have sufficient research skills to be able to critically evaluate and participate in outcome studies that will relate to their clinical practice.

Clinical Guidelines

- Standards of practice are devised from research by experts in the field to guide and standardize practice across the nation. Nurse practitioners should know how to analyze clinical guidelines to determine those that are written by objective scholars and are without organizational, professional, or pharmaceutical bias. See the National Guideline Clearinghouse at www.guideline.gov.
- Factors to consider in evaluating guidelines include source of guideline, appropriateness of methodology used to develop guideline, use of expert opinion/clinical experience in decision making, public policy issue considerations, feasibility issues, use of peer preview, congruence with other practice guidelines, timeliness, and funding source.

Critical Thinking/Decision Making

- Critical thinking involves acquisition of knowledge with an attitude of deliberate inquiry. Part of critical thinking may be innate, but most people can learn to think critically.
- Decision making is a higher level of critical thinking. It involves making decisions based on an understanding of the different options, and the possible desirability of the outcomes of each option in the mind of the clinician and the patient.
- Pattern recognition, similarity recognition, common-sense understanding, skilled know-how, sense of importance, and deliberative rationality are all important aspects that influence decision making.

Communication

- The written and oral transfer of information regarding the structure, process, and outcome of healthcare encounters. Good communication is a necessity for healthcare providers for interviewing and teaching patients, recording information and decisions, and sharing or clarifying information with others involved in the patient's care. All communication is privileged and confidential, and written documentation is subject to specific standards and audits.
- Types of special communication:
  - Triage: The prioritization and sorting of patients according to a preexisting standard; used in disaster and emergency settings
  - Case management: A system of controlled oversight and authorization of services and benefits provided to patients

CASE STUDIES

Case 1: Emily, 2 months old, is coming to the clinic for her well-baby exam. Her birth history is unremarkable, with a birthweight of 7 pounds, 8 ounces (16.5 kg) and length of 20.5 inches. She is breastfed on demand, about every 3–4 hours. She has not had any immunizations.

1. What vaccines will Emily need today?
2. What developmental milestones will you assess for in a 2-month-old?
3. There is no fluoride in the tap water; when should you start Emily on fluoride? How much will you give her per day?
4. Emily's mother is thinking about discontinuing breastfeeding and starting infant formula. What information should you provide to her that might encourage her to continue to breastfeed?

Case 2: Travis, a 4-year-old, comes to the clinic for a school physical. His last check-up was at 3 years of age. He is 40 pounds and 39 inches. His immunization records indicate he has had 4 DtaP, 3 IPV, 1 MMR, 2 hepatitis B, and 3 Hib vaccine shots.

1. What vaccines will he need today?
2. What safety issues will you discuss with Travis and his parents?

Josh, Travis's 14-year-old brother, needs a pre-participation sports physical. Josh weighs 225 pounds and is 5 feet, 8 inches tall.

3. What will your assessment examination focus on?
4. What counseling does Josh need?
5. What immunizations might Josh need?

Case 3: You have been asked to set up a health fair for a large computer company. The company would like to focus on the employees, their families, and the retired workers. You research the company and find out that there are equal numbers of employees with young children, single employees, and retired employees planning to attend the health fair.

1. What primary prevention topics will you address for parents of young children?
2. What secondary prevention topics will you address for adults ages 18–50?
3. What secondary prevention topics will you address for adults 50 and older?
4. How would you educate the participants about stress management?

REFERENCES

Agency on Healthcare Research and Quality. (2007). *Guide to clinical preventive services* (AHRQ Pub. No. 07-05100). Washington, DC: U.S. Department of Health and Human Services. Available at http://www.ahrq.gov/clinic/pocketgd.htm

American Academy of Pediatrics. (2004). *Pediatric nutrition handbook.* Elk Grove, IL: Author.

American Academy of Pediatrics. (2006). *The 2006 red book: Report of the Committee on Infectious Disease.* Elk Grove, IL: Author.

American Academy of Family Physicians. (2005). *Advance directives and do not resuscitate orders.* Retrieved January 14, 2008, from www.familydoctor.org/handouts/003.html

Bandura, A. (1986). *Social foundations of thought and action.* Englewood Cliffs, NY: Prentice-Hall.

Becker, M. (1972). The health belief model and personal health behavior. *Health education monographs, 2,* 326–327.

Behrman, R., Kliegman, R., & Jenson, H. (2004). *Nelson textbook of pediatrics.* Philadelphia: W.B. Saunders.

Berul, C. (2000). Cardiac evaluation of the young athlete. *Pediatric Annals, 29*(3), 163.

Brownson, R. C. (2001). *Applied epidemiology: Theory to practice* (2nd ed.). London: Oxford University Press.

Burke, M., & Laramie, J. (2003). *Primary care of the older adult: A multidisciplinary approach.* Philadelphia: Elsevier Health Sciences.

Burns, E. E., Dunn, M., & Brady, A. (2004). *Pediatric primary care: A handbook for nurse practitioners* (3rd ed.). Philadelphia: Elsevier Health Sciences.

Centers for Disease Control and Prevention. (2008). Immunization schedule. *MMWR: Morbidity and mortality weekly report.* Retrieved September 22, 2008, from http://www.cdc.gov/vaccines/ed/default.htm

Erikson, E. (1963). *Childhood and society* (2nd ed.). New York: Norton.

Friedman, M. (2003). *Family nursing: Research, theory and practice* (5th ed.). Norwalk, CT: Appleton & Lange.

Hay, W. W., Levin, M. J., Sondheimer, J. M., & Deterding, R. R. (2006). *Current pediatric diagnosis & treatment.* Norwalk, CT: Appleton & Lange.

Hernandez, C., Singleton, J., & Aronzon, D. (2001). *Primary care pediatrics.* Philadelphia: Lippincott.

Heron, M. (2007). Deaths: Leading causes for 2004. *National Vital Statistics Report, 56*(5). Retrieved February 15, 2008, from http://www.cdc.gov/nchs/data/nvsr/nvsr56/nvsr56_05.pdf

Hockenberry, M. J. (2006). *Whaley & Wong's nursing care of infants and children* (86th ed.). St. Louis, MO: Mosby Year Book, The National Center for Health Statistics.

Goroll, A., & Mulley, A. (2006). *Primary care medicine: Office evaluation and management of the adult patient.* Philadelphia: Lippincott Williams & Wilkins.

Illingworth, R. (1987). *The development of the infant and young child.* London: Churchill Livingstone.

Jarvis, C. (2007) *Physical examination and health assessment.* St. Louis, MO: Elsevier Health Sciences.

Kerr, M. E., & Bowen, M. (1988). *Family evaluation: An approach based on Bowen Theory.* New York: W. W. Norton & Co.

Kliegman, R. M., Marcdant, K. .J., Jenson, H. B., & Behrman, R. E. (2006). *Nelson essentials of pediatrics* (5th ed.). Philadelphia: Elsevier.

Look after the whole family using this blood pressure reading chart. (2006). Retrieved September 19, 2008, from http://www.highbloodpressureinfo.org/blood-pressure-reading-chart.html

Maslow, A. (1954). *Motivation and personality.* New York: Harper & Row.

National Cholesterol Education Program. (2002). *Third report of the expert panel on detection, evaluation, and treatment of high blood cholesterol in adults.* Washington, DC: National Heart, Lung, and Blood Institute.

National Heart, Lung, and Blood Institute. (2001). *Obesity education initiative.* Retrieved September 22, 2008, from http://www.nhlbisupport.com/bmi/

National Institute on Aging. (2008). *Health disparities toolbox.* Retrieved February 9, 2008, from http://www.nia.nih.gov/ResearchInformation/outreach.htm

Nelms, B., & Mullins, R. (1982). *Growth and development: A primary health care approach.* Englewood Cliffs, NJ: Prentice Hall.

Pender, N., Murdaugh, C. L., & Parsons, M. A. (2001). *Health promotion in nursing practice* (4th ed.). Upper Saddle River, NJ: Prentice Hall.

Piaget, J. (1969). *The theory of stages in cognitive development.* New York: McGraw-Hill.

Prochaska, J. O., & DiClemente, C. C. (1984). *The trans-theoretical approach: Crossing traditional boundaries of change.* Homewood, IL: Dow-Jones-Irwin.

Selye, H. (1974). *Stress without distress.* Philadelphia: JB Lippincott.

Tanner, J. M. (1962). *Growth of adolescents* (2nd ed.). Oxford: Blackwell Scientific.

Uphold, C. R., & Graham, M. V. (2003). *Clinical guidelines in family practice* (4th ed.). Gainesville, FL: B. Barmarrae Books.

U.S. Census Bureau. (2008). *Statistical abstract of the United States.* Retrieved February 9, 2008, from http://www.census.gov/compendia/statab/

U.S. Department of Health and Human Services. (1996). *Healthy people 2000* (pp. 479–510). Washington, DC: U.S. Public Health Service.

U.S. Department of Health and Human Services, Office of Disease Prevention and Health Promotion. (2001). *Healthy people 2010.* Retrieved September 22, 2008, from http://www.health.gov/healthypeople/default.htm

U.S. Preventive Services Task Force. (2007). *Guide to clinical preventive services, 2007.* Retrieved February 15, 2008, from http://www.ahrq.gov/clinic/pocketgd07/index.html

Whaley, L., & Wong, D. (1999). *Nursing care of infants and children* (6th ed.). St. Louis, MO: Mosby.

4

Infectious Diseases

Elizabeth Petit de Mange, PhD, MSN, BSN, NP-C, RN

GENERAL APPROACH

- Making the correct diagnosis of infectious disease in the family setting requires familiarity with the infectious organisms commonly seen in each age group.
- Mild illness is common in children, particularly upper respiratory infection in infants and toddlers.
- A fever is a temperature greater than 38°C (100.4°F) rectal, 37.5°C (99.5°F) oral, and 37°C (98.6°F) axillary. The normal temperature varies throughout the circadian rhythm, being lowest in the early morning and higher in the afternoon.
- Transmission of infection is influenced by the organism: its mode of transmission; its viability in the environment; number of organisms present in the environment; resistance of the potential host to the organism; and frequency of asymptomatic or carrier state.

Assessment
- Obtain thorough history of symptoms of present illness as well as possible contacts and exposure to infectious illness. Inquire about patient smoking or secondhand smoke.
- Factors indicating possible bacterial infection: loss of appetite, dehydration, high fever, chills, significant weakness or malaise
- Perform a physical exam for signs of infection including vital signs; skin, noting rash; eyes, noting conjunctivitis; head, noting nuchal rigidity, adenopathy; ears, nose, and throat, noting erythema and drainage; lungs, noting adventitious sounds; heart, noting murmurs; abdomen, noting tenderness, change in bowel sounds, organomegaly; musculoskeletal, noting tenderness, warmth, swelling, and erythema.

- Neurological exam including mental status may be needed to rule out central nervous system (CNS) infection or complication.
- Gram stain may be used as initial screen to help determine best antibiotic: gram positive organisms stain deep violet; gram negative organisms appear red.
- Culture to determine causative organism: obtain culture first, treat second to prevent false negative
- Sensitivity testing helps clarify the most appropriate antibiotics to use.

Management
- Assess for allergies to medications and clarify type of reaction to previous antibiotic use.
- Be aware of drug resistance patterns in the community, often caused by overuse of antibiotics.
- Avoid treating a viral illness with an antibiotic "just in case," or because parent states "She always needs an antibiotic or she won't get better."
- Improvement with antibiotics occurs in 2–3 days for most infections. Beyond this time frame, consider reassessing the patient and treatment plan.
- It is important to educate and document criteria for reevaluation if patient is not improving.
- Adequate hydration is important in the treatment of infectious illnesses, especially in children.
- 90% of respiratory infections are viral.
- Do not prescribe or administer aspirin or products containing aspirin to patients under 19 years of age for viral infections to avoid risk of developing Reye's syndrome.
- Due to decreased immune response, elderly have increased risk of secondary bacterial infections.
- If pregnant, use antibiotics in pregnancy category B; most antibiotics pass into breast milk.
- Know local health department guidelines for reporting communicable diseases.
- Seek referral to infectious disease specialists early rather than later in the course of unknown or unusual infection.
- Be alert to endemic diseases.
- Be alert to diseases that may be a result of bioterrorism.

Red Flags
- The very young and very old are at special risk for severe infections; also those with a compromised immune system, such as history of splenectomy, or concomitant illness such as diabetes.
- Recognize the unique physiologic and psychological responses of older patients to infectious disease and therapy.
- A fever with listlessness or flaccidity requires an aggressive evaluation, no matter the age.
- Bacteremia and sepsis may present with fever or hypothermia, chills, tachycardia, tachypnea, hypotension, altered mental status; mortality is nearly 50% in septic shock.
- Consult with physician or refer to specialist if illness does not respond to initial therapy or presentation is unusual; may need hospitalization if patient is unable to take oral medication or keep hydrated, or for severe infection requiring IV antibiotics.
- Know and recognize "classic" diagnostic features of certain illnesses, such as Koplik spots in measles (rubeola), subcutaneous nodules in rheumatic fever, etc.

- Educate the patient and caregiver, document recommendations, and follow up with patient and caregiver when infection is not resolving as expected.

Pediatric Issues

- All infants with fever who are younger than 3 months of age, or 3–12 months of age with no focal sign of infection, may require admission with a work-up including urine and blood cultures, lumbar puncture, and chest x-ray.
- Frequent (up to 10) viral illnesses, especially upper respiratory illnesses, per year are common in infants and toddlers.
- The family nurse practitioner should educate the caregivers of children between newborn and 19 years of age and educate adolescents to not take over-the-counter medications and other products that contain salicylates and other related compounds to avoid risk of Reye's syndrome. Instruct the caregiver and patients to check with pharmacist or healthcare provider.
- Transmission of infections in older infants and toddlers is mainly through droplet secretions on hands and through sharing toys in group settings.
- Children are contagious long before they are symptomatic. While it is important to exclude sick children from group settings and contact with other children, parents and day care workers need to understand that this will not necessarily reduce the spread of infection to others.
- Good handwashing is the single most effective tool in the prevention of illness.
- Washing toys may prevent the spread of illness.

2007–2008 Child Care Exclusion List

For children in out-of-home day care, child care settings for grades K–5, and medically fragile children:
- Illness requiring more care than the staff can reasonably provide
- Illness with fever, lethargy, irritability, persistent crying, difficulty breathing
- Diarrhea with blood or mucus
- Vomiting that has not been determined to be of noninfectious origin
- Mouth sores with drooling (unless determined to be noninfectious)
- Rash with fever or behavioral change (unless determined to be noninfectious)
- Purulent conjunctivitis
- Impetigo, until 24 hours after initiation of treatment
- Tuberculosis, until determined to be no longer infectious
- Streptococcal pharyngitis, until 24 hours after initiation of treatment
- Pediculosis, until after first treatment given
- Scabies, until after treatment given
- Varicella, until all lesions have crusted over
- Measles, until 4 days after rash began
- Mumps, until 9 days after parotid or other salivary gland swelling began
- Pertussis, until after 5 days of antibiotic therapy (of 14-day course)
- Hepatitis A, until 1 week after illness or jaundice began, unless disease is causing more severe symptoms
- E. coli (O157:H7) or Shigella, until diarrhea resolves and two negative stool cultures have been obtained

NOTE: Requirements for adult staff and nonimmunized children exposed to infections diseases can be found at the Centers for Disease Control and Prevention website, at www.scdhec.gov/health/disease/docs/2007-2008_Childcare_Exclusion_List.pdf.

VIRAL INFECTIONS

Fifth Disease (Erythema Infectiosum)

Description
• Mild, self-limiting viral disease characterized by erythematous, macular rash first appearing on the cheeks and ears, leading to a "slapped cheek" appearance

Etiology
• Caused by human parvovirus B19
• Transmitted via droplet, most often through contact with infected saliva, nasal secretions, sputum, and sometimes blood
• Communicable prior to the onset of symptoms; not infectious after onset of rash
• Incubation period 4–14 days up to 21 days; rash and joint symptoms occur 2–3 weeks after acquiring the infection

Incidence and Demographics
• Cases often occur as part of community outbreaks during late winter and early spring; may also occur sporadically.
• Spread to household contacts is common.

Risk Factors
• Institutional style day care setting
• School age
• Adults without immunity
• Contact with saliva, nasal secretions, and sputum of infected persons

Prevention and Screening
• May reduce transmission through rigorous handwashing and careful handling of used facial tissues

Assessment
HISTORY
• Prodrome usually absent; if present includes mild fever, malaise, headache, mild pruritus, and myalgias 7–10 days prior to rash
• Rash, beginning on the face and ears, with circumoral pallor, leading to "slapped cheek" appearance; progressing to an erythematous, maculopapular, "lacy" rash (often pruritic) beginning on the trunk and moving to arms, buttocks, and thighs; mild pruritus
• Arthralgias and arthritis may also be present; more common in infected adults, especially women

PHYSICAL EXAM
- Fever is low grade if present
- Note characteristic appearance of rash on face and body (see above)
- Rash fluctuates in intensity with environmental changes up to weeks and months after appearance; may increase or reappear following sunlight exposure, warm bath, vigorous play
- No lymphadenopathy or focal signs of infection
- May also see evidence of arthralgias and arthritis; more common in infected adults, especially women

DIAGNOSTIC STUDIES
- None usually performed in uncomplicated cases
- White blood count (WBC) usually normal; anemia with decreased reticulocytes is possible
- Detection of parvovirus B19-specific immunoglobulin (Ig) M antibody is possible to confirm diagnosis in complicated cases (persists for 2–4 months); IgM is usually detectable 3 days after infection. IgG is usually detectable 7 days after infection. A positive IgG antibody in the absence of IgM indicates previous infection and immunity
- Pregnant women exposed to fifth disease in the first trimester should be serologically tested for IgM and IgG antibodies; if a susceptibility or positive infection, weekly ultrasounds are indicated for 4–8 weeks after exposure or 2–4 weeks after infection to detect fetal hydrops

Differential Diagnosis
- Undifferentiated viral syndrome prior to rash appearance
- Other viral infections with rash

Management
NONPHARMACOLOGIC TREATMENT
- Symptomatic
- Isolation not indicated but avoid pregnant women and the immunocompromised

PHARMACOLOGIC TREATMENT
- Acetaminophen or ibuprofen for fever, myalgia, arthralgia in patients under 19 years of age
- Antipruritics, if necessary
- Intravenous immunoglobulin for chronic infection in immunocompromised patients
- If there is evidence of fetal hydrops, fetal transfusion may be considered

LENGTH OF TREATMENT
- As long as symptomatic

Special Considerations
- Infections during pregnancy may cause fetal hydrops and death, though risk is relatively low.

- Highest risk is if the mother is exposed during the first 20 weeks of pregnancy.
- B19-infected fetuses may be treated with intrauterine blood transfusions.
- Individuals with sickle cell disease or other chronic anemias are at risk for developing severe anemia if infected.
- Immunocompromised persons are at risk of serious illness if infected.
- Aspirin and aspirin-containing products should not be administered to anyone under 19 years of age for a viral illness to avoid risk of developing Reye's syndrome.

When to Consult, Refer, Hospitalize
- Refer to hematologist for complications—aplastic crisis, chronic anemia

Follow-Up
- None necessary in low-risk patients
- Closely follow immunocompromised patients or those experiencing aplastic crisis
  COMPLICATIONS
    - Aplastic crisis, chronic anemia
    - Arthritis, arthralgias in adults

Herpangina

Description
- Acute viral illness causing fever, ulcerative mouth lesions, cough, coryza, pharyngitis

Etiology
- Enterovirus (Coxsackie A and B)
- Transmitted by fecal–oral and oral–oral route
- Incubation 3–6 days

Incidence and Demographics
- Seen more frequently in temperate climates (summer and fall)
- Affects primarily children, day care through school age

Risk Factors
- More frequent in low socioeconomic groups

Prevention and Screening
- Good handwashing

Assessment
  HISTORY
    - Prodrome of fever as high as 106°F, pharyngitis, malaise, headache, backache, anorexia, drooling, vomiting, diarrhea

  PHYSICAL EXAM
    - 1–2 mm vesicles and ulcers on the anterior tonsillar pillars, soft palate, uvula, tonsils, pharyngeal wall, and posterior buccal surfaces

DIAGNOSTIC STUDIES
- Throat culture to rule out streptococcal pharyngitis

Differential Diagnosis
- Herpes simplex gingivostomatitis
- Aphthous stomatitis
- Hand, foot, and mouth disease
- Vincent's angina
- Streptococcal pharyngitis

Management
NONPHARMACOLOGIC TREATMENT
- Symptomatic—rest and fluids

PHARMACOLOGIC TREATMENT
- Acetaminophen or ibuprofen for fever and discomfort in patients under 19 years of age
- Variety of solutions consisting of viscous lidocaine 2%, diphenhydramine, and either Maalox or Kaopectate can be applied to lesions to relieve discomfort

LENGTH OF TREATMENT
- As long as symptomatic

Special Considerations
- None

When to Consult, Refer, Hospitalize
- Consult with a physician or infectious disease specialist if symptoms persist longer than 2 weeks or if child is unable to drink or eat

Follow-Up
- None usually needed

EXPECTED COURSE
- Resolves in 3–5 days

COMPLICATIONS
- Rarely myocarditis, meningitis, or encephalitis

Infectious Mononucleosis

Description
- Acute viral illness with fever, fatigue, pharyngitis, and adenopathy; some risk of complications

Etiology
- Epstein-Barr virus (EBV) is causative organism
- Transmission oropharyngeal route (saliva) or blood
- Communicability: Respiratory tract viral shedding can occur for months after infection
- Incubation 30–50 days

Incidence and Demographics
- Common in high school and college-age
- Transmitted via saliva

Risk Factors
- Living in group settings

Prevention and Screening
- Handwashing
- Avoid sharing eating or drinking utensils
- Avoid close personal contact

Assessment

HISTORY
- Fatigue, fever, swollen glands, and sore throat occur in most people
- Fever lasts about 10 days, fatigue may linger for several weeks
- Malaise and headache also occur frequently

PHYSICAL EXAM
- Lymphadenopathy may be significant and includes the posterior cervical and occipital nodes; lasts up to 4 weeks
- Exudative pharyngitis is often confused with streptococcal pharyngitis
- Petechiae of the palate and eyelid edema may occur; body rash occurs in a few
- Hepatomegaly or splenomegaly may occur in about 40% of people; lasts about 4 weeks
- Jaundice evident in a few

DIAGNOSTIC STUDIES
- Monospot is usual screening test; a rapid, nonspecific test for heterophile antibody agglutination
- Complete blood count (CBC) with differential shows atypical lymphocytosis
- Abnormal liver function tests: Aminotransferases (ALT, AST) and gamma glutamyl transferase (GGT) levels are elevated in 85% of cases; may need to follow in severe infection
- Consider throat culture to R/O group A streptococcal infection
- Consider EBV antibody titer (viral capsid antigen, early antigen) if diagnosis is in doubt, especially in older patients

Differential Diagnosis
- Other viral syndromes: rubella, adenovirus, toxoplasmosis, cytomegalovirus
- Serum sickness
- Leukemia
- Hepatitis
- Group A streptococcal or viral pharyngitis

Management

NONPHARMACOLOGIC TREATMENT
- Symptomatic, no isolation required, see prevention

- Warm salt water gargles for pharyngitis
- No contact sports, heavy lifting, strenuous activity for first 2–3 weeks and as long as splenomegaly persists
- Realistic schedule of rest
- Increased fluid intake

PHARMACOLOGIC TREATMENT
- Acetaminofen or ibuprofen for fever and discomfort in patients under 19 years of age
- Do not prescribe ampicillin or amoxicillin unless comorbid streptococcal pharyngitis exists; if needed, treatment may cause rash
- Steroids may be given to treat pharyngitis that leads to airway obstruction or hematologic complications (5–7-day taper)

Special Considerations
- Patients with recent EBV infection should not donate blood.

When to Consult, Refer, Hospitalize
- Refer to hematologist, neurologist, hepatologist, etc., early if any complications suspected.
- Hospitalization may be necessary for complications.

Follow-Up
- Based on clinical course; no follow-up may be necessary if fever and symptoms resolve after 10 days; follow up if jaundice, hepatosplenomegaly, or complications develop.
  EXPECTED COURSE
  - Duration variable, 3–4 weeks

COMPLICATIONS
- Tend to occur in younger or older patients
- CNS disorders such as aseptic meningitis, encephalitis, seizures, Guillain-Barré syndrome, optic neuritis, coma, transverse myelitis, Bell's palsy
- Hematologic complications such as hemolytic anemia, aplastic anemia, thrombocytopenia, hemolytic uremic syndrome
- Other rare complications: Splenic rupture (LUQ pain), myocarditis, pericarditis, pleural effusion, pneumonitis, hepatitis, erythema multiforme, nephrotic syndrome, uveitis, monoarthritis

Influenza

Description
- Acute viral illness that occurs in epidemics, usually in the fall and winter

Etiology
- Caused by an orthomyxovirus that appears in antigenic types A and B
- Frequent mutations produce new strains each flu season

Incidence and Demographics
- Very common
- Frequently leads to pneumonia in the elderly, contributing to the fifth leading cause of death in the elderly; young children also commonly affected

Risk Factors
- Close contact with infected persons
- Nursing home resident
- Elderly patients residing with children

Prevention and Screening
- Influenza vaccine provides immunity to 85% of those inoculated.
- Protection begins about 2 weeks after vaccination and lasts a few months.
- Vaccination recommended for all children between 6 months and 5 years of age, all adults >50 years old, and all others at risk of complications or exposure such as having a chronic illness, nerve or muscle disorders, respiratory compromise, immunosuppression, residence in a nursing home, pregnant during flu season, healthy caregivers of infants < 6 months, healthcare providers, and individuals traveling during influenza season or traveling to the tropics in an organized group.
- No influenza vaccines are approved for children <6 months.
- Administer antivirals such as amantadine or rimantadine shortly after exposure to influenza A.
- Administer antivirals such as oseltamivir and zanamivir after exposure to influenza A or B.
- LAIV (FluMist, a flu vaccine nasal spray) may be used in all healthy persons between 2 years and 49 years old without a history of asthma or wheezing; not to be administered to pregnant women, children and adolescents on aspirin therapy, individuals with history of Guillian-Barré syndrome, or people with allergy to chicken eggs or nasal spray components.

Assessment
HISTORY
- Acute onset
- Malaise
- Headache
- Nausea
- Muscle aching
- Nasal stuffiness

PHYSICAL EXAM
- Fever, chills
- Mild pharyngeal injection
- Conjunctival redness

DIAGNOSTIC STUDIES
- CBC: leukopenia is common
- Nasal or throat swab for identifying the influenza antigen

Differential Diagnosis
- Colds
- Bronchitis
- Pneumonia
- Other acute febrile illnesses

Management

NONPHARMACOLOGIC TREATMENT
- Rest
- Encourage fluids

PHARMACOLOGICAL TREATMENT
- Analgesics
- Cough syrup (NOTE: over-the-counter cough syrups are not recommended for children <2 years of age)
- Antivirals must be started within 2 days of symptom onset to be effective
- Amantadine (Symmetrel) 100 mg qd or bid or rimantadine (Flumadine) 100 mg po bid for 7 days for influenza A
- Oseltamivir (Tamiflu) 75 mg po bid or zanamivir (Relenza) 2 inhalations BID for 5 days for influenza A or B

When to Consult, Refer, Hospitalize
- Patients at either extreme of age are very vulnerable and should be referred to an infectious disease specialist.

Follow-Up

EXPECTED COURSE
- Usual duration is 1–7 days
- Often a longer and more severe course in the elderly

COMPLICATIONS
- Pneumonia
- Death

Measles (Rubeola)

Description
- Acute viral disease with fever (higher than 101°F); erythematous, maculopapular rash; cough; coryza; conjunctivitis; and a characteristic rash of the oral mucus membranes known as Koplik spots

Etiology
- Measles virus (RNA virus, Paramyxovirus family)
- Transmitted by direct contact with infectious droplets, or less commonly by airborne spread; highly contagious
- Incubation period 8–12 days
- Communicable 1–2 days before symptoms begin; 3–5 days before rash to 4 days after rash onset

Incidence and Demographics
- Greater than 99% reduction in the reported incidence of measles since vaccination began in 1963
- Most new cases secondary to importation from other countries

Risk Factors
- Lack of immunization; up to 5% of cases secondary to vaccine failure

Prevention and Screening
- Vaccine, usually given as MMR (measles, mumps, rubella) subcutaneous per routine schedule with first dose at 12–15 months, booster at 4–6 years of age

Assessment
HISTORY
- Prodrome of fever >101°F, malaise; cough, coryza, and/or conjunctivitis—the 3 Cs of measles

PHYSICAL EXAM
- Red, maculopapular rash beginning on face and neck; progressing slowly down trunk and extremities between second and fourth days and lasting 5–7 days
- Rash begins as discrete lesions, then becomes confluent and salmon-colored (morbilliform rash); lesions initially blanch with pressure
- When fever subsides, rash fades to faint brown stain; skin may desquamate
- Koplik spots are tiny, bluish-white spots on an erythematous base, clustered on the buccal mucosa near the molars, and are pathognomonic for measles. Appear 1–2 days before onset of rash and may last up to 12–15 days

DIAGNOSTIC STUDIES
- Acute (when rash appears) and convalescent (2–4 weeks) antibody titers
- Serum IgM antibodies peak 10 days after onset of rash, disappear after 20–60 days
- Measles virus detected from nasopharyngeal secretions, conjunctiva, blood, or urine

Differential Diagnosis
- Rubella
- Scarlatina
- Roseola

Management
NONPHARMACOLOGIC TREATMENT
- Symptomatic: Rest and fluids
- Isolation for 4 days after appearance of rash
- Avoid bright lights (photosensitivity)

PHARMACOLOGIC TREATMENT
- Acetaminophen or ibuprofen for fever and discomfort in patients under 19 years of age
- Consider vitamin A (200,000 IU po if >12 months old; 100,000 IU PO for infants 6–12 months old) in children at high risk for complications such as pneumonia (e.g., immunodeficiency, malabsorption, malnutrition); repeat in 24 hours and in 4 weeks if any ophthalmologic evidence of vitamin A deficiency.
- Give in all children in communities with vitamin A deficiency, particularly in developing countries.
- Live measles vaccine given within 72 hours of exposure may provide protection in some cases.
- Immune globulin may be given within 6 days of exposure; do not give with live vaccine. Susceptible household contacts should receive immune globulin since identification of the index case usually occurs after 72 hours (American Academy of Pediatric [AAP], 2006).
- Immune globulin dosing: 0.25 mL/kg body weight, IM; immunocompromised children should receive 0.5 mL/kg body weight. Maximum dose is 15 mL.
- Wait for 5 months after Ig 0.25 mL/kg body weight administered before giving the measles vaccine; wait 6 months after Ig 0.5 mL/kg body weight administered.

Special Considerations
- Do not prescribe or administer aspirin or aspirin-related products for a viral infection or syndrome due to the risk of Reye's syndrome in patients under 19 years of age.
- Children between 6 and 11 months traveling outside of the United States should be administered monovalent measles vaccine or MMR if unavailable before traveling if possible. The dose administered before 12 months of age should not count towards the MMR series (Centers for Disease Control and Prevention, 2007a).
- Children older than 12 months of age traveling outside the United States should receive two doses of MMR at least 28 days apart before departing (Centers for Disease Control and Prevention, 2007a).

When to Consult, Refer, Hospitalize
- No reason to refer in uncomplicated cases.

Follow-Up
- Daily during acute phase, 3–4 days after onset of rash; more often if indicated (high-risk individual, infant, presence of complications)
    EXPECTED COURSE
    - Recovery within 3–4 days after onset of rash, resolves in 10 days

    COMPLICATIONS
    - Otitis media, pneumonia, croup, diarrhea, acute encephalitis (1 in 1,000 cases); subacute sclerosing panencephalitis (SSPE) very rare, may develop years after measles infection

Mumps (Parotitis)

Description
- Acute viral disease affecting the salivary glands, primarily the parotid gland

Etiology
- Caused by a paramyxovirus
- Transmitted via the respiratory route (direct contact)
- Communicable 1–2 days prior to 5 days after the onset of parotid swelling
- Incubation period 16–18 days, but cases may occur 12–25 days after exposure

Incidence and Demographics
- Fewer than 1,000 cases per year; dramatic decline since implementation of vaccination
- Most reported cases in children 5–14 years of age; declining since introduction of second MMR vaccine in early childhood
- May see outbreaks in immunized populations; however, most cases of parotitis in immunized children are not due to mumps

Risk Factors
- Unimmunized persons

Prevention and Screening
- Primary prevention through vaccination; vaccine, usually given as MMR subcutaneous per routine schedule with first dose at 12–15 months, booster at 4–6 years of age. Postexposure vaccination is not effective.
- Exclusion from school or day care until 9 days from onset of parotid gland swelling.
- During outbreaks, exclusion of unimmunized children from school or day care for 26 days after onset of parotid gland swelling of the last person with mumps in the affected school or day care

Assessment
HISTORY
- Fever, malaise, pain in or behind the ear during chewing or swallowing
- "Classic" symptom is extreme pain when ingesting tart or sour substances

PHYSICAL EXAM
- Tender, swollen parotid glands, which typically covers angle of jaw; may also see submaxillary and sublingual gland involvement. Parotid glands may not be involved; approximately 1/3 of mumps cases do not have clinically apparent salivary gland swelling
- Tenderness persists 1–3 days; swelling persists 7–10 days
- Openings of the ducts of the involved salivary glands may be red and swollen.
- Fever may be normal, slight, or high (up to 104°F).

DIAGNOSTIC STUDIES
- WBC may show leukopenia and lymphocytosis
- Isolation of mumps virus in cell culture, best collected from saliva
- Rise in serum IgG titers or positive mumps IgM antibody test

- Serum amylase level increased in approximately 90% of patients with parotitis, not specific to mumps; helpful in differentiating parotitis from cervical adenopathy

Differential Diagnosis
- Parotitis from other causes, including infectious, tumor, or parotid duct obstruction
- Tooth infection or abscess
- Cervical adenitis

Management
NONPHARMACOLOGIC TREATMENT
- Supportive, push fluids, bed rest, warm or cold compresses to swollen areas (whichever is more soothing)
- Avoid tart, sour, acidic food and drink, and mucous membrane irritants such as peppermint
- Wash mouth with fat-free broth or saline solution
- Isolation until swelling is gone

PHARMACOLOGIC TREATMENT
- Acetaminophen or ibuprofen for fever and discomfort in patients under 19 years of age

When to Consult, Refer, Hospitalize
- Refer to specialist with any suggestion of complications

Special Considerations
- International travelers are at risk for exposure to mumps. Immunization is recommended if unsure of immunity status. Evidence of presumptive immunity includes documentation of physician-diagnosed disease; laboratory evidence of immunity; documentation of administration of two doses of live mumps vaccine; or birth date before 1957 (Centers for Disease Control and Prevention, 2007b).

Follow-Up
EXPECTED COURSE
- Duration up to 10 days

COMPLICATIONS
- Meningitis, which is symptomatic in approximately 10% of patients
- Other CNS involvement, including cerebellar ataxia
- Orchitis is common in infection after puberty, but sterility is rare
- Rare: Arthritis, thyroiditis, mastitis, glomerulonephritis, oophoritis, pancreatitis, myocarditis, transverse myelitis, thrombocytopenia, paresis of the facial nerve, hearing impairment

Roseola

Description
- Acute viral disease of infants and young children characterized by significant fever for 7–10 days that resolves by crisis, followed by faint, erythematous, maculopapular rash that lasts hours to days

Etiology
- Caused by human herpesvirus 6 (HHV-6)
- HHV-6 is a common cause of febrile illness in infants and young children, with or without rash.
- Roseola-like illnesses may be caused by a variety of different viruses, such as coxsackie viruses, echoviruses, adenoviruses, and parainfluenza virus.
- Transmission is by droplets and fecal-oral route.
- Incubation period is 9–10 days.

Incidence and Demographics
- Affects children ages 3 months–4 years; peak age 6–24 months

Risk Factors
- Institutional-style day care setting

Prevention and Screening
- Prevention difficult; should institute droplet and secretion precautions in institutionalized patients
- Remove from day care until afebrile (no infectious risk after afebrile even if rash is still present).

Assessment
HISTORY
- Sudden onset of fever (may be sustained or spiking); fever may be as high as 106°F; fever is what usually prompts parents to seek medical attention; lasts 3–7 days
- Cough, sore throat; faint rash that appears when the fever begins to drop

PHYSICAL EXAM
- Presence of fever up to 106°F
- Faint blanching, erythematous, maculopapular rash beginning on day 4 (lasts 1–2 days)
- May have lymphadenopathy (suboccipital, posterior cervical, postauricular), mild pharyngitis

DIAGNOSTIC STUDIES
- None indicated; if blood counts done, may see leukopenia and lymphocytosis

Differential Diagnosis
- Other viral, febrile illnesses with rash
- Drug reaction rash

Management
NONPHARMACOLOGIC TREATMENT
  • Supportive; push fluids in febrile phase

PHARMACOLOGIC TREATMENT
  • Acetaminophen or ibuprofen for fever and discomfort in patients under
    19 years of age

LENGTH OF TREATMENT
  • While symptomatic

Special Considerations
• None

When to Consult, Refer, Hospitalize
• No reason to refer in uncomplicated cases

Follow-Up
EXPECTED COURSE
  • Mild, self-limiting

COMPLICATIONS
  • Seizures (probably associated with high fever as opposed to viral invasion of
    cerebrospinal fluid [CSF] or cerebral structures), aseptic meningitis, encephalitis,
    thrombocytopenia purpura

Rubella (German Measles)

Description
• Mild viral disease with low-grade fever and generalized erythematous, maculopapular
  rash; generalized lymphadenopathy, most commonly suboccipital, postauricular,
  cervical; high risk if contracted during pregnancy

Etiology
• Rubella virus (RNA virus, Togaviridae family)
• Transmitted by direct or droplet contact with nasopharyngeal secretions
• Incubation period 14–23 days
• Communicable a few days before rash onset and for 5–7 days after rash appears
• Infants with congenital rubella may shed virus for 1 year or more.

Incidence and Demographics
• Incidence has declined by 99% since onset of vaccination; most cases now occur
  in young unimmunized or inadequately immunized adults (outbreaks in colleges or
  occupational settings).

Risk Factors
• Unimmunized or inadequately immunized young adults

Prevention and Screening
- Administer live attenuated vaccine, usually in the form of MMR, to unimmunized individuals, especially women of childbearing age. Vaccine, usually given as MMR subcutaneous per routine schedule with first dose at 12–15 months, booster at 4–6 years of age.
- Active immunization after exposure will not prevent infection; initiation of passive immunity with immune globulin not helpful
- Females of childbearing age should be tested for rubella antibody titer and if titer is low, should receive vaccine and avoid pregnancy for at least 28 days after vaccination

Assessment
   HISTORY
   - History of cough, coryza, malaise, fever, headache, possibly stiff joints

   PHYSICAL EXAM
   - Maculopapular rash, beginning on the face and spreading rapidly to the trunk; second day, rash begins to disappear in same pattern, usually resolved by third day
   - Fever, lymphadenopathy (suboccipital, postauricular, cervical), conjunctivitis, pharyngitis

   DIAGNOSTIC STUDIES
   - Rubella virus can be detected on nasal smear
   - Acute (7–10 days) and convalescent (2–3 weeks) serum titers (> 4-fold increase)
   - To determine immune status, order latex agglutination immunoassay

Differential Diagnosis
- Other viral diseases characterized by fever and rash

Management
- Symptomatic—rest and fluids
- Isolation if in an institution
- Stay home from work or school for 7 days after onset of rash

Special Considerations
- Maternal infection associated with high incidence of congenital anomalies and/or fetal demise
- Follow droplet precautions when caring for infants with congenital rubella until 3 or more successive negative nasopharyngeal and urine cultures are obtained

When to Consult, Refer, Hospitalize
- No reason to refer in uncomplicated cases

Follow-Up
   EXPECTED COURSE
   - Usually an acute, self-limiting illness
   - Arthritis and/or neuritis may occur in young children, more common in older children and adults

COMPLICATIONS
- Congenital rubella is associated with congenital anomalies and/or fetal demise
- Rare complications of postnatally acquired rubella include encephalitis, thrombocytopenia

Severe Acute Respiratory Syndrome (SARS)

Description
- Severe febrile viral lower respiratory tract illness

Etiology
- Caused by SARS-associated coronavirus (SARS-CoV)

Incidence and Demographics
- First reported in Asia in February 2003
- Spread to North America, South America, Europe
- According to CDC: 8,089 cases of SARS and 774 deaths worldwide
- In United States, 8 people with lab evidence of SARS; all had traveled to SARS areas
- Incubation period 2–10 days with median of 4–6 days
- Spread by close (within 3 feet) respiratory droplet transmission or fomites

Risk Factors
- Recent travel to mainland China, Hong Kong, Singapore, or Taiwan
- Close contact with persons ill with SARS
- Occupations at high risk: Healthcare workers, laboratory technicians
- Cluster of atypical pneumonia without other diagnosis

Prevention and Screening
- Avoid travel to high-risk areas
- Isolation of persons with possible SARS infection

Assessment
HISTORY
- History of exposure to SARS patient or SARS location

PHYSICAL EXAM
- Fever >100.4°F, headache, body aches, mild respiratory symptoms; headache and myalgia may precede fever
- 10%–20% have diarrhea
- After 2–7 days, dry cough develops with dyspnea and pneumonia

DIAGNOSTIC STUDIES
- No specific clinical or lab test available
- Obtain CBC with differential (70%–90% with lymphopenia), blood cultures
- Chest x-ray (CXR) and/or chest CT scan; chest CT may show infiltrate before CXR. Obtain CT if positive epidemiological link to known SARS case and negative CXR 6 days after symptoms develop; repeat CXR on day 9 of illness.

- Pulse oximetry
- Sputum for Gram stain and culture
- Viral respiratory testing for Influenza A and B and respiratory syncytial virus (RSV)
- Lab tests available through state health department: RT-PCR for SARS-CoV on blood, stool, and respiratory secretions; serology for SARS-CoV antibodies and viral culture for SARS-CoV. Obtain signed consent; due to the possibility of false-positive results, lab studies should only be obtained on patients meeting certain criteria. See CDC website for information: www.cdc.gov/ncido/sars/index.htm

Differential Diagnosis
- Influenza
- RSV
- Mycoplasma
- Bacterial pneumonia
- Viral pneumonia

Management
NONPHARMACOLOGIC TREATMENT
- Supportive care

PHARMACOLOGIC TREATMENT
- No specific treatment for SARS
- Appropriate treatment for complications

Special Considerations
- Persons with possible SARS must be quarantined in the home for 10 days or until fever resolved and person is free from respiratory symptoms

When to Consult, Refer, Hospitalize
- Refer SARS patients to an infectious disease specialist as soon as possible.
- Hospitalize any patient with worsening illness.
- Consult with state health department and/or CDC for lab testing and management of possible SARS cases.

Follow-Up
EXPECTED COURSE
- Mild cases resolve without complication

COMPLICATIONS
- 10% fatality rate overall, with >50% older than 60 years

Varicella (Chickenpox)

Description
- Usually mild acute viral disease characterized by generalized, pruritic, vesicular rash and fever

Etiology
- Caused by varicella zoster virus (herpesvirus family)
- Highly contagious; transmitted by airborne respiratory secretions from infected persons
- Rarely spread through contact with fluid from vesicles
- Contact with patients with herpes zoster (shingles) can cause chickenpox in susceptible individuals.
- Communicable 1–2 days before rash until vesicles are crusted, approximately 5 days after onset of rash
- Incubation period usually 14–16 days but may be 10–21 days

Incidence and Demographics
- Seen in all ages; most frequent in young schoolchildren, children attending day care

Risk Factors
- Unimmunized person

Prevention and Screening
- Vaccination is the best form of prevention (refer to the most current CDC- and AAP-recommended childhood and adult immunization schedule in Chapter 3)
- Isolate infected persons
- Children should not return to school or day care and adults should not return to work until all lesions are crusted over

Assessment
HISTORY
- Headache, mild fever, malaise

PHYSICAL EXAM
- Rash in various stages; progresses from macules to papules to vesicles on erythematous base within 6 hours after onset
- Vesicles crust in 4–6 days
- Some medical authors note vesicles appearing first on scalp and mucus membranes; others report vesicles appearing first on the trunk and back simultaneously with mucus membranes, and then spreading to scalp and extremities
- Vesicles may be seen in the conjunctivae, mouth, throat, esophagus, trachea, rectum, and vagina; little scarring occurs
- Vesicles rarely appear on the palms and soles
- Pruritus present in areas of crusted vesicles
- Usually appear in 3 crops on 3 successive days

DIAGNOSTIC STUDIES
- None indicated
- May see leukopenia
- May see WBC elevation with secondary infection
- May perform acute and convalescent titers
- Virus can be detected in vesicular scrapings during the first 3–4 days of the eruption

Differential Diagnosis
- Herpes simplex
- Papular urticaria
- Multiple insect bites
- Allergic skin reaction
- Scabies
- Smallpox
- Other viral fever and rash diseases
- Impetigo

Management

NONPHARMACOLOGIC TREATMENT
- For pruritus: Calamine or Cetaphil lotion, baths with baking soda or oatmeal

PHARMACOLOGIC TREATMENT
- May administer varicella vaccine to exposed, susceptible children within 72 hours (up to 120 hours) after varicella exposure; may prevent or modify the disease.
- Acetaminophen or ibuprofen for fever and discomfort for persons under 19 years of age
- Antipruritics such as diphenhydramine 5mg/kg/day, divided q6h
- Consider oral acyclovir (Zovirax) or other antivirals for persons at high risk of severe infection (older than age 12, chronic disease, immunocompromised, long-term salicylate therapy) if can initiate within 24 hours of onset of rash
- Administer varicella zoster immune globulin (VZIg) within 72–96 hours after exposure in immunocompromised children

Special Considerations
- Varicella zoster virus remains latent in nerve roots and may emerge later in life as herpes zoster (shingles).
- Do not prescribe or administer aspirin or aspirin-related products to persons under 19 years of age due to associated risk of Reye's syndrome.
- Due to increased risk of severe disease and complications in children over 12, adolescents without reliable history of disease should be immunized.

When to Consult, Refer, Hospitalize
- No reason to refer in uncomplicated cases

Follow-Up
- Return to day care, school, or work only after all lesions are crusted.

COMPLICATIONS
- Secondary, bacterial infection of skin (impetigo)
- Scarring, which may be a cosmetic concern
- Encephalitis, nephritis, hepatitis, glomerulonephritis
- Reye's syndrome
- Thrombocytopenia
- Pneumonia

West Nile Virus (WNV)

Description
- Viral infection causing febrile illness, rash, arthritis, myalgias, weakness, lymphadenopathy, and meningoencephalitis

Etiology
- The WNV is caused by the Arbovirus of family Flaviviridae. The transmission cycle if spread by infected mosquitoes to birds and from infected birds to feeding mosquitoes.
- Human infection is primarily from the bite of an infected mosquito.
- Horses and domestic animals are sometimes infected by the bite of an infected mosquito. However, there is no documentation of spread of the disease from animal to animal or animal to human.
- Although rare, infection can be spread through blood transfusions, organ transplantation, and prenatal transmission.

Incidence and Demographics
- Reported in Asia, Africa, Europe, and United States (first in 1999)
- As of March 2008, 3,598 cases of WNV reported in United States with ~60% having mild disease and ~30 % severe disease, including 121 deaths
- Incubation period 5–15 days
- 20% of infected people develop mild illness lasting 3–6 days
- 1 in 150 develop severe neurological disease, encephalitis more than meningitis
- Adults >50 years at greatest risk for serious illness
- Mortality 5%, with most deaths in older adults

Risk Factors
- Outdoor activities when mosquito activity is high
- Outdoor occupation
- Blood transfusion and organ transplant recipients
- Elderly

Prevention and Screening
- Avoidance of mosquito bites: Minimize outdoor activity, wear protective clothing, and protect home and yard from breeding mosquitoes by draining standing water and maintaining window screens
- When outdoors, apply insect repellent containing DEET (up to 50% strength), Picaridin, or oil of lemon eucalyptus; Permethrin is also recommended for use on clothing, shoes, and other gear.
- Pediatric Note: Oil of lemon eucalyptus products should not be used on children under 3 years. The American Academy of Pediatrics does not recommend the use of DEET on infants <2 months.
- Apply repellent to clothing and exposed skin, avoiding eyes and mouth; do not apply to skin under clothing. Efficacy of repellent is affected by concentration, perspiration, and getting wet. Reapply repellent as needed.
- Control of vectors by public health spraying against mosquitoes
- Wear gloves when disposing of dead birds
- Report dead birds to local health department
- Blood donations screened for WNV using nucleic acid-amplification test

Assessment

HISTORY
- Determine exposure to mosquitoes
- History of blood transfusion or organ transplantation

PHYSICAL EXAM
- Nondescript fever with maculopapular or morbilliform rash on neck, trunk, arms, and legs
- Arthritis, myalgias, generalized weakness, and lymphadenopathy
- Meningitis: Fever, headache, and nuchal rigidity
- Encephalitis: Fever, headache, and altered mental status ranging from confusion to coma, with or without additional signs of brain dysfunction (paresis, flaccid paralysis, ataxia, sensory deficits, optic neuritis, seizures, and abnormal reflexes)

DIAGNOSTIC STUDIES
- CSF with IgM antibody for WNV is confirmative; CSF with pleocytosis (increased number of lymphocytes)
- WNV antibody in serum is presumptive of recent infection in patients with acute CNS infection; a >4-fold increase in antibody titers 2–4 weeks apart is confirmative
- Pleocytosis: Increased number of lymphocytes in CSF

Differential Diagnosis
- California encephalitis
- Eastern equine encephalitis
- Western equine encephalitis
- Powassan encephalitis
- St. Louis encephalitis
- Colorado tick fever
- Dengue fever

Management

NONPHARMACOLOGIC TREATMENT
- Supportive care
- Monitor for complications

PHARMACOLOGIC TREATMENT
- Appropriate treatment of complications

LENGTH OF TREATMENT
- Continue supportive care until improvement

Special Considerations
- CDC website for West Nile virus: www.cdc.gov/ncidod/dvbid/westnile/background.htm

When to Consult, Refer, Hospitalize
- Report West Nile virus encephalitis cases to the state health department
- Immediately refer patients to an infectious disease specialist

- Patients with deteriorating mental status should be referred immediately to a physician for hospitalization

Follow-Up
- Majority have very minor illness and recovery without complications
    COMPLICATIONS
        - Central nervous system abnormalities
        - Death

BACTERIAL AND OTHER INFECTIONS

Lyme Disease

Description
- Tick-borne infection from a spirochete transmitted via the deer tick bite that often begins with rash (erythema migrans), then headaches, arthritis, and neurologic sequelae. While up to 20% of patients have complications, most do not have permanent sequelae.

Etiology
- Caused by the spirochete *Borrelia burgdorferi*; most common vector-borne disease in the United States
- Transmitted to humans by *Ixodes scapularis* tick (deer tick); not transmitted by larger dog tick
- Size of tick is 2–9 mm
- Painless bite; ticks usually drop off unnoticed in 2–4 days; must be embedded >24 hours to transmit disease
- Incubation period from bite to appearance of erythema migrans is 3–31 days; usually 7–14 days

Incidence and Demographics
- 90% of cases Mid-Atlantic, Northeastern, and North Central areas of the United States: New York, New Jersey, Connecticut, Rhode Island, Maryland, Massachusetts, Pennsylvania, and Wisconsin
- In 2006, 19,931 reported cases yielding an incidence of 8.2 cases/100,000 (CDC, 2008b)
- Incidence is 30.2/100,000 in the 10 states with the most reported number of cases
- Occurs during tick season, spring through the first frost

Risk Factors
- Live in endemic region
- Spend time outdoors for recreation or occupation
- Exposed skin
- No use of repellants
- 30%–50% of cases occur in children and adolescents

Prevention and Screening

- Reduce exposed skin: Wear light-colored clothing to see ticks; wear long pants and long sleeves; tuck shirts into pants, tuck pants into socks. When outdoors, apply insect repellent containing DEET (up to 50% strength), Picaridin, or oil of lemon eucalyptus; Permethrin is also recommended for use on clothing, shoes, and other gear
- **Pediatric Note:** Oil of lemon eucalyptus products should not be used on children under 3 years. The American Academy of Pediatrics does not recommend the use of DEET on infants <2 months.
- Apply repellent to clothing and exposed skin, avoiding eyes and mouth; do not apply to skin under clothing. Efficacy of repellent is affected by concentration, perspiration, and getting wet; reapply repellent as needed.
- Walk in middle of path; avoid walking near tree branches, bushes, or grass; inspect skin, hair, and scalp after spending day outside; examine clothing before coming into house.
- Examine pets for ticks regularly.
- Lyme disease vaccine was withdrawn from the market in 2002 by manufacturer due to low sales and is no longer commercially available.
- Prophylactic antibiotics are not routinely used following tick bites. However, factors to take into consideration include: Was the tick on the individual for 24 hours before being removed or falling off? Has it been at least 3 days since the individual removed the tick or it fell off? Is Lyme disease common in the location where the individual was exposed to the tick?

Table 4–1. Stages of Lyme Disease

Stage	Symptoms
Stage 1: Early localized disease (3–30 days post-exposure)	• Flu-like symptoms of fever, chills, myalgia, arthralgia, headache • 50%–90% of patients develop a distinctive rash termed erythema migrans within about 1 week of tick bite: begins as red macule or papule, expands rapidly over several days to annular, erythematous patch with central clearing, >5 cm and may be as large as 30 cm • Resolves in 3–4 weeks without treatment; usually in area of tick bite but may occur anywhere
Stage 2: Early disseminated disease (weeks to months post-exposure)	• Begins roughly 3–5 weeks after initial infection, as spirochete spreads • Wide variety of symptoms, most notably persistent fatigue • Migratory arthralgia common • Cranial nerve palsies (especially facial nerve) common • Meningitis, conjunctivitis may occur; carditis with heart block rare • Most common manifestation is multiple erythema migrans, usually smaller than initial lesion
Stage 3: Late disease (months to years later)	• Months to years after initial infection, characterized by recurrent pauciarticular arthritis, usually affecting large joints (knees) • Central and peripheral nervous system affected, may develop subacute encephalopathy, distal paresthesias • Memory, mood, sleep problems may be noted • Cardiac involvement

Assessment

HISTORY
- Most unable to identify tick bite, but have history of possible exposure.

PHYSICAL EXAM
- Complete physical exam should be done.
- Characteristic rash (target lesion); may find tick or tick remnant in Stage 1.
- Signs of cranial nerve palsies, meningeal signs, pericarditis, monoarthritis in Stage 2.
- Late in disease may be recurrent tendonitis, bursitis, synovitis; memory loss; motor or sensory deficits; iritis, optic neuritis, and other eye manifestations (see Table 4–1 for descriptions of each stage of the disease).

DIAGNOSTIC STUDIES
- Lyme disease is primarily a clinical diagnosis; serology has uncertain sensitivity but is used to confirm the presence of specific antibodies to B. *burgdorferi* in serum (see Table 4–2).
- Step 1: ELISA method is preferred: more sensitive and specific. If positive, proceed to step 2.
- Step 2: Western blot assay can detect both IgM and IgG and is used as a confirmatory test.
- Serologic tests are not necessary if patient has classic presentation of exposure to endemic area and erythema migrans; tests often negative early in course.
- For late disease, patient must have specific symptoms and objective signs prior to testing.
- Patients with Lyme disease may not have elevated titers during the first several weeks of illness (false negative test result).
- Do not test patients with nonspecific symptoms for Lyme disease as there is a relatively high incidence of false positives in the general population.

Table 4–2. Laboratory Findings in Lyme Disease

Serum Test	Early Findings	Midcourse	Late Findings
	2–4 weeks after erythema migrans	6–8 weeks	4–6 months
IgM	Appears	Peaks	Declines to low levels
IgG	Negative	Appears	Peaks; remains elevated but at lower level

Differential Diagnosis
- Rocky Mountain spotted fever
- Rheumatic fever
- Viral disease
- Fibromyalgia
- Other forms of arthritis

Management

NONPHARMACOLOGIC TREATMENT
- Hydrate patients; keep skin well-lubricated
- Remove tick using firm tension, fine tweezers, and clean site. Do not squeeze or puncture the tick. If the tick head or other parts are not removed, clean with antimicrobial as removing head can cause tissue damage and has no effect on risk of Lyme disease.

PHARMACOLOGIC TREATMENT
- Adults
  - Early disease: Doxycycline (Vibramycin) 100 mg bid po 14–21 days
  - Late disease: Same as early disease but treatment is 21–28 days
  - Persistent or recurrent arthritis, carditis, meningitis, or encephalitis:
    » Cetriaxone (Rocephin) 2 g qd or 1 g bid IV or IM 14–21 days
    » OR Penicillin G IV 20 million units in 4 divided doses
- Pediatric
  - Early disease: <8 years of age Amoxicillin (Amoxil) 25–50 mg/kg/day po divided into 2 doses daily not to exceed 2 g/day for 14–21 days
  - Early disease: 8 years of age Doxycycline (Vibramycin) 100 mg bid po 14–21 days
  - Late disease: Same as early disease except treatment is 21–28 days
  - Persistent or recurrent arthritis, carditis, meningitis, or encephalitis:
    » Ceftriaxone (Rocephin) 75–100mg/kg qd, not to exceed 2 g/day for 14–21 days
    » OR Penicillin G IV 300,000 U/kg/day in four divided doses not to exceed 20 million U/day

---

Box 4-1. Management of Lyme Disease

Early localized disease
- Children <8 years old: Amoxicillin 25–50 mg/kg/day ÷ into 2 doses daily, po x 14–21 days; max 2 g/day
- Children ≥8 years old: Doxycycline 100 mg po bid x 14–21 days (drug of choice)
- PCN allergy or intolerance to tetracycline: May use cefuroxime axetil or erythromycin

Early disseminated and late disease
- Multiple erythema migrans: Amoxicillin or doxycycline at doses appropriate for age for 21 days
- Isolated facial palsy: Amoxicillin or doxycycline at doses appropriate for age for 21–28 days
- Arthritis: Amoxicillin or doxycycline at doses appropriate for age for 28 days
- Persistent or recurrent arthritis, carditis: Ceftriaxone 75–100 mg/kg IV or IM qd x 14–21 days; max 2 g/day; or penicillin 300,000 U/kg/day ÷ into 4 doses daily for 14–28 days, IV, max 20 million U/day
- Meningitis or encephalitis: Ceftriaxone or penicillin for 30–60 days

---

Adapted from *Red Book 2006: Report of the Committee on Infectious Diseases* (26th ed.), by American Academy of Pediatrics, 2006, Elk Grove Village, IL: Author.

Special Considerations
- Amoxicillin is recommended for children and for pregnant and lactating women.

When to Consult, Refer, Hospitalize
- Refer to infectious disease specialist and/or to other specialist as soon as diagnosis is suspected. Monitor for central nervous system or cardiac involvement, uncertain diagnosis, or failure to respond to po medication.
- Consult with physician if IV therapy required.
- Lyme disease must be reported to CDC.

Follow-Up
EXPECTED COURSE
- Most respond promptly; complete resolution of symptoms in 4 weeks
- Long-term outcome not clear. In one study, many had residual symptoms; however, treatment had often been delayed or patients were undertreated.

COMPLICATIONS
- Recurrent arthritis, chronic neurologic symptoms, congestive heart failure, cardiomyopathy

Pertussis

Description
- Upper respiratory illness characterized by progressive cough that can become severe and spasmodic

Etiology
- *Bordetella pertussis*
- Transmission is respiratory
- Incubation 6–20 days
- Communicable until 5 days after treatment initiated

Incidence and Demographics
- The number of cases reported to the CDC has increased since 1980; in 2005, 25,000 cases were reported (a 40-year high)
- Majority of cases occur in children between 6 months and 5 years old
- 27% of cases were among adults

Risk Factors
- Lack of immunization

Prevention and Screening
- See Chapter 3 for pertussis immunizations for children and adults

Assessment
HISTORY
- Catarrhal stage: Mild upper respiratory symptoms with cough and mild conjunctival injection (most contagious stage); indistinguishable from the common cold

- Paroxysmal stage: severe bursts of cough with inspiratory whoop followed by vomiting; fever is absent or low grade (less than 101°F). Cough is forceful, rapid, staccato sequence; child unable to breath between coughing, which is often accompanied by emesis.

PHYSICAL EXAM
- Depending on stage, patient may appear tired; apnea may occur in young infants
- Obtain vital signs, eyes, ears, nose, throat, respiratory, and cardiac exam to rule out other illnesses

DIAGNOSTIC STUDIES
- Nasopharyngeal cultures in the catarrhal stage or IgA testing for B. pertussis to confirm diagnosis
- CBC will show leukocytosis

Differential Diagnosis
- Bronchiolitis
- Bronchitis
- Pneumonia
- Other viral and bacterial upper respiratory infections
- Cystic fibrosis
- Foreign body

Management

NONPHARMACOLOGIC TREATMENT
- Symptomatic—rest and fluids
- Admission for infants less than 6 months old

PHARMACOLOGIC TREATMENT
- Erythromycin 40 to 50 mg/kg/day in 4 divided doses
- Or trimethoprim/sulfamethoxazole (Bactrim) 8mg/kg/day (trimethoprim component) given bid
- Beta-2 agonists to control paroxysmal cough
- Corticosteroids for severely ill patients

LENGTH OF TREATMENT
- 14 days

Special Considerations
- Antibiotics do not significantly shorten the disease; they do reduce transmission.
- Do not use cough suppressants.

When to Consult, Refer, Hospitalize
- Consult with physician for infants younger than 6 months and others who present with potentially severe disease; often require hospitalization for supportive care.
- Pertussis must be reported to CDC.

Follow-Up
- Follow via telephone contact; discourage clinic visits
    EXPECTED COURSE
    - May be 10 weeks in uncomplicated cases

    COMPLICATIONS
    - Pneumonia, seizures, encephalopathy, death

Rheumatic Fever (Rf)
Description
- Serious inflammatory systemic immune process occurring 1 week to 6 months after group A *beta-hemolytic streptococcal pharyngitis*

Etiology
- Anti-streptococcal antibodies cross-react with human cardiac myocytes, cartilage, and thalamic and subthalamic nuclei of the CNS, causing carditis, arthritis, and chorea.
- Heredity may play a role, causing a particular immune response to strep.

Incidence and Demographics
- Frequency and severity has decreased due to better treatment of pharyngitis.
- Remains an important cause of cardiac death in 5–25-year-olds.
- Many older patients have valvular disease caused by rheumatic fever.

Risk Factors
- Immigrants to the United States
- Genetic predisposition
- Age 5–15
- More common in girls and African Americans
- Living in the Midwest or Intermountain West in the mid- to late 1980s

Prevention and Screening
- Timely antibiotic treatment of *group A beta hemolytic streptococcal* upper respiratory infection

Assessment
    HISTORY
    - May have history of recent sore throat
    - Presents with gradual onset of fever, malaise, and joint pain (classically migratory pain and possible inflammation of large joints; disappears in 3–4 weeks)
    - Other symptoms are fatigue, irritability, abdominal pain, epistaxis (rare)

    PHYSICAL EXAM
    - Heart murmurs indicating mitral valve 75%, aortic valve 30%, tricuspid or pulmonic <5% involvement; occur within 2 weeks, may be permanent
    - Pericarditis, myocarditis may last 6 weeks to 6 months
    - Subcutaneous nodules (painless, freely movable over extensor surfaces of elbows, knees, and wrists)

- Neuro: Facial grimaces and tics, chorea (purposeless, involuntary, rapid movements of trunk and/or extremities) are late findings
- Rash is rare; present with red macular lesions with rounded or serpiginous margins and pale centers; transient and migratory, occurs mainly on trunk and proximal extremities
    - Guidelines for diagnosis of rheumatic fever, Jones criteria
    - Required for diagnosis: Evidence of a preceding streptococcal infection such as elevated or increasing antistreptolysin-O titer or other streptococcal antibodies, positive throat culture for group A streptococcus, or recent scarlet fever
    - Two major symptoms or one major and two minor are required for diagnosis (see Table 4–3)

Table 4-3. Jones Criteria for Rheumatic Fever

Major Symptoms	Minor Symptoms
Carditis (common)	Clinical: Fever (101°F –102°F), arthralgias, previous RF
Polyarthritis (common)	or preexisting rheumatic heart disease
Chorea (uncommon)	Laboratory: Acute phase reaction (leukocytosis,
Erythema marginatum (uncommon)	elevated erythrocyte sedimentation rate (ESR),
Subcutaneous nodules (uncommon)	abnormal c-reactive protein or
	Prolonged PR interval or other electrocardiographic changes

DIAGNOSTIC STUDIES
- To diagnose current strep throat: Throat culture may or may not be positive
- To document preceding strep infection: Streptococcal antibody titers—obtain acute and convalescent serum titers (2–4 weeks)
- To confirm diagnosis of RF and evaluate severity of illness
    - ESR elevation
    - C-reactive protein elevation
    - Prolonged PR interval on ECG

Differential Diagnosis
- Rheumatoid arthritis
- Systemic lupus erythematosus
- Lyme disease

Management
NONPHARMACOLOGIC TREATMENT
- Strict bed rest until C-reactive protein has been normal for 2 weeks, ESR and temperature are normal

PHARMACOLOGIC TREATMENT
- Depends on specific symptoms and severity of disease; refer to specialist
- For pain, use codeine rather than nonsteroidal anti-inflammatory drugs (NSAIDs)

- Carditis is treated with inotropic agents, diuretics, vasodilators, and corticosteroids as indicated
- Chorea is treated with sedatives and benzodiazepines

LENGTH OF TREATMENT
- Bedrest until temperature, lab results, pulse rate (<100/min in adults), and ECG return to normal
- Antibiotics as above

Special Considerations
- Educate regarding meticulous oral hygiene to prevent bacterial seeding.
- Educate patient to notify healthcare providers about cardiac condition prior to any procedure.
- Treat patients who have history of rheumatic fever prophylactically to prevent recurrent rheumatic fever (secondary prevention). Usual antibiotic is penicillin. These patients should take a full course of antibiotic followed by continuous prophylactic dose for 10 years if the patient had carditis; 5 years if patient did not have carditis.
- Prophylaxis prior to procedures that may cause bacteremia is important indefinitely (see Table 4–4)
- Patients who should receive prophylaxis:
  - High-risk patients
    - Prosthetic valve, previous bacterial endocarditis, complex, cyanotic congenital heart disease, surgically constructed systemic pulmonary shunts or conduits
  - Medium-risk patients
    - Acute rheumatic fever (ARF) patients who have acquired valvular dysfunction but NOT for patients with previous ARF without valvular dysfunction
    - Other moderated risk patients include those with uncorrected cardiac congenital defects, hypertrophic cardiomyopathy, mitral regurgitation, mitral valve prolapse with murmur, and possibly men greater than 45 with mitral valve prolapse without murmur

When to Consult, Refer, Hospitalize
- Refer to rheumatologist and/or cardiologist for all suspected cases
- Hospitalize for acute carditis and chorea

Table 4-4. Prophylaxis for Recurrent Rheumatic Fever

Procedures For Which Indicated	Prophylactic Regimen Needed
Dental and Respiratory Tract, Esophagus	
Periodontal surgery, scaling, professional teeth cleaning; tonsillectomy, adenoidectomy; respiratory tract surgery, bronchoscopy	*Adults:* Amoxicillin 2 g po 1 hour before the procedure; if unable to take oral: Ampicillin 2 g IV or IM 30 minutes before procedure *Children:* Amoxicillin 50mg/kg; po 1 hour before procedure; if unable to take oral: Ampicillin 50 mg/kg IV or IM 30 minutes before procedure *Penicillin Allergic:* • Clindamycin (Cleocin): Adults 600 mg, children 20 mg/kg, po 1 hour before or IV 30 minutes before procedure • Cefadroxil (Duricef) or cephalexin (Keflex): Adults 2 g, children 50 mg/kg, po 1 hour before procedure • Azithromycin (Zithromax) or clarithromycin (Biaxin): Adults 500 mg, children 15 mg/kg, po 1 hour before procedure *Penicillin Allergic, Unable to Take Oral:* Cefazolin (Kefzol): Adults 1 g, children 25 mg/kg, IM or IV 30 minutes before procedure
Gastrointestinal and Genitourinary Tract	
Sclerotherapy of esophageal varices, esophageal stricture dilation, endoscopic retrograde cholangiography, biliary tract surgery, surgery associated with intestinal mucosa; prostatic surgery, cystoscopy, urethral dilation	Amoxicillin: Adults 2 gm, children 50 mg/kg, po 1 hour before procedure; IV or IM 30 minutes before *Penicillin Allergic:* • Vancomycin (Vancocin): Adults 1 g, children 20 mg/kg, IV over 1–2 hours, completed within 30 minutes of procedure *If Patient Is High-Risk:* *Adults:* Ampicillin 2 g IM or IV and gentamicin 1.5 mg/kg (not to exceed 120 mg) within 30 minutes of starting the procedure; 6 hours later, ampicillin 1 g IV/IM or amoxicillin 1 g orally *Children:* Ampicillin 50 mg/kg IM or IV (not to exceed 2.0 g) and gentamicin 1.5 mg/kg within 30 minutes of starting the procedure; 6 hours later ampicillin 25 mg/kg IM/IV or amoxicillin 25 mg/kg orally *High-Risk, Penicillin Allergic:* • Adults: Vancomycin 1g IV over 1–2 hours and gentamicin 1.5 mg/kg (not to exceed 120 mg), 30 minutes before procedure • Children: Vancomycin 20 mg/kg IV over 1–2 hours and gentamicin 1.5 mg/kg IV/IM 30 minutes before procedure

Adapted from *The Sanford Guide to Antimicrobial Therapy* (37th ed.), by D. N. Gilbert, R. C. Moellering, & M. A. Sande, 2007, Hyde Park, VT: Antimicrobial Therapy, Inc.

Follow-Up
- Usually followed by cardiologist to monitor C-reactive protein and reevaluate every 4–6 weeks when patients present for prophylaxis

   EXPECTED COURSE
   - Initial episodes may last months in children and weeks in adults

   COMPLICATIONS
   - Recurrent acute rheumatic fever secondary to streptococcal reinfection
   - Cardiomegaly, heart failure, pericarditis, mitral regurgitation, aortic insufficiency
   - Death in 1%–2%

Rocky Mountain Spotted Fever (Rmsf)

Description
- Moderate systemic febrile illness with rash caused by vasculitis of small vessels; systemic symptoms including fever, characteristic rash; risk of severe complications and death

Etiology
- *Rickettsia rickettsii* transmitted by bite of infected tick
- Tick must attach and feed for 4–6 hours to transmit infection
- No person-to-person transmission; disease confers immunity
- Incubation 2–14 days

Incidence and Demographics
- More than 50% of cases occur in South Atlantic region; occurs predominantly in southeastern and central states; also upper Rocky Mountain states, Canada, Mexico, and South and Central America
- Approx 250 to 1200 cases reported annually in the United States; peaks in late spring and summer
- $2/3$ of patients are age <15 years

Risk Factors
- Exposure to tick bites; camping or yard work; exposed skin due to short pants, sleeves; no repellant

Prevention and Screening
- Avoid tick bites; see Lyme disease

Assessment
   HISTORY
   - Triad: Fever, rash, and history of tick bite, although not all are present at time of initial assessment
   - Presents with sudden onset of fever higher than 104°F in nearly 100% patients
   - Severe headache unrelieved by analgesics; myalgia (particularly in calf and thigh)
   - Nausea and vomiting, abdominal pain, lymphadenopathy, cough, confusion are possible
   - History of possible tick bite or exposure

PHYSICAL EXAM
- Characteristic maculopapular rash usually appears before the sixth day of illness, spreads from wrists and ankles to trunk, neck, and face
- If untreated, rash becomes petechial in about 4 days, then progresses to purpuric and coalesced
- Moderate to high fever, conjunctival injection
- Splenomegaly occurs in approximately 50% of patients

DIAGNOSTIC STUDIES
- Titers; acute and convalescent sera (a fourfold increase in antibody titer) may not rise for 10–14 days
- Routine blood work may show nonspecific changes, identify complications: CBC with differential (thrombocytopenia, variable WBC count, mild anemia), PT and PTT (prolonged), BUN and creatinine (elevated in renal insufficiency), electrolytes (mild hyponatremia), LFTs (elevated in hepatitis)

Differential Diagnosis
- Systemic viral infection
- Bacterial sepsis
- Meningitis
- Meningococcemia
- Lyme disease
- Rubella
- Scarlet fever
- Mononucleosis
- Rheumatic fever
- Drug reaction
- Erythema multiforme
- Ehrlichiosis

Management
NONPHARMACOLOGIC TREATMENT
- Rest and fluids
- Isolation not indicated

PHARMACOLOGIC TREATMENT
- **Important to treat promptly;** treatment before day 5 of illness in children affords highest likelihood of good outcome
- Doxycycline (Vibramycin) is the treatment of choice in adults who are not pregnant and children of all ages unless hypersensitive to tetracyclines
- Adults
  - Doxycycline (Vibramycin) 100 mg bid after loading dose of 200 mg
  - If patient is sensitive to tetracyclines use
    » Amoxicillin 500 mg tid or
    » Cefuroxime (Ceftin) 500 bid
  - Late stage: Ceftriaxone (Rocephin) 2 g IV qa
- Pediatric
  - ≤ 45 kg: Doxycycline (Vibramycin) 2–4 mg/kg/day po in 2 divided doses
  - ≥ 45 kg: Doxycycline (Vibramycin) 100 mg po bid

- Pregnant women
    - Chloramphenicol (Chloromycetin) 500 mg q 6 hours

LENGTH OF TREATMENT
- 5–10 days or until afebrile 2–5 days

Special Considerations
- Educate patient on the tick associated with RMSF and ways to avoid the infection.

When to Consult, Refer, Hospitalize
- Consult with infectious disease specialist as soon as possible for possible hospitalization, any signs of complications.
- Rocky Mountain spotted fever must be reported to CDC.

Follow-Up
- See patient for follow-up every 2–3 days if not hospitalized, until symptoms resolved.
    EXPECTED COURSE
    - Follow up 1–2 days after initial visit; inform patients to return at first sign of complications
    - Most cases resolve without complication if treated promptly; can persist for 3 weeks
    - Refer for tertiary care as soon as complications develop or if petechial rash on first visit

    COMPLICATIONS
    - Central nervous system, cardiac, pulmonary, gastrointestinal, and renal involvement; disseminated intravascular coagulation, shock, death

Scarlet Fever (Scarlatina)

Description
- An acute infectious disease usually associated with streptococcal pharyngitis and characterized by a vascular response to bacterial exotoxin

Etiology
- Toxin produced by group A hemolytic streptococcus (GAS) and occasionally produced by certain strains of staphylococci.
- Strep toxin usually has a pharyngeal source.
- A rare source is strep or staph infections from wounds or burns
- Transmitted by direct projection of large droplets or physical transfer of respiratory secretions
- Incubation 3–5 days
- Communicable during incubation and clinical illness, 10 days; no longer communicable after 24 hours of antibiotic

Incidence and Demographics
- Usually occurs in children 6–12 years, but also occurs in adults

Risk Factors
- Outside-the-home day care setting
- School-age children

Prevention and Screening
- Early identification of GAS by throat culture and removal from school or child care for 24 hours after initiation of antibiotic
- Good handwashing
- Household contact screening for GAS or prophylaxis treatment is not effective

Assessment

HISTORY
- Prodrome: 1–2 days of fever, sore throat, headache; also may be abdominal pain and vomiting
- Rash appears in 1–5 days

PHYSICAL EXAM
- Initial pharyngitis is beefy red with or without exudate; also white coating on tongue on days 1–2, sheds by day 4–5 (shiny red with prominent papillae)
- Rash presents as fine eruptions on an erythematous bases, texture of sandpaper, blanches with pressure; initially on chest and axilla, spreads to abdomen and extremities
- Red streaks in skin folds of axillae and antecubital fossa (Pastia's lines)
- Flushed face with circumoral pallor
- Rash becomes generalized; desquamation begins on face after 7–10 days

DIAGNOSTIC STUDIES
- Rapid antigen test or throat culture for strep
- Antistreptolysin O (ASO) titer to confirm recent infection with group A strep (not useful in management of acute streptococcal pharyngitis)

Differential Diagnosis
- Viral syndromes
- Mononucleosis
- Drug reaction

Management

NONPHARMACOLOGIC TREATMENT
- Rest and fluids

PHARMACOLOGIC TREATMENT
- Prompt therapy is imperative to prevent rheumatic fever and other complications
- Penicillin V (Pen VEE K) 500 mg bid; erythromycin 250 q6h, or cefadroxil (Duricef) 500 bid
- For staphylococcal scarlet fever, dicloxacillin (Dynapen)

LENGTH OF TREATMENT
- 10 days

Special Considerations
- Recurrence of GAS pharyngitis may be treated with prophylactic penicillin during times of increased risk of infection (spring, late fall, and winter).

When to Consult, Refer, Hospitalize
- Chronic GAS pharyngitis
- Evidence of pneumonia, bacteremia, shock, or other severe complications

Follow-Up
- Repeat throat culture indicated for patients at risk for rheumatic fever.
  EXPECTED COURSE
  - Improvement should be seen 2–3 days after starting antibiotic

  COMPLICATIONS
  - Otitis media, sinusitis, bacteremia, rheumatic fever, and glomerulonephritis
  - Risk is reduced with prompt diagnosis and treatment

HIV-RELATED ISSUES

Healthcare Worker Exposures To Blood And Other Body Fluids That May Contain HIV

Description
- "Exposure" may place a healthcare worker (e.g., an employee, student, contractor, attending clinician, public safety worker, volunteer) at risk for HIV infection, and therefore requires consideration for postexposure prophylaxis (PEP).
- Exposure is defined as a percutaneous injury, contact of mucous membrane or nonintact skin, or contact with intact skin when the duration of contact is prolonged (i.e., several minutes or more) or involves an extensive area with blood, tissue, or other body fluids.
- Any direct contact with concentrated HIV in a research laboratory or production facility

Etiology
- Fluids with known risk of HIV transmission: blood, bloody fluids, semen, vaginal fluids, concentrated HIV materials in research labs
- Fluids with suspected risk of HIV transmission: pleural fluid, cerebrospinal fluid, peritoneal fluid, synovial fluid, pericardial fluid, amniotic fluid
- Materials with doubtful risk of HIV transmission: feces, vomitus, urine, saliva, sweat, tears (unless bloody)

Incidence and Demographics
- Factors that may increase risk for HIV transmission after an exposure include a device visibly contaminated with the patient's blood, a procedure that involved a needle placed directly in a vein or artery, or deep injury.
- Risk of HIV transmission after a percutaneous exposure to HIV-infected blood is approximately 0.3%; mucous membrane exposure is 0.09%; skin exposure less.

Risk Factors
- Contact with blood or other body fluids from patients in a healthcare or laboratory setting

PREVENTION AND SCREENING
- Healthcare workers should always follow CDC recommendations for universal or standard precautions
- Wear gloves when contact with blood or bodily fluids is possible
- Use of "personal protective equipment" (masks, goggles, gowns) when engaging in procedures that involve blood or bodily fluids
- Prevention of needle injuries, use of puncture-proof containers, use of "safety" needles, refrain from resheathing or post-use manipulation of needles

Assessment
HISTORY
- Evaluate exposure: Type of fluid, type of exposure (needle gauge, depth of needlestick, visible blood, mucous membrane), and duration of exposure
- Evaluate exposure source person: Prior HIV testing results, CD4 levels, history of possible HIV exposures, and risk for HIV (IV drug use, sexual contact, acute HIV syndrome)
- If source person is HIV-positive, document current HIV RNA levels, CD4 levels, and current or previous antiretroviral treatment

PHYSICAL EXAM
- Assess site or wound, anxiety level of healthcare worker

DIAGNOSTIC STUDIES
- Source person: If HIV serologic status unknown, request HIV antibody after incident, provide pretest counseling and consent form; also test for hepatitis B and C
- If consent cannot be obtained, follow local and state laws
- If source person is HIV-seronegative, no testing of worker is needed
- Exposed healthcare workers: HIV antibody testing offered for baseline evaluation with worker consent
- Also test healthcare workers for hepatitis B immune status
- Pregnancy testing should be offered to all women of childbearing age
- Maintaining confidentiality of test results and documentation is critical

Management
NONPHARMACOLOGIC TREATMENT
- Immediately following exposure:
  - Skin: Wash thoroughly with soap and water
  - Eyes: Irrigate immediately with saline or water. Tilt head back, hold eyelid open, pour water or saline over eye, and pull eyelid up and down to cleanse entire area. If wearing contact lenses, do not remove while irrigating eye. After flushing the affected eye, remove contact lenses and clean thoroughly.
  - Mouth, nose: Clean water rinse/flush

- Consider and discuss risks and benefits of postexposure prophylaxis, based on type of fluid, source risk, and type of exposure
- Counsel exposed worker to follow measures to prevent secondary transmission especially the first 6–12 weeks: sexual abstinence or use of condoms; refrain from donating blood, plasma, organs, tissue, or semen; refrain from breastfeeding if applicable

PHARMACOLOGICAL TREATMENT

- Tetanus-diphtheria (Td) vaccine should be given if the patient has not been vaccinated within the past 5 years. Patients >65 years of age who have never received tetanus toxoid-diphtheria and accellular pertussis (TDaP) should receive a dose of TDaP instead of Td. If the patient has completed the primary series of three doses Td or a dose of tetanus-diphtheria and acellular pertussis (TDaP) vaccine should be substituted for Td as a booster. If the patient has not received the primary series of Td, the patient should begin the primary series of three doses of Td with the first two doses administered 4 weeks apart and the third dose administered 6–12 months later. A dose of TDaP can be substituted for any of the three doses of Td.
- Hepatitis B vaccine series (if not already vaccinated and no evidence of immunity)
- Hepatitis B immune globulin (if source antigen positive or high risk for hepatitis B and healthcare worker not immune)
- After evaluation/assessment of HIV infection risk, determine need for postexposure prophylaxis (see Tables 4–5 and 4–6)
- Postexposure chemoprophylaxis with a combination of drugs using a nucleoside reverse transcriptase inhibitor (NRTI) or a nonnucleoside reverse transcriptase inhibitor (NNRTI) and, if appropriate, a protease inhibitor (PI)
- Data support zidovudine (ZVD) efficacy for postexposure prophylaxis; in a case control study, the risk for HIV infection was decreased to 79% among healthcare workers who used ZDV.

LENGTH OF TREATMENT

- PEP should be administered for 4 weeks if worker can tolerate

Table 4-5. Basic and Expanded Postexposure Prophylaxis Regimens in HIV

Percutaneous Exposure type	HIV Status Class I (Low viral load and asymptomatic)	HIV Status Class II (Symptomatic, acute sero-conversion, or high viral load, known drug resistance)	Source Known/ HIV Status Unknown	Source Unknown
Less Severe (solid needle, superficial)	Recommended: Basic 2-drug regimen	Recommended: Expanded 3-drug PEP	No regimen unless the source has significant risk factors, then consider 2-drug therapy	No regimen unless the setting has significant exposure to HIV-infected patients, then consider 2-drug therapy
More Severe (hollow needle, deep injury, with visible blood or used in source's artery or vein)	Recommended: Expanded ≥3 drug PEP	Recommended: Expanded ≥3 drug PEP	No regimen unless the source has HIV risk factors, then consider 2-drug therapy	No regimen unless the setting has significant exposure to HIV-infected patients, then consider 2-drug therapy

Note: Initiate all therapies as soon as possible and continue for 4 weeks. If source is known to be HIV-negative, then no regimen necessary.
From "Updated U.S. Public Health Service guidelines for the management of occupational exposure to HBV, HCV, and HIV: Recommendations for postexposure prophylaxis" by Centers for Disease Control, 2007, *MMWR: Morbidity and Mortality Weekly Report*, 56(49), pp. 1291–1292.

Table 4-6A. HIV Drug Classification and Potential Side Effects

Drug Name and Class	Side Effects and Recommended Testing	Comment
NRTI NNRTI PI	All associated with hepatotoxicity and skin rash	
PI AND HEP C	Associated with hyperglycemia Some PIs are associated with hyperlipidemia leading to pancreatitis	Have fasting blood glucose tested every 3–4 months during first year of PI
PI AND NRTI	Combination associated with lipodystrophy	

Table 4–6. Possible Side Effects of Currently Available Drugs for Postexposure Prophylaxis

Drug Name and Class	Drug Dosage	Side Effects and Recommended Testing	Comment
Zidovudine ZDV; AZT; Retrovir (NRTI)	200 mg PO q8h or 300 mg PO q12h	Associated with lactic acidosis and hepatic steatosis Nausea, vomiting, headache, fatigue, insomnia, anemia, and neutropenia (rare); all side effects are reversible Get CBC at baseline, and 2 and 4 weeks	Intolerance is common; marrow suppression is rare; for GI intolerance, take with meals or multiple small doses; for severe intolerance, substitute d4T (40 mg po bid)
Lamivudine Epivir or 3TC (NRTI)	<50 kg: 2 mg/kg bid >50 kg: 150 mg PO bid	Peripheral neuropathy, pancreatitis, fatigue, fever, chills, sore throat, rash, GI intolerance, muscle and joint pain; get pancreatic enzymes	Usually well-tolerated Never use as a monotherapy
Combivir Lamivudine and Zidovudine (NRTI)	1 tablet bid (150 mg of Lamivudine and 300 mg Zidovudine)	Side effects seen in Zidovudine and Lamivudine	Well-tolerated and chosen for compliance issues especially in healthcare workers
Stavudine Zerit, d4T (NRTI)	>60 kg: 40 mg q12h <60 kg: 30 mg PO q12h	Associated with lactic acidosis and hepatic steatosis Peripheral neuropathy, headache, diarrhea, nausea, insomnia, anorexia, pancreatitis, increased LFTs, anemia and neutropenia Get CBC at baseline, LFTs	Take with Lactaid tablets if lactose intolerant Avoid alcohol
Didanosine Videx; ddI (NRTI)	Adults >60 kg: tablets, 200 mg PO q12h; powder, 250 mg PO q12h; >60 kg: tablets, 125 mg PO q12h; powder, 167 mg PO q12h	Associated with lactic acidosis and hepatic steatosis Pancreatitis, neuropathy, diarrhea, abdominal pain, and nausea Get periodic amylase and lipase	Take on an empty stomach

Table 4–6. Possible Side Effects of Currently Available Drugs for Postexposure Prophylaxis (cont.)

Drug Name and Class	Drug Dosage	Side Effects and Recommended Testing	Comment
Abacavir Ziagen, ABC (NRTI)	300 mg po bid	Headache malaise, abdominal pain, diarrhea, rash, elevated LFTs, rare hypersensitive reaction Get periodic LFTs	May be taken with or without food If a hypersensitivity reaction occurs, never rechallenge
Indinavir IDV Crixivan (PI)	800 mg po q8h or 1200 mg po q12h	Renal calculi or nephrotoxicity, GI intolerance, hepatitis, glucose intolerance/ diabetes Get LFTs, U/A, renal function, and glucose at baseline, and 2 and 4 weeks	Must ingest >1.5 L/ day of fluids; must take every 8 hours on empty stomach or with small low-fat snack
Ritonavir Norvir, RTV (PI)	300 mg po q12h increasing by 100 mg po q12h to a maximum of 600 mg po q12h	Diarrhea, weakness, nausea, circumoral paresthesia, taste alteration, increased cholesterol and triglycerides Get periodic lipid panel	Never use as a monotherapy In solution that has a bitter taste Tobacco decreases serum levels
Nelfinavir Viracept, NFV (PI)	750 mg po tid or 1250 mg po bid	Diarrhea, nausea, abdominal pain, weakness, and rash Get periodic glucose, lipid panel	Never use as a monotherapy Use loperamide for diarrhea Take with food
Saquinavir Fortovase, Invirase, SQV (PI)	Fortovase 1200 mg po tid Invirase 600 mg po tid	Diarrhea, abdominal pain, nausea, hyperglycemia, increased LFTs, photosensitivity Get periodic glucose, LFTs	Lactose-intolerant patients will need to take Lactaid tablets before taking Saquinavir Take with food Ingesting grapefruit helps bioavailability Use sunscreen
Amprenavir Agenerase, AMP (PI)	1200 mg po bid	Nausea, diarrhea, rash, circumoral paresthesia, taste alteration, and depression	
Lopinavir/Ritonavir Kaletra (PI)	1 tablet bid (400 mg of Lopinavir and 100 mg of Ritonavir)	Diarrhea, fatigue, headache, nausea, increased cholesterol and triglycerides Get periodic lipid panel	

Table 4-6. Possible Side Effects of Currently Available Drugs for Postexposure Prophylaxis (cont.)

Drug Name and Class	Drug Dosage	Side Effects and Recommended Testing	Comment
Delavirdine Rescriptor, DLV (NNRTI)	200 mg po tid for 14 days then 400 mg tid	Rash, nausea, diarrhea, headache, fatigue, increased LFTs Get periodic LFTs	No food issues
Efavirenz EFV, Sustiva (NNRTI)	600 mg QHS	Rash including Stevens-Johnson syndrome, insomnia, somnolence, dizziness, poor concentration Get periodic LFTs	
Nevirapine Viramune, or NVP (NNRTI)	Adults: 200 mg po x 14 days then 200 mg po bid	Associated with hepatitis and hepatic necrosis Rash including Stevens-Johnson syndrome, fever, nausea, diarrhea, headache, and increased LFTs, glucose intolerance/ diabetes	No food requirement Never use as a monotherapy

Adapted from "Updated U.S. Public Health Service guidelines for the management of occupational exposure to HBV, HCV, and HIV: Recommendations for postexposure prophylaxis" by Centers for Disease Control and Prevention, 2007, MMWR: Morbidity and Mortality Weekly Report, 56(49), pp. 1291–1292.

Special Considerations
- Pregnant women
- Consider the short- or long-term effects on the fetus and newborn when offering postexposure prophylaxis to pregnant workers
- Counsel regarding potential risk for HIV transmission based on the type of exposure, the stage of pregnancy (first trimester being the period of maximal organogenesis and risk for teratogenesis), and safety of drug combinations
- Breastfeeding: Consider temporary discontinuation of antiretroviral therapy
- Resistance of the source virus to antiretroviral drugs; if resistance is known or suspected, add extra antiretroviral drug, protease inhibitor

When to Consult, Refer, Hospitalize
- Consult with HIV expert; refer to U.S. Department of Health and Human Services's current guidelines

Follow-Up
- Advise exposed healthcare workers to seek medical evaluation for any acute illness occurring during the follow-up period; illness characterized by fever, rash, myalgia, fatigue, malaise, or lymphadenopathy may indicate acute HIV infection.

- For patients at high risk or exposed to HIV+ source: HIV antibody testing at 6 weeks, 12 weeks, and 6 months

    EXPECTED COURSE
    - In some situations, modifying the dose interval while administering a lower dose of drug will help promote adherence to regimen

    COMPLICATIONS
    - HIV seroconversion
    - Side effects from antiretroviral therapy such as nausea/vomiting, nephrolithiasis, hemolytic anemia, hyperglycemia, or worker unable to finish medication
    - All FDA-approved NRTIs, NNRTIs, and PIs are associated with hepatotoxicity

Human Immunodeficiency Virus (HIV) Infection and Acquired Immunodeficiency Syndrome (AIDS)

Description
- Viral infection with the human retrovirus, HIV, that destroys cells with critical immune system functions. The HIV-1 virus can infect all cells expressing the T4 (CD4+) antigen, which serves as a receptor for HIV; once in the cell, it replicates and causes cell fusion or death. The virus depends on reverse transcriptase for replication and, because the CD4+ lymphocyte directs many other cells in the immune network, infection of the CD4+ lymphocyte allows for disorder of virtually all body systems.
- AIDS: Disease characterized by opportunistic infections; or HIV+ persons with CD4 cell counts <200/mL or a CD4 ratio <14%.
- Criteria for HIV infection:
    - Persons 13 years or older with repeatedly (2 or more) reactive screening tests (ELISA) plus specific antibodies identified by a supplemental test (e.g., Western blot)
    - Other specific methods of diagnosis of HIV-1 include virus isolation, antigen detection, and detection of HIV genetic material by PCR or branched DNA assay (bDNA)

Etiology
- Viral transmission; HIV usually transmitted through sexual intercourse (homosexual/heterosexual); IV drug use; transfusions of blood or blood products; needle stick or mucous membrane exposures in healthcare workers; injections with unsterilized, used needles such as acupuncture, tattooing, or medical injection; perinatal; breastfeeding (mother to child)
- Seroconversion takes an average of 3 weeks from transmission; using standard serologic tests, >95% of patients seroconvert within 5.8 months following HIV transmission.
- Median time from infection with HIV to AIDS is 10 years.
- Stages of HIV infection include viral transmission, primary HIV infection (acute retroviral syndrome), seroconversion, asymptomatic chronic infection, symptomatic HIV infection, AIDS, advanced HIV infection.

Incidence and Demographics
- The cumulative number of AIDS cases reported to CDC through December 2007 is 1,000,000.
- 25% of infected persons are unaware of status.
- 1% of AIDS cases are pediatric, most acquired perinatally.
- Sexual intercourse is most common method of transmission, followed by intravenous drug use.
- Male and female African American rate of infections remains higher than in any other ethnic group.
- Highest incidence in 20–49-year-olds.
- Women 15–44 years old are fastest growing group of U.S. epidemic.
- Mortality declining in United States since 1994 because of highly active antiretroviral therapy.

Risk Factors
- Unprotected anal, oral, or vaginal sex with multiple partners
- Unprotected sex with an HIV-positive person or IV drug abuser
- IV drug abuse or needle-stick exposure
- Blood transfusion outside of the U.S., or in U.S. during the period 1977–1985
- Unprotected sex with a person with recent or past history of sexually transmitted diseases
- Sexually transmitted disease
- Children born to HIV+ women
- Persons sustaining occupational exposure to blood or bodily fluids
- Incarceration; high rates in prison populations who take infection back to community upon release

Prevention and Screening
- Promote sexual abstinence or decrease number of sexual partners; reduce unsafe sexual behavior; encourage condom use
- Treat sexually transmitted diseases
- Prevent/treat IV drug users
- HIV antibody testing of plasma, organ, and tissue donors
- Postexposure antiretroviral prophylaxis treatment for healthcare workers
- Counsel HIV+ mothers about the risks of vertical transmission of HIV to their infant associated with breastfeeding.
- Routine perinatal screening recommended in U.S.
- Antiretroviral treatment for HIV+ women during pregnancy and labor, and for newborn after delivery, to prevent perinatal transmission
- Refer to http://aidsinfo.nih.gov/contentfiles/PerinatalGL.pdf for current guidelines.

Assessment
HISTORY
- Index of suspicion is raised by obtaining a complete history of symptoms, risk factors, personal medical history; may remain asymptomatic for years
- Complaints causing parents to seek care for their child are generalized lymphadenopathy, failure to thrive, recurrent or persistent thrush, recurrent infections

- Adolescents may present with sexually transmitted disease, persistent vaginal candidiasis, persistent "colds"
- Adults may present with variety of complaints at any stage of HIV

PHYSICAL EXAM
- A complete physical exam is necessary
- Infant born to infected mother may be entirely normal for 1 year or more
- Infant/child may show failure to gain weight (failure to thrive), generalized lymphadenopathy, hepatosplenomegaly, recurrent or persistent thrush, recurrent or chronic parotitis, recurrent infections or infections that fail to respond to treatment; Pneumocystis carinii infection may be first manifestation
- Adolescents and adults may show wide variety of physical findings related to STDs, serious infections, malignancies, cardiac and neurologic dysfunction
- Hairy leukoplakia of the tongue, Kaposi's sarcoma highly linked to HIV infection

DIAGNOSIS BY STAGE OF HIV
- Primary HIV infection ("acute HIV infection"): Time of exposure to onset of symptoms usually 2–4 weeks
  - Typical symptoms include fever (96%), adenopathy (74%), pharyngitis (70%), rash (erythematous maculopapular; 70%), myalgias or arthralgias (54%), diarrhea (32%), headache (32%), nausea and vomiting (27%), hepatosplenomegaly (14%), and thrush (12%)
- Asymptomatic infection: Clinically asymptomatic or in some cases persistent generalized lymphadenopathy
- Early symptomatic HIV infection (AIDS-Related Complex, "ARC" or "Stage B"): Conditions that are more common and more severe in HIV infection but are not AIDS-indicator conditions
- Examples: Thrush, oral hairy leukoplakia, peripheral neuropathy, cervical dysplasia, constitutional symptoms (fever, weight loss), recurrent herpes zoster, idiopathic thrombocytopenic purpura, and listeriosis
- AIDS (CDC definition): HIV+ persons with CD4 cell counts <200mm or a CD4 ratio <14% or a variety of conditions such as candidiasis of esophagus, trachea, bronchi or lungs; invasive cervical cancer; recurrent bacterial pneumonia; Kaposi's sarcoma (KS); pneumocystic pneumonia; wasting syndrome due to HIV; and others

FOR DIAGNOSIS IN INFANTS AND CHILDREN
- Infants <18 months
  - Positive results on two separate specimens (excluding cord blood) using one or more of the following HIV virologic (nonantibody) tests:
    » HIV nucleic acid (DNA or RNA detection)
    » HIV p24 antigen test, including neutralization assay in a child ≥1 month of age
    » HIV isolation (viral culture)
- Presumptive diagnosis for children <18 months may be based on positive results of HIV virologic tests on 1 serum specimen and no subsequent negative tests OR diagnosis of HIV infection based on laboratory criteria and documented in

the medical record by a physician **OR** the presence of AIDS-defining conditions as defined by CDC

- Children <18 months born to HIV-infected mother categorized as "not infected with HIV" if child does not meet the criteria for infection **AND** has at least 2 negative HIV antibody screening tests from separate specimens at ≥6 months of age **OR** at least 2 negative HIV virologic tests from separate specimens at ≥1 month of age and ≥4 months of age **AND** no other laboratory or clinical evidence of HIV infection (definitive criteria)
- Presumptive criteria for children <18 months born to HIV-infected mother categorized as "not infected with HIV" if child does not meet definitive criteria but has 1 negative EIA HIV antibody test at ≥6 months of age and no positive HIV virologic tests **OR** has 1 negative HIV virologic test performed at ≥4 months of age and no positive virologic tests **OR** 1 positive HIV virologic test with at least 2 subsequent negative virologic tests, at least 1 of which is ≥4 months of age or negative HIV antibody results, at least 1 of which is at ≥6 months of age **AND** no other laboratory or clinical evidence of infection **OR** designation by a physician to be "not infected" and the physician has noted the testing results in the medical record **AND** no other laboratory or clinical evidence of HIV infection is noted.
  - Children <18 months born to HIV+ mothers and not meeting the above criteria for HIV infection or "not infected with HIV" categorized as having perinatal exposure
- Children >18 months and adolescents:
  - Diagnosed as having HIV infection if they have a positive screening test for HIV antibody and positive result on a confirmatory test for HIV antibody (e.g., Western blot) **OR** positive result of HIV virologic test **OR** diagnosis of HIV infection based on laboratory tests and recorded in the medical record by a physician **OR** presence of AIDS-defining conditions

DIAGNOSTIC STUDIES

- ELISA screening test; Western blot assay or IFA to confirm
- Negative antibody test does not guarantee person seronegativity; window of time (1–3 months) from transmission to seroconversion; retesting recommended 6 months to a year from last high-risk exposure
- In acute HIV infection, ELISA will be negative; must repeat test to confirm seroconversion for diagnosis
- Can directly detect viral antigens or nucleic acids (plasma HIV RNA, HIV DNA/PCR, p24 antigen); used to diagnose early infection, determine when to initiate treatment, and assess treatment response
- CD4 count used to assess damage to immune system and monitor effectiveness of treatment
- Maternal antibodies may remain present for up to 15 months; therefore, antibody tests unreliable in infants
- HIV blood culture more reliable in infants >4 weeks old

Differential Diagnosis

- Cancer
- Endocrine diseases
- Malabsorption syndromes
- Tuberculosis
- Other infections
- Hepatic disease
- Enterocolitis
- Endocarditis
- Renal disease

Management

NONPHARMACOLOGIC TREATMENT

- Counsel regarding prevention of transmission through use of condoms, cleaning up blood spills, not sharing razor blades or needles
- Stress that patients must adhere to drug regimen if it is to be helpful
- Encourage a healthy lifestyle: balanced diet, smoking cessation, substance abuse cessation, decrease stress, adequate sleep
- Discuss protection from contagious disease; wash hands after contact with soil; avoid cleaning litter box (toxoplasmosis), rough play with kittens (cat scratch disease); food safety
- Health maintenance referral: dental exam every 6 months, ophthalmology examination at diagnosis and annually. When CD4 count is less than 75, refer to ophthalmologist or optometrist trained in CMV retinitis for screening every 4–6 months.
- Tests to determine concomitant diseases, immunity status; Mantoux PPD, rapid plasma regain serum (RPR), Pap smear every 6–12 months, HBsAg, hepatitis C serology, toxoplasmosis serology, cytomegalovirus IgG, varicella IgG, chest x-ray
- Baseline labs before drug therapy: chemistry, liver function, renal profile, CBC with differential and platelets
- Immunizations: Annual inactivated influenza vaccine for patients with CD4 count >100; Pneumovax every 5 years, consider hepatitis B (HBV; 3-dose schedule unless evidence of immunity) and H. influenzae B vaccines; tetanus-diphtheria (Td) vaccine should be given if the patient had not been vaccinated within the last 5 years. Patients older than 65 years of age who have never received tetanus toxoid-diphtheria and acellular pertussis (TDaP) should receive a dose of TDaP instead of Td. If the patient has completed the primary series of 3 doses Td or a dose of tetanus-diphtheria and acellular pertussis (TDaP), vaccine should be substituted for Td as a booster. If the patient has not received the primary series of Td, the patient should begin the primary series of 3 doses of Td with the first 2 doses administered 4 weeks apart and the third dose administered 6–12 months later. A dose of TDaP can be substituted for any of the 3 doses of Td. Give inactivated polio, mumps, rubella, measles vaccines the same as HIV-negative patients, hepatitis A (HAV; 2-dose schedule unless serologic evidence of previous disease), HBV (unless evidence of immunity); Varicella zoster (consider for asymptomatic patients with high CD4 counts and no evidence of immunity or significant exposure); human papillomavirus vaccine (HPV) recommended for all females who have not received the

3-dose series. The second dose should be given 2 months after the first and the third dose given 6 months later. Do not administer live vaccines to any patient severely immunocompromised (CD4 counts <200 cells/µL): polio, varicella, zoster, BCG, LAIV, Flumist. MMR and varicella and zoster are also contraindicated in pregnant women.

- All 50 states, Washington, DC, and U.S. territories require reporting of AIDS cases to local health authorities.

PHARMACOLOGIC TREATMENT
- Initiate antiretroviral treatment when CD4+ count <350/µL or viral load >30,000 copies/mL by DNA or 55,000 copies by PCR
- Four therapeutic interventions have been shown to prolong survival
  - Antiretroviral therapy: Combination of three or more medications from different classes known as highly active antiretroviral therapy (HAART)— two nucleoside reverse transcriptase inhibitors (NRTIs) with a third agent of any category recommended by the CDC. (Review current recommended combination therapies at http://aidsinfo.nih.gov.) As of February 2008, there are six classes of FDA-approved antiretroviral medications: NRTIs, NNRTIs, PIs, entry inhibitors, fusion inhibitors, and integrase inhibitors.
- P. carinii prophylaxis
- M. avium prophylaxis
- Care by a specialist with HIV-care experience
- Treat concurrent infections of tuberculosis or hepatitis

When to Consult, Refer, Hospitalize
- All HIV-infected infants, children, adolescents, pregnant women, and adults should be referred and followed by an HIV specialist knowledgeable for that age group.
- Refer HIV patients to appropriate support groups.
- Refer to current guidelines at http://www.aidsinfo.nih.gov.

Special Considerations
- Always maintain patient confidentiality.
- In older HIV patients, it is important to differentiate between geriatric and HIV symptoms and be aware of potential drug interactions.

Follow-Up
- See CDC publications for a list of AIDS-defining conditions.
- Treat for opportunistic infections.
- Assess for mental health issues and social isolation.

Illnesses Of Unknown Origin Fever Without Localizing Signs

Description
- Fever 38.4°C (101.1°F) or higher at least once in 24 hours with no source of infection or cause for hyperthermia; also known as fever without focus. For children with fever >10 days' duration, the term fever of unknown origin (FUO) is used; some experts suggest that fever should be present for 3 weeks as an outpatient or 1 week as an inpatient before the term FUO is applied.

Etiology
- The principal causes of FUO are rheumatologic disease, infection, and neoplasm; drug fever is uncommon.
- Most FUOs result from atypical presentations of common diseases.

Incidence and Demographics
- Fever without localizing signs or symptoms, usually of acute onset and present for less than 1 week, is a common diagnostic dilemma in children <36 months of age.
- An infectious agent, usually viral, is identified in 70% of infants <3 months of age with fever.

Risk Factors
- Independent of age, fever with petechiae with or without localizing signs indicates high risk for life-threatening bacterial infections such as bacteremia, sepsis, and meningitis.

Prevention and Screening
- Routine wellness exams
- Avoid infected persons
- Seek medical attention if fever does not resolve with rest, fluids, and antipyretics within 24 hours of onset

Assessment
HISTORY
- Note onset of fever, degree, duration, diurnal variation
- Changes in environment, foods, and/or lifestyle changes around the time of fever onset, particularly history of exposure to animals (domestic and wild), travel history
- Uncommon dietary habits or pica, tick bites, ethnic background, and family history of disease
- Recent sick contacts (healthcare workers or day care)
- Medication and transfusion history
- Number of school days missed
- Family stresses
- Review of systems; particularly note intermittent rashes, arthralgias, weight loss, behavior changes

PHYSICAL EXAM
- May be entirely normal, or demonstrate mild findings such as clear rhinorrhea
- Absence of sweating may indicate familial dysautonomia

DIAGNOSTIC STUDIES
- CBC with differential and platelets; blood, urine, and CSF cultures should be obtained, as indicated
- Consider ESR, chest x-ray and TB skin testing
- Course of action and diagnostic studies performed should be individualized based on presentation and child's age

Differential Diagnosis
- Inflammatory disease
- Viral illness
- Bacterial infections
- Neoplasm
- Abscess
- Familial dysautonomia
- Hypothalamic dysfunction
- Drug fever

Management

NONPHARMACOLOGIC
- Maintain hydration, good nutrition, adequate sleep
- Treat symptomatically

PHARMACOLOGIC
- See Box 4–2

Box 4–2. Guidelines for Management of Fever

Infants <1 month of age

Infants may acquire community pathogens; also at risk for late-onset neonatal bacterial diseases and perinatally acquired herpes simplex virus infection.

CBC, blood culture, urine culture, consider lumbar puncture and culture.

Always treated aggressively in hospital; maintain on prophylactic antibiotics for 3 days pending culture results. Some practitioners hospitalize infants <4 months of age if no focus of infection found on PE in office.

Infants between 1 and 3 months of age

Serious bacterial disease occurs in 10%–15%, including bacteremia in 5%, of febrile infants <3 months old.

Infants who appear generally well, have been previously healthy, have no focus for infection, total WBC 5,000–15,000 cells/mm3, absolute band count <1,500 cells/mm3, and normal urinalysis are unlikely to have a serious bacterial infection. Negative predictive value of these criteria for serious bacterial infection is >98%, and >99% for bacteremia.

CBC, blood culture, urine culture, consider lumbar puncture.

Usually treated aggressively with hospitalization and prophylactic antibiotics.

If CBC is within normal limits and adequate follow-up assured, consider treatment with IM ceftriaxone pending culture results.

Children >3 months of age/Adults

Low-grade fever: Give antipyretics and observe.

Acetaminophen 15mg/kg/dose no more than q4h and no more than five doses in 24 hours.

Ibuprophen 10 mg/kg/dose if >6 months old; no more than q6h and no more than four doses in 24 hours.

Fever >102°F, obtain a CBC. If WBC is >15,000/mm3, obtain a blood culture and administer IM Ceftriaxone. Obtain urine culture in males <6 months and females <2 years; some providers obtain urine cultures on all children with high fever and no focus for infection found on exam

Special Considerations
- Do not prescribe or administer aspirin or aspirin-related products to patients under 19 years of age.

When to Consult, Refer, Hospitalize
- All HIV-infected infants, children, adolescents, pregnant women, and adults should be referred and followed by an HIV specialist knowledgeable for that age group/circumstance.

Follow-Up
- If not hospitalized, follow up in 1–3 days depending on age of child, degree of fever; occasionally, source of infection will become identifiable in time.
- If blood or CSF cultures are positive and child not hospitalized, admit and treat with IV antibiotics.
    - COMPLICATIONS
        - Children with FUO have a better prognosis than do adults; dependent on primary disease process, which is usually an atypical presentation of a common childhood illness
        - In many cases, no diagnosis can be established and fever abates spontaneously
        - In as many as 25% of cases in which fever persists, cause of fever remains unclear, even after thorough evaluation

Kawasaki Disease

Description
- Acute, self-limiting, multisystem vascular illness with rash and fever; also known as mucocutaneous lymph node syndrome. Leading cause of acquired heart disease in children in the United States.

Etiology
- Unknown, though most likely infectious

Incidence and Demographics
- 80% of cases in children <5 years old (peak age 18–24 months); 5% of cases in children >10 years old; rare over age 15
- 1.5:1 male-to-female ratio
- Recurrence low
- No clear genetic pattern, though incidence is lowest among White Americans and highest among Americans of Asian and Pacific Island descent
- Epidemics in the U.S. seem to occur during the winter and spring in 2–3 year intervals
- No person-to-person spread, although siblings seem to be affected at a higher rate

Risk Factors
- Unknown

Prevention and Screening
- Unknown

Assessment

HISTORY
- May report recent history of cold, cough, or ear infection
- Persistent fever, red mouth and lips, and swollen hands with rash

PHYSICAL EXAM
- Erythematous mouth and pharynx with "strawberry tongue" and red, swollen, and cracked lips
- Bulbar conjunctivitis without exudate
- Cervical lymphadenopathy—usually unilateral, involves at least one node swollen to >1.5 cm diameter
- Polymorphous, generalized, erythematous rash
- Induration of hands and feet
- Periungual and groin desquamation may occur

DIAGNOSTIC CRITERIA
- Persistent fever plus four of the five criteria listed in Box 4–3
- **OR** persistent fever plus three of the criteria in Box 4–3 **AND** evidence of coronary artery abnormalities
- Infants may have atypical Kawasaki disease; irritability, abdominal pain, diarrhea, vomiting may be apparent with coronary artery disease

Box 4–3. Diagnostic Criteria for Kawasaki Disease

Persistent fever >5 days without an identifiable source, presence of four of five other clinical criteria, and unresponsive to antibiotics; diagnosis can be made if fever and only three criteria are met along with documented coronary artery disease.

(1) Mucous membrane involvement (erythematous mouth, pharynx; strawberry tongue; dry, fissured lips)
(2) Nonpurulent bilateral conjunctivitis
(3) Polymorphous, erythematous, generalized rash
(4) Cervical lymphadenopathy involving at least one node ≥1.5 cm in diameter
(5) Polymorphous exanthema

Adapted from *Red Book*, by American Academy of Pediatrics, 2006, Elk Grove Village, IL: Author.

Diagnostic Studies
- None available; nonspecific tests include ESR, platelet counts, serum C-reactive protein
- CBC with differential: WBC usually elevated with a left shift (increased band forms); thrombocytosis develops in second week
- ECG, echocardiogram indicated to assess presence of cardiac or coronary artery disease

Differential Diagnosis
- Rickettsial diseases
- Rubella
- Rubeola
- Scarlet fever
- Rheumatic fever

- Epstein-Barr virus
- Drug reaction (Stevens-Johnson syndrome)
- Juvenile rheumatoid arthritis
- Scalded skin syndrome
- Toxic shock syndrome

Management

NONPHARMACOLOGIC TREATMENT
- Supportive: Rest, fluids, protection of skin (lubrication, good hygiene)
- No tart or acidic beverages
- Bland diet (secondary to mouth ulceration)

PHARMACOLOGIC TREATMENT
- High-dose aspirin as anti-inflammatory (80–100 mg/kg/day qid); dose reduced after acute phase to prevent coronary thrombosis. If coronary artery abnormalities present, continue low-dose aspirin therapy (3–5 mg/kg) indefinitely.
- High-dose immune globulin intravenous (IGIV) therapy (2 g/kg as single dose)—initiate as soon as possible; efficacy questionable if initiated after 10th day of illness.
- Initiation of aspirin and IGIV within 10 days of fever onset substantially reduces prevalence of coronary artery dilation and aneurysms.
- Hold measles and varicella immunizations for 11 months after IGIV therapy; if at high risk for measles exposure, may immunize and repeat immunization after 11 months.

Special Considerations
- Aspirin therapy in patients under 19 years of age should be monitored closely due to risk of Reye's syndrome.

When to Consult, Refer, Hospitalize
- All suspected cases of Kawasaki disease are managed in hospital, in conjunction with physician.
- Refer all suspected cases to cardiologist.

Follow-Up
- Long-term management dependent on degree of cardiac involvement; echocardiogram in 6–8 weeks.

EXPECTED COURSE
- Without treatment, fever resolves in 12 days; other symptoms, 6–8 weeks after onset
- Myocardial infarction and sudden death may occur months to years later

COMPLICATIONS
- Bacterial superinfections (desquamating skin)
- Coronary aneurysms
- Pericardial effusion
- Myocarditis

- Myocardial infarction
- Arthritis and arthralgias
- Jaundice, liver and gall bladder problems
- Aseptic meningitis

Infections From Bioweapons (BW)

Description
- Biological agents with bioweapons potential are characterized as Category A agents. These agents can be easily disseminated or transmitted from person to person, cause high mortality with potential for major public health impact, and require prompt action. Numerous viruses, several bacteria, and toxins may be used as weapons, but those that are known to have been weaponized, have effective dispersal methods, and be environmentally stable include anthrax, botulism, plague, smallpox, tularemia, and viral hemorrhagic fevers (Ebola, Marburg, Lassa, dengue, yellow fever, and others).

Etiology
- Naturally occurring organisms that have been altered to increase lethality

Incidence and Demographics
- Smallpox is no longer found in wild form; all other potential bioagents occur naturally. Inhalation anthrax is rare, though dermatologic infection is still found fairly often in farm workers. Large scale outbreaks of botulism have never occurred.

Risk Factors
- Any population can be at risk, though bioweapons attacks are more likely to occur in densely populated, urban areas or at large, crowded events, such as football games.

Prevention and Screening
- Primary care providers must maintain an elevated level of suspicion.
- Family nurse practitioners must be aware of modes of transmission, incubation periods, and communicable periods of these diseases; an excellent source of information is the CDC Emergency Preparedness and Response website: http://www.bt.cdc.gov/index.asp.

Assessment
HISTORY
- Symptoms for most agents may initially mimic those of common viral illnesses and include fever, fatigue, malaise, muscle aches, headache, cough, vomiting, diarrhea, rashes
- For most agents, symptoms will quickly increase in intensity and severity
- First indication of unannounced biologic attack will likely be an unusual increase in number of persons seeking care

PHYSICAL EXAM
- Ill-appearing patient, often out of proportion to degree of illness prevalent in the community

Table 4-7. Potential Bioweapons Agents

Biological Agent	Transmission/Incubation	Clinical Presentation	Diagnosis	Management
Anthrax (bacillus anthracis): Gram-positive, spore-forming aerobic rod that causes cutaneous or pulmonary infection. Cutaneous anthrax does not have BW potential.	• Inhalation of aerosolized spores; person-to-person transmission does not occur. • Incubation 1–7 days	• Biphasic, with initial prodrome of nonspecific febrile flu like illness. May be followed by brief period of improvement, then rapid onset of high fever, severe respiratory distress. • Shock, death within 24–36 hours	• Chest x-ray shows mediastinal widening; gram-positive bacilli on unspun peripheral blood smear.	• Ciprofloxacin or doxycycline; standard contact precautions. Prophylaxis should be offered with the same agents. A vaccine is available, but supply is limited.
Botulism Caused by neurotoxin produced by Clostridium botulinum, a spore-forming, obligate anaerobe found in soil. Botulinum toxin is the most lethal natural poison known.	• Toxin can be aerosolized; sources of entry include wounds, GI and respiratory tracts. It can also be dispensed in food. There is no person-to-person transmission. • Incubation 12–36 hours.	• Symmetric cranial neuropathies (e.g., drooping eyelids, weakened jaw clench, difficulty swallowing, speaking), blurred vision or diplopia, symmetric descending weakness in a proximal to distal pattern, respiratory dysfunction	• Routine laboratory tests usually unremarkable. Definitive diagnostic testing for botulism available only at the CDC; diagnosis is primarily clinical.	• Supportive care, including ventilator support • Passive immunization with equine antitoxin

Table 4–7. Potential Bioweapons Agents (cont.)

Biological Agent	Transmission/Incubation	Clinical Presentation	Diagnosis	Management
Plague (Yersinia pestis): Nonmotile bacillus	• Bubonic: Transmitted by bites from infected fleas; most common type • Pneumonic: Inhalation of respiratory droplets from a human or animal with respiratory plague; may be aerosolized • Secondary cases would occur from contact with infected individuals. A BW attack most likely to produce pneumonic plague. • Incubation 2–4 days	• Bubonic: Enlarged, painful, regional lymph nodes (buboes), fever, chills, and prostration • Pneumonic: Fever, weakness, and rapidly developing pneumonia with shortness of breath, chest pain, cough, and sometimes bloody or watery sputum	• Clinical diagnosis important as treatment must begin in <24 hours. Large numbers of patients with severe pneumonia, particularly if accompanied by hemoptysis, must trigger prompt presumptive treatment and isolation. • Prophylaxis of close contacts	• Streptomycin, gentamicin, tetracycline, or chloramphenicol begun within 24 hours greatly improves prognosis; isolation and supportive care necessary • Prophylactic therapy begun within 7 days is very effective in preventing infection. • No vaccine is available.
Smallpox Caused by a DNA virus in the orthopox-virus family	• Person-to-person transmission; spread by inhalation of air droplets or aerosols. Smallpox virus is specific for humans; animal infection does not occur. • Weaponized smallpox can be spread by aerosol or by bombs or missiles. • Secondary infection would occur from direct person-to-person spread, via both droplet and infected fomites (clothing, bedding). • Incubation 12–14 days	• High fever, malaise, severe aching pains, prostration • Later, a papular rash develops over the face and spreads to the extremities, soon becomes vesicular and later, pustular. • Rash is most dense on face.	• Patients are most contagious from time of onset of rash until scabs form. • Initial diagnosis must occur at a military facility. • After confirmation of community disease, subsequent diagnoses made on basis of clinical presentation.	• No known effective antiviral agents • Treatment is supportive. • All potentially infected persons should be hospitalized in their homes. • In event of widespread outbreak, specific hospitals would be designated for treatment of smallpox patients. • Widespread vaccination would be indicated; smallpox vaccine is effective only if administered within 4 days of exposure. • Vaccine is available, though supply is government-controlled.

Table 4–7. Potential Bioweapons Agents (cont.)

Biological Agent	Transmission/Incubation	Clinical Presentation	Diagnosis	Management
Tularemia (Francisella tularensis) Gram-negative coccobacillus. Type A most virulent and likely to be weaponized. Very small amount (10–50) organisms can produce disease.	• Naturally occurring in temperate areas of North America, Europe, and Asia. • Weaponized tularemia can be delivered via aerosol, with infection occurring secondary to inhalation, skin or mucus membrane contact, or GI exposure from contaminated soil, water, food or animals. • Person-to-person transmission is not known to occur. • Incubation 1–4 days, depending on virulence of strain, site, and size of inoculum	• Presentation dependent on route of administration. • Inhalation most likely • Symptoms include abrupt onset of fever with progression to pneumonia and respiratory. disease, hilar lymphadenopathy and pleuritis Inhalation can also cause sepsis without respiratory symptoms; this syndrome has a high fatality ratio	• No means of rapid testing is widely available.e • Diagnosis is initially clinical. F. tularensis may be identified by culture done in biological safety level (BSL) 3 labs.	• Streptomycin IM or gentamicin IV for infection • Ciprofloxacin or doxycycline at usual doses recommended for mass casualties or post-exposure. • Vaccine is not widely available and immunity is incomplete.

Table 4–7. Potential Bioweapons Agents (cont.)

Biological Agent	Transmission/Incubation	Clinical Presentation	Diagnosis	Management
Viral Hemorrhagic Fevers (VHF) A group of illnesses caused by several distinct RNA viruses (Arenaviridae, Bunyaviridae, Filoviridae, Flaviviridae), including Ebola hemorrhagic fever, Marburg virus, Lassa fever, hantavirus pulmonary syndrome (HPS)	• Humans are not the natural reservoir of these viruses and are infected when they come into contact with secretions of infected hosts. • However, with some viruses, after the accidental transmission from the host, humans can transmit the virus to one another. • Naturally occurring human cases occur sporadically. • Incubation dependent on virus	• Specific signs and symptoms vary by the type of VHF; initial signs and symptoms include marked fever, fatigue, dizziness, muscle aches, loss of strength, and exhaustion. • Patients often show signs of bleeding under the skin, in internal organs, or from body orifices (mouth, eyes, ears, etc.). • Full-blown VHF evolves to shock and generalized bleeding from the mucous membranes.	• High index of suspicion, detailed travel history important. • Lab findings supportive of infection vary; typically leucopenia, thrombocytopenia occur • Immunoglobulin (Ig) M antibody by enzyme linked immunosorbent assays (ELISA) during the acute illness • Diagnosis by viral cultivation requires 3–10 days and can only be done at BSL 4 labs (CDC, military facilities) illness; leucopenia, thrombocytopenia occur.	• There is no cure or established drug treatment for VHFs, though ribavirin has been tried with Lassa fever. • Therapy is supportive and barrier isolation techniques should be initiated. • No vaccines are available.

DIAGNOSTIC STUDIES
- Blood cultures, CBC, electrolytes
- Other studies dictated by clinical picture

Differential Diagnosis
- Common wild virus agents (Fifth disease, Coxsackie, varicella)
- Other potential biological agents

Management
NONPHARMACOLOGIC TREATMENT
- Rapid isolation of patient and contacts
- Refer to infectious disease specialists
- Rapidly notify public health authorities
- Psychological and mental health problems brought on by the event will require significant expertise

PHARMACOLOGIC TREATMENT
- See Table 4–7
- Empiric therapy may be indicated if large numbers of individuals present with a nonspecific febrile illness in a limited time frame and location under credible threat of attack. Empiric therapy is ciprofloxacin or doxycycline po or IV at routine recommended doses.

Special Considerations
- Appropriate management of postexposure prophylaxis and its complications will be critical in containing spread of infection.

Follow-Up
COMPLICATIONS
- Dependent on agent
- Most potential agents have high lethality, 30%–100%

CASE STUDIES

Case 1. 18-year-old male freshman complains of losing weight and fatigue x 1 month. He states he is chronically tired, can't get enough sleep, and feels feverish, but he doesn't have a thermometer in his dorm room. He has occasional aching joints. Of note is a cold a few weeks ago with a sore throat. He went to the university clinic at that time, had a rapid strep test done, and was told it was negative. He is concerned because he has missed more than 8 classes this month.

PMH: Usually healthy. Few occasional colds. Was told he had a heart murmur but not sure if he still does. Chickenpox at age 8. No past surgeries or hospitalizations; not sure of his immunizations status. No current medications, NKDA.

1. Should you be concerned about measles, mumps, rubella, polio, diphtheria, and pertussis because he does not know whether his immunizations are up-to-date?
2. What other history is needed?

Exam: No lymphadenopathy, pharynx pink without exudate, systolic murmur best heard over the 2nd ICS, no joint swelling or tenderness, no rash or skin lesions.

3. What is your differential diagnosis?
4. What initial diagnostic and management plan is appropriate?

Case 2. 6-year-old male with both parents who are quite worried because his "hands are swollen and his eyes are red." Has had a low-grade fever for over 1 week; highest 101°F. Also had runny nose so mother thought he had a cold. Yesterday, his eyes were red, but didn't notice anything about the hands. Today, eyes are very red, lips are red and swollen, and hands are swollen and beginning to peel.

PMH: No childhood illnesses; occasional colds; 1 or 2 ear infections as a baby. Bilateral hernia repair at age 9 months. Immunizations up to date.

1. What are you looking for on physical exam?
2. What do you suspect from this child's presentation?
3. What is your management plan?

Case 3. 14-month-old female with father who states, "She had a high fever a few days ago. Now she has a rash."

HPI: Visited 4 days ago for persistent fever of 2-day history. Fever as high as 104°F. Diagnosed with viral syndrome and sent home with instructions for fever management and to push fluids. Now returns, afebrile today, but has a light red rash on chest and back. Appetite poor, drinking liquids. Her face was flushed when she had the fever, but now face is pale.

PMH: History of recurrent otitis media, 4 episodes in 9 months. Immunizations up to date. No current medications.

1. What other history is needed?
2. What screening tests need to be done?
3. What is the likely diagnosis and what management is appropriate?

REFERENCES

Agency on Healthcare Research and Quality. (2007). *Guide to clinical preventive services.* Retrieved June 6, 2008, from http://www.ahcpr.gov/clinic/uspstfix.htm

American Academy of Pediatrics. (2006). *Red book 2006: Report of the Committee on Infectious Diseases* (26th ed.). Elk Grove Village, IL: Author.

Centers for Disease Control and Prevention. (2007a). *Health information for international travel. 2008.* Atlanta: U.S. Department of Health and Human Services, Public Health Service 2007. Retrieved July 7, 2008, from http://wwwn.cdc.gov/travel/yellowBookCh4-Mumps.aspx

Centers for Disease Control and Prevention. (2007b). Recommended adult immunization schedule— United States—October 2007–September 2008. *MMWR: Morbidity Mortality Weekly Report, 56*(41), Q1–Q4. Retrieved June 6, 2008, from http://www.cdc.gov/mmwr/pdf/wk/mm5641-Immunization.pdf

Centers for Disease Control and Prevention. (2007c). Updated U.S. Public Health Service guidelines for the management of occupational exposure to HBV, HCV, and HIV: Recommendations for postexposure prophylaxis. *MMWR: Morbidity and Mortality Weekly Report 56*(49), 1291–1292. Retrieved February 7, 2008, from http://www.cdc.gov/mmwr/mmwrhtml/mm5649a4.htm

Centers for Disease Control and Prevention. (2007d). West Nile virus update: United States, January 1–September 11, 2007. *MMWR: Morbidity and Mortality Weekly Report 56*(36), 936–937. Retrieved January 21, 2008, from www.cdc.gov/ncidod/dvbid/westnile/index.htm

Centers for Disease Control and Prevention. (2008a). *Preparation and planning for bioterrorism emergencies.* Retrieved March 1, 2008, from http://www.bt.cdc.gov/agent/index.asp

Centers for Disease Control and Prevention. (2008b). *Reported cases of Lyme disease by year, United States,* 1991–2006. Retrieved February 28, 2008, from http://www.cdc.gov/ncidod/dvbid/lyme/ld_UpClimbLymeDis.htm

Centers for Disease Control and Prevention. (2008c). Summary of notifiable diseases. *MMWR: Morbidity and Mortality Weekly Report 57*(7), 179–183. Retrieved February 25, 2008, from http://www.cdc.gov/mmwr/preview/mmwrhtml/mm5707a4.htm

Centers for Disease Control and Prevention, Division of Global Migration and Quarantine. (2008a). *Lyme disease.* Retrieved February 20, 2008, from http://wwwn.cdc.gov/travel/yellowBookCh4-LymeDisease.aspx

Centers for Disease Control and Prevention, Division of Global Migration and Quarantine. (2008b). *Protection against mosquitoes, ticks, fleas and other insects and arthropods.* Retrieved February 20, 2008, from http://wwwn.cdc.gov/travel/yellowBookCh2-InsectsArthropods.aspx

Centers for Disease Control and Prevention, National Center for Immunization and Respiratory Diseases. (2008). Notice to readers: Expansion of use of live attenuated influenza vaccine (FluMist®) to children ages 2–4 years and other FluMist changes for the 2007–08 influenza season. *MMWR: Morbidity and Mortality Weekly Report 56*(46), 1217–1219. Retrieved February 21, 2008, from http://www.cdc.gov/mmwr/preview/mmwrhtml/mm5646a4.htm

Centers for Disease Control and Prevention, National Center for Infectious Disease. (2008). *Parvovirus B19 (fifth disease).* Retrieved March 1, 2008, from http://www.cdc.gov/ncidod/dvrd/revb/respiratory/parvo_b19.htm.

Centers for Disease Control and Prevention, SC Division of Acute Disease Epidemiology. (2008). *Childcare exclusion list.* Retrieved March 10, 2008, from http://www.scdhec.gov/health/disease/docs/2007-2008_Childcare_Exclusion_List.pdf

Edmunds, M. W., & Mayhew, M. S. (2004). *Pharmacology for primary care providers* (2nd ed.). St. Louis, MO: Mosby.

Gilbert, D. N., Moellering, R. C., & Sande, M. A. (2007). *The Sanford guide to antimicrobial therapy* (37th ed.). Hyde Park, VT: Antimicrobial Therapy.

Goroll, A. H., & Mulley, A. G. (2006). *Primary care medicine* (4th ed.). Philadelphia: Lippincott, Williams & Wilkins.

Kleigman, R. M., Marcdante, K. J., Jensen, H. B. , & Behrman, R. E. (2006). *Nelson essentials of pediatrics* (5th ed.). Philadelphia: Saunders.

Kretsinger, K., Broder, K. R., Cortese, M. M., Joyce, M. P., Ortega-Sanchez, I., Lee, G. M., et al. (2006). Preventing tetanus, diphtheria, and pertussis among adults: Use of tetanus toxoid, reduced diphtheria toxoid and acellular pertussis vaccine. *MMWR: Morbidity and Mortality Weekly Report* RR17, 1–33. Retrieved March 1, 2008, from http://www.cdc.gov/MMWR/preview/mmwrhtml/rr5517a1.htm

Mayo Clinic Staff. (2007). *Lyme disease.* Retrieved February 18, 2008, from http://www.mayoclinic.com/health/lyme-disease/DS00116/DSECTION=8#

Newburger, J. W., Takahashi, M., Gerber, M. A., Gewitz, M. H., Tani, L. Y., Burns, J. C., et al. (2004). Diagnosis, treatment, and long-term management of Kawasaki disease: A statement for health professionals. *Circulation, 110,* 2747–2771. Retrieved February 20, 2008, from http://www.circ.ahajournals.org/cgi/content/abstract/110/17/2747

Rakel, R. E., & Bope, E. T. (2006). *Conn's current therapy.* Philadelphia: Saunders Elsevier.

McPhee, S. J., Papdakis, M. A. & Tierney, L. M. (Eds.). (2008) *Current medical diagnosis and treatment* (47th ed.). New York: Lange Medical Books/McGraw-Hill.

U.S. Department of Health and Human Services. (2005). *Side effects of anti-HIV medications.* Retrieved June 6, 2008, from http://aidsinfo.nih.gov/ContentFiles/SideEffectAnitHIVMeds_cbrochure_en.pdf

U.S. Department of Health and Human Services. (2008). *2007–2008 childcare exclusion list.* Retrieved June 5, 2008, from http://www.scdhec.net/health/disease/docs/2007-2008_School_Exclusion_List.pdf

U.S. Department of Health and Human Services, Food and Drug Administration. (2008). *Public health advisory: Nonprescription cough and cold medicine use in children.* Retrieved January 20, 2008, from http://www.fda.gov/CDER/drug/advisory/cough_cold_2008.htm

U.S. Department of Health and Human Services, Panel on Antiretroviral Guidelines for Adults and Adolescents. (2008). *Guidelines for the use of antiretroviral agents in HIV-1-infected adults and adolescents.* Retrieved June 6, 2008, from http://aidsinfo.nih.gov/contentfiles/AdultandAdolescentGL.pdf

Common Problems of the Skin

Deborah Gilbert-Palmer, EdD, FNP-BC

GENERAL APPROACH

- Dermatologic complaints can be indicative of a dermatological disorder or may prove to be symptomatic of a systemic problem.
- Dermatologic disorders can have a profound impact on the patient's self-image; psychological assessment needs to be included in the history-taking and addressed in the treatment plan.
- Use proper terminology to describe dermatologic lesions (see Tables 5–1 and 5–2).

Table 5–1. Morphologic Definitions for Primary Skin Lesions

Term	Definition and Example	Size
Macule	Flat, nonpalpable colored spot (freckle)	Up to 5 mm
Papule	Solid, elevated, circumscribed lesion (acne)	Up to 5 mm
Nodule	Solid, elevated, circumscribed lesion (erythema nodosum)	0.5–1.2 cm
Vesicle	Fluid-filled, elevated, circumscribed lesion (herpes simplex)	Up to 5 mm
Cyst	Encapsulated, fluid-filled mass (epidermoid cyst)	Variable
Bulla	Fluid-filled, elevated, circumscribed lesion (second-degree burn, severe poison ivy)	Larger than 5 mm
Pustule	Pus-filled, elevated, circumscribed lesion (acne)	Up to 5 mm
Wheal	A suddenly occurring transient elevation of the skin, circumscribed, may or may not be erythematous (hives, urticaria)	0.5 to 10 cm diameter
Tumor	Solid, elevated mass	Larger than 1 cm

Table 5-2. Morphologic Definitions for Secondary Skin Lesions

Lesion	Definition	Example
Scale	Dry, greasy fragment of dead skin	Psoriasis
Crust	Dry mass of exudate	Impetigo
Ulcer	Sharply-defined, deep erosion	Decubitus ulcer
Scar	Permanent skin change as a result of newly formed connective tissue	Burn scar
Lichenification	Induration and thickening of skin resulting from chronic scratching or rubbing	Eczema
Fissure	Linear split through dermis and epidermis	Cheilitis

- The most important part of the assessment is a thorough history.
- Physical exam is best performed in a well-lit room with a penlight for illumination and shadowing (to determine if lesion is raised), a Wood's lamp for fluorescing certain types of lesions, a magnifying lens, glass slides for diascopy (to determine blanching) and skin scrapings, potassium hydroxide (KOH) solution (to illuminate hyphae), 5% acetic acid for acetowhitening (to illuminate human papilloma virus lesions), mineral oil for suspected scabies, Giemsa or Wright stains, and a regular microscope.
- Assessment should also include appearance of the patient (comfortable, agitated, toxic) and vital signs, with referral to an ER for the toxic patient.

Dermatologic Signs to Be Assessed and Documented
- Distribution of lesion (generalized or localized, central or peripheral, symmetric or asymmetric, predilection for certain body areas such as extensor or flexor surfaces and intertriginous areas, sun-exposed or pressure areas)
- Arrangement of lesions (discrete, confluent, scattered, linear, zosteriform, polycyclic, grouped, patchy, accurate, reticular, scarlatiniform)
- Shape or configuration of the primary lesion (annular, oval, nummular, iris, pedunculated, verrucous, umbilicated, gyrate, serpiginous)
- Color of lesions (erythematous, violaceous, hypomelanotic, depigmented, flesh-colored, hypermelanotic, variegated)
- Borders or margins of lesions (well-demarcated or ill-defined)
- Palpable qualities (soft, firm, mobile, fixed, hard, fluctuant, tender, hot/warm/cool, smooth, rough, indurated)
- Measured dimensions (diameter, width, length, elevation, depression)
- Descriptive terms (lichenified, atrophied, sclerosed, pigmented, friable, hyperkeratotic, weeping, crusted, mobile or nonmobile, hypertrophic/keloidal, excoriations)
- Morphology of primary and secondary lesions (see above)
- Associated symptoms involving hair, vision, nails, mucous membranes, lymphatic system, hepatosplenomegaly, and/or neurologic changes

Changes Associated With Aging
- Should be identified and recognized as normal, such as dermatoheliosis or photoaging of the skin evidenced by wrinkles and drying, pigment changes, pseudo scars, senile purpura, solar lentigines, alopecia, seborrheic keratoses.

- Seborrheic keratoses are benign epithelial growths that occur with aging and become darkened in color; have a warty, greasy surface; and are raised papules or plaques, 1–3 cm in size, with a characteristic "stuck on" appearance. No treatment is necessary unless skin cancer cannot be ruled out, then biopsy and excise.

Health Maintenance and Screening Guidelines
- Skin cancer is the most common cancer in the United States today.
- Sun exposure, especially early in life, has been identified as a risk factor.
- Primary prevention involves counseling patients to avoid sun exposure and to protect themselves with appropriate sunscreen and clothing.
- Secondary prevention involves screening for skin lesions with premalignant or malignant characteristics during routine health exams and referring patients at increased risk for melanoma to specialists.
- Tertiary prevention involves removal of precancerous lesions, such as suspicious moles and actinic keratoses.
- Actinic (solar) keratoses are due to sun exposure and may be precursors to squamous cell carcinoma. They are single or multiple, discrete, flat or slightly raised, dry, scaly, brownish or reddish lesions up to 1.5 cm in size. They should be biopsied if inflamed or indurated and can be removed by liquid nitrogen, curettage, or fluorouracil cream application.

Use of Topical Steroids
- Steroid medications should be ordered in the lowest dosage and duration.
- Table 5–3 ranks the topical steroids by potency.
- Fluorinated steroids cause thinning of the tissue; avoid using on the face and genital region.

Red Flags
- *Anaphylaxis* may evolve rapidly from a variety of exposures including drugs, exercise, food, insect stings, and latex; rapidly evolving symptoms may include hives, pruritus, flushing, shortness of breath, wheezing, tachycardia, difficulty swallowing, nausea, vomiting, abdominal cramping, and possible shock. Epinephrine (1:1000) 0.3 to 0.5 mL for adults and 0.01 mL/kg for children should be administered immediately and every 20 minutes as needed, along with supportive care.
- *Necrotizing fasciitis* is a rapidly progressing deep infection of the subcutaneous tissue that presents as a large erythematous, edematous plaque with a central area of necrosis, pain out of proportion to the degree of cellulitis, fever, and crepitation; caused by beta-hemolytic streptococcus and/or staphylococcus. Urgent hospitalization for debridement and IV antibiotics is necessary.
- *Malignant melanoma:* The five cardinal signs are asymmetry; border is irregular and often scalloped; color is mottled with variegated display of brown, black, gray, and/or pink; diameter is large (greater than 6.0 mm); elevation is almost always present with subtle or obvious surface distortion and best assessed by side-lighting of the lesion.

Table 5-3. Common Topical Steroids (Ranked by Potency, Most to Least)

Group	Example
Group 1	Augmented betamethasone dipropionate ointment 0.05% (Diprolene)
	Clobetasolpropionate cream, ointment 0.05% (Topicort)
Group 2	Augmented betamethasone dipropionate cream (Diprosone)
	Desoximetasone cream, gel, ointment 0.25% (Topicort)
	Fluocinonide cream, gel, lotion, ointment 0.05% (Lidex)
	Betamethasone valerate ointment 0.1%
Group 3	Triamcinolone acetonide cream, lotion, ointment 0.05% (Kenalog)
	Flurandrenolide cream, lotion, ointment 0.05% (Cordran)
	Fluocinolone acetonide cream 0.2% (Synalar-HP)
	Betamethasone valerate cream 0.1%
Group 4	Desonide cream 0.05%
	Fluocinolone acetonide cream 0.025% (Synalar)
	Hydrocortisone valerate cream 0.2% (Westcort)
	Hydrocortisone cream, ointment, lotion 2.5% (Hytone)

ALLERGY

Contact Dermatitis

Description
- Cutaneous reaction to an external substance—either irritant or allergen—that may appear as an asymmetric distribution of red, raised, and/or inflamed rash, or rash only on exposed areas.
- Includes metal, plant, chemical or food substances

Etiology
- 80% of cases due to universal irritants (soap, detergents, organic solvents). Irritant contact dermatitis due to direct injury of the skin (e.g., from detergent).
- Allergic contact dermatitis results from previous immunosensitization; see poison ivy, oak, antimicrobials, adhesive tape, latex.

Incidence and Demographics
- Less common in African-Americans
- Common in all ages. Age has no influence on sensitization; however, allergic contact dermatitis is less common in young children.
- Occupational sensitization is a common cause of disability in industry.

Risk Factors
- Exposure to irritant or allergen
- Prior sensitization to allergen

Prevention and Screening
- Protective clothing in presence of potential exposure
- Avoidance of known irritants/allergens

Assessment

HISTORY

- Pruritic rash in unnatural pattern on exposed skin
- Known exposure to irritant or allergen
- May include systemic symptoms of toxicity if extensive involvement

PHYSICAL EXAM

- Morphology: Erythematous papules, vesicles, or bullae on inflamed background; scaling, erythema, edema; thickened skin and weepy, encrusted lesions in chronic phase; local area hot and swollen
- Location/distribution: Exposed skin surfaces in unnatural pattern, mimicking possible path of irritant
- Particular irritant or allergen may be obvious by location of symptomse
- Metal allergy: Most common offender is nickel in jewelry and clothing
- Distribution: Neck, wrists, waist, strap line, ear lobes
- Generally mild and chronic with scaling, pigmentation changes, and pruritus
- Plant dermatitis
- Distribution and arrangement: Often linear pattern
- Most commonly caused by poison ivy, poison oak, and poison sumac
- Secondary signs: weeping, scaling, edema, crusting, and excoriation

DIAGNOSTIC STUDIES

- Clinical diagnosis but patch testing may be warranted for severe or recurrent episodes with unclear etiology

Differential Diagnosis

- Atopic dermatitis
- Impetigo
- Scabies

Management

- See Table 5–4

NONPHARMACOLOGIC TREATMENT

- Remove offending irritant or allergen within 20 minutes; may require patch testing after episode is resolved
- Wash potentially contacted clothing
- Bathe in tepid water with soap to wash allergen/irritant off skin
- Cool compresses with astringent (Domeboro solution) or colloidal oatmeal suspension (Aveeno) to treat pruritus

PHARMACOLOGIC TREATMENT

- Oral antihistamines (diphenhydramine or hydroxyzine) for pruritus
- Topical steroids applied bid
- Systemic steroids for severe or extensive involvement
  - Prednisone: Begin at 60 mg and taper over 2–3 weeks, depending upon severity of symptoms
  - Medrol Dosepak considered inadequate dose for this condition
- Oral antibiotics for secondarily infected lesions
- UVA-UVB or PUVA treatments

Table 5–4. Pruritus Control Using Pharmacologic and Nonpharmacologic Methods

Treatment	Specific Recommendatons
Nonpharmacologic treatments	Lukewarm or cool baths with or without colloidal oatmeal or baking soda Cool compresses

Pharmacologic treatments	Medications
Oral antihistamines	Diphenhydramine (Benadryl) 12.5 mg/5 mL syrup, chewables 12.5 mg, tablets 25 mg OTC Children: 5 mg/kg/day divided q6–8h Hydroxyzine (Atarax) 10 mg/5mL syrup; tablets of 10, 25, and 50 mg Children: 5 mg/kg/day divided q6–8h Adolescents and adults: 25–50 mg qid prn Caution that topical Benadryl given to very small children taking oral product may result in overdose due to absorption through skin
Oral antihistamines (less sedating)	Loratadine (Claritin) for children 2–5 yrs, 5 mg per day (syrup); >6 yrs, 10 mg qd (tabs, Redi-tabs) OTC Alavert >6 yrs, 10 mg qd (tabs, oral-disintegrating tabs) Cetirizine (Zyrtec) in children over 6 months 6–23 mos, 2.5 mg qd–bid 2–5 yrs, 2.5–5 mg qd >6 yrs, 5–10 mg qd Preparations: Zyrtec syrup 5 mg/tsp, 5–10 mg tabs
Topical antipruritic agents	OTC products: Prax lotion, Itch-X, Aveeno Anti-itch Cream Rx products: Cetaphil with menthol 0.25% and phenol 0.25%

Adapted from *Clinical Guidelines in Child Health* by M. Graham & C. Uphold, C. 2003, Gainesville, FL: Barramae Books, Inc.

LENGTH OF TREATMENT
- Length of treatment determined by extent of involvement and response; often 1–2 weeks

Special Considerations
- Steroids are contraindicated in pregnancy unless clinically warranted.
- Distribution of symptoms may help determine causative agent.

When to Consult, Refer, Hospitalize
- Consultation/referral to allergist for patch testing if indicated
- Hospitalization should be considered for toxic or unstable patients (infants, elderly).

Follow-Up
EXPECTED COURSE
- Course is usually dictated by irritant or allergen and extent of involvement
- Metal allergies tend to be low-level and chronic, with possible lichenification and hyperpigmentation

COMPLICATIONS
- Toxicity and secondary infection

Urticaria

Description
- Represents a reaction in the dermis and subcutaneous tissues to various stimuli; characterized by erythematous wheals that appear on any part of the body.
- The lesions may be round, oval, or form rings or arcs; often pruritic.
- In acute urticaria, hives, or wheals, appear abruptly and may last 24–36 hours.
- In chronic urticaria, lesions persist for longer than 6 weeks.
- Urticaria may occur along with angioedema or with generalized anaphylaxis.

Etiology
- May be allergic or nonallergic, IgE-mediated or non-IgE–mediated hypersensitivity in which there is release of chemical mediators (histamine, prostaglandins, serotonin, kinins) from cutaneous mast cells that leads to increased vascular permeability.
- Fluid extravasates from small blood vessels, causing typical lesions.
- Many and varied causes include foods, medicines, inhalants, infectious agents, physical factors (heat, cold, exercise, sunlight).

Incidence and Demographics
- Experienced by up to 20% of population at some point.
- Can occur at any age; more common in children and adolescents.

Risk Factors
- History of allergies, asthma, atopic diseases

Prevention and Screening
- Allergen avoidance
- Sunscreen or protective clothing if solar urticaria

Assessment
HISTORY
- Complete review of recent exposure to possible causative factors, such as medications, foods, injections, infections, inhalations, animals
- Family or personal history of previous episodes of urticaria, atopic disease
- Exposure to sun, cold, stress, water, exercise
- Chronic health problems
- Extent of pruritus
- Assess for any lip and hand swelling, shortness of breath, or signs of a more generalized reaction

PHYSICAL EXAM
- Mildly erythematous, blanching, flat-topped lesions with pale centers
- Lesions may be 2 mm–20 cm in diameter, scattered or coalesced, generalized or localized distribution
- May appear and fade within 24 hours; later may reappear
- Heat may intensify lesions
- Evaluate mucous membranes and airway
- Evaluate lungs for wheezing, BP for hypotension

DIAGNOSTIC STUDIES
- If fever, assess for infectious underlying cause and perform appropriate diagnostic tests as needed

Differential Diagnosis
- Erythema multiforme
- Contact dermatitis
- Juvenile rheumatoid arthritis
- Mastocytosis
- Pityriasis

Management
NONPHARMACOLOGIC TREATMENT
- Avoid suspected offending agent

PHARMACOLOGIC TREATMENT
- Oral antihistamines such as diphenhydramine (Benadryl) 5 mg/kg/day in 4 divided doses or hydroxyzine (Atarax) 2 mg/kg/day in 3–4 divided doses
- Topical steroids not useful; systemic steroids are used for severe or extensive reactions
- Epinephrine (1:1,000) 0.01 mL/kg subcutaneously for signs of anaphylaxis; Epi-pen or Ana-kit for prophylaxis of bee sting by patient

LENGTH OF TREATMENT
- As long as needed to resolve symptoms

Special Considerations
- Angioedema and anaphylaxis occur by the same mechanism as urticaria.
- Angioedema occurs in up to 50% of children with urticaria, and usually involves the face, hands, and feet.
- Anaphylaxis may evolve rapidly with the hives, accompanied by airway edema, pruritus, flushing, wheezing, tachycardia, difficulty swallowing, nausea, vomiting, abdominal cramping, and possible shock.
- A precise cause of the urticaria is often not found.

When to Consult, Refer, Hospitalize
- Refer to allergist or immunologist if urticaria persistent for >6 weeks.
- Immediately transfer to an emergency facility for signs of anaphylaxis with emergency care en route.

Follow-Up
- Recheck if symptoms persist beyond 36 hours.
    COMPLICATIONS
        • Angioedema, anaphylaxis, or secondary infection of site as a result of scratching

ECZEMATOUS CONDITIONS

Atopic Dermatitis

Description
- Chronic skin condition characterized by inflammation and intense itching along a typical pattern of distribution; presentation frequently varies according to the age and race of the patient. Pruritus is most characteristic finding.
- Scratch-itch-scratch cycle perpetuates and exacerbates problem.
- Infantile atopic dermatitis is usually erythematous and vesicular and is a frustrating scratch-itch-rub cycle seen in infants, usually on the face, antecubital and popliteal fossae, and lateral legs.
- Childhood-type atopic dermatitis is more often papular with lichenified plaques and appears as erosions and crusts as the child scratches the sites.

Etiology
- IgE-mediated inherited dermatitis that involves abnormality in the cell-mediated immune system.
- Often a manifestation of multisystem atopy, which includes asthma, allergic rhinitis, and atopic dermatitis.

Incidence and Demographics
- Common condition; 66% have positive family history of atopic problems; inherited IgE-mediated hypersensitivity; frequent onset in infancy or early childhood (60% by 1 year).
- 10% of infants are affected; 90% of those affected have onset between ages 6 weeks and 5 years.
- 75%–85% of those with atopic dermatitis will develop allergic rhinitis; 50% of these will develop asthma.

Risk Factors
- Positive family history of atopic problems; past medical history (PMH) of asthma, allergic rhinitis, or atopic dermatitis
- Dry environment; repetitive skin abrasion
- Emotional stress; hormonal factors (pregnancy, menses, thyroid); infections

Prevention and Screening
- Environmental controls
- Coping skills
- Management of pruritus

Assessment

HISTORY
- Pruritic rash in classic distribution
- PMH or family history of asthma or allergic rhinitis/dermatitis

PHYSICAL EXAM
- Morphology: Initially poorly defined erythematous patches, papules, or patches, with or without scales
- Develops into red, weeping, crusted patches; eventually become lichenified
- Distribution: Extensor and exposed surfaces of infants
- Flexor folds: Antecubital and popliteal fossae; wrists, neck, and forehead of older children and adults; upper trunk
- Associated findings: Lichenification, excoriations, fissures and erosions, periorbital hyperpigmentation, rhinitis and/or asthma, dermatographism, keratosis pilaris, ichthyosis vulgaris, cataracts in up to 10% of patients
- African-Americans may lose pigmentation in lichenified areas

DIAGNOSTIC STUDIES
- Mainly a clinical diagnosis
- Increased serum IgE, eosinophilia; allergy testing
- Bacterial cultures to rule out S. aureus; viral cultures to rule out herpes simplex

Differential Diagnosis
- Seborrheic dermatitis
- Nummular eczema
- Psoriasis
- Dermatophytosis
- Scabies
- Contact dermatitis

Management

NONPHARMACOLOGIC TREATMENT
- Acute weeping lesions: humidify environment; decrease use of hot water, soap, and abrasive clothing
- Take long, soaking baths in warm water. Pat dry; don't use abrasive towels/rubbing.
- Liberal use of emollients and/or lubricating lotions after bathing; oatmeal baths for pruritus
- Relaxation techniques, behavior modification may be helpful in severe cases.
- Patients need to learn stress management techniques to control flare-ups as well.

PHARMACOLOGIC TREATMENT
- Oral antihistamines such as diphenhydramine (Benadryl) for pruritus
- Topical steroids bid sparingly, potency based on response
- Immunomodulators: Pimecrolimus or tacrolimus
- Montelukast (Singulair): May use in children older than 2 years and adults
- Systemic steroids (prednisone) are sometimes warranted in severe flare-ups; begin at 60 mg and taper down over 2–4 weeks
- Oral antibiotics may be necessary for secondarily infected lesions

- UVA-UVB and PUVA treatments for recalcitrant cases
- Tar preparations in those unresponsive to steroids

LENGTH OF TREATMENT
- Prednisone treatment should be limited to a 2-week tapered course.
- Topical preparations are used intermittently as symptoms warrant.
- Treat acute flares until controlled while maintaining and then continuing nonpharmacologic treatment; may require occlusive dressings at night for 2–6 weeks.

Special Considerations
- Systemic steroids are usually contraindicated in pregnancy and lactation.
- Geriatric patients are predisposed to atrophic skin and steroids exacerbate atrophy; use topical steroids of lower potency.
- *Nummular eczema* is a chronic, pruritic, inflammatory dermatitis in coin-shaped plaques of 4–5 cm; usually on anterior aspects of lower legs but may also appear on trunk, hands, and fingers; pruritus often intense.
  - Secondary skin changes include exudative crusting, scaling, excoriation, lichenification, and postinflammatory hyperpigmentation
  - Treatment is the same as for atopic dermatitis
- *Dyshidrotic eczema* is an acute, chronic, or recurrent dermatosis of palms, fingers, and/or soles characterized by a sudden onset of deep pruritic rash on hands and feet, which may last for weeks.
  - Initially clear vesicles in clusters on palms and soles; later scaling, lichenification, painful fissures
  - Pruritus is treated with wet dressings of Domeboro solution, oatmeal, high-potency corticosteroid cream bid, oral antihistamines
  - May need dermatology referral for intralesional steroid injections for small, localized involvement; systemic steroids for severe or extensive involvement; oral antibiotics for secondarily infected lesions; or possible PUVA treatments

When to Consult, Refer, Hospitalize
- Consult or refer patients with suboptimal response to above regimen to dermatologist or for PUVA, UVA-UVB treatment.

Follow-Up
- Every 2 weeks until well controlled
  EXPECTED COURSE
  - Chronic condition with subacute phases and acute flares
  - Usually more symptomatic during winter months

  COMPLICATIONS
  - Secondary infection and/or cellulitis
  - Skin atrophy, striae from overuse of topical steroids

Seborrheic Dermatitis

Description
- Chronic, recurrent and sometimes pruritic inflammatory disease of skin where sebaceous glands are most active (face, scalp, body folds)

Etiology
- Unknown with questionable role of *Pityrosporum ovale*

Incidence and Demographics
- 2%–5% of population affected; males more than females
- Infancy ("cradle cap") and adults between 20 to 50 years

Risk Factors
- Family history
- HIV infection; zinc or niacin deficiency; Parkinson's disease

Prevention
- Daily cleansing of skin with soap, water, and cloth

Screening
- None

Assessment
HISTORY
- Gradual onset of greasy, scaly rash on face and scalp
- Possibly associated with *slight* pruritus

PHYSICAL EXAM
- Usually see fine, dry, white, or yellow scale on erythematous base, or
- Dull red plaques with thick, white, or yellow, scaly, greasy lesions
- Morphology: Lesions are yellowish-red, greasy, moist, sharply marginated, 5–20 mm scaling macules and papules; in dark-skinned children, hypopigmentation may be present
- Distribution: Scalp, eyebrow, eyelids, nasolabial folds, cheek, behind ears, intertriginous areas
- Secondary signs: Possible inflammatory base, sticky crusting (more common on ears), fissures (more common at ear attachments to scalp)

DIAGNOSTIC STUDIES
- Diagnosis is usually made clinically

Differential Diagnosis
- Psoriasis
- Impetigo
- Dermatophytosis

Management
NONPHARMACOLOGIC TREATMENT
- For infant scales: Antiseborrheic shampoo used 3 times per week; leave on for 5 minutes before rinsing. For stubborn infant scales, apply warm mineral or baby oil for 10 minutes before shampoo.
- Adolescents: Avoid cold creams and moisturizers, which may plug sebaceous glands
- Remove scaling of eyelashes with baby shampoo

PHARMACOLOGIC TREATMENT
- Frequent shampooing with selenium sulfide (Selsun or Exsel), tar (Polytar, T-Gel or Tegrin), or zinc (Head & Shoulders) shampoos
- Salicylic acid may be helpful in removing crusts
- Hydrocortisone lotion for stubborn areas, and/or ketoconazole (Nizoral) cream
- Treatment of face includes sulfur-based soap
- Topical steroids (1% hydrocortisone lotion with sulfur)
- **No fluorinated steroids on the face**

LENGTH OF TREATMENT
- Chronic condition requires initial therapy until symptoms resolve, followed by maintenance therapy of ketoconazole shampoo, lotions, and/or topical steroids qd

Special Considerations
- Systemic steroids contraindicated in pregnancy and lactation unless clinically warranted

When to Consult, Refer, Hospitalize
- Consult or refer for unresponsive cases

Follow-Up
- Visits every 1–2 months during maintenance phase to monitor disorder and for signs of skin atrophy

EXPECTED COURSE
- Chronic condition requiring initial treatment phase and maintenance therapy

COMPLICATIONS
- Secondary infection
- Skin atrophy, striae from chronic topical steroids

ACNE

Acne Vulgaris and Nodulocystic Acne

Description
- A polymorphic disorder of the pilosebaceous unit characterized by inflammation and a variety of lesions ranging from comedones to inflamed cysts on the face, upper torso, and back.
- Acne vulgaris consists of open and closed comedones, inflamed papules, and pustules.
- Nodulocystic acne or acne conglobata consists of cysts, abscesses, and sinus tracts.
- Acne fulminans is most severe form; suppuration of lesions, may have systemic symptoms such as fever and arthritis

Etiology
- Five factors usually involved:
  - Excess keratin plugging of the sebaceous follicles
    - Increased androgen production during puberty; some pathologic conditions such as polycystic ovarian syndrome (POS) affect sebum production
    - Pore-blocking cosmetics and trauma from harsh scrubbing may affect keratinization and blocking of the sebaceous duct; retention of sebum, overgrowth of *Propionibacterium acnes*
  - Bacterial colonization with *Propionibacterium*; *P. acnes* commonly is found in the pilosebaceous unit of healthy skin but proliferates in the impacted sebaceous duct
  - Sebum overproduction and increased androgenic production; disordered functioning of the pilosebaceous unit includes excessive sebum production, abnormal follicular keratinization (comedogenesis)
  - Inflammation due to the distention of the hair follicle with *P. acnes* and sebum
  - Genetics

Incidence and Demographics
- Most common skin condition; present in 80%–85% of all adolescents due to increased androgen production
- Males more than females; light-skinned more than darker-skinned
- May persist into the second decade of life; then more common in women
- Flare in perimenopausal women due to elevated unopposed adrenal androgens

Risk Factors
- Elevated circulating androgen hormones as described above
- Use of follicle-blocking cosmetics and hair spray
- Oral contraceptives with high progestin component; anticonvulsants; systemic or topical steroid use
- Genetic predisposition, male

Prevention and Screening
- Good skin hygiene, avoidance of follicle-blocking cosmetics

Assessment
HISTORY
- Onset associated with puberty or androgen excess
- May include history of use of oil-based cosmetics and/or harsh scrubbing

PHYSICAL EXAM
- Mild to moderate acne, or acne vulgaris
  - Presence of comedones, inflamed papules, pustules and cysts on face, upper torso and back
    - » Open comedones, or "blackheads" (follicular orifice is dilated)
    - » Closed comedones, or "whiteheads" (plug in the sebaceous duct enlarges)
- Inflamed papules and pustules result from the proliferation of *P. acnes*
- Severe acne or nodulocystic acne
  - Cysts and nodulocystic lesions develop as the plug enlarges and may result in sinus tracts forming under the skin; inflamed cysts develop as abscesses
  - Possible presence of scarring from healed lesions

DIAGNOSTIC STUDIES
- None are necessary unless the patient has acne fulminans and appears toxic, then CBC and blood cultures are appropriate; bacterial culture may be indicated to rule out folliculitis; serologic testing

Differential Diagnosis
- Rosacea
- Abscess
- Cutaneous manifestations of systemic lupus erythematosus (SLE)
- Furunculosis
- Tinea barbae
- Folliculitis

Management
NONPHARMACOLOGIC TREATMENT
- Gentle washing bid with mild soap such as Dove, Basis, or Neutrogena, or noncomedogenic cleanser
- Avoid oil-based cosmetics and hairsprays as these plug follicles
- Avoid picking or squeezing lesions as this may lead to scarring

PHARMACOLOGIC TREATMENT
- Acne vulgaris
  - Keratolytic topical agents including benzoyl peroxide 5% and 10% qd to bid or salicylic acid 0.5%–10% in many OTC preparations
  - Topical antibiotics including erythromycin 1%–2% gel qd or bid or clindamycin 1% gel or solution qd or bid
  - Antibacterial/keratolytic agent azelaic acid (Azelex) 20% cream qd x 2 weeks then bid
  - Topical comedolytic agent tretinoin (Retin-A) 0.025% to 0.1% cream or gel bid or adapalene (Differin) 0.1% gel qd to bid
  - Antiandrogen therapy through oral contraceptives such as Ortho-TriCyclen

- Nodulocystic acne and widespread acne or acne resistant to other therapies
  - Oral antibiotics such as tetracycline 250 mg qd to tid; erythromycin 250 mg qd to tid; minocycline 50 to 100 mg qd to bid
  - Systemic isotretinoin (Accutane) 0.5–2 mg/kg/day in 2 divided doses

LENGTH OF TREATMENT
- Treatment is long term and may continue for years. Topical agents should be started individually or with a combined keratolytic and antibiotic such as Benzamycin gel qd and increased to bid after 1–2 week to avoid excessive drying from these products.
- Start oral antibiotics bid to tid and taper over time to qd after improvement is achieved.
- Systemic isotretinoin should be used for 15–20 weeks; may restart after 2 months off the drug.

Special Considerations
- Patients need to be advised that minimal response is to be expected in the first 4–6 weeks of therapy and optimal response may take several months on the various regimens.
- Patients should be started on a single agent with the addition of other agents as tolerated.
- Because all of the topical treatments can be drying, it is important to start slowly (qd with one agent) and increase to bid, adding second and third agents one at a time.
- Gender: Females with polycystic ovaries or other hyperandrogenism and females with late-onset acne may benefit from the use of oral contraceptives with low androgenic activity.
- Race: Darker-skinned people are more likely to develop post-inflammatory hyper-pigmentation. Azelaic acid cream possesses hypopigmentation properties and may be useful in limiting post-inflammatory hyperpigmentation.
- Most anti-acne drugs (topical and oral) cause photosensitivity reactions; sun exposure should be limited and liberal use of oil-free sunscreen gel is advised.
- Pregnancy and lactation: Isotretinoin is a teratogen and must be avoided. **Women of childbearing age must be strongly counseled to use reliable contraception for 1 month prior to, during, and 1 month following use of this drug.**
- Laboratory monitoring for patients on isotretinoin includes lipid panel, CBC, liver function tests (LFT), glucose.

When to Consult, Refer, Hospitalize
- Referral to a dermatologist is appropriate if a suboptimal response is achieved after adequate trial on 2 or 3 of the above drugs and if isotretinoin is being considered.

Follow-Up
- Initial follow up every 2 months until stable regimen established with successful control.
  EXPECTED COURSE
  - Long-term management often necessary for several years

  COMPLICATIONS
  - Excess drying of the skin from topical agents
  - Potentially severe side effects with isotretinoin, such as pseudotumor cerebri

(increased risk with tetracycline), pancreatitis, hepatotoxicity, corneal opacities, blood dyscrasias, premature epiphyseal closure; pregnancy category X

Acne Rosacea

Description
- Chronic acneform inflammation of central third of face
- Does not involve any comedones, the classic lesion of acne vulgaris

Etiology
- Cutaneous vascular disorder of unknown etiology with increased reaction of capillaries to heat ("flushing")
- Sebaceous gland hyperplasia
- Ocular manifestations such as conjunctivitis, blepharitis, and episcleritis occur

Incidence and Demographics
- Predominantly affects women in 35–50-year age range
- Severe form with rhinophyma is seen almost exclusively in men older than 40

Risk Factors
- Found more commonly in individuals with fair skin who burn and rarely tan
- Positive family history of rosacea is a risk factor; more common in those with migraine headaches
- Excessive ETOH consumption is associated with flares

Prevention and Screening
- None

Assessment
HISTORY
- History of abnormal flushing of the central portion of the face after drinking hot or alcoholic beverages or eating spicy foods

PHYSICAL EXAM
- 2–3 mm papular and pustular discrete and clustered lesions on the central portion of the face on an erythematous base; rosy coloration of nose, chin, cheeks; no comedones
- Dilatation of the superficial capillaries causes flushing and eventually leads to telangiectasia
- Ocular symptoms such as blepharitis or keratitis may be associated
- Chronic symptoms can lead to lymphatic changes causing cellulitis
- Irreversible hypertrophy of the nose (rhinophyma) is a result of chronic inflammation and is seen almost exclusively in men older than 40

DIAGNOSTIC STUDIES
- Based on clinical presentation; culture or biopsy is not necessary

Differential Diagnosis
- Acne vulgaris
- Butterfly rash of SLE
- Cellulitis
- Folliculitis

Management
NONPHARMACOLOGIC TREATMENT
- Includes avoidance of triggers that cause facial flushing such as hot beverages, ETOH, highly spicy foods, exposure to sun and wind, emotional stress, and certain medications such as niacin

PHARMACOLOGIC TREATMENT
- Topical metronidazole (MetroGel) 0.75%, erythromycin 2%, or clindamycin (Cleocin T) gel bid
- Tetracycline 250 mg orally tid or bid
- Doxycycline (Vibramycin) 100 mg orally bid
- Minocycline (Minocin) 50–100 mg orally bid
- Erythromycin 250 mg orally tid or bid

LENGTH OF TREATMENT
- Long-term initially at bid or tid dosing, tapering down to qd maintenance dosing
- If no improvement with above regimens, a trial of trimethoprim-sulfamethoxazole (TMP-SMX), oral metronidazole (Flagyl), dapson, or isotretinoin (Accutane) may be considered

Special Considerations
- Pregnant and lactating women, use erythromycin
- Menopausal women who are experiencing flushing associated with hormonal fluctuations may benefit from hormone replacement therapy (HRT) or clonidine (Catapres) if HRT is contraindicated

When to Consult, Refer, Hospitalize
- If response is suboptimal, refer to dermatologist

Follow-Up
- 2–4 weeks initially; once patient responds to therapy, self-management is appropriate with family nurse practitioner follow-up visits annually

EXPECTED COURSE
- Initial response usually within 3 weeks, maximum response by 9 weeks

COMPLICATIONS
- Rhinophyma as described above; may require surgical debulking

Hidradenitis Suppurativa

Description
- Chronic suppurative disease of the apocrine gland region of the axillae, anogenital region, breasts, and scalp with development of sinus tracts and scarring

Etiology
- Unknown, but there may be genetic predisposition toward occlusion of the follicular orifice leading to retention of secretions, nodular formation, abscesses, draining sinuses, and eventual scarring

Incidence and Demographics
- Race: All, but with more extensive involvement in African-Americans
- Age: Puberty to climacteric
- Gender: More commonly found in axillae in females, in anogenital region in males

Risk Factors
- Family history
- Nodulocystic acne
- Obesity
- Apocrine duct obstruction (antiperspirant use)

Prevention and Screening
- Management of obesity
- Avoidance of antiperspirants in people who have had previous problems with them

Assessment
HISTORY
- Recurrent painful lesions with suppuration in the axillae and/or anogenital area

PHYSICAL EXAM
- Abscess of axillae and/or anogenital region, erythematous nodules
- Seropurulent/purulent drainage from single or multiple openings on skin
- Hypertrophic scarring, keloid and sinus tract formation
- Dilated open comedones, often double comedones which are characteristic
- Lymphedema possible

DIAGNOSTIC STUDIES
- Cultures not usually indicated because multiple pathogens colonize

Differential Diagnosis
- Furuncle or carbuncle
- Cat-scratch disease
- Ruptured inclusion cyst
- Lymphadenitis

IN ANOGENITAL INVOLVEMENT
- Sinus tracts and fistulas associated with ulcerative colitis and enteritis
- Lymphogranuloma venereum

Management
NONPHARMACOLOGIC TREATMENT
- Use of local heat; keep the area clean and dry
- Weight loss; avoidance of antiperspirants

SURGICAL TREATMENT
- Initially incise and drain acute abscesses
- Excision of nodules or marsupialization of sinuses in chronic cases
- Complete excision of axillae or involved anogenital area to the fascia with split skin grafting for extensive, chronic disease

PHARMACOLOGIC TREATMENT
- Oral antibiotics until resolution (may take weeks)
  - Erythromycin 250–500 mg qid
  - Tetracycline 250–500 mg qid
  - Minocycline (Minocin) 100 mg bid
- Intralesional triamcinolone (Aristospan; 5 mg/mL) diluted with lidocaine injected into wall of lesion, followed by incision and drainage
- Oral prednisone taper (70 mg qd initially, tapered over 14 days)
- Oral isotretinoin (Accutane) 0.5–2 mg/kg/day in two divided doses

LENGTH OF TREATMENT
- Chronic and recurrent disease: Treat episodic flares with oral antibiotics; steroids as above
- For frequent flares or extensive involvement, continuous antibiotics are indicated pending surgical intervention

Special Considerations
- Erythromycin is recommended for pregnant women

When to Refer, Consult, Hospitalize
- Referral to a surgeon is indicated for extensive and/or chronic involvement

Follow-Up
- Weekly during flare

EXPECTED COURSE
- Usually recurrent flares, but may be resolved after surgery
- Often spontaneous remission towards the end of the third decade of life

COMPLICATIONS
- Fistulas to urethra, bladder, and/or rectum
- Anemia of chronic disease

PAPULOSQUAMOUS ERUPTIONS

Pityriasis Rosea

Description
- Common, maculopapular, red scaly, sometimes pruritic rash appearing on trunk and proximal extremities; self-limiting with spontaneous remission

Etiology
- Unclear but most likely viral

Incidence and Demographics
- More common in spring and fall months and in temperate climates
- Age 10–35 years; 50% more common in women; young adults most commonly affected

Risk Factors
- Sharing a household with an affected individual

Prevention and Screening
- None

Assessment
HISTORY
- Single, large herald patch appearing most commonly on trunk, followed in 1–2 weeks by generalized exanthem; mild to moderate pruritus
- No systemic symptoms but may have been preceded by viral-like illness

PHYSICAL EXAM
- Initial lesion is "herald patch": 2–6 cm, round, scaly plaque usually on trunk
- Generalized fine, oval, 3–7 mm papules and plaques with fine "collarette" scale
- Distribution on trunk, often in Christmas tree pattern, following skin lines

DIAGNOSTIC STUDIES
- None; clinical diagnosis; may do KOH scraping to rule out tinea

Differential Diagnosis
- Drug eruptions
- Secondary syphilis
- Guttate psoriasis
- Tinea corporis
- Tinea versicolor
- Seborrheic dermatitis
- Erythema migrans

Management

NONPHARMACOLOGIC TREATMENT
- UV or natural sunlight exposure

PHARMACOLOGIC TREATMENT
- None usually necessary, but may use oral antihistamines or topical corticosteroids to relieve pruritus

LENGTH OF TREATMENT
- Spontaneous remission in 6–8 weeks

Special Considerations
- None

When to Consult, Refer, Hospitalize
- No need

Follow-Up
- For patient reassurance or when diagnosis is in question
- Complications rare but may be postinflammatory hypo- or hyperpigmentation

FUNGAL AND YEAST INFECTIONS

Fungal (Dermatophyte) Infections

Description
- Persistent superficial fungal infection of the keratinized layer of the skin, including the stratum corneum (epidermomycosis), nails (onychomycosis), and hair (trichomycosis)
- Infections are named by the body part involved or, in the case of tinea versicolor, for the multicolored appearance.

Etiology
- Caused by several dermatophytes with regional predominance
- In the U.S. there are three common dermatophytes: *Microsporum, Trichophyton*, and *Epidermophyton.*
- Can be spread by direct contact with an active lesion on an animal or another human; with fomites such as clothing, linens, or gym mats; or, rarely, from the soil.

Incidence and Demographics
- Affects all ages, races, genders; African-American adults believed to have lower incidence.
- More common in tropical climates, warmer months in temperate climates
- More common in immunocompromised, including when secondary to prolonged use of topical steroids, with greater risk of intractable infection

Risk Factors
- Heat and humidity
- Obesity
- Immunocompromise: decreases host resistance to fungal infection
- Diabetes

Prevention and Screening
- Climate control as appropriate: Air conditioning; loose, cotton clothing
- Management of obesity
- Air drying or using an electric hair dryer to completely dry intertriginous areas
- Completely dry athletic shoes between wearings
- Frequently changing shoes, white cotton socks during day; wearing sandals
- Do not share combs, brushes, or hair ornaments
- Avoid occlusive ornaments: acrylic nails; synthetic jewelry, belts, shoes

Assessment
HISTORY
- Known exposure to others with tinea or high-risk population
- Mild to moderately pruritic localized "rash" or isolated lesion

PHYSICAL EXAM
- Presentation differs based on location of lesion: Tinea corporis (scalp), tinea manus (hand), tinea facialis (face); exposed areas, commonly known as ringworm
  - Scaling erythematous plaque ranging from <1 cm up to 20 cm
  - Varying shapes: Annular (round), arciform, or polycyclic
  - With or without pustules/vesicles
  - Usually has an elevated, sharp border with central clearing
  - Color is erythematous or hyperpigmented
  - Tinea manuum may be bilateral (50%), may occur with tinea pedis or tinea cruris
  - May be confused with granuloma annulare, which is similar in appearance, but is a self-limiting condition of the hands, feet, elbows, and knees
- Tinea cruris (groin), commonly known as jock itch
  - Similar but usually arciform or polycyclic and duller red in coloring
  - Often coexists with tinea pedis; infection transferred from feet to groin
  - Maceration common in intertriginous areas
- Tinea pedis (foot), commonly known as athlete's foot
  - Erythema, maceration between toes
  - Diffuse desquamation with superficial white scales and possible bulla formation
  - Hyperkeratosis of soles
  - Painful fissuring/cracking along lateral borders of the soles and toe webs
  - Usually bilateral foot involvement
- Tinea versicolor (trunk and neck)
  - Superficial *Pityrosporum orbiculare* yeast that colonizes all human skin
  - Clinically significant only in some individuals
  - Hypo- or hyperpigmented nummular macules

– Discrete, scattered, or confluent patches
– Usually asymptomatic but may be mildly pruritic
- Trichomycosis (hair): Tinea capitis (head) and tinea barbae (beard)
    – Involve dermatophyte invasion of the hair follicle by *trichophyton* dermatophytes
    – Inflammation of the hair follicle, alopecia
    – Painful, boggy, suppurative nodules with crusting/scabs
- Onychomycosis (nail): Tinea unguium
    – Nails become white, brown, yellow, or black; thicken and surface becomes roughened; eventually separate from the nail bed

DIAGNOSTIC STUDIES
- Wood's lamp: Tinea capitis fluoresces green
    – Tinea versicolor fluoresces faint yellow-green scales
    – Tinea cruris does not fluoresce, but Wood's lamp exam can differentiate erythrasma, a bacterial infection that fluoresces coral-red
- KOH mount: Skin scrapings placed on a slide in 10%–30% KOH solution with a cover slip, viewed under a microscope after warming for 30–60 seconds, will demonstrate mycelia and hyphae.
    – Tinea versicolor appears as long hyphae and few buds ("spaghetti and meatballs")
- Fungal cultures can identify a fungus but usually take weeks to grow.
    – Indicated only when an infection is resistant to treatment

Differential Diagnosis
Based on location of lesions; includes many scaling skin disorders such as:
- Psoriasis
- Erythrasma
- Candidiasis
- Contact dermatitis
- Seborrhea
- Dyshidrotic eczema
- Atopic dermatitis
- Lichen simplex chronicus
- Lichen planus
- Pityriasis rubra pilari
- Pityriasis rosea
- Erythema migrans
- Polymorphic light eruption
- Phototoxic drug eruption
- SLE
- Beard folliculitis
- Scabies
- Impetigo
- Ecthyma

Management

NONPHARMACOLOGIC TREATMENT
- Treat chronic, immunocompromising conditions
- Follow preventive measures described above

PHARMACOLOGIC TREATMENT
- Initial treatment with topical antifungal preparations such as clotrimazole 1% (Lotrimin), ketoconazole 2% (Nizoral), terbinafine 1% (Lamisil): Apply to affected area including a 2-cm peripheral border and rub in bid.
- Topical selenium sulfide 2.5% shampoo to skin for 30 minutes, then wash off for tinea versicolor; repeat 2 weeks later.
- Systemic antifungal agents for widespread, recurrent, or resistant infections, as well as onychomycosis
- Ciclopirox (Penlac) 8% topical solution (nail lacquer) applied to nail and 5 mm surrounding skin daily (remove with alcohol weekly) for up to 48 weeks for onychomycosis.
- Dosage
  - Griseofulvin 250 – 500 mg bid (children >30 lbs: 5 mg/lb of body wt/day)
  - Ketoconazole (Nizoral) 200 mg qd (children >2 yrs: single dose of 3.3 to 6.6 mg/kg)
  - Terbinafine (Lamisil) 250 mg qd (not indicated in children)
  - Itraconazole (Sporanox) 200 mg qd (may use pulsing dose of 200 mg bid x 1 week, no meds x 3 weeks then repeat; not indicated in children)

LENGTH OF TREATMENT
- Resolution is slow and treatment length depends on the location of the dermatophytosis; all take several weeks
  - Tinea capitis and tinea barbae: 8–16 weeks
  - Tinea corporis, tinea manuum, tinea facialis: 4–6 weeks
  - Tinea cruris: 4–6 weeks
  - Tinea versicolor: 4–6 weeks
  - Tinea pedis: 4–12 weeks
  - Tinea unguium: 8–12 months

Special Considerations
- Side effects from systemic antifungal agents include hepatotoxicity and lowering of serum testosterone. LFTs should be evaluated prior to starting oral agents and q 4–6 weeks thereafter.
- Most antifungals are pregnancy category C; terbinafine is category B.
- Breastfeeding not recommended with antifungal use.

When to Consult, Refer, Hospitalize
- Refer to dermatologist for extensive involvement or unresponsive infection.
- Consider hospitalization for immunosuppressed patients with extensive disease.

Follow-Up
- Q 4 weeks for reevaluation and LFTs

EXPECTED COURSE
- Relapse is common

COMPLICATIONS
- Loss of hair, nail

Candidiasis (Moniliasis)

Description
- Yeast-like superficial fungus that causes pruritic rash on moist cutaneous and mucosal sites in vulnerable individuals when local immunity is interrupted.

Etiology
- *Candida* species (*Candida albicans* [most common], *Candida glabrata*, *Candida tropicalis*) that are normal inhabitants of mucosal surfaces and intestinal tracts of healthy individuals.
- Infection occurs when local or systemic immunity of the host is disrupted.

Incidence
- All ages, both sexes equally, and all races can be affected.
- In babies, most commonly occurs in the diaper region.

Prevention and Screening
- None

Risk Factors
- Predisposing factors that alter immunity; immunocompromised states: HIV and chronic debilitation
- Chemotherapy or broad-spectrum antibiotic therapy; diabetes or poly endocrinopathies
- Maceration from repeated immersion in water, skin folds
- Occlusive clothing that traps moisture such as diapers or rubber boots; diapers' plastic outer covering
- Hyperhidrosis (excessive sweating); obesity with redundant skin folds
- Corticosteroid use
- Pregnancy and oral contraceptives

Assessment
HISTORY
- Pruritic and/or burning sensation and rash in characteristic locations such as intertriginous areas, anogenital region, and redundant skin folds
- Painful or sensitive white, "stuck on" lesions of the oral mucosa with decreased taste and odynophagia ("thrush")
- White curd-like vaginal discharge usually associated with pruritus, external dysuria, and dyspareunia (vulvovaginitis)
- Painful fissuring of the foreskin of uncircumcised males with dysuria
- Painful, inflamed nail folds, discolored nails and a creamy discharge (paronychial candidiasis)
- Painful, congested ear canal with moist exudate (otitis externa)

PHYSICAL EXAM
- Bright red, smooth macules
- Maceration is typical of all intertriginous infections
- Scaling elevated border
- "Satellite" lesions: Similar macules outside main lesion
- Oral and vaginal candidiasis: White, stuck on but removable plaques on inflamed mucosa
- Balanoposthitis: Flattened pustules, edema, erosions, fissuring on erythematous surface of penis
- Candida otitis externa: Edematous ear canal with macerated appearance and moist, white, scaly exudate

DIAGNOSTIC STUDIES
- 5% KOH preparation under microscope demonstrates buds and pseudohyphae in clusters
- Cultures may be done to identify specific species but this is *usually* not done because it takes 1–2 weeks for results

Differential Diagnosis
ORAL CANDIDIASIS
- Hairy leukoplakia
- Pernicious anemia
- Geographic tongue
- Bite irritation

GENITAL CANDIDIASIS
- Bacterial vaginosis
- Lichen planus
- Condyloma acuminatum
- Scabies
- Inverse pattern psoriasis
- Erythrasma

INTERTRIGINOUS AREAS
- Eczema
- Atopic dermatitis
- Contact dermatitis
- Dermatophytosis

PARONYCHIAL CANDIDIASIS
- Herpetic whitlow
- *S. aureus* paronychia

Management
NONPHARMACOLOGIC TREATMENT
- Management of underlying predisposing factors such as obesity, diabetes
- Air exposure of affected areas, such as diaper region in infants
- Careful drying of intertriginous areas and redundant skin folds
- Wear cotton undergarments; avoid tight, synthetic clothing

PHARMACOLOGIC TREATMENT
- Oral (thrush)
  - Nystatin (Mycostatin) oral suspension 4–6 mL (adults), 2 mL (children), swish and swallow qid
  - Clotrimazole (Mycelex) 10 mg troches 3–5x/day (3 years and older), dissolve in mouth
  - Systemic ketoconazole (Nizoral) 200 mg po qd to bid (adults, usually not recommended in children), fluconazole (Diflucan) 100 mg po qd to big (adults; check manufacturer literature for children), itraconazole (Sporanox) 100 mg po qd (adults, not recommended for children)
  - Amphotericin B 3 mg/kg/day IV for resistant cases in immunocompromised hosts
- Intertriginous and anogenital infections
  - Castellani paint x 1
  - Topical antifungal: Clotrimazole 1% cream, miconazole (Monistat) 2% cream, ketoconazole 2% cream, econazole (Spectazole) 1% cream, terconazole (Terazol) 0.4 or 0.8% cream, terbinafine (Lamisil) 1% cream or solution bid, tolnaftate (Tinactin) 1% cream, solution, powder applied bid
  - Nystatin cream or ointment applied bid to tid to diaper area in infants
  - Oral antifungal treatment as described above may be necessary in extensive or recurrent infections or when host immunity is suppressed
  - Oral fluconazole (Diflucan 150 mg) x 1 has been successful in the treatment of vaginal candidiasis (see Chapter 13)

LENGTH OF TREATMENT
- Oral candidiasis: 10–14 days
- Intertriginous and anogenital candidiasis: One to several weeks, depending on extent of the infection and the immune status of the host
- Paronychial candidiasis: 2–4 weeks

Special Considerations
- Immunosuppressed patients are subject to extensive and recurrent infections and may require a daily maintenance dose to limit recurrences.

When to Refer, Consult, Hospitalize
- Immunosuppressed patients with extensive or severe candidiasis, particularly oral/esophageal candidiasis, may require hospitalization or home IV infusion therapy of amphotericin B and nutrition supplementation.

Follow-Up
- Patients should be seen in 2–4 weeks and PRN to evaluate progress.

EXPECTED COURSE
- Resolution can be expected in patients without immunosuppression but predisposing factors such as obesity and poorly controlled diabetes mellitus may make recurrences common

COMPLICATIONS
- Secondary infection of excoriated lesions
- Weight loss secondary to odynophagia with esophagitis

BACTERIAL INFECTIONS OF THE SKIN

Cellulitis

Description
- Acute bacterial infection of the dermis and subcutaneous tissues; spreads in rapid, diffuse manner
- Erysipelas is a type of cellulitis, usually of the face, caused by beta-hemolytic streptococci and accompanied by fever and malaise

Etiology
- Usually caused by beta-hemolytic streptococci and *Staphylococcus aureus*; may also be caused by *Haemophilus influenzae* in children, *Pseudomonas aeruginosa* from hot tubs, and *Pasteurella* from animal bite wounds, especially cats
- Occurs when a break in the skin allows bacteria to enter, most common in children <3 years and older adults

Incidence and Demographics
- Common in all age groups

Risk Factors
- Breaks in the skin from lacerations, abrasions, excoriations; underlying dermatosis; previous cellulitis
- Diabetes mellitus; hematologic malignancies
- IV drug use; immunocompromise; chronic lymphedema (after mastectomy or coronary artery grafting)

Prevention and Screening
- Discourage scratching; maintain short, clean nails
- Meticulous diabetic foot care

Assessment
HISTORY
- May be unaware of original break in skin
- Possible history of fungal infection or dermatitis of the affected area
- Possible fever, malaise, anorexia, pain increased with weight-bearing
- Possible airway occlusive symptoms if cellulitis involves the face (erysipelas)

PHYSICAL EXAM
- Puncture wound, fissure, or laceration may be visible
- Erythematous plaque that is edematous, hot, and tender with sharply defined, irregular border
- Vesicles, bullae, abscesses may be seen within the plaque

- Possible erythematous streaking (lymphangitis)
- Regional lymphadenopathy
- Toxic signs may be present, especially if the involved area is large or if the patient is immunocompromised or a child
- *Necrotizing fasciitis*, a deep infection of the subcutaneous tissue, appears as a large erythematous plaque with a central area of necrosis; beta-hemolytic streptococcus is usually the invading organism; staphylococcus may or may not be involved

DIAGNOSTIC STUDIES
- Culture lesion; blood cultures (false negatives in about 75% of the cases)
- In facial cellulitis, culture of cerebrospinal fluid
- Bone scan if lesion on heel or hand to rule out osteomyelitis
- CBC, WBC, and sedimentation rate are indicated if the patient appears toxic

Differential Diagnosis
- Deep vein thrombosis or thrombophlebitis
- Early contact dermatitis
- Giant urticaria
- Fixed drug eruption
- Necrotizing fasculitis
- Swelling over septic joint
- Erythema migrans
- Early herpes zoster

Management
NONPHARMACOLOGIC TREATMENT
- Rest, immobilization, and elevation of the involved extremity (bedrest if leg is involved)
- Application of hot, moist compresses x 20–30 minutes qid

PHARMACOLOGIC TREATMENT
- Oral antibiotics that cover Gram-positive organisms:
  - Dicloxacillin (Dynapen) 250–500 mg qid x 5–10 days (children: 12.5–25 mg/kg/day qid x 10 days)
  - Erythromycin 250–500 mg x 5–10 days (children: 30–50 mg/kg/day qid x 10 days)
  - Cephalexin (Keflex) 250–500 mg qid x 5–10 days (children: 25–50 mg/kg/day qid x 10 days)
- For human bites, amoxicillin/clavulanate (Augmentin) 875/125 mg bid (adults; see manufacturer recommendations for children)
- Ceftriaxone (Mefoxin) 250 mg to 1 g IM qd (same in children)
- Ceftriaxone 1 g IV qd for more severe infections (same in children)
- NSAIDs prn for analgesia, fever treatment, and to decrease inflammation

LENGTH OF TREATMENT
- 5–10 days, depending on the extent of involvement

Special Considerations
- Young children, immunocompromised patients, and patients with synthetic heart valves are at greater risk of toxicity and may warrant hospitalization.
- Medical management of predisposing conditions such as diabetes, IV drug use, malignancies, or chronic lymphedema will augment the treatment of the cellulitis.

When to Consult, Refer, Hospitalize
- Hospitalize if toxic symptoms, facial cellulitis, or debridement necessary
- Refer to surgeon or infectious disease specialist if the patient is not responding to therapy.

Follow-Up
- The erythematous plaque should be outlined with an indelible pen on initial assessment and the patient should return daily for first few days to monitor progression or regression of the involved area.

  EXPECTED COURSE
  - Resolution is expected in 5–10 days

  COMPLICATIONS
  - Toxicity or septicemia
  - Patients with diabetes may lose leg following severe cellulitis
  - Lymphedema may result from recurrent erysipelas

Impetigo

Description
- Primary or secondary superficial bacterial infection of the skin leading to nonbullous or bullous impetigo or to ecthyma, a deeper infection involving the dermis
- Characteristic skin lesion is a honey-colored crust
- Characterized by its autoinoculable nature

Etiology
- *S. aureus*, group A beta-hemolytic streptococci (GAS), or mixed bacteria
- Organism gains access through breaks in the integrity of the skin caused by trauma, scratching, scaling, or inflammation
- Secondarily infected preexisting dermatitis is "impetiginization"

Incidence and Demographics
- Accounts for 10% of all skin problems in general outpatient pediatrics
- More prevalent in urban areas with poverty and overcrowding
- More common in young children ages 2–7 years

Risk Factors
- Young age; may be endemic in day care centers or schools; contact sports
- Poor hygiene, crowded living conditions

Prevention and Screening
- Good hygiene, including keeping children's nails cut short

Assessment

HISTORY
- Rash that may or may not be pruritic that has been present for days to weeks
- Possible history of underlying dermatitis (atopic, contact)
- Possible exposure to household members or school/sports exposure

PHYSICAL EXAM
- Lesions can appear on skin in which the integrity has been disturbed
- Commonly found on the face, torso, and extremities
- Nonbullous: Small vesicles, pustules that rupture causing erosion and superficial honey-colored crusting often caused by *Streptococcus pyogenes*; regional lymphadenopathy present with fever
- Bullous: Large transparent flaccid vesicle or bullae containing clear yellow fluid on erythematous base; rupture easily and are often caused by *S. aureus*; rupture leaves a rim surrounding a moist shallow ulcer; often found in clothing-covered areas

DIAGNOSTIC STUDIES
- Diagnosis is primarily clinical; cultures may be warranted if diagnosis is in doubt or if the lesions fail to respond to an appropriate course of antibiotics
- Possible gram stain
- May want to perform serology for anti-DNAse beta to look for prior strep infection

Differential Diagnosis

- Excoriations
- Perioral dermatitis
- Seborrheic dermatitis
- Contact dermatitis
- Herpes simplex or zoster
- Dermatophytosis
- Scabies
- Stasis or atherosclerotic ulcers
- Varicella
- Staphylococcal scalded skin syndrome

Management

NONPHARMACOLOGIC TREATMENT
- Wash area with soap to remove crusts prior to applying topical antibiotic
- Wash all linens, wash cloths, etc., separately from other clothing
- Meticulous handwashing

PHARMACOLOGIC TREATMENT
- Mupirocin (Bactroban) 2% tid ointment topically to lesions (if limited) x 7–10 days
- Beta-lactamase–resistant oral antibiotics if widespread lesions (>0.3) or if topical treatment undesired

- Penicillin VK 250–500 mg qid x 10 days (children: 30–60 mg/kg/day qid x 10 days)
    - Erythromycin 250–500 mg qid x 10 days (children: 30–50 mg/kg/day qid x 10 days)
    - Dicloxacillin 500 mg qid x 10 days (children: 12.5–25 mg/kg/day qid x 10 days)
- If Pen VK or erythromycin is the drug of choice, cultures are warranted to ensure sensitivity to S. *aureus*
- If culture demonstrates methicillin-resistant S. *aureus*, vancomycin (Vancocin) is an alternative

LENGTH OF TREATMENT
- 10-day treatment is usually adequate; if patient is not responding to initial course, cultures should be done to demonstrate antibiotic sensitivity

Special Considerations
- Penicillin VK or erythromycin are drugs of choice in pregnant and lactating women.

When to Consult, Refer, Hospitalize
- Hospitalization is warranted in toxic-appearing patient.

Follow-Up
EXPECTED COURSE
- Generally resolved with 10-day course of antibiotics
- Patients should be instructed to return sooner if symptoms do not appear to be resolving or if condition appears to be spreading

COMPLICATIONS
- With nontreatment or noncompliance with medication regimen, infection may progress to lymphangitis, cellulitis, erysipelas, bacteremia, or septicemia
- GAS complications include guttate psoriasis, scarlet fever, glomerulonephritis
- Scarring often occurs after healing of ecthyma

Folliculitis, Furuncle, and Carbuncle

Description
- Folliculitis is the local inflammation of hair follicles by infection or irritation; usually self-limiting.
- A furuncle (boil or abscess) is an infection deep in a hair follicle.
    - Furunculosis refers to several discrete furuncles.
- A carbuncle is a deeper abscess, involves subcutaneous tissue, arising in several contiguous hair follicles, interconnected by sinus tracts; may have several pustular openings onto skin; may be associated with systemic symptoms of fever and malaise.

Etiology
- Usually S. *aureus*, rarely other bacteria; hot tub folliculitis caused by P. *aeruginosa*
- Most common in hairy areas exposed to friction, pressure, and moisture

Incidence and Demographics
- Age: More common in children, adolescents, and young adults

Risk Factors
- Chronic staphylococcus carrier state (nares, axillae, anogenital, intestine)
- Obesity, poor hygiene, injection of drugs
- Metabolic abnormalities (chronic granulomatosis, high serum IgE), diabetes mellitus, HIV

Prevention and Screening
- Good hygiene, improvement in underlying factors such as diabetes and obesity

Assessment
HISTORY
- Folliculitis appears as single or multiple small pustules with possible mild erythema
- Furuncle and carbuncles present as painful, warm, erythematous lesions with central pustulation developing over days
- Carbuncles are sometimes accompanied by systemic symptoms of fever and malaise
- History of predisposing factors or prior boils

PHYSICAL EXAM
- Furuncle: Firm, tender nodule with a central necrotic plug. The nodule becomes fluctuant below the necrotic plug, usually with a pustule over the plug
- Carbuncle: Several adjacent, coalescing furuncles with multiple, loculated abscesses, draining pustules, and necrotic plugs
- Vital signs may indicate fever and tachycardia
- Local lymphadenopathy

DIAGNOSTIC STUDIES
- Laboratory studies are usually not indicated
- Gram staining usually demonstrates Gram-positive cocci with multiple neutrophils
- Culture and sensitivity may be done to confirm S. aureus or identify methicillin-resistant S. aureus or other bacteria that may be resistant to treatment
- Blood cultures are indicated if the patient remains febrile or appears toxic

Differential Diagnosis
- Ruptured epidermal or pilar cyst
- Hidradenitis suppurativa
- Necrotizing HSV

Management
NONPHARMACOLOGIC TREATMENT
- Warm, moist compresses or sitz baths x 10 minutes q 2–3 hours (usually all that is necessary for folliculitis)

• Incision and drainage required for furuncle and carbuncle if large or pointing (pustule looks "ripe"); sterile packing is often necessary to allow the incision to continue to drain
• Washing daily with antibacterial soap; clean razors and personal items; change towels daily

PHARMACOLOGIC TREATMENT
• Topical antibiotics usually are not effective
• Mupirocin ointment (Bactroban) tid to nares is helpful in eliminating chronic S. aureus carrier state, or applied after shower to prevent recurrence
• Systemic antibiotics usually indicated for multiple furuncles and carbuncles, marked inflammation, or immunocompromised
    − Dicloxacillin (Dynapen) 250–500 mg qid; children: 12.5–50 mg/kg/day in divided doses
    − Cephalexin (Keflex) 250–500 mg qid; children: 25–50 mg/kg/day in divided doses
    − Amoxicillin and clavulanic acid (Augmentin) 250–500 mg; children: 20–40 mg/kg/day in divided doses
    − EES 400 mg tid; children: 30–50 mg/kg/day in divided doses
    − Clarithromycin (Biaxin) 250–500 mg bid
    − Azithromycin (Zithromax) 250 mg qd
    − Clindamycin (Cleocin) 150–300 mg qid
• Methicillin-resistant S. aureus (MRSA)
    − Minocycline (Minocin) 100 mg bid (adults); 4 mg/kg initially, then 2 mg/kg bid (children >8 years)
    − Trimethoprim-sulfamethiazole DS (Bactrim or Septra) bid; 8 mg/kg/day based on trimethoprim divided bid (children >2 months)
    − Ciprofloxacin (Cipro) 500 mg bid (18 and older only)
    − Rifampin (Rifadin) may be added to one of the above antibiotics
    − Vancomycin IV for severe infections

LENGTH OF TREATMENT
• 7–10 days

Special Considerations
• Erythromycin should be used in pregnant or lactating women.

When to Consult, Refer, Hospitalize
• Consult with physician if large furuncle or carbuncle requiring incision and drainage.
• Referral to general surgeon is indicated for extensive abscess involvement or recurrent.

Follow-Up
• Daily follow-up initially to monitor response and to remove packing from surgical site
    ### COMPLICATIONS
    • Bacteremia and possible seeding of heart valves, joints, spine, long bones, and viscera
    • Cavernous venous thromboses and meningitis

VIRAL SKIN INFECTIONS

Herpes Simplex Virus (HSV)

Description
- Recurrent viral mucocutaneous infection spread by skin-to-skin, skin-to-mucosa, or mucosa-to-skin contact; only known to affect humans
- Sites of involvement include the vermillion border of the lips, buccal mucosa, gingiva, cheeks, distal tips of fingers (herpetic whitlow), anogenital region
- Genital HSV infection is a sexually transmitted disease
- Requires break in normal skin integrity for initial cutaneous infection; asymptomatic until provoked

Etiology
- Herpes simplex virus type 1 and type 2. HSV replicates within epithelial cells, lyses them, and then produces a thin-walled vesicle.
- HSV type 2 usually associated with genital lesions.
- The virus migrates within several hours along sensory neurons to nerve root ganglia, where it then resides in a latent state.
- Viral reactivation occurs during periods of physical or emotional stress, although the exact mechanism of stimulating reactivation is unclear.
- When reactivated, it migrates back to the skin along sensory nerves, producing typical lesions.

Incidence and Demographics
- Most often affects young adults, but can affect any age

Risk Factors
- Intimate skin-to-skin or skin-to–mucous membrane contact with an infected person during stages of viral shedding; the virus is not stable at room temperature and therefore is unlikely to be spread through fomites or aerosol
- Contagious during the prodromal and vesicular stages
- Sun exposure to face; viral upper respiratory infection
- Altered hormonal status (menstruation)
- Immune status alteration (HIV, malignancy, chemotherapy, systemic corticosteroids, irradiation)

Prevention and Screening
- Safe sex practices; avoidance of close contact while symptomatic

Assessment
HISTORY
- May not be aware of contact with infected person (incubation period 2–20 days; average 6 days)
- The initial or primary outbreak of HSV may range from very minor to severe, with grouped vesicles at the site of exposure
- Commonly associated with regional lymphadenopathy, malaise, muscle pain, headaches, and possible fever

- In childhood, most often presents as acute gingivostomatitis with multiple shallow, painful ulcers; fever; hyper-salivation; and lymphadenopathy
- Recurrences preceded by prodromal tingling or aching at the site of previous lesions; may be less severe, no systemic symptoms

PHYSICAL EXAM
- Thin-roof, grouped vesicles on erythematous bases, often at border of lips, penis, labia, buttocks
- Vesicles burst, with shallow ulcer exposed with crusting and ulcerations, then crust and dry over 1 week
- Regional lymphadenopathy, malaise, muscle pain, headaches, and possible fever

DIAGNOSTIC STUDIES
- Tzanck smear microscopic exam (Wright's or Giemsa's stain) would demonstrate giant, multinucleated epidermal cells
- Herpes culture or DNA probe of exudate from pierced vesicle or scraping from crusted ulcer (may get false-negative results from crusted lesions or after the initial 24–48 hours of an outbreak when viral shedding has slowed or ceased)
- Little clinical value from HSV serology

Differential Diagnosis
- Aphthous stomatitis
- Herpangina
- Chancroid
- Syphilis
- Pyoderma
- Trauma
- Hand, foot, and mouth disease
- Impetigo
- Herpes zoster
- Erythema multiform

Management
NONPHARMACOLOGIC TREATMENT
- Sitz baths, cool compresses, Burrow's solution for comfort
- Safe sex practices of limited value; condoms do not reduce risk of transmission as viral shedding occurs along a wide area of the groin/perineal region
- Sunscreen may prevent outbreaks in infected persons

PHARMACOLOGIC TREATMENT
- Oral antivirals are usually not indicated for adults unless infection is genital (see Chapter 13 for genital herpes treatment)
- Acyclovir (Zovirax) 15 mg/kg per day in divided in 5 doses x 7 days in children with gingivostomatitis; for adults, 200 mg 5 times daily or 800 mg tid or valacyclovir 1000 mg bid or famciclovir 250 mg tid
- Topical 5% acyclovir q2h (only approved indication is for treatment of initial outbreak in immunocompromised patients) x 5 days
- Penciclovir (Denavir) cream q2h x 4 days (indicated for treatment of recurrent oro-labial herpes; has only been shown to reduce average attack from 5 to 4.5 days)

- Prophylactic acyclovir 400 mg bid; valacyclovir 500 mg qd or Famciclovir 125–250 mg bid when risk of triggers high (UV light exposure, dental or oral surgery)

Special Considerations
- Treatment of an initial outbreak of herpes genitalis during pregnancy is recommended because the risk to the fetus of complications from a severe and prolonged outbreak outweighs the risk of complications from medications.
- Patients with frequent outbreaks should be evaluated for other STDs, including HIV.
- HIV+ patients with CD4 <50 should be on prophylactic oral therapy; topical therapies not effective.

When to Consult, Refer, Hospitalize
- Consult with physician if hospitalization required for IV therapy if immuno-compromised with widespread disease.

Follow-Up
- Routine follow-up not necessary unless severe
    - EXPECTED COURSE
        - Usual resolution of symptoms within 2 weeks for first occurrence, 5–7 days for recurrences
        - Recurrences become less frequent with passage of time

    - COMPLICATIONS
        - Secondary infection of lesions
        - Post-inflammatory hyperpigmentation
        - Erythema multiforme

Herpes Zoster

Description
- "Shingles;" acute, painful, unilateral, localized vesicular cutaneous infection in a dermatomal pattern

Etiology
- Varicella zoster virus (VZV), usually contracted in childhood as chickenpox
- Lies dormant in a nerve ganglion; reactivation of virus causes eruption along course of the nerve; cause of reactivation unclear

Incidence and Demographics
- Occurs most often in persons older than 50; less than 10% of cases occur under age 20

Risk Factors
- Immunosuppression, advanced age; previous infection with varicella
- Trauma to the sensory ganglia

Prevention and Screening
- Varicella vaccine now included in routine childhood immunization schedule may prevent development of herpes zoster in later life.
- Varicella vaccine later in life when anti-VZV antibodies are declining may be effective in preventing development of herpes zoster; now recommended at age 60+ years.

Assessment

HISTORY
- Pain (piercing, stabbing, boring), paresthesias (tingling, burning, itching), and allodynia (heightened sensitivity to mild stimuli) along neuronal pathway preceding eruption by 3–5 days; may mimic internal pathology
- Generalized malaise, fever, and headache in about 5%

PHYSICAL EXAM
- Initially grouped vesicles along a unilateral dermatomal pathway, followed by bullae within 2 days (more than one contiguous dermatome may be involved but noncontiguous dermatome involvement is rare)
- By day 4, vesicles become pustules, followed by crusting in 7–10 days
- Lesions occur on erythematous, edematous cutaneous base

DIAGNOSTIC STUDIES
- Diagnosis can be made clinically
- Tzanck smear, serum VZV antibodies, viral culture

Differential Diagnosis
- Herpes simplex
- Contact dermatitis
- Erysipelas
- Bullous impetigo
- Poison ivy or oak
- Necrotizing fasciitis

Management

NONPHARMACOLOGIC TREATMENT
- Moist dressings (water, normal saline, or Burrow's solution) may decrease pain

PHARMACOLOGIC TREATMENT
- Acyclovir (Zovirax) 800 mg 5 times daily
- Valacyclovir (Valtrex) 1000 mg tid
- Famciclovir (Famvir) 500 mg tid
- IV acyclovir 10 mg/kg tid
- IV foscarnet (Foscavir) for acyclovir-resistant strains
- Pain management with narcotic pain medications or NSAIDs

LENGTH OF TREATMENT
- 7 to 10 days

Special Considerations
- Most common risk factor is the decreasing immunity, putting those with advancing age and immunocompromised conditions most at risk.

When to Consult, Refer, Hospitalize
- Disseminated infection may require hospitalization or in-home IV therapy
- Patients with corneal involvement require ophthalmology evaluation

Follow-Up
- Follow up in 2 weeks to ensure it is resolving.
  - EXPECTED COURSE
    - Initial course generally resolved in 2–3 weeks

  - COMPLICATIONS
    - Postherpetic neuralgia
    - Local hemorrhage, gangrene, or secondary infection
    - Systemic meningoencephalitis, cerebral vascular syndrome, cranial nerve syndromes (ophthalmic, trigeminal, facial, and auditory), peripheral motor weakness

Human Papilloma Virus/Verruca/Warts

Description
- Discrete, benign, epithelial hyperplasia on skin and mucous membranes
  - Vulgaris: Common wart, no particular location
  - Plantaris: Plantar wart, plantar surface of foot; plana: flat wart

Etiology
- Infection caused by human papillomaviruses, DNA viruses of which at least 70 types have been described; have incubation period of 1–6 months; 65% have spontaneous resolution in 12–24 months, but some persist for years
- Many varieties identified with specific morphology and predilection for different anatomical sites
- Most warts are benign; subtypes that infect the cervix known to have oncogenic potential; also sexually transmitted

Incidence and Demographics
- Occurs in all ages and races, most frequently seen in 10% of school-age children and 5% of adults
- Immunocompromised persons at greater risk for clinically widespread disease

Risk Factors
- Skin-to-skin contact
- Household contact
- HIV+

Prevention and Screening
- Education about contagious nature of virus and avoidance of contact

Assessment

HISTORY
- Painless skin lesion present from days to months, possibly with known exposure (incubation period 2–9 months)
- Plantar warts generally become painful with weight bearing
- Warts may bleed if disrupted by shaving or scratching
- May be mildly pruritic, especially if secondarily infected

PHYSICAL EXAM
- Verruca vulgaris or "common warts": Firm, hyperkeratotic 1–10mm papules with surface cleft
  - Usually flesh-colored and discrete
  - May be vegetative
  - Characteristic black puncta, or "dish-brown dots," are thrombosed capillary loops, best seen with hand lens; may only be apparent after paring callused surface
  - Common on hands, fingers, and knees (sites of trauma), pressure points on feet
- Verruca plantaris or "plantar warts": Flesh-colored, rough, hyperkeratotic papules or plaques (possible mosaic configuration) with black puncta on plantar surface of feet
- Verruca plana or "flat warts": Small, skin-colored, flat-topped ("mesa-like") 1–5 mm papules
  - Usually round or oval
  - Always discrete and closely set multiple lesions that sometimes appear in a linear configuration (autoinoculation from scratching)
  - Found on face, hands, or shins

DIAGNOSTIC STUDIES
- Clinical with black puncta pathognomonic; suspicious lesions should be sent for pathology evaluation

Differential Diagnosis
- Molluscum contagiosum
- Seborrheic keratosis
- Actinic keratosis
- Clavus or callus of feet
- Condylomata lata
- Squamous cell carcinoma
- Imbedded foreign body

Management

NONPHARMACOLOGIC TREATMENT
- Warts of the hand: Laser surgery, electrodesiccation, cryotherapy (liquid nitrogen)
- Apply opaque (duct) tape to verruca plantaris or planus, change weekly (shown to be as effective as other treatments)

PHARMACOLOGIC TREATMENT
- Verruca vulgaris: Keratolytic agents (salicylic or lactic acids); OTC salicylic acid (Compound W, DuoPlant) preparations applied nightly; soak in warm water 10 minutes, dry and "sand" lesion with emery board before applying product; cover with bandaid or tape to increase effectiveness; apply daily
- Verruca plantaris: Same as with vulgaris, except use higher potency product
- Verruca planus: Retinoic acid A or salicylic acid applied daily
- Anogenital warts: Podophyllin topical application every 1–2 weeks ; bi- or trichloroacetic acid topical application every 1–2 weeks; imiquimod 5%
- Systemic H-2 blockers such as cimetidine (Tagamet) or ranitidine (Zantac) bid for persistent warts in children that are along the vermillion border of lip or eyelid, are very extensive, or treatment is painful

LENGTH OF TREATMENT
- 4–12 weeks

Special Considerations
- Podophyllin is contraindicated in pregnant and lactating women.
- *Molluscum contagiosum* is another cutaneous viral infection (poxvirus) with characteristic pearly white papules 1–2 mm in size with umbilicated center.
  - Spontaneous regression occurs in 6 months unless immunocompromised
  - Widespread involvement in the immunocompromised; requires treatment as above

When to Consult, Refer, Hospitalize
- Consult with dermatology for inadequate resolution with above regimens.

Follow-Up
- For treatment in office as indicated

EXPECTED COURSE
- 50%–60% spontaneously regress within 2 years
- 65% of patients have recurrences regardless of treatment

COMPLICATIONS
- Scarring, postinflammatory hyperpigmentation

PARASITIC INFESTATIONS AND BITES

Scabies

Description
- Infestation by scabies mite, spread by direct contact; leads to generalized pruritus, a hypersensitivity reaction to the scabies excretions

Etiology
- *Sarcoptes scabiei* that thrive and multiply only on human skin; spread by human-to-human contact; may live up to 2 days on clothing and bed linens

- Sensitization to S. *scabiei* must occur prior to developing the generalized pruritus associated with an infestation. For persons with an initial infestation, sensitization takes about 10 days; subsequent infestations progress to the pruritic stage much more quickly.

Incidence and Demographics

- Common in young children under the age of 5 through direct contact; in young adults, usually through sexual contact; and in the elderly and infirm in residential facilities; worldwide distribution
- Epidemics occur in cycles; incubation 4–6 weeks

Risk Factors

- Institutional living
- Immunocompromised status

Prevention and Screening

- Prompt treatment and washing of linens, etc.

Assessment

HISTORY
- Usually can give history of close contacts with similar symptoms
- Severe generalized pruritus sparing head and neck, with initial infestation about 1 month after exposure; with reinfestation, pruritus begins immediately
- Pruritus and scratching often interfere with sleep

PHYSICAL EXAM
- Characteristic scattered vesicles, burrows, or nodules: gray or skin-colored ridge, serpiginous or straight, 2 mm to a few cm in length; with excoriations
- Common distribution: axillae, anogenital region, wrists, hands (webs of fingers), waist, and flexor surfaces of elbows
- May develop generalized erythroderma; may also develop lichen simplex chronicus
- In atopic individuals, an eczematous dermatitis is common
- Postinflammatory hyperpigmentation may occur; secondary infections to denuded sites are common
- Crusted vesicles or burrows result after infestation of several months

DIAGNOSTIC STUDIES
- Serum eosinophilia
- Microscopic identification by placing a drop of mineral oil over a burrow and scraping the burrow with a blade. Mites, eggs, or fecal droppings can be identified on slide

Differential Diagnosis

- Drug eruption dermatitis
- Atopic or contact dermatitis
- Pityriasis rosea
- Herpetiform dermatitis
- Pediculosis dermatitis
- Insect bites

- Impetigo
- Delusions of parasitosis
- Metabolic pruritus

Management

NONPHARMACOLOGIC TREATMENT

- Wash all bedding and clothing in washing machine with hot soapy water and hot dry cycle at time of treatment; seal nonwashable clothing and articles in plastic bag for 1 week
- Lubricants may help reduce itching

PHARMACOLOGIC TREATMENT

- Management of pruritus relies on pharmacologic treatment for eradication of the mites and their eggs, and pharmacologic treatment of pruritus
- Lindane 1% cream overnight (8–12 hours) x 1; avoid in children and pregnant women
- Permethrin (Elimite) 5% cream overnight (8–14 hours) x 1 (able to be used on infants from 2 months and older and by pregnant women)
- A tapered course of systemic steroids starting at 70–80 mg qd and tapering by 5 mg qd is often necessary to treat wide spread pruritus
- Topical steroids bid to severely pruritic areas
- Systemic antihistamines such as diphenhydramine (Benadryl) 25–50 mg q 4–6 hours for treatment of pruritus

LENGTH OF TREATMENT

- One-time treatment with lindane or permethrin may be effective, but a repeat treatment in 14 days is often necessary to eliminate infestation
- Systemic steroids are generally tapered over 10–14 days
- Systemic antihistamines are used on an as-needed basis

Special Considerations

- Lindane contraindicated if pregnant, lactating, or child under 2 years of age.
- Lindane known to cause seizures if used just after a bath or in patients with extensive dermatitis.
- Lindane-resistant cases may occur; try permethrin.

When to Consult, Refer, Hospitalize

- Refer to dermatologist when resolution is not achieved with above regimens.

Follow-Up

- Patients should be brought back for follow-up in 1–2 weeks, then at weekly intervals if there is extensive dermatitis.

EXPECTED COURSE

- Mites may be eradicated with one or two treatments, but the generalized pruritus may persist for several weeks since it is a hypersensitivity reaction to the mite

COMPLICATIONS

- Secondary infection, abscesses, and/or cellulitis due to scratching

Insect Bites and Stings

Description
- Very common injury in children and all ages, caused by flying or crawling insects
- Kinds of insects include ticks, bees or wasps, fleas, and chiggers
- Two U.S. spiders are known to bite humans and are capable of producing severe reactions: brown recluse and black widow

Etiology
- Spider venom is composed of enzyme-spreading factor and a toxin distributed by the enzyme (not an allergic reaction); causes toxic reaction with possible systemic symptoms
- Many bites cause allergic reactions with local or systemic symptoms, immediate or delayed
- Anaphylaxis is possible
- Mosquitoes are the most common insects that afflict children, usually cause local reactions

Incidence and Demographics
- More common in the late spring or summer months
- Flea bites occur year round
- Spiders live in dark areas such as closets, under porches, and in wood piles; are most common in southern regions, but can be found anywhere in U.S.

Risk Factors
- Playing or walking in grassy or wooded areas
- Wearing bright-colored clothing or perfumed products

Prevention and Screening
- Avoid infested areas
- Apply insect repellents (containing less than 10% diethyltoluamide [DEET] or permethrin) before going outside
- Wear neutral-colored clothing, avoid scented products
- Apply permethrin to clothing
- Wear protective clothing such as long pants and shirts
- Carefully check for ticks after a hike in potentially tick-infested areas
- Eliminate fleas from living areas with powders or spray

Assessment
HISTORY
- Recent exposure to insect-infested areas; report of feeling a bite or sting
- Swelling, pain, or pruritus of affected area
- May be complaints of nausea, vomiting, diarrhea, headache, fever, lightheadedness, flushing, hives, dyspnea, wheezing

PHYSICAL EXAM
- Presentation varies due to different insects and individual reaction
- Mosquitoes: scattered erythematous pruritic wheals with central punctum

- Fleas: Irregularly grouped or linear urticarial wheals or papules with central punctum
- Bees and wasps: Redness, edema, pain, pruritus, induration
- Chiggers: Discrete bright red papules on legs and belt line
- Distribution usually on exposed areas of skin, except fleas (areas where clothing is snug)
- Spiders: Swelling and erythema at site, and may develop more severe reactions in areas of fatty subcutaneous tissue; necrosis can develop in 4 hours
- Wheezing, hypotension, change in mental status may present in anaphylaxis

DIAGNOSTIC STUDIES
- None

Differential Diagnosis
- Varicella
- Impetigo
- Scabies

Management
NONPHARMACOLOGIC TREATMENT
- Cool compresses or ice; colloidal oatmeal baths
- Remove stinger or tick if visible

PHARMACOLOGIC TREATMENT
- Symptomatic treatment of pruritus: Pramoxine (topical anesthetic), topical steroids, oral antihistamines
- Oral corticosteroids if more severe pruritus and swelling
- Update tetanus prophylaxis as needed
- Epinephrine and other emergency measures for anaphylactic reactions
    - Dose of epinephrine 1:1,000 (aqueous) 0.01 mL/kg per dose administered subcutaneously; infants/children: 0.01 mg/kg, max 0.5mg/dose; adults: 0.1–0.5 mg, max dose 1 mg
    - If life-threatening systemic anaphylaxis occurs, call 911 and emergency transport; give epinephrine as above; start IV, oxygen, inhaled albuterol (Proventil) nebulizer if bronchospasm severe

LENGTH OF TREATMENT
- Until symptoms relieved, usually 48 hours

Special Considerations
- Papular urticaria, a hypersensitivity reaction, may develop secondary to bites from mosquitoes, fleas, or other insects—grouped urticarial papules with a central punctum, vesicles, pustules, bullae. This reaction usually occurs in the first decade of life, and may last for 1–2 years.
- Secondary infection may develop.

When to Consult, Refer, Hospitalize
- Transfer to acute care facility for anaphylactic reaction

Follow-Up
- None usually necessary unless urticaria or more serious reaction
  COMPLICATIONS
  - Spider bites by brown recluse or black widow can cause tissue necrosis

Pediculosis Capitis And Pubis

Description
- An infestation with one of the three species of parasitic lice that affect humans: *Pediculus humanus capitis*, *Pediculus humanus corporis*, or *Pthirus pubic*, which are wingless, blood-sucking insects
- Infestation of the scalp, body, or pubic hair causing mild pruritus and excoriation

Etiology
- Incubation period from egg to hatching is 6–10 days; lice mature in 2–3 weeks and then lay eggs
- Lice need to ingest blood every few hours; can survive on fomites >2 days

Incidence and Demographics
- All ages, but pediculosis capitis more common in children (estimated up to 10 million children in the U.S. infected annually); pediculosis pubis more common in young adults, spread through close physical or sexual contact, sharing bed linens
- Head lice uncommon in African-American population

Risk Factors
- Shared hats, combs, head–head contact; epidemics of head lice in schools
- Sexual promiscuity and poor personal hygiene for pubic lice

Prevention and Screening
- Education of parents, children, and school personnel about the modes of transmission and to avoid sharing hats, combs, etc.
- Educating young adults about the modes of transmission and to avoid sexual promiscuity

Assessment
  HISTORY
  - Mild pruritus of scalp and nape of neck, pubis, or axilla for days to weeks
  - Only symptom in child may be restlessness
  - Sexual contact with affected individual; poor personal hygiene

  PHYSICAL
  - Pediculosis capitis
    - 2–5 mm mobile lice are often difficult to find; usually fewer than 10 lice per infestation
    - More commonly found are the small (1.0 mm), creamy, yellowish-white nits adherent to shaft of hair as it emerges from the scalp; anywhere from a few to thousands of nits may be found on one scalp
    - White nits farther from the scalp indicate a longer-standing infection (hair grows approximately 0.5mm/day)

– Excoriations, crusting, purulent exudate (plica polonica), eczematous dermatitis, or papular urticaria and lichen simplex chronicus along nape of neck
– Regional lymphadenopathy may be found with long-standing infestation or extensive excoriations and crusting
• Pediculosis pubis
  – Lice appear as 1–2 mm brownish-gray adherent dots on hair in the pubic region, perineum, axillae, and torso
  – Nits: Whitish-gray dots on hair shaft
  – Papular urticaria: Slate-gray or bluish-gray 0.5–1 cm nonblanching macules
  – Excoriations, crusting, purulent exudate, regional adenopathy

DIAGNOSTIC STUDIES

• Mainly a clinical diagnosis, but may be confirmed by microscopic exam of lice, which demonstrates a 1–4 mm 6-legged insect with a gray-white body that may be engorged with blood, or nits which are <0.5 mm yellowish-white eggs or, in the case of an older nit, an empty, translucent white egg
• Wood's lamp demonstrates pearly fluorescence of live nits
• Bacterial cultures confirm secondary infection and sensitivity

Differential Diagnosis

• Hair spray/lacquer
• Eczema
• Tinea cruris
• Dandruff
• Neurotic excoriation
• Impetigo
• Contact or seborrheic dermatitis
• Scabies

Management

NONPHARMACOLOGIC TREATMENT

• Vacuuming carpets and furniture; washing clothing and linens in hot water and using hot dryer; and soaking combs, brushes, and hair ornaments in rubbing alcohol are all effective means of controlling the environment to prevent spread or reinfection with lice
• The hair should be combed with a fine-toothed comb after treating to remove adherent nits
• Wetting the hair with white vinegar prior to combing loosens the nits to facilitate removal
• In resistant cases, applying an oily substance such as mayonnaise, leaving on overnight, and shampooing out in morning may be effective
• Children may return to day care or school the day after treatment
• Seal unwashable articles in a plastic bag for 10 days

PHARMACOLOGIC TREATMENT

• Permethrin shampoo (Nix) or pyrethrin shampoo (RID), worked well into the hair and scalp and left on for 10 minutes; re-treat in 1 week
• Lindane 4% shampoo left on for 4 minutes

   – Ovide lotion, 0.5% malathion in an alcohol and pine needle solution, may
      be used as alternative
   • Secondarily infected lesions should be treated with appropriate antibiotics
   • Treat nits on eyebrows and eyelashes with petroleum jelly; apply tid 8–10 days
      and comb out nits

   ### LENGTH OF TREATMENT
   • Once, with retreatment in 1 week

Special Considerations
• Lindane not recommended for pregnant and lactating women or children under 2 years.

When to Consult, Refer, Hospitalize
• Usually not necessary

Follow-Up
• Patients should be reevaluated in 1 week and retreated if any nits or lice remain.
   #### EXPECTED COURSE
   • Reinfection is likely if schools are not notified and other children are not
      evaluated and treated, or if sexual contacts or bed partners are not treated

   #### COMPLICATIONS
   • Secondary infection, excoriated lesions

TUMORS

Basal Cell Carcinoma

Description
• Slow-growing carcinoma that most commonly presents as a papule or nodule that may
   have central umbilication, progressing to significant ulceration; no risk of metastasis,
   but can produce significant cosmetic deformity. Most commonly seen skin cancer,
   arising on sun-exposed areas.

Etiology
• Excess sun exposure, particularly in fair-skinned individuals
• Slow-growing, common skin cancer that is a result of proliferating atypical basal cells
   with various amounts of stroma; requires a hair follicle to develop.
• Can become invasive if located on the face, in the ear canal, or in the posterior
   auricular sulcus; metastasis is rare

Incidence and Demographics
• Age >40; male > female
• 400,000 cases per year
• Dark skin rarely affected

Risk Factors
- Excess sun exposure (especially sunburns in youth), fair skin with poor tanning ability
- Prior treatment with x-ray for facial acne

Prevention and Screening
- Education about risk of excess sun exposure, should start with young children
- Monthly skin self-exam, yearly clinical exam

Assessment
HISTORY
- Patients may or may not be aware of suspicious lesions

PHYSICAL EXAM
- Waxy or "pearly" appearing firm, round, or oval papules or nodules on sun-exposed skin (80% on the face and neck); visible telangiectasia
- "Ulcer" or "sore" with a rolled border ("rodent bite ulcer"); central umbilication possible
- Crusting may be present; pink or red; pigmented lesions may be brown, blue, or black

DIAGNOSTIC STUDIES
- Biopsy demonstrating atypical basal cells

Differential Diagnosis
- Molluscum contagiosum
- Warts
- Cysts
- Scarring
- Other benign lesions
- Squamous cell carcinoma

Management
- Excision, cryosurgery, or electrosurgery
- Mohs surgery: Microscopically controlled surgery for lesions in the danger zones of nasolabial folds, around eyes, in ear canal and posterior auricular sulcus
- Radiation therapy is alternative in areas of possible cosmetic disfigurement
    LENGTH OF TREATMENT
    - Retreat if reoccurs

Special Considerations
- Reoccurrence or development of new lesion may occur within 5 years

When to Consult, Refer, Hospitalize
- Refer all suspected skin cancer to dermatologist or provider with experience in skin cancer assessment for biopsy.

Follow-Up

EXPECTED COURSE
- Resolution with above therapies is the norm, but at-risk patients should be followed to monitor for new lesions

COMPLICATIONS
- Cosmetic disfigurement

Squamous Cell Carcinoma

Description
- A skin malignancy that occurs on sun-exposed areas and may arise out of actinic keratoses on exposed parts in individuals who burn easily; develops in the course of a few months; approximately 5% potential for metastasis. Second most common type of skin cancer.
- Bowen's disease is carcinoma-in-situ arising on any area of skin.

Etiology
- Skin exposure to exogenous carcinogen such as sunlight, ionizing radiation
- Also arises from arsenic ingestion, tobacco, human papilloma virus
- Malignant growth of epithelial keratinocytes developing on skin and mucous membranes

Incidence and Demographics
- Higher incidence in Sunbelt states
- Age >55; male > female

Risk Factors
- Fair skin with poor tanning ability
- Sun exposure—outdoor workers and sportsmen
- Arsenic ingestion, tobacco use, radiation exposure
- Preexisting solar keratosis
- Organ transplant patients
- Cases around oral cavity and surrounding region and genitalia have greater risk of metastasis

Prevention and Screening
- Sun precautions; monthly skin self-exam, yearly clinical exam

Assessment

HISTORY
- Suspicious lesion developing over months to years
- Most often on sun-exposed skin (face, lips, hands, and forearms)

PHYSICAL EXAM
- Originate with small red nodule, papule, or plaque; progresses to induration
- Thick, adherent, keratotic scale
- Honey-colored exudate extruded from periphery
- May be eroded, crusted, ulcerated, hard, erythematous, isolated or multiple

DIAGNOSTIC STUDIES
- Biopsy demonstrating atypical squamous cells

Differential Diagnosis
- Basal cell carcinoma
- Malignant melanoma
- Actinic keratosis
- Paget's disease
- Other benign lesions

Management
- Immediate surgery or radiation depending on the size, shape, and location of the tumor
- Strict sun precautions for rest of life; lesions 2 cm or greater prone to recur
    LENGTH OF TREATMENT
    - Retreat if recurs

Special Considerations
- Any slowly evolving isolated keratotic lesion in a high-risk patient that persists for over 1 month is to be considered carcinoma until proven otherwise with a biopsy.

When to Consult, Refer, Hospitalize
- Refer all suspected skin cancer to dermatologist or provider with experience in skin cancer assessment for biopsy

Follow-Up
    EXPECTED COURSE
    - Remission achieved in 90% of cases
    - Follow up to monitor for reoccurrence annually and if patient reports change in any existing lesion; photographs of lesions can be kept for comparison of appearance

    COMPLICATIONS
    - Scarring and disfigurement

Malignant Melanoma

Description
- Least common but most lethal of all skin cancers; has a high risk of metastasis
- Classifications: Superficial spreading melanoma (most common), nodular melanoma (poorer prognosis), lentigo maligna melanoma, acral lentiginous melanoma (African-Americans and dark-skinned Caucasians), desmoplastic melanoma, and melanoma of the mucous membranes

Etiology
- Malignant growth of melanocytes
- Widely metastatic

Incidence and Demographics

- Only 3% of all skin cancers; accounts for two-thirds of skin cancer deaths
- Cases with lymph node involvement at time of diagnosis have a 5-year survival rate of 30%; those with distant metastasis, <10%
- More common in Sunbelt states

Risk Factors

- Positive family history, congenital nevi, familial dysplastic nevi syndrome
- Excessive sun exposure, outdoor occupation or sports
- Severe sunburn, particularly at an early age; fair skin

Prevention and Screening

- Sun exposure precautions
- Monthly skin self-exams and yearly clinical exams

Assessment

HISTORY

- New pigmented lesion or recent change in longstanding skin lesion
- Lesion that burns, itches, hurts, or bleeds

PHYSICAL EXAM

- Macule, papule, or nodule
- Colors ranging from pink to brown, blue, or black
- Borders most often irregular
- Size may vary from a few millimeters to centimeters
- The five cardinal signs of malignant melanoma are
    - **A**: Asymmetry
    - **B**: Border is irregular and often scalloped
    - **C**: Color is mottled with variegated display of brown, black, gray, and/or pink
    - **D**: Diameter is large (greater than 6.0 mm)
    - **E**: Elevation is almost always present with subtle or obvious surface distortion; best assessed by side-lighting of the lesion
- Five histopathologic types:
    - Superficial spreading malignant melanoma (most common)
    - Nodular malignant melanoma
    - Acral-lentiginous melanoma (palms of hands, soles of feet, nail beds)
    - Malignant melanomas of mucous membranes
    - Melanomas arising from blue or congenital nevi

DIAGNOSTIC STUDIES

- Biopsy including margins and depth of invasion assessment
- Lymph node biopsy is often also indicated

Differential Diagnosis

- Benign nevi
- Seborrheic keratosis
- Vascular skin lesions
- Squamous cell or basal cell carcinoma

Management
- Aggressive surgical management by excision with margins intact
- Chemotherapy for patients with high-risk melanomas to be managed by oncology specialist
  - LENGTH OF TREATMENT
    - To be determined by oncologist

Special Considerations
- Persons with skin phototype 1 or 2 should NEVER sunbathe and should always use sunscreens with a sun protection factor (SPF) of >30 (see Table 5–5 for skin phototype classifications).

Table 5–5. Skin Phototype Classifications

Skin Phototypes

1	Pale white	Does not tan; burns easily
2	White	Tans poorly; burns easily
3	White	Tans after initial burn
4	Light brown	Tans easily
5	Brown	Tans easily
6	Dark brown	Blackens

When to Consult, Refer, Hospitalize
- All suspected malignant melanomas should be referred to a dermatologist for biopsy.

Follow-Up
EXPECTED COURSE
- Prognosis based on staging of initial lesion
- Monthly skin self-exam; dermatology follow-up every 6 months for suspicious lesions
- All patients should be monitored annually for newly appearing and changing lesions; any lesion that is itchy or tender for more than 2 weeks needs to be evaluated

COMPLICATIONS
- Lung, liver, brain, bowel metastasis

OTHER INTEGUMENTARY CONDITIONS

Alopecia Areata

Description
- Sudden loss of hair in discrete oval patches
- Severity varies; may affect eyelashes, eyebrows, body hair, and nails
- Alopecia areata totalis involves the whole scalp; alopecia areata universalis involves all the body hair.

Etiology
- Not fully known, but most likely an autoimmune process

Incidence and Demographics
- Rarely occurs before age 4 years
- Of childhood and adult cases, half occur before age 20
- Recurrence is common

Risk Factors
- Positive family history in 20%
- Associated with trisomy 21, atopy, other autoimmune disorders

Prevention and Screening
- Screen during annual exam
- Prevention: None

Assessment

HISTORY
- Usually is asymptomatic except for the sudden (overnight or over a few days) loss of hair
- Occasionally there is burning or itching of the scalp just prior to the hair loss

PHYSICAL EXAM
- One or more well-circumscribed patches of hair loss appear suddenly
- Scalp is generally clear and unaffected, occasionally is slightly inflamed
- Hair at the periphery of the patches is easy to pull out
- "Exclamation point hairs" are pathognomonic; short hairs at the periphery with an attenuated bulb
- Fine nail pitting in approximately 20% of cases

DIAGNOSTIC STUDIES
- Usually none except to exclude other diagnoses: fungal cultures, KOH, scalp biopsy

Differential Diagnosis
- Tinea capitis
- Systemic disease, drugs, and toxins
- Trichotillomania
- Traumatic alopecia from cosmetic treatments
- Traction alopecia-tight braids, rollers
- Androgenic (male-pattern hair loss)

Management

NONPHARMACOLOGIC TREATMENT
- Education of child and parents about disease and course
- Support groups
- Hair pieces, hats, or head coverings
- Psychological counseling

PHARMACOLOGIC TREATMENT
• Controversial, as spontaneous resolution often occurs, but may include topical, systemic, or intralesional steroids, or topical minoxidil or anthralin

LENGTH OF TREATMENT
• Monitor and reassure for regrowth in 6–12 months

Special Considerations
• More diffuse, nonscarring hair loss may occur due to androgen hormonal changes, postpartum factors, systemic disease, weight loss, a wide variety of drugs and toxins, thyroid disease, lupus, and congenital syndromes.
• Scarring hair loss can occur with connective tissue diseases, skin diseases, burns, radiation, congenital disorders, and tumors.
• Trichotillomania is a type of traction alopecia due to self pulling of hair.

When to Consult, Refer, Hospitalize
• Refer to dermatologist if diagnosis is uncertain or scarring occurs.

Follow-Up
• Routine health maintenance exams

EXPECTED COURSE
• Course and prognosis is extremely variable, though there is often some resolution within 1–2 years
• Hair that regrows is often hypopigmented and fine; reoccurrence may occur

COMPLICATIONS
• Usually none

Psoriasis

Description
• A common benign, acute, or chronic skin disease with scaling papules and plaques in characteristic distribution

Etiology
• Alteration in cell kinetics of keratinocytes with shortening of cell turnover rate, resulting in increased production of epidermal cells; normal maturation of the skin cells cannot take place, keratinization develops.
• Unknown etiology and pathophysiology with genetic link

Incidence and Demographics
• Age: 75% type 1 early onset (age 16 years in females, 22 years in males); 25% type 2 late onset (56 years males and females)
• Race: 1%–2% of Caucasian population affected
• Rare in West Africans, Japanese, Alaskan Natives, and very rare in North and South American Indians
• Polygenic heredity

Risk Factors
- Trauma (Köbner's phenomenon—lesions develop in areas of trauma)
- Infections (streptococcal) can lead to Guttate psoriasis
- Drugs: Corticosteroids, lithium, interferon, beta-adrenergic blockers, and possibly alcohol can cause psoriasis drug eruptions
- Stress can lead to exacerbations
- Genetic predisposition

Prevention and Screening
- Stress management

Assessment

HISTORY
- Skin lesions usually with insidious onset, but may be acute
- Pruritus may or may not be present
- May be associated with acute systemic illness with fever and malaise
- May be associated with arthralgias/arthritis

PHYSICAL EXAM
- Morphology: Silvery-white scaling papules and plaques
- Distribution: Usually symmetrical; involves scalp, extensor surfaces, and areas subject to trauma (Köbner's phenomenon)
- Associated symptoms: May involve pitting of nails
- Characteristic scale attaches to skin at only one point and there is a drop of blood where scale peels off (Auspitz sign)
- Variations: Guttate psoriasis (drop-like lesions), pustular psoriasis, psoriatic arthritis

DIAGNOSTIC STUDIES
- None usually needed except to rule out other conditions
- Rheumatoid factor is negative in psoriatic arthritis

Differential Diagnosis
- Seborrheic dermatitis
- Tinea and candida
- Drug eruptions
- Eczema
- Lichen simplex chronicus

Management

NONPHARMACOLOGIC TREATMENT
- Avoid rubbing or scratching lesions
- Oatmeal baths for pruritus
- Avoid excessive sun exposure

PHARMACOLOGIC TREATMENT
- Topical fluorinated steroids with occlusive dressing (Cordran tape) for limited area
- Interlesional steroids
- Avoid general use of systemic steroids, which can cause rebound flares
- 2%–3% salicylic acid to peel off scales
- Systemic therapy: Methotrexate, Anthralin, oral retinoids, or hemodialysis
- UVB light with coal tar or psoralens; PUVA if UVB therapy fails
- Occlusive therapy with DuoDERM or Tegaderm for at least 7 days
- Calcipotriene ointment 0.005%; Tazarotene gel for mild to moderate involvement
- May require cyclosporin or sulfasalazine

LENGTH OF TREATMENT
- Treatment duration depends on type of psoriasis diagnosed, but primarily until flare-up subsides

Special Considerations
- Von Zumbusch acute pustular psoriasis is a life-threatening problem with acute onset. There is no known precipitating factor and the patient may or may not have had stable plaque-like psoriasis in the past.
- Requires emergency hospitalization

When to Consult, Refer, Hospitalize
- All patients should be referred to a dermatologist for confirmation of diagnosis and assistance in developing plan of care.

Follow-Up
- Routine follow-up with laboratory monitoring if systemic medications used.
  EXPECTED COURSE
  - Chronic condition requiring initial treatment phase and maintenance therapy

  COMPLICATIONS
  - Secondary infection

Burns

Description
- Thermal, electrical, or chemical injury causing damage to the epidermis, dermis, and/or subcutaneous tissue

Etiology
- Exposure to intense heat of fire or steam or to damaging chemicals or electrical voltage; the longer the contact with the skin, the greater the burn injury

Incidence and Demographics
- Approximately 1.25 million burn injuries annually in U.S.
- Flame burns most common in adults; scald burns more common in children
- Scald, tar, chemical, and electrical burns more common in the workplace

Risk Factors
- Firefighters
- Unsupervised children
- Workplace exposure to scalding liquids (tar, steam) and chemicals or electricity

Prevention and Screening
- Education on fire safety and safe handling of hot liquids, chemicals, and electricity in the community and workplace
- Remove from source and apply cold to stop the burning process

Assessment
HISTORY
- Exposure to fire, chemicals, scalding liquids, or electricity
- Intense pain at site of exposure, but third-degree burns are usually painless

PHYSICAL EXAM
- Burns are classified by extent and depth of tissue involvement, patient age, and associated illness or injury
- Patient's age and health status is critical; even minor burn on infant or elderly patient may be fatal
- Extent of involvement can be measured by using the "rule of nines"
    - Anterior head and neck = 4.5%
    - Posterior head and neck = 4.5%
    - Torso and abdomen = 18%
    - Back = 18%
    - Anterior arms = 4.5% each
    - Posterior arms = 4.5% each
    - Genitalia = 1%
    - Anterior legs = 9% each
    - Posterior legs = 9% each
    - Another estimate of extent of involvement is to equate the patient's palm size as 1% of total body size

- Depth of injury described as first-, second-, or third-degree burns
  - First degree burns: Superficial burns involving the epidermis only; redness and blanching erythema (demonstrating capillary refill) of affected area with no initial blistering
  - Second degree burns: Partial-thickness burns involve entire epidermis and variable portions of the dermis; red, moist, and edematous skin with small or large bullae
  - Third degree burns: Full-thickness burn involving entire dermis and subcutaneous tissue; pale, white, tan, or charred wound that may appear dry and depressed below surrounding skin; skin may feel tight and leathery

DIAGNOSTIC STUDIES
- Immediate clinical triage is essential to allow patients to be treated in most appropriate setting

Differential Diagnosis
- Contact dermatitis
- Herpes zoster
- Atopic dermatitis
- Child abuse
- Scalded skin syndrome

Management
- Office management: First-degree burns (e.g., sunburn)
  - Superficial second-degree burns of up to approximately 5%–6% total body surface area (TBSA) that do not affect areas of function or cosmesis
  - Selected deeper second-degree burns if not on lower extremities, hands, face, areas of function or cosmesis, or genitals that probably do not cover more than 1% to 2% TBS
  - Patient or family must be reliable and the home situation functional
- Emergency stabilization of serious burn patients following the advanced trauma life support (ATLS) guidelines including establishing and maintaining an airway, establishing vascular access, and instituting fluid resuscitation
  NONPHARMACOLOGIC TREATMENT
    - Burns involving the eye should be irrigated with water, saline, or lactated Ringer's solution
    - The wound should be cleaned and debrided using plain soap and water, Betadine diluted with water, or saline solution; remove any dead skin
    - Elevate involved extremities

  PHARMACOLOGIC TREATMENT
    - Topical silver sulfadiazine (Silvadene) in a 1/16-inch layer over entire surface, covered with nonabsorbent gauze (Kerlix or Telfa) and wrapped in at least a 3-inch thick nonadhesive wrap
    - Analgesia with narcotics or NSAID as needed
    - Tetanus prophylaxis
    - Antibiotic coverage for secondary infection

LENGTH OF TREATMENT
  • Dressing changes bid with frequent reevaluation until resolution

Special Considerations
• Very young, elderly, or debilitated patients are at higher risk for hemodynamic compromise.

When to Consult, Refer, and Hospitalize
• Refer patients with the following burn characteristics to a burn center:
  – Deep second-degree or third-degree burns
  – Burns of greater than 10% TBSA in patients <10 years and >50 years
  – Burns of greater than 20% TBSA in all other patients
  – Burns of the face, hands, and feet; over a joint or of the perineum; or burns that are circumferential
  – Burns resulting from child or adult abuse
  – Inhalation injury, electrical burns, chemical burns
  – Suspected toxic epidermal necrolysis syndrome

Follow-Up
• Within several days to ensure proper home wound management and evaluate for signs of infection; then possibly weekly until healed
    EXPECTED COURSE
      • Depends on the extent and location of the burn

    COMPLICATIONS
      • Hemodynamic compromise, multi-organ failure, sepsis
      • Scarring
      • Posttraumatic stress
      • Increased photosensitivity of healed skin

CASE STUDIES

Case 1. A 6-year-old male child presents to your clinic after playing outside all week while parents worked to clear a vacant adjacent lot. Within 2 days, the mother noticed the child to be scratching at legs. Upon close examination, an erythematous linear rash was noted on both lower extremities.
PMH: Asthma
Medications: Montelukast 5 mg po q pm and Albuterol inhaler prn

1. What pertinent history is it important to ask?
2. What is the most likely diagnosis based on this history?
3. What would you expect to find on physical exam?
4. Is he contagious?
5. How would you treat this patient?

Case 2. A 26-year-old White male comes in with a complaint of a "funny rash" on his back and across his shoulders that has resulted in "brown and white patches." He reports to you that he has had this rash for 6 months; however, his girlfriend noticed that the rash was spreading.
Social History: Works in an automobile factory and enjoys playing volleyball in his off time. Recently joined a church volleyball league.
PMH: Healthy, does not smoke, drinks 2–3 nights per week with friends

1. What pertinent history is it important to ask?
2. You note discrete, scattered, or confluent patches. Wood's lamp exam reveals faint yellow-green scales. What is the most likely diagnosis?
3. What laboratory tests would you order to confirm the diagnosis?
4. How would you treat this patient?

Case 3. A 5-year-old girl presents to the clinic with skin lesions that the mother reports were at first vesicular by description and have now become honey-crusted. They are in various stages of healing on her face, arms, and legs. Nothing itches at all. Has had no fever. Attends day care.
PMH: No hospitalizations, 2–3 bouts of otitis media per year

1. What pertinent history is it important to ask?
2. What is the most likely diagnosis given this presentation?
3. What would you look for on physical exam?
4. Is she contagious?
5. What laboratory tests would you order?
6. How would you treat this patient?

REFERENCES

Balin, A. K. (2006). *Seborrheic keratoses.* Retrieved January 15, 2008, from http://www.emedicine.com/derm/topic397.htm

Berger, T. G. (2005). Skin, hair and nails. In L. M. Tierney, S. J. McPhee, & M. A. Papadakis (Eds.), *Current medical diagnosis and treatment* (44th ed.). New York: Lange Medical Books/McGraw Hill.

Blount, B. W. (2002). Rosacea: A common, yet commonly overlooked, condition. *American Family Physician, 66*(3), 435–440.

Bower, M. G. (2007). Confronting the "flesh-eating" infection. *Nursing, 37*(6), 48hn1–48hn4.

Domino, F. J. (2008). *The 5 minute clinical consult.* Philadelphia: Lippincott, Williams & Wilkins.

Edmunds, M. W., & Mayhew, M. S. (2004). *Pharmacology for the primary care provider* (2nd ed.). St. Louis, MO: Mosby.

Facts and Comparisons. (2008). *Drug facts and comparisons* 2008. St. Louis, MO: Wolters Kluwer Health.

Fisher, D. (2001). Common dermatoses: How to treat safely and effectively during pregnancy, part 2. *Consultant, 41*(8), 1174–1177.

Gilbert, D. N., Moellering, R. C., Jr., Eliopoulus, G. M., Sande, M. A., & Chambers, H. F. (2007). *The Sanford guide to antimicrobial therapy.* Hyde Park, VT: Antimicrobial Therapy.

Goroll, A. H., & Mulley, A. G. (2006). *Primary care medicine* (4th ed.). Philadelphia: Lippincott, Williams & Wilkins.

Graham, M., & Uphold, C. (2003). *Clinical guidelines in child health.* Gainesville, FL: Barramae Books, Inc.

Hall, J. C. (2000). *Sauer's manual of skin diseases* (8th ed.). Philadelphia: Lippincott, Williams & Wilkins.

Hay, W. W., Levin, M. J., Sondheimer, J. M., & Deterding, R. R. (2006). *Current pediatric diagnosis & treatment.* New York: McGraw-Hill.

Kaplan, D. L. (2001). Dermclinic: Cutaneous conundrums, dermatologic disguises. *Consultant, 41*(4), 523–525, 529–530, 571–579.

Marghoob, A. A. (2002). Dermatologic look-alikes: Skin cancer concerns. *Clinical Advisor, 5*(4), 121–122, 127.

Rees, M. T. (2002). Managing atopic eczema. *Primary Health Care, 12*(8), 27–32.

Tierney, L. M., McPhee, S. J., & Papadakis, A. (2005). *Current medical diagnosis and treatment* (44th ed.). Norwalk, CT: Appleton & Lange.

U.S. Preventive Services Task Force. (2007). *Guide to clinical preventive services.* Retrieved December 12, 2007, from http://www.ahrq.gov/clinic/uspstfix.htm

Witman, P. M. (2001). Concise review for clinicians: Topical therapies for localized psoriasis. *Mayo Clinic Proceedings, 76*(9), 943–949.

Wolff, K., Johnson, R. A., & Suurmond, D. (2005). *Color atlas & synopsis of clinical dermatology* (4th ed.). New York: McGraw-Hill.

6

Eye, Ear, Nose, and Throat Disorders

Lisa Neri, MSN, CRNP

GENERAL APPROACH

- Testing of visual acuity is the single most important test in evaluation of eye complaints in primary care.
- With the emergence of increasingly resistant organisms, it is imperative to be more judicious in the choice to prescribe antibiotics for upper respiratory infections, sinusitis, and acute otitis media.
- The most important treatment is to obtain a good history of illness and make a correct diagnosis.
- Proper equipment, including a hermetically sealed otoscope with a pneumatic attachment, is critical to performing a proper physical exam.

Red Flags

Eyes
- A case of a sudden onset of vision change is an emergency.
- Use caution in differentiating between viral conjunctivitis and herpetic keratitis, two distinctly different problems with different treatments that share a similar presentation. DO NOT use topical steroid eye preparations. Significant damage can occur with their use in the presence of early stage herpetic lesions, which are not immediately visible.

- With ocular chemical burns, irrigate immediately and copiously before evaluation.
- If the history suggests a projectile ocular foreign body but the physical exam is unrevealing, refer to an ophthalmologist immediately for further evaluation.
- *Know when to refer*: Many eye problems require evaluation and management by a specialist. See Table 6–1 for signs and symptoms that should be referred immediately to an ophthalmologist.
- *Acute angle closure glaucoma* results in permanent vision loss if not treated *immediately*.
- *Retinoblastoma* (malignant tumor of retina) may present as white pupils (leukocoria), esotropia, exotropia, or anisocoria; refer to ophthalmologist for prompt evaluation.
- *Macular degeneration* is the leading cause of irreversible vision loss; incidence increases with age. Progressive deterioration of central vision and macular damage can be classified into two categories: atrophic (dry), which is associated with ischemia; or exudative (wet), which is associated with leakage of fluid from blood vessels. Complaints of visual changes such as patchy blurry spots or distortion in central visual field should be promptly evaluated by an ophthalmologist. Treatment is aimed at stabilization of vision through laser surgery and visual aids.

Table 6-1. Indicators of Vision-Threatening Disorders

Symptoms	Signs
Blurred vision that does NOT clear with blinking	Ciliary flush
	Abnormal pupils
Acute loss or decreased vision	Increased intraocular pressure
Halos around sources of lights	Shallow anterior chamber
Flashing lights	Proptosis (forward displacement of the eye globe within the orbit of the eye)
Sudden floating spots or sensation of "cobwebs" across field of vision	Severe green-yellow discharge, eye erythema, chemosis, and lid edema
Photophobia	Absent red reflex
Periocular headache	
Ocular pain	
Nystagmus	
Corneal damage (opacities, trauma)	

Ears
- *Complications of ear infections*: Otitis media or externa with spreading infection, mastoid tenderness, lymphadenopathy and neurologic abnormalities. URGENT REFERRAL
- Suspected *perforated tympanic membrane* is a contraindication for removal of cerumen impaction by irrigation; refer to a specialist.

Nose and Sinuses
- Important, serious findings pointing to complications of sinusitis include external facial swelling, erythema, or cellulitis over an involved sinus (periorbital or forehead); vision changes such as diplopia; difficulty moving eyes (extraocular muscles [EOMs]); proptosis; and any abnormal neurologic signs. URGENT REFERRAL

Throat
- *Epiglottal spasm*: In cases of suspected epiglottitis, attempting to examine the oral cavity or insert a tongue blade for visualization of the pharynx can result in acute airway obstruction and potential asphyxiation.
- Consider *peritonsillar abscess* when the patient with severe tonsillitis (usually more pronounced unilaterally) appears toxic with fever, trismus, "hot potato" voice, palatal bulge, and uvula deviation.

DISORDERS OF THE EYES

Blepharitis

Description
- An acute or chronic problem of the eyelid margins, characterized by redness, crusting, and scaling of the lid margin at the base of the lashes and often producing eye irritation.
- Anterior blepharitis involves the eyelid skin, eyelashes, and associated glands.
- Posterior blepharitis involves the meibomian glands.

Etiology
- Squamous form: Most commonly associated with seborrheic dermatitis; may be caused by inflammation or hypersecretion of sebaceous glands
- Infectious or ulcerative form: Most commonly due to *Staphylococcus aureus*; rarely may be caused by other bacteria, viruses, fungi, scabies, or lice
- Meibomian gland dysfunction
- Inflammation or infection of the eyelid margins causes edema, redness, tenderness, and discharge

Incidence and Demographics
- One of the most common eye disorders; not common in children
- Affects predominately adult population, males and females equally
- Mixed (seborrheic and infectious) blepharitis most common type

Risk Factors
- History of skin problems: Seborrheic dermatitis, contact dermatitis, acne rosacea
- Poor hygiene, including improper cleaning of the face, using old and/or contaminated eye makeup, contact lens use
- Immunocompromised: Chemotherapy, diabetes, HIV

Prevention and Screening
- Maintenance of lid hygiene can decrease risk of reoccurrence

Assessment
HISTORY
- Common complaints are eyelids itching, burning, and crusting with redness of the lid margin
- Symptoms are worse upon awakening (typically in the morning)

- Additional complaints of purulent drainage if infection has developed (conjunctivitis, stye)
- History of recurrent stye

PHYSICAL EXAM
- All types: Eyelid erythema, change in eyelash pattern (broken, missing, misdirected)
- Seborrheic type: Dandruff-like flaking, scaling, waxy surface of lid margin
- Infectious: Purulent discharge, concurrent papules or pustules, punctate ulcerations
- Mixed: All signs listed above
- Chronic: Thickening of lid with or without above concurrent symptoms
- Conjunctiva may be injected
- Visual acuity unaffected, exam of cornea and pupil normal

DIAGNOSTIC STUDIES
- Rarely, a culture of secretions may be indicated if treatment failure with usual antibiotics

Differential Diagnosis
- Cancer: Initial presentation is similar to blepharitis, styes, and chalazion; consider if no response to treatments after 1 month

Management
NONPHARMACOLOGIC TREATMENT
- Warm, moist compresses qid x 15 minutes
- Daily lid hygiene using dilute tear-free shampoo with warm, damp cotton tip (cotton swab or ball)
- No use of contact lens or eye makeup while symptomatic or being treated

PHARMACOLOGIC TREATMENT
- Topical ophthalmic antibiotics: Choice of bacitracin, sodium sulfacetamide, erythromycin, ofloxacin (Ocuflox), depending on sensitivities, allergies. Applied 1–4 x daily, as indicated by severity
- Consider oral antibiotics for ocular symptoms associated with rosacea (doxyclycline 100 mg bid, Oracea 40 mg once daily, or tetracycline 250 mg qid)

LENGTH OF TREATMENT
- Antibiotics 1–2 weeks, then reduce to every afternoon or evening x 4–8 weeks; should continue 1 month past symptom resolution
- Lid hygiene as maintenance for control, possibly with antibiotic ophthalmic ointment, as it is often chronic
- Ocular Rosacea, 12 weeks and reassess

Special Considerations
- Herpes simplex infection of eyelid may appear very similar to staphylococcus blepharitis, but has acute onset.

When to Consult, Refer, Hospitalize
- Refer to ophthalmologist if failure to respond to treatment, or if concurrent or additional symptoms develop requiring surgical treatment (meibomian gland drainage or extraction)

Follow-Up
> EXPECTED COURSE
> - Chronic inflammatory symptoms maintained with lid hygiene
> - Infectious component should resolve with treatment as above

> COMPLICATIONS
> - Infection spread to conjunctiva, cornea

Nasolacrimal Duct Obstruction

Description
- "Blocked tear ducts" with tear drainage cut off between the lacrimal sac and nose

Etiology
- Blockage caused by residual epithelial membranes; canalization of the nasolacrimal duct is incomplete
- Generally not completely occluded

Incidence and Demographics
- Approximately 5%–7% of newborns have some degree of blockage

Risk Factors
- None known

Prevention and Screening
- No known prevention

Assessment
> HISTORY
> - Parent reports excessive tearing and crusting of lashes or mucus discharge from one or both eyes
> - Crusting of eyelashes in the morning

> PHYSICAL EXAM
> - Note presence of watery or mucus discharge; may be purulent if infected; eyes look wet, tearing over lid
> - Maceration of eyelids from excessive tearing; crusting on lashes
> - Rubbing eyes, reddened conjunctiva

> DIAGNOSTIC STUDIES
> - None indicated; if infected, may perform culture and sensitivity
> - May perform fluorescein study (dye disappearance test)

Differential Diagnosis
- Congenital glaucoma
- Dry eye reflex tearing
- Entropion
- Ectropion
- 7th nerve palsies
- Imperforate puncta
- Dacryocystitis
- Canaliculitis

Management

NONPHARMACOLOGIC TREATMENT
- Observe for up to 1 year if asymptomatic other than watery eyes
- Lacrimal sac massage: Apply downward pressure on lacrimal sac to expel build-up
- Probing and irrigation: Done by ophthalmologists, usually if unresolved by 12 months of age; may be done sooner if repeated infections or excessive discharge

PHARMACOLOGIC TREATMENT
- Treat secondary infections with antibiotic ointment as indicated

LENGTH OF TREATMENT
- Secondary infections for 5–7 days

Special Considerations
- None

When to Consult, Refer, Hospitalize
- Reevaluate at 12 months; refer to ophthalmologist if patient remains symptomatic

Follow-Up

EXPECTED COURSE
- 95% of cases will resolve by 12 months

COMPLICATIONS
- Dacryocystitis
- Secondary infection of conjunctivae or eyelids due to excessive drainage

Hordeolum (Stye) and Chalazion

Description
- Inflammatory disorders of the lubricating glands of the eyelids and eyelashes
- Hordeolum (stye) is an infected and inflamed area of the Zeis or Moll glands that lubricate the skin and eyelashes, located at the eyelid margin and pointing to the skin surface (external hordeolum).
- Chalazion is a granulomatous inflammation of the meibomian glands on the conjunctival aspect of the eyelid (internal hordeolum).

Etiology

- Obstructed glands (Zeis, Moll, or meibomian) causes inflammatory papule, pustule, or granulomatous papule
- Hordeolum: 75%–90% caused by infection with S. aureus
- Chalazion: Meibomian gland dysfunction that may occur after a stye

Incidence and Demographics

- Extremely common in all ages, especially children and adolescents

Risk Factors

- Poor hygiene, use of contaminated eye makeup
- Blepharitis, wearing of contact lens

Prevention and Screening

- Eyelid hygiene

Assessment

HISTORY

- Patient complains of a sudden onset of localized tenderness, swelling, or redness of the eyelid

PHYSICAL EXAM

- Localized or generalized erythema of the eyelid
- Erythematous papule or pustule may be visible on outer or conjunctival aspect of the eyelid
- May be ulceration at base of lash follicle where infectious head has ruptured
- Conjunctiva may be injected
- Visual acuity unaffected; exam of cornea and pupil normal

DIAGNOSTIC STUDIES

- None indicated

Differential Diagnosis

- Cancer
- Trauma
- Blepharitis

Management

NONPHARMACOLOGIC TREATMENT

- Warm compresses up to 4x daily for 15–20 minutes
- Lid hygiene until resolved (see section on blepharitis)
- Surgical drainage by ophthalmologist for persistent chalazion localized to one meibomian gland

PHARMACOLOGIC TREATMENT

- Ophthalmic antibiotics on eyelid margin: erythromycin ointment (ilotycin) 2–4x daily

LENGTH OF TREATMENT
- Lid hygiene and warm compresses continued until resolution
- Antibiotic ointment for 7 days
- May require oral Dicloxacillin or Cephalexin if topical ineffective

Special Considerations
- None

When to Consult, Refer, Hospitalize
- Refer nonresponding conditions to an ophthalmologist for excision and drainage or curettage.
- Though rare, the initial presentation of cancer is similar to blepharitis, styes, and chalazion; consider if no response to treatments after 1 month and refer to ophthalmology.

Follow-Up
EXPECTED COURSE
- Resolves with treatment
- May be recurrent or develop in clusters that do not heal well; consider diabetes mellitus
- Should be seen after eyelid quiets to assess need for surgical treatment

COMPLICATIONS
- Cellulitis of the eyelid

Strabismus

Description
- Misalignment of the eye; commonly referred to as "crossed eyes"
  - Described as "esotropia" when the eyes are crossed; "exotropia" when the eyes are divergent; "hypertropia" or "hypotropia" when the eyes are up or down
  - Uncorrected, may result in amblyopia (permanent loss in visual acuity). When eyes are misaligned, the brain will receive two images instead of the normal one; the brain manages this by "shutting down" or not processing one of the images. Left untreated, this eventually becomes permanent, leading to loss of depth perception.

Etiology
- More than 100 different types; 50% of cases are esotropia
- May be paralytic (paralysis of one or more ocular muscles) or nonparalytic (unequal muscle tone)
- May be congenital or disease-induced; diseases that may cause strabismus include retinoblastoma, neurologic disorders such as cerebral palsy, and certain genetic conditions
- Viral infections can affect the cranial nerves, causing the development of strabismus; in the case of viral illness, the strabismus may resolve spontaneously.
- Results from an inability of the visual cortex to use the eyes together or to a disorder of the cranial nerves (3, 4, or 6) or the extraocular muscles

- An intermittent phoria—esophoria or exophoria—is common in the first 6 months of life. It may be noted by parents particularly when infant is tired; may report that child's eyes are "crossed" for a few seconds to minutes. Phorias resolve spontaneously by 6 months of life and do not require referral prior to that time.

Incidence and Demographics
- Genetic: Parents with strabismus have a 12%–17% chance of having a child with strabismus
- 4% of the population affected

Risk Factors
- Family history of strabismus
- Head or eye trauma, infections, eye disorders
- Large refractive errors
- Lid abnormalities
- Down syndrome
- Prematurity

Prevention and Screening
- Alignment of eyes should be assessed on all well-child check-ups; visual acuity should be assessed in routine exams as soon as children are capable of using eye charts (sooner if indicated).

Assessment
HISTORY
- Parent reports the child's eyes "don't move together," "are crossed," "look strange," etc.
- Other subjective statements regarding the child's ability to see may be offered
- Note age at onset; amount of waking hours that eye deviation is noticed (may be worse in the afternoon and evening when the child is more fatigued); note pre-, peri- and postnatal history
- Note if sudden onset
- Note history of trauma, presence of other acute or chronic illnesses
- Note family history of strabismus, other eye disorders

PHYSICAL EXAM
- The four tests used to assess ocular alignment are:
  - EOMs: Six cardinal positions of gaze would detect primarily a paralytic strabismus, but in each position, the corneal light reflex can be used to assess for nonparalytic strabismus.
  - Corneal light reflex (Hirschberg): Demonstrates a nonparalytic tropia
  - Perform cover–uncover test by having the patient stare at a fixed point. A cover is then placed over one eye for a few seconds and then rapidly removed. The eye that was under the cover is carefully observed for movement or deviation, if detected latent strabismus is present.
  - Perform Bruckner's test by standing about 20" from child in darkened room and looking at both eyes through ophthalmoscope; note symmetry of red reflexes bilaterally.
- Note presence of nystagmus or other involuntary eye movements

- Perform funduscopic exam; note fullness of red reflex
- Assess general developmental level
- Perform complete neurologic exam (strabismus is more common in children who are developmentally delayed or who have central nervous system [CNS] pathology)

DIAGNOSTIC STUDIES
- CAT scan and MRI studies of the orbits and head may be helpful to exclude an intracranial mass (bleed or tumor) if onset is acute with deviation between the eyes changing with changing gaze positions (incomitancy) or if associated with trauma, craniofacial abnormalities, or neurologic disease
- Visual evoked response (VER), electroretinogram (ERG), and electro-oculography (EOG) may be helpful if a neurological etiology is suspected

Differential Diagnosis
- Amblyopia
- Refractive error
- Pseudostrabismus
- CNS or orbital tumor

Management
NONPHARMACOLOGIC TREATMENT
- Eyeglasses may be sufficient to induce binocular function and correct refractive errors
- Surgery on the eye muscles is successful up to 80% of the time; some patients (20%–25%) may require a second surgery
- Patching the unaffected eye may be done, alone or prior to glasses or surgery
- Visual training exercises have limited usefulness

PHARMACOLOGIC TREATMENT
- Topical miotic drops may be helpful in some forms of esotropia; this is done only by the ophthalmologist

Special Considerations
- None

When to Consult, Refer, Hospitalize
- Refer to an ophthalmologist *as soon as strabismus is observed*, especially in infancy; in an infant <1 year, amblyopia can occur with as little as 1 week of abnormal visual input

Follow-Up
EXPECTED COURSE
- Depends on type and treatment modality employed; once alignment is achieved, patients are followed every 3–12 months (depending on age and type of strabismus)
- Decompensation and reappearance of strabismus may occur in up to 40% of patients in adulthood

COMPLICATIONS
- Amblyopia, loss of depth perception, blindness, disfiguring eye appearance

Retinoblastoma (RB)

Description
- Tumor of the retina of congenital origin

Etiology
- Originates in retinoblasts following loss, mutation, deletion, or rearrangement of the retinoblastoma gene on chromosome 13

Incidence and Demographics
- 45% inherited; 55% of retinoblastomas noninheritable type
- Overall uncommon; occurs in 1:16,000–1:25,000 live births; about 200–300 new cases per year
- Most common primary intraocular tumor in childhood; represents 3% of all childhood malignancies

Risk Factors
- Family history of retinoblastoma or retinomas (nonmalignant)

Prevention and Screening
- None known; genetic testing can identify individuals with the retinoblastoma mutation only about 5% of the time (not helpful)
- Red reflex checks at all well-baby and well-child visits
- Siblings and children of parents with RB should have thorough ophthalmic examinations (may do under anesthesia)

Assessment
HISTORY
- If disease is unilateral, may present itself at ages 6 months–5 years; mean age of 2 years
- Bilateral disease usually presents by 12–13 months of age
- Parents may note crossed eyes or outward deviation of eyes
- Leukocoria may be noticed in a photograph
- Pain and redness are rare; usually no complaints of visual problems because unaffected eye maintains the vision
- Note family history of malignancies, particularly of the eyes

PHYSICAL EXAM
- "Cat's eye reflex" (leukocoria): White pupil seen when observing the red reflex, may be unilateral or bilateral (~60% are bilateral)
- Other findings may include the presence of esotropia, exotropia, anisocoria, or proptosis (late finding)

DIAGNOSTIC STUDIES
All studies should be done by ophthalmologist and oncologist
- Aqueous cytology
- CT scan of the head and orbits
- Ocular ultrasonography

Differential Diagnosis
- Retinopathy of prematurity
- Coats' disease
- Hypopyon
- Iritis
- Uveitis
- Toxoplasmosis, other ocular infections

Management
- By ophthalmology and oncology; treatment will depend on extent of disease and may include chemotherapy, radiation, and/or surgery (enucleation)

When to Consult, Refer, Hospitalize
- All children with RB are referred immediately to ophthalmology

Follow-Up
- Frequent follow-up by ophthalmology
- Future evaluations for
  - Contralateral eye developing RB (in about 15%)
  - Metastasis: Occurs before 5 years
  - Evaluate for second malignancies; may include osteosarcoma (most common) and melanoma; occurs in about 10% of children
    EXPECTED COURSE
    - Mortality from RB is approximately 8%
    - Vision is salvageable in a large percentage of children diagnosed at early stages

    COMPLICATIONS
    - Death
    - Blindness

Conjunctivitis

Description
- Acute inflammation of the palpebral and bulbar conjunctival layer of the eyes
  - Commonly referred to as "pink eye" or "red eye"; may be bilateral or unilateral
  - Conjunctivitis in the first month of life is most commonly caused by infections passed via vaginal delivery; known as ophthalmia neonatorum

Etiology
- Many causative organisms; *Chlamydia trachomatis* and *Neisseria gonorrhoeae* most common in newborns
- Viral: Adenoviruses (most common), herpes zoster, herpes simplex virus
- Bacterial: *S. aureus* (common in adults), streptococci (common in children), *N. gonorrhea, N. meningitides, H. influenzae, Pseudomonas,* or *Moraxella*
- Chlamydial: Can lead to blindness (rare in United States); associated with genital infection
- Dacrocystitis in the newborn

- Allergic: Exposure to seasonal allergens such as hay fever, pollen, trees, grass
- Chemical exposure (splash or gas), UV light exposure, smoke, contaminated eye makeup, eye drops, contact lens, or solutions for lens wear
- Systemic disease manifestation: Reiter syndrome, thyroid exophthalmos, varicella, measles, psoriasis, and autoimmune disorders (e.g., Sjögren syndrome)
- Inflammatory process causes dilation of blood vessels, edema, and exudate of conjunctival membrane

Incidence and Demographics
- Common eye disorder in all ages
- Increased incidence in fall due to higher incidence of viral infections and exposure to seasonal allergens

Risk Factors
- Exposure to infectious agents, chemical agents, wind, extreme temperatures, allergens

Prevention and Screening
- Avoidance of known allergens, irritants, and others with conjunctivitis
- Occupational precautions such as wearing goggles in high-risk situations
- Frequent handwashing and good hygiene to reduce risk of transmission
- Gonorrhea prophylaxis for newborns: 1% silver nitrate, 0.5% erythromycin, or 1% tetracycline ointment

Assessment
HISTORY (SEE TABLE 6–2)
- Irritated eyes with redness, mild pain, or itching in one or both eyes, or spread from one to the other
- Watery or purulent drainage, crusting on eyelashes upon awakening
- Visual complaints limited to c/o blurry vision that clears with blinking
- Assess for associated symptoms that may indicate systemic disease such as rash, lesions, joint pain, fever, genitourinary complaints, constitutional symptoms

Table 6–2. Differentiating Characteristics of Conjunctivitis

Cause	Symptoms
Bacterial	Often starts in one eye, spreads to both
	May follow a viral conjunctivitis as a secondary infection
	Crusty or mucoid discharge
N. gonorrhea	Copious amounts of purulent discharge
Chlamydia	Pre-auricular lymphadenopathy
	Genitourinary symptoms may be evident
	Photophobia (indicator of advanced infection)
Viral	Profuse tearing
	Pre-auricular lymphadenopathy
	Herpetic type may be associated with cold sores
Allergic	Stringy discharge; usually bilateral
	Itchy eyes
	+/- associated allergy type symptoms (rhinitis, sneezing)
	"Cobblestone" appearance of conjunctival edema

PHYSICAL EXAM
- Vision, pupillary reaction, and EOMs intact
- Edema of eyelids and matted eyelashes
- Injected appearance limited to conjunctiva
- NOTE: Ciliary flush, corneal changes, pupil abnormalities, and photophobia are not associated with simple conjunctivitis; must rule out keratitis, iritis, or other serious conditions through urgent referral (see Box 6–1)

DIAGNOSTIC STUDIES
- None routinely ordered; may consider culture of discharge if severe, copious
- May consider fluorescein staining to assess for epithelial integrity (keratitis, ulcer)
- Enzyme immunoassays for chlamydia organisms if suspected as etiology

DIFFERENTIAL DIAGNOSIS
- Acute uveitis
- Foreign body
- Acute glaucoma
- Scleritis, episcleritis
- Corneal disorders
- Keratitis

Management
NONPHARMACOLOGIC TREATMENT
- Eye compresses 15 minutes qid: cool for itching or irritation, warm for crusting
- Saline irrigation of eye for viral, gonococcal, irritant, or chemical etiology
- Discontinue wearing contact lens and eye makeup until resolved
- Replace eye makeup
- Avoid contact lens wear until resolved and consider replacement with new lenses
- Hygiene measures: Wash pillowcases, fresh washcloth with each use, handwashing
- NO patch

PHARMACOLOGIC TREATMENT
- Allergic: OTC topical ophthalmic vasoconstrictors, antihistamines, or combination products such as naphazoline 0.05% (Albalon, Naphcon-A) or antazoline 0.5% (Vasocon-A); antihistamine/mast cell stabilizer like olopatadine 0.1% (Patanol)
- Bacterial: Antibiotic drops or ointment such as sulfacetamide sodium (Sodium Sulamyd) 10%, tobramycin (Tobrex) 0.3%, or gentamicin (Garamycin) 1–2 drops q4h x 5 days or erythromycin (Ilotycin) ointment 2–3 x daily for 7–10 days
- Chlamydial: Doxycycline (Vibramycin) 100 mg po bid x 3 weeks in adult; in children, erythromycin 50 mg/kg/d po/4 doses x 14 days; if other bacteria suspected, base treatment on culture and sensitivity results
- NO ophthalmic steroid preparations
- If gonococcal, hospitalize and treat with systemic ceftriaxone (Rocephin) 25–50 mg/kg/d IV or IM, or cefotaxime (Claforan) 25–50 mg/kg/d IV or IM q 12h x 7 days
- Herpes simplex virus: Refer to ophthalmologist for treatment

LENGTH OF TREATMENT
- Initiate treatment and reexamine within 24–48 hours if no improvement
- Length of treatment determined by etiology and responsiveness to treatment

SPECIAL CONSIDERATIONS
- Geriatrics: Greater chance of systemic diseases associated with conjunctivitis
- Pregnancy or lactation: Do not use doxycycline

When to Consult, Refer, Hospitalize
- Hospitalization for hyperacute bacterial conjunctivitis requiring IV antibiotics
- Immediate referral to ophthalmologist if severe pain, ciliary flush, changed visual acuity, abnormal eye exam, or signs of herpetic etiology
- Referral to ophthalmologist if worsening of symptoms within 24–48 hours

Follow-Up
EXPECTED COURSE
- Bacterial conjunctivitis typically lasts 2–4 days with treatment, or 2 weeks without treatment
- Chlamydial symptoms will last 3–9 months if left untreated
- Viral conjunctivitis can last from 10 days to 4 weeks depending upon type

COMPLICATIONS
- Potential for spread of infection to surrounding areas (blepharitis, keratitis, iritis)
- Superinfection
- Scars on cornea, lids, with eyelids or lashes misdirected
- Hypopyon

Iritis/Uveitis/Keratitis

Description
- Iritis: Inflammation of the iris
- Keratitis: Corneal inflammation or infection that is potentially vision-threatening; result of infection or direct irritation
- Uveitis: Inflammation of one or more of the components of uveal tract (iris, ciliary body, choroids, and retina)
  - Anterior uveitis: Iritis, iridocyclitis, or cyclitis
  - Posterior uveitis: Choroiditis or chorioretinitis
  - Panuveitis: All components affected
- May be acute or chronic

Etiology
- Most cases of anterior uveitis are associated with a number of inflammatory conditions, particularly HLA-B27–related diseases including juvenile rheumatoid arthritis, ankylosing spondylitis, Reiter syndrome, psoriasis, ulcerative colitis, and Crohn's disease; and other conditions such as sarcoidosis, tuberculosis, syphilis, collagen vascular disease

- Posterior uveitis: Usually occurs as a result of certain organisms, particularly toxoplasmosis, histoplasmosis, cytomegalovirus, herpes simplex, herpes zoster, mycobacterium, *Cryptococcus*, Lyme disease, West Nile virus, cat scratch disease
- Infection is frequently the cause in immunocompromised patients

Risk Factors
- Immunocompromised status
- Autoimmune and inflammatory systemic conditions
- Contact lenses

Prevention and Screening
- High-risk groups: Screened routinely by ophthalmology

Assessment

HISTORY
- Anterior uveitis: Acute onset of eye pain, redness, photophobia, visual loss. Eye pain can be incapacitating.
- Posterior uveitis: Gradual loss of vision or blurry vision, floating black spots; typically no pain or redness

PHYSICAL EXAM
- Anterior (iritis): Tenderness to palpation, diffuse redness with perilimbal erythema; pupil may be small and irregular
- Iritis: Opacities or haziness on the cornea and within the aqueous (may hinder funduscopic exam). If visualized, funduscopic findings may include keratic precipitates ("mutton fat"), nodules on the iris, hypopyon, macular changes (lesions, edema), and optic neuropathy (rare)
- Posterior uveitis: Funduscopic findings will vary with the offending organism

DIAGNOSTIC STUDIES
- Usually unnecessary, but may need studies to determine if an undiagnosed underlying cause exists

---

Box 6–1. Characteristics of Keratitis/Iritis/Uveitis

Keratitis

Corneal inflammation or infection that is potentially vision-threatening; due to infection or direct irritation

Contact lens use is most common cause of bacterial keratitis (sleeping with lenses in eyes)

Findings include ciliary injection, watery or purulent discharge, sensitivity to light

Possible corneal clouding or lesions, lower visual acuity and pupillary response, or extraocular herpetic rash

Refer to ophthalmologist

Iritis/Uveitis

Inflammation of the uveal tract including the iris and the ciliary body (anterior) and/or choroid (posterior)

Usually associated with immunologic disorders; infection with TB, syphilis, CMV, toxoplasmosis, herpes, Lyme disease; or may be idiopathic

Presents as deep eye pain, ciliary flush, photophobia, possible decreased vision

Work-up for associated condition such as HLA-B27, ANA, PPD, Lyme serology, RPR if severe or recurrent

Refer to ophthalmologist

Differential Diagnosis
- Retinal detachment
- Intraocular tumors
- CNS lymphoma
- See Table 6–3

Table 6-3. Selected Differential Diagnoses of the Red Eye

	Allergic Conjunctivitis	Infectious Conjunctivitis	Iritis	Glaucoma
Symptoms	Itchy	Eyes "stick together" in morning	Pain, photophobia	Often no symptoms
Redness	Diffuse; not associated with perilimbal erythema	Diffuse redness, greater towards fornices	Circumcorneal (perilimbal erythema)	Diffuse redness of bulbar conjunctiva
Discharge	Watery	Moderate to heavy mucoid or mucopurulent	None	None or tearing
Pupils	Normal	Normal	Constricted	Large pupils
Visual acuity	Normal	Normal	Decreased, blurred vision	Decreased
Associated Findings	Other allergic symptoms may be noted (sneezing, nasal congestion, wheezing)			Increase intraocular pressure; eyeballs may seem firm
Comments	Seasonal, uncommonly seen age < 3 years Often family history of allergies	Known contact or current URI symptoms	Common complication of autoimmune disorders, especially juvenile rheumatoid arthritis (JRA)	Usually congenital Very rare but can cause blindness Treatable

Adapted from *Current Pediatric Diagnosis and Treatment* (18th ed., p. 364), by W. Hay, M. J. Levin, J. M. Sondheimer, & R. R. Deterding, 2006, New York: Lange Medical Books/McGraw-Hill.

Management
PHARMACOLOGIC TREATMENT (UNDER THE MANAGEMENT OF AN OPHTHALMOLOGIST)
- Corticosteroids
- Other treatments may include antimicrobials, systemic immunosuppression, chemotherapy

When to Consult, Refer, Hospitalize
- All patients are referred immediately to an ophthalmologist

Follow-Up
EXPECTED COURSE
- Variable depending on underlying disease and tolerance to medications

COMPLICATIONS
- Loss of vision

Glaucoma

Description
- Conditions producing increased intraocular pressure (IOP) from obstruction of the flow of aqueous humor in the anterior chamber of the eye. Acute angle-closure glaucoma refers to the sudden obstruction of flow of humor. Increased intraocular pressure may result in optic nerve atrophy, decreased peripheral vision, and vision deterioration that can lead to blindness if left untreated.
- Glaucoma may be chronic open-angle (most common and includes subacute), or acute angle-closure.

Etiology
- An altered eye structure with an anatomically narrow anterior chamber angle predisposes patients to developing glaucoma.
- Chronic open-angle glaucoma develops because there is partial obstruction to the aqueous outflow at the trabecular meshwork.
- In acute angle-closure glaucoma, the iris occludes the trabecular meshwork, causing progressively increasing IOP.

Incidence and Demographics
- Acute angle-closure glaucoma: Estimated 0.5% of population; 3%–4% of those >70 years of age
- Acute angle-closure glaucoma occurs more commonly (500/100,000) in African-Americans and Asians; in Caucasians, 100/100,000. Females have a greater incidence than males. Typical age of onset 55–70 years
- Chronic glaucoma affects 4% of those age >40; 10% of those >age 80

Risk Factors
- Family history (2%–5% lifetime risk)
- Diabetes
- African-American and Native Alaskan ancestry
- Altered anatomy of eye: Small cornea, hyperopia, shallow anterior chamber
- Hyperopia, which is associated with a narrowed angle

- Pathology of the eye: Cysts of the iris or ciliary bodies, cataracts
- Use of medications with cholinergic inhibition or prolonged use of high-dose oral and topical corticosteroids
- History of ocular trauma
- Acute angle-closure glaucoma is precipitated by sudden pupil dilation correlating with events such as stress, anxiety, sudden hypervolemia, or sudden darkness

Prevention and Screening
- Screening eye exam starting at age 40 biannually; sooner if high-risk
- IOP screening after age 65 (per U.S. Preventive Task Force; controversial)
- Prophylactic laser treatment to second eye for prevention of damage

Assessment

HISTORY
- Variable presentation depending on type; see Table 6–4
- Thorough history to identify precipitating events, other medical problems, medications

PHYSICAL EXAM
- Findings are presented in Table 6–4 as they correlate to the classifications of glaucoma
- Screening exams include visual acuity, peripheral vision by confrontation, inspection of outer eye and sclera, pupillary response, funduscopic to assess optic cup-to-disc ratio
- Further examination by a specialist is required to assess with slit lamp

Table 6–4. Presentations of Glaucoma

	Acute angle-closure	Chronic	Subacute
Symptoms	Pain around eyes/brows Tearing, no discharge Vision blurred Halos seen around lights Frontal headache Nausea and vomiting	Asymptomatic (early stage) OR similar to subacute OR Vision loss in late stage	Dull ache in one eye Mild blurring of vision Symptoms worse with activity (TV in the dark, reading) Symptoms improve with sleep or rest
Physical exam findings	IOP 40–80 mmH Diffuse conjunctival injection g Ciliary flush Pupil sluggish, mid-dilated, often oval shape Lid and corneal edema Shallow anterior chamber	Normal or increased IOP Increased cup-to-disc ratio Normal pupil Multiple peripheral anterior synechiae (iris adheres to cornea)	IOP 10–23 mmHg Pupil dilated Shallow anterior angle +/- peripheral anterior synechiae

DIAGNOSTIC STUDIES

- Intraocular pressure measurement is performed as part of the work-up, but elevation is not necessary to precipitate glaucoma pathology. There can be damage over time in chronic glaucoma with IOP within normal range, as well as with elevation.
- IOP normal range is 10–20 mmHg; >20 indicates need for further specialist evaluation.
- Gonioscopy performed by a specialist is required for evaluation and diagnosis

Differential Diagnosis

- Anterior uveitis
- Variant types of glaucoma
- Conjunctivitis
- Eye trauma
- Neurologic disease

Management

NONPHARMACOLOGIC TREATMENT

- Laser iridotomy or incisional iridectomy is the definitive treatment for acute glaucoma after medical stabilization. Bedrest is maintained in the acute case pending surgical treatment.
- Risk of precipitating an acute angle-closure attack is reduced with patient education regarding medications to avoid (such as OTC cold preparations), overhydration via sudden intake of large volumes, and instructions on signs of acute attack to be reported immediately.

PHARMACOLOGIC TREATMENT

- Acute angle-closure glaucoma medical management consists of the use of agents including alpha-adrenergic agonists: apraclonidine (Iopidine); beta-adrenergic blockers—timolol (Timoptic); carbonic anhydrase inhibitors—acetazolamide (Diamox); miotics—pilocarpine (Pilocar); and/or systemic hyperosmotic agents—mannitol (Osmitrol)
- Chronic open-angle glaucoma is managed with maintenance medications to reduce IOP via several mechanisms:
  - Enhance aqueous outflow parasympathomimetics, topical miotics (pilocarpine), topical prostaglandins (Lantanprost)
  - Decreased production of aqueous humor: beta blockers—timolol, betaxolol (Betoptic), or carbonic anhydrase inhibitors—acetazolamide

LENGTH OF TREATMENT

- Medical management is ongoing for subacute or chronic glaucoma

Special Considerations

- Medications must be used with caution in patients who are on diuretics; or who have renal failure, concomitant pulmonary (COPD), endocrine (diabetes), cardiovascular (CHF), or metabolic disease (acidosis)

When to Consult, Refer, Hospitalize
- Acute angle-closure glaucoma requires immediate initiation of medication and referral to an ophthalmologist for surgical treatment.
- Chronic or subacute glaucoma requires consult/referral to an ophthalmologist for examination and monitoring of the condition.

Follow-Up
- Followed every 3 months by ophthalmologist
    - EXPECTED COURSE
        - Course varies greatly depending on severity, duration, early/late diagnosis
        - If treated surgically, recurrence of acute attack is rare
        - Medical management of chronic glaucoma may prevent visual loss if initiated early and treated adequately

    - COMPLICATIONS
        - Loss of visual fields and visual acuity leading to blindness if untreated
        - Cornea damage: Chronic edema, fibrosis, vascularization, or cataracts
        - Atrophy of the iris, malignant glaucoma, central retinal vein occlusion

Cataract

Description
- Progressive, painless clouding of the lens of the eye resulting in localized or generalized vision loss and blindness

Etiology
- 90% due to the aging process
- Other causes: Eye trauma, congenital, corticosteroid use, infectious or inflammatory conditions, physical causes (radiation, infrared heat), systemic disease (diabetes mellitus, thyroid, parathyroid, sarcoid, others)
- Protein changes occur in the normally transparent lens, causing opacity and scattering of light

Incidence and Demographics
- Leading cause of blindness in the world with 17 million affected
- Cataracts are present in 92% of those age >75 years; females > males

Risk Factors
- Aging
- Cigarette smoking
- Alcohol consumption if heavy quantities
- Infection/inflammatory conditions
- Predisposing systemic diseases and exposure to conditions as listed above

Prevention and Screening
- No definite measures to prevent cataract formation
- Theoretical measures to slow the process include use of glasses with ultraviolet protection in sunny conditions, use of antioxidants such as vitamins C or E
- Screening for cataract is part of every routine, annual eye exam after age 40–50

Assessment
HISTORY
- May be asymptomatic; vision change is gradual and may go unnoticed due to adaptation
- Visual complaints range from clouding of vision that is patchy and peripheral, vision loss centrally or all-encompassing of the visual field
- Early symptoms directly attributed to the eyes include worsened vision, blurring, or difficulty with night driving due to bright lights
- Symptoms associated with worsening vision are related to falls, injuries, or accidents
- Non–aging-related cataracts have several etiologies; the history must be thorough

PHYSICAL EXAM
- Visual acuity testing will establish baseline; follow-up visits to track changes.
- Funduscopic exam reveals altered red reflex (dark spots or generally diminished) and clouding of the lens. At the highly advanced stage, the pupil will appear white.
- All other aspects of the outer eye exam are unremarkable.
- Funduscopic exam may detect other age-related changes that also affect vision (macular degeneration, diabetic or hypertensive retinopathies).

DIAGNOSTIC STUDIES
- In work-up by ophthalmologist, special studies may be done, including glare test, contrast sensitivity, retinal or macular function assessment.

Differential Diagnosis
- Corneal scarring
- Tumor
- Retinal detachment
- Lens opacities
- Retinal scar

Management
NONPHARMACOLOGIC TREATMENT
- Vision correction with corrective lenses in early stages or after surgery for some patients
- Surgery necessary when cataract markedly decreases visual acuity (i.e., cataract extraction and artificial lens implant)

PHARMACOLOGIC TREATMENT
- No drugs will halt the progression of the aging process in the eye
- Postoperatively, topical antibiotic and ophthalmic steroids under direction of an ophthalmologist

Special Considerations
- The presence of other diseases (e.g., macular degeneration, diabetic or hypertensive retinopathy) influences decision to perform corrective surgery.

- Make surgeon aware if patient is taking an alpha-1 antagonist (tamsulin, doxazosin, terazosin, or alfuzosin) prior to surgery due to the increased risk of intraoperative floppy iris syndrome.

When to Consult, Refer, Hospitalize
- All patients with cataracts should be referred to an ophthalmologist for eye assessment, management, and treatment.

Follow-Up
EXPECTED COURSE
- The natural course of cataracts is to progressively worsen until vision is lost
- Surgical extraction with lens implant improves vision in the absence of other diseases in 95% of the cases

COMPLICATIONS
- Blindness
- Incomplete correction with residual altered vision (i.e., pupil damage)
- Retinal detachment, glaucoma, hemorrhage, post-operative infection

OCULAR TRAUMA

Subconjunctival Hemorrhage

Description
- Bleeding beneath the conjunctiva

Etiology
- May occur spontaneously or by minimal trauma, increased intrathoracic pressure, or Valsalva
- Rupture of a conjunctival blood vessel causes a bright red, sharply delineated area surrounded by normal appearing conjunctiva

Risk Factors
- Presence of clotting disorder
- Raised venous pressure: Coughing, sneezing, straining

Prevention and Screening
- None

Assessment
HISTORY
- Report of sudden appearance of blood in the eye
- May or may not be history of trauma
- Sometimes noticed upon awakening
- No reports of pain, blurred vision, or other related symptoms

PHYSICAL EXAM
- Normal-appearing external eye; PERRLA (pupils equal, round, reactive to light and accommodation) and normal funduscopic exam
- Blood noted under part or the entire conjunctiva; usually unilateral but may be bilateral

DIAGNOSTIC STUDIES
- Usually none if suspected
- Fluorescein stain to r/o corneal abrasion
- Work up for bleeding disorder if repeated episodes

Differential Diagnosis
- Hyphema
- Corneal abrasion

Management
NONPHARMACOLOGIC TREATMENT
- None indicated

PHARMACOLOGIC TREATMENT
- None indicated unless associated infectious findings (conjunctivitis)

Special Considerations
- May be seen in hypertension and in neonates or their mothers as a result of labor and delivery

When to Consult, Refer, Hospitalize
- Refer to ophthalmologist if suspicious or associated with history of blunt trauma
- Refer to hematologist if recurrent

Follow-Up
EXPECTED COURSE
- Hemorrhages resorb in 1–2 weeks

Hyphema

Description
- Hemorrhage into the anterior chamber of the eye

Etiology
- Blunt or penetrating injury to eye such as from a rock, BB gun pellet, dart, stick, fists, or baseballs; or from a fall
- Child abuse
- Infrequently: Tumors, vascular abnormalities, coagulation disorders, leukemia
- Spontaneous (uncommon)

Risk Factors
- Blunt trauma to the eye, especially penetrating type
- Anticoagulant therapy
- Hemophilia
- Sickle cell anemia

Prevention and Screening
- Use of protective eyewear in high-risk situations
- Maintenance and control of hematologic disorders

Assessment

HISTORY
- Obtain details regarding precipitating event
- Eye pain usually is present from trauma or increased intraocular pressure
- Decrease in visual acuity may or may not be noticeable to the patient
- History of hemophilia, blood disorders (including sickle cell disease), medications (especially those that would affect clotting such as aspirin, NSAIDs, and herbal preparations such as ginkgo biloba)
- History of sickle cell disease or trait increases risk of rebleeding and the development of complications; usually needs more aggressive management
- Children, especially young children, often are somnolent; needs to be differentiated from decreased level of consciousness associated with a head injury

PHYSICAL EXAM
- Check visual acuity in both eyes; typically decreased in affected eye
- Blood in the anterior chamber is visible to varying degrees, from partial filling seen as a visible fluid level line to completely filled chamber. (Bleeds are graded according to the amount of blood in the anterior chamber with grade 4 being the worst—entire chamber filled. Incidence of complications increases with higher grades.)
- May have increased ocular pressure (eye is firm on palpation) or decreased (soft eye)
- Pupillary response may be sluggish
- Obtain a neurological exam if patient is somnolent
- Assess for other signs of bleeding (e.g., bruising)

DIAGNOSTIC STUDIES
- Clotting times; CBC with differential if indicated
- Possible sickle cell prep (African, Hispanic, or Mediterranean descent)

Differential Diagnosis
- Globe trauma
- Eye contusion
- Systemic disease

Management

NONPHARMACOLOGIC TREATMENT
- Apply bilateral eye patches to limit additional injury or blinking during transport to emergency facility or ophthalmologist (put no pressure on the globe)
- Keep patient in an upright position during transfer
- Bedrest at home or in hospital for 5–7 days with head of bed elevated 30°–45°
- No TV viewing or reading
- If severe or developing complications, surgery may be done to evacuate blood

PHARMACOLOGIC TREATMENT
- Acetaminophen with or without codeine may be used as needed for pain

Special Considerations
- Aspirin products, miotics, mydriatics should be not be used
- May need sedation to ensure complete rest

When to Consult, Refer, Hospitalize
- Immediate referral to emergency facility, hospital, and/or ophthalmologist
- If at home, must follow up daily to check intraocular pressure and check for rebleeds

Follow-Up

EXPECTED COURSE
- Variable, dependent on severity; ophthalmology may manage at home or as an inpatient
- Blood usually resorbs in 5–10 days (if no rebleeding)

COMPLICATIONS
- Vision loss
- Recurrent bleeding (~25%): Most common time is 5 days postinjury; increases risk of complications
- Permanent corneal staining (from the hemorrhage) and subsequent haziness
- Glaucoma (immediately or later in life)

Corneal Abrasion

Description
- An interruption in the superficial or epithelial layer of the cornea

Etiology
- Trauma (scratch, foreign body or object hits the eye)
- Denuded cornea causes symptoms

Incidence and Demographics
- Common in all ages; occurs in 80% of persons older than 75 years

Risk Factors
- Lack of use of eye protection during activities such as painting, carpentry, drilling, hobby, or working with tools

- Participation in dance or sports without hair appropriately secured (occasionally long hair swings into the eyes and causes abrasion)
- Contact lens wear

Prevention and Screening
- Use of eye protection during high risk activities

Assessment
HISTORY
- Complaints of sudden sensation of a foreign body and variable degree of pain in the eye along with photophobia, watery eyes

PHYSICAL EXAM
- Eye appears injected (red), sensitive to light, with increased lacrimation
- Altered integrity of normally smooth cornea seen as irregular light reflex; actual abrasion may be visible with the naked eye or only upon fluorescein staining
- Vision is unchanged, pupils are reactive, and funduscopic exam is normal

DIAGNOSTIC STUDIES
- Fluorescein staining will reveal epithelial disruption on the cornea

Differential Diagnosis
- Foreign body
- Keratitis
- Corneal ulcer
- Contact lens roughing
- Herpes ulcer of cornea
- Acute angle glaucoma

Management
NONPHARMACOLOGIC TREATMENT
- Irrigation with normal saline to flush any particles, foreign body
- Patching of eye no longer recommended
- Avoid wearing contact lenses

PHARMACOLOGIC TREATMENT
- Analgesics for pain (systemic)
- Prophylactic antibiotic ointment or drops to prevent infection; avoid aminoglycosides due to delayed healing (polymixin); preparations with steroid are contraindicated
- Tetanus booster if indicated

LENGTH OF TREATMENT
- Topical antibiotics for 5–7 days

Special Consideration
- Topical analgesics are used for evaluation of the eye in a clinic setting only and should not be prescribed for pain management at home
- Advise patients of risk of severe complications and need for follow-up next day

When to Consult, Refer, Hospitalize
- Referral to an ophthalmologist if injury extensive, signs of infection, or if not improved in 24 hours

Follow-Up
- Should be observed in 24 hours
    - EXPECTED COURSE
        - Variable depending on severity; simple corneal abrasion resolves in 48 hours

    - COMPLICATIONS
        - Infection, ulceration
        - Loss of vision

Ocular Foreign Body

Description
- An abnormal substance on the epithelium of the eye surface such as dust, a piece of dirt, or other foreign object

Etiology
- Foreign bodies in the eye occur with an incident such as the wind blowing airborne particles or sand toward the eye or a projectile from equipment use (e.g., carpentry, mechanical work, hobby, lawn mowing)
- Disruption in the epithelial integrity of the cornea causes symptoms
- If foreign body penetrates further than the epithelial surface, ophthalmologist referral is indicated

Incidence and Demographics
- Commonly occurring condition

Risk Factors
- Lack of or improper use of protective eyewear during at-risk activities
- Living or playing in dusty or sandy environment (e.g., desert, beach)

Prevention and Screening
- Use of protective eyewear in appropriate or at-risk situations

Assessment
    HISTORY
- Foreign body sensation; degree of additional signs or symptoms is dependent on what the foreign body is and how long it has been there
- Associated complaints include lacrimation, pain, sensation of need to rub eyes, redness of the eye, photophobia if on the corneal or pupillary areas of the eye
- Determine event; some projectiles puncture the eye and become lodged in the deeper layers, leaving only a relatively minor injury apparent; if history suggests this, immediate referral is advised

PHYSICAL EXAM
- Complete a thorough examination of the eye; include visual acuity, inspection of the outer eye, and both the outer and inner aspect of the upper and lower eyelids; check pupillary response, EOMs; funduscopic examination
- Evert the eyelids for visualization of inner aspect of the eyelids
- Findings may include a quiet eye (no tearing, discharge, injection, or edema), dark specks on the iris, "rust ring" at site of entry of steel or iron projectile, diffuse injection, abrasion or tear of the epithelial layer

DIAGNOSTIC STUDIES
- Fluorescein staining will detect defects on the epithelial lining of the conjunctiva and cornea
- Slit lamp exam to assess inner eye thoroughly if no foreign body found

Differential Diagnosis
- Corneal abrasion
- Herpetic ulcer
- Intraocular penetration of foreign body
- Infection
- Glaucoma
- Other keratitis

Management
NONPHARMACOLOGIC TREATMENT
- Irrigation of the eye with normal saline solution for 10 minutes or more
- After application of eye anesthetic drops (proparacaine HCL, [e.g., Ophthaine]), foreign bodies that are superficial may be dislodged with irrigation alone, or gentle touch with a moistened cotton-tipped applicator; evert the eyelid to remove foreign bodies under eyelids
- NOTE: Use moistened cotton-tipped applicator ONLY if object is not embedded
- Application of patch to injured eye is no longer recommended

PHARMACOLOGIC TREATMENT
- Use of topical ophthalmic anesthetic is reserved for examination ONLY, not treatment
- Topical antibiotics are applied for prophylaxis; avoid aminoglycosides (polymixin)
- Tetanus booster if indicated

DIAGNOSTIC STUDIES
- Fluorescein staining will detect a concurrent corneal abrasion
- Slit lamp exam may be necessary to assess for intraocular penetration of foreign body

LENGTH OF TREATMENT
- Depends on extent of injury; patient seen by ophthalmologist for follow-up if necessary

Special Considerations
- Do not prescribe ophthalmic anesthetics for home pain control, use systemic analgesics (acetaminophen with codeine prn)

When to Consult, Refer, Hospitalize
- All incidents of foreign body in the eye are referred to an ophthalmologist within 24 hours unless patient reports symptoms are completely resolved
- All penetrating injuries, with or without the object remaining, must be referred to an ophthalmologist immediately
- Presence of a rust ring requires referral to ophthalmologist for treatment

Follow-Up
EXPECTED COURSE
- Depends on type of foreign body and severity of the injury

COMPLICATIONS
- Penetration of foreign body
- Infection, corneal abrasion
- Glaucoma secondary to intraocular inflammation, cataract formation

PROBLEMS OF THE EARS

Hearing Loss

Description
- Diminished or absent sense of hearing due to mechanical obstruction of sound transmission, neurological impairment, or both

Etiology
- *Conductive*: Decreased hearing via air conduction; interference of transmission of sound through the external auditory canal or transmission of vibrations from the tympanic membrane through the ossicular chain to the oval window
- *Sensorineural*: Hearing via bone conduction is impaired; the malfunction is in the cochlea, the cochlear portion of the eighth cranial nerve, or both
- *Mixed*: Both air and bone conduction impaired
- *Presbycusis*: Hearing loss due to the aging process; it is a nonpathologic, high-frequency hearing loss

Incidence and Demographics
- Approximately 1 of every 1,000 infants is born deaf
- Incidence of congenital hearing loss in 1 per 600 live births
- Congenital hearing loss typically diagnosed around 30 months of age, when language and developmental skills may already be delayed
- In adults, incidence of hearing loss is 140/100,000 per year with males = females
- Hearing loss of handicapping severity seen in 4% of persons age <45 years and in 29% of those age >65 years
- Loss occurs at any age, but more prominent in the elderly
- Otosclerosis most common cause of progressive hearing loss in the young adult

Risk Factors

- Hereditary (otosclerosis—immobility of the ossicles of the middle ear)
- Occupational exposure to loud noises
- Allergy or eustachian tube dysfunction
- In children, acute otitis media and otitis media with effusion, also genetic
- Ototoxic antibiotics: Streptomycin, gentamicin (Garamycin), vancomycin (Vancocin)
- Ototoxic diuretics: Ethacrynic acid and furosemide (Lasix)
- Ototoxic miscellaneous: Salicylates, platinum-based antineoplastic agents (cisplatin, carboplatin)

Prevention and Screening

- In 1993, the National Institutes of Health (NIH) recommended universal screening of neonates; many states have now mandated neonatal screening
- Otitis Media Guidelines Panel recommends audiometry after 3 months of chronic middle ear fluid
- Routine screening after age 65 (U.S. Preventive Task Force, 2007)
- Aggressive treatment of infections such as meningitis, or upper respiratory infection (URI) and eustachian tube dysfunction when there are known problems with ear infections
- Use of ear protection when exposed to loud noises (occupationally, home, such as mowing lawn)
- Avoidance of known ototoxic medications
- Avoidance of flying or diving (changes in barometric pressure) if URI present

Assessment (see Table 6–5)

DIAGNOSTIC STUDIES

- Tympanometry assessing tympanic membrane (TM) mobility
- Sedimentation rate to screen for autoimmune disease if indicated
- Audiometric evaluation for all chronic hearing loss, for acute hearing loss of unknown etiology
- Vestibular testing if tinnitus or vertigo involved
- CT if suspect tumors/bony lesions
- MRI if suspect acoustic neuroma

Table 6-5. Characteristics of Hearing Loss

	Conductive	Sensorineural	Presbycusis
Etiology	Congenital Impaction with wax or foreign body Infection Perforated TM Trauma Tissue overgrowth: otosclerosis, cholesteatoma Tumor	Prolonged exposure to loud noises Ototoxic substances Inner ear infections Ménière's disease Metabolic diseases: Diabetes, myxedema, thyroid Infectious: Syphilis, viral Trauma: Temporal bone injury or fracture Autoimmune disease	Aging Associated with smoking
Pattern of Loss	Decreased low tones, vowels; may have 60–70 dB deficit	Decreased high-frequency pitch, consonant discrimination, and background noise	Gradual loss of all tones; begins with highs then progresses to lows
History	Unilateral loss	Unilateral or bilateral Hears better in quiet room Associated with tinnitus and dizziness Sudden loss: assess for acoustic neuroma	Develops tinnitus, sensitive to loud and high pitches
Exam	Speaks softly Variable findings: Normal, foreign body, wax impaction, edema, obstruction, fluid behind TM; stiff, retracted or bulging TM Rinne: BC > AC in affected ear Weber lateralizes to poor ear	Speaks loudly Exam normal Rinne: AC > BC bilaterally Weber lateralizes to the better ear	Exam normal Nonspecific Weber or Rinne findings

Differential Diagnosis

- Presbycusis
- Infectious, vascular, metabolic, problems
- TB of temporal bone
- Acoustic neuromas
- Medications including aminoglycosides, loop diuretics (e.g., furosemide), antineoplastics, salicylates

- Conductive problems: obstruction of canal, TM impairment, otosclerosis, cholesteatoma, cochlear damage

Management

NONPHARMACOLOGIC TREATMENT

- Depends on etiology; remove obstructing wax or foreign body (Cerumenex and irrigation), treat underlying infections, discontinue ototoxic medications, surgical treatment (e.g., cochlear implants), hearing aids, adaptive measures (lip-reading, sign language)

PHARMACOLOGIC TREATMENT

- Antibiotics if indicated (acute otitis externa or media)
- Steroid therapy may be indicated for sudden sensorineural loss of unknown etiology

LENGTH OF TREATMENT

- Variable depending on underlying cause

Special Considerations

- Sign language interpreters should be considered in the primary care office for communication with patients with hearing impairments.
- Infants with one or more of the following factors are at risk for hearing loss and should be referred for comprehensive auditory testing: birthweight <1500 g; Apgar score of 5 or less at 5 minutes; developmental delay; more than 24 hours in NICU; severe hyperbilirubinemia; seizures or other neurologic abnormalities; physical abnormalities of skull, ears, nose, or throat at birth; history of maternal or neonatal infection or sepsis; history of head injury at birth; family history of hereditary hearing loss.

When to Consult, Refer, Hospitalize

- Refer to an otolaryngologist for any hearing loss of unknown etiology
- Refer cases not amenable to simple care such as wax removal, treatment of uncomplicated otitis
- Referral to audiologist for audiometric testing and consult

Follow-Up

EXPECTED COURSE

- Presbycusis and sensorineural loss may not be reversed; progression may be slowed or halted
- Temporary hearing alterations are reversible when related to minor problems such as congestion, otitis, wax, or foreign body obstruction that are responsive to treatment

COMPLICATIONS

- Potential for serious sequelae with cholesteatoma including balance problems, facial nerve paralysis, meningitis, brain abscess
- Neurologic abnormalities, perforations, cholesteatoma, tinnitus, vertigo, deafness

Impacted Cerumen

Description
- Obstruction of the external auditory canal due to accumulation of cerumen (ear wax), a naturally occurring lubricant that serves as a protective lining of the canal

Etiology
- Excessive production of ear wax beyond what can be cleared by natural mechanisms
- Manipulation of canal (e.g., introduction of cotton-tipped applicator) that pushes cerumen deeper into canal, resulting in a build-up that is beyond the ability of the natural process of clearing

Incidence and Demographics
- Farmers and industrial workers around grains, powders, and textiles; and the elderly have a greater incidence of impacted cerumen

Risk Factors
- Ear hygiene practices that pack cerumen in, e.g., Q-tips
- Age, occupation (wearing headphones, ear plugs), use of hearing aids

Prevention and Screening
- None

Assessment
HISTORY
- Hearing loss
- Feeling of fullness or pressure, itching
- Pain if pushed against tympanic membrane

PHYSICAL EXAM
- Dark brown wax, may be moist or dry
- Partial or complete obstruction of ear canal
- Visualization of the canal and TM may be partially or completely blocked by the wax

Differential Diagnosis
- Foreign body in canal
- Otitis media
- Otitis externa

Management
NONPHARMACOLOGIC TREATMENT
- Removal of the cerumen can be achieved by the use of a curette, or by irrigation with warm water to dislodge and rinse it out of the canal
- Contraindications for irrigation: Tympanostomy tube, perforated tympanic membrane, organic foreign body (e.g., legumes swell in contact with water)

PHARMACOLOGIC TREATMENT
  • Treatment to soften hardened cerumen may be achieved by instilling 1–2 drops of baby oil or solvents (Cerumenex) for 10–30 minutes prior to irrigation
  • Maintenance to avoid recurrent buildup can be done with the use of 3 drops of hydrogen peroxide and water (1:1), mineral oil or baby oil 1–2 drops, 1–2 x weekly; and by warm water rinsing of ear with a bulb syringe monthly

LENGTH OF TREATMENT
  • May require ongoing maintenance indefinitely

Special Considerations
• Provide education about proper ear hygiene

When to Consult, Refer, Hospitalize
• Referral to a specialist is required if the affected ear is the only ear with intact hearing, if there is suspected perforation of the TM, or if coexisting problems of the ear are present, such as severe infection, unexplained hearing loss, or hearing loss that did not clear with treatment of the impaction

Follow-Up
EXPECTED COURSE
  • Acute impaction is generally resolved completely following treatment
  • Ongoing potential for repeated impaction is minimized by maintenance

COMPLICATIONS
  • Pain, bleeding

Otitis Externa

Description
• Inflammation or infection of the external ear and auditory canal
• Commonly called "swimmer's ear"

Etiology
• Trauma to skin lining external auditory canal (as with cotton-tipped swab)
• Localized infected hair follicle (furuncle) in outer third of the canal
• Bacterial: *Staphylococcus aureus, Streptococcus pyogenes, Pseudomonas aeruginosa*
• Fungal secondary to prolonged otic antibiotic use: Aspergillus or Candida infection
• Viral infection
• Eczematous conditions: Seborrheic dermatitis, atopic dermatitis, psoriasis, neurodermatitis

Incidence and Demographics
• Affects 3%–10% of those seeking otologic care
• Commonly occurring problem in the general population
• More common in summer and warmer climates

Risk Factors
- Immunocompromised states
- Diabetes, especially in the elderly
- Predisposition to retaining moisture in the ear canal (small canal) after swimming or bathing
- Eczema
- Hearing aids

Prevention and Screening
- Use of ear plugs while swimming for those predisposed to otitis externa
- Completely drying ear canal after water exposure (blow dryer on cool setting)
- Application of 2% acetic acid solution (OTC) 1–2 drops after swimming
- Treatment of underlying conditions

Assessment

HISTORY
- Typical presentation includes pain of auricle which is often worsened by jaw movement, discharge of varying color from the ear canal, itching, sense of fullness

PHYSICAL EXAM
- Furunculosis is specifically localized to the one spot, which may or may not have extended erythema around it
- Tenderness of the auricle, pinna with movement. Auricle may appear normal, or reveal scaling, erythema, and edema; displacement of the external ear indicates mastoiditis
- External auditory canal lumen often narrowed by edema, accumulation of cellular debris and discharge, with TM visualization affected
- TM normal or dull
- Indicators of advanced infection or necrotizing malignant otitis externa: Ulcerations, facial nerve palsy, mastoid tenderness, cellulitis, fever, chills, malaise; requires **immediate referral**

DIAGNOSTIC STUDIES
- For general uncomplicated otitis externa, no diagnostic studies are indicated
- Resistant infections may warrant culturing, and an erythrocyte sedimentation rate (ESR) will be significantly increased in malignant otitis externa

Differential Diagnosis
- Acute otitis media
- Bullous myringitis
- Wisdom tooth eruption
- Mastoiditis
- TMJ problems
- Malignant otitis externa
- Foreign bodies
- Neoplasms
- Chronic suppurative otitis media

Management
NONPHARMACOLOGIC TREATMENT
- Removal of debris for enhancing examination by cleansing with curette or cotton-tipped swab with hydrogen peroxide/water solution (1:1; NOTE: do not irrigate)
- Placement of a wick or gauze strip in canals with greatly narrowed lumen to draw in otic drops
- Incision and drainage of furuncles
- Application of local heat (water bottle, warm pack) to outer ear for pain relief
- Avoid swimming while active infection

PHARMACOLOGIC TREATMENT
- OTC pain management (acetaminophen, NSAIDS); may need opioids.
- Topical otic antibiotic: Ofloxacin (Floxin), polymyxin B sulfate/neomycin sulfate/hydrocortisone (Cortisporin); or antifungal: acetic acid (VoSoL HC) to fight infection in combination with a corticosteroid to decrease inflammation
- Topocal acidifying agent such as acetic acid to inhibit growth of bacteria and fungi (Vosol)
- Oral antibiotics may be used in addition to topical medications in severe cases and in the immunocompromised: ciprofloxacin (Cipro) 750 mg q 12 hours, ofloxacin (Floxin) 400 mg q 12 hours, dicloxacillin (Dynapen) 500 mg q 6 hours, or cephalexin (Keftab) 500 mg q 6 hours if coexisting otitis media or severe infection (*P. aeruginosa*, *S. aureus*)

LENGTH OF TREATMENT
- Typical application dose of solutions to ears 3–4 drops 3–4x daily for 1–2 weeks
- Complicated case or malignant otitis externa requires prolonged therapy, 6–8 weeks

Special Considerations
- Necrotizing malignant otitis externa is typically found in those who are older than age 65, diabetic, or immunocompromised and requires **immediate specialist referral**
- 90% of adults with infection have been found to have some form of glucose intolerance

When to Consult, Refer, Hospitalize
- Referral to a specialist is indicated for those who do not respond to treatment, with severe infections, systemic involvement, cellulitis, malignant external otitis

Follow-Up
EXPECTED COURSE
- Simple cases will resolve with treatment; however, reoccurrence or chronic problems will require ongoing monitoring and prophylactic measures (ear plugs, acetic acid 2% after bathing or swimming).
- Patient should return for reevaluation after 1 week if not improved

COMPLICATIONS
- Mastoiditis, malignant external otitis, cellulitis

Otitis Media

Description
- Infection and/or inflammation of middle ear space with accumulation of fluid/pus
- Acute otitis media (AOM): Presence of fluid in the middle ear associated with signs or symptoms of acute local or systemic illness
- Otitis media with effusion (OME) may be asymptomatic but also may cause apparent decreased hearing, problems in balance, and discomfort at night when lying flat; it is an accumulation of serous fluid that remains for 2–3 months without indications of acute infection.

Etiology
- Acute otitis media:
  - Typically follows an upper respiratory infection
  - Eustachian tube (ET) may become obstructed from chronic negative pressure, leading to accumulation of fluid or effusions in the middle ear
  - *Streptococcus pneumoniae, H. influenzae, Moraxella catarrhalis*, Group A ß-hemolytic *Streptococcus, S. aureus*, and *Enterobacteriaceae*: Organisms gain access from the nasopharynx to the normally sterile middle ear, creating purulent exudate and increased pressure
  - Viral: Respiratory syncytial virus (RSV), influenza
- Otitis media with effusion:
  - Residual fluid in middle ear following acute otitis media
  - Eustachian tube dysfunction: The typically short, narrow, flexible, and horizontal eustachian tube found in children predisposes them to accumulation of nasopharyngeal secretions in the ET and middle ear; supine bottling and sucking may also contribute to reflux of fluid from the nasopharynx

Incidence and Demographics
- Most common in children under 6 years, but occurs in all ages
- Peak incidence is in the first 2 years of life

Risk Factors
- Eustachian tube dysfunction
- Recent URI, allergies
- Anatomic anomaly (adenoid hypertrophy, cleft palate)
- Cigarette use (as smoker or exposure to secondhand smoke)
- Native American, Caucasian, or Alaskan Native heritage
- Males > females
- Family history of AOM
- Day care attendance, under age 2

Prevention and Screening
- Avoid cigarette smoking and secondhand exposure
- Limit day care attendance

Assessment

HISTORY
- Acute otitis media:
  - Rapid onset
  - Symptoms: Otalgia, ear pulling, fever, irritability, otorrhea, sleeplessness, hearing loss, balance problems, anorexia, vomiting and/or diarrhea
  - May report extreme pain that is suddenly relieved with popping sensation, indicative of a ruptured tympanic membrane
- Otitis media with effusion:
  - Symptoms are variable, ranging from none to severe with pain, vertigo, and ataxia
  - Typically c/o a sense of fullness in the ear and decreased hearing in the affected ear; popping or crackling sounds in the ear with yawning, chewing, swallowing, or blowing nose
  - May report recent history of URI

PHYSICAL EXAM
- Acute otitis media:
  - Decreased TM mobility, discoloration of TM (white, yellow), fullness or bulging of TM, opacification of TM
  - Erythema of the TM may be present; erythema alone does not indicate AOM
  - Increased vascularity of tympanic membrane
  - Mobility of the TM is reduced on pneumatic otoscopy when there is fluid in the middle ear (70%–90% accuracy)
  - Bullae on the TM is indicative of M. *pneumoniae*
  - Fluid in external auditory canal may be noted with perforation of the TM
  - May be preauricular or cervical lymph node tenderness and enlargement
  - An entirely normal exam warrants further examination of related structures for conditions that may present with referred ear pain (e.g., TMJ dysfunction, sinusitis, cranial nerve abnormalities, dentition problems, nasopharyngeal carcinoma)
- Otitis media with effusion:
  - TM retracted with blunting of landmarks and a diffuse light reflex on inspection
  - Pneumatic otoscopy will detect decreased movement of TM
  - TM opaque, dull, pale golden yellowish color (not red), with or without air bubbles

DIAGNOSTIC STUDIES
- Tympanometry to confirm tympanic membrane mobility
- Audiometry to evaluate effect on hearing
- No routine testing is indicated, although CBC may be done if complicated or systemic infection suspected
- In severe cases, such as with immunosuppression or mastoiditis, culture of aspirated fluid from middle ear may be indicated and is performed by ENT

Differential Diagnosis

- Otitis externa
- Barotrauma (flying)
- Tonsillitis
- Mumps
- Mastoiditis
- Dental abscess
- Anatomic abnormalities
- Foreign body
- Sinusitis
- TMJ dysfunction
- Trauma
- Nasopharyngeal carcinoma

Management

NONPHARMACOLOGIC TREATMENT
- Valsalva maneuver or chewing gum to facilitate opening of eustachian tubes for draining middle ear

PHARMACOLOGIC TREATMENT
- Acute otitis media:
  - Pain management with OTC preparations such as acetaminophen or NSAIDS; codeine additionally if needed; may use topical analgesics such as Auralgan
  - Decongestants for the associated congestion of the nose or sinuses (NOTE: Does not affect otitis media, but provides symptom relief for congestion)
  - Antihistamines ONLY if allergies with increased watery secretions
  - Antibiotic therapy: Penicillins, cephalosporins, sulfonamides, macrolides (see Table 6–6)
  - CDC guidelines for antibiotic therapy:
    » First-line therapy: Amoxicillin 90 mg/kg/day, in divided doses in children <40 kg for 10 days <2 years of age; >2, 5–7 days; if >40 kg, dose as adults, i.e., 500 mg tabs tid
    » Consider use of sulfa or macrolide in event of penicillin allergy
  - If there is a TM perforation or patient has tubes, may use an antibiotic otic suspension such as ofloxacin (Floxin Otic) or Ciprodex Otic
  - When choosing antibiotic, consider risk of infections with resistant strains of bacteria
  - For clinically defined treatment failures after 3 days of therapy, an alternative agent should be selected after considering risk of infection with resistant strains; choose drug effective against drug-resistant *S. pneumoniae* (DRSP) and beta-lactamase–producing pathogens such as oral amoxicillin-clavulanate (Augmentin XR), cefuroxime axetil (Ceftin), or intramuscular ceftriaxone (Rocephin) x 3 days
  - Otitis media with effusion:
    - Antibiotic therapy is not routinely indicated for serous otitis media

LENGTH OF TREATMENT
- Antibiotic therapy is generally for 10 days with the exception of azithromycin (Zithromax), cefpodoxime (Vantin), and cefdinir (Omnicef), which are 5 days

Special Considerations

- Accurate diagnosis is essential to avoid overuse of antibiotics.
- Based on the 2004 American Academy of Pediatrics/American Academy of Family Physicians guidelines, observation without the use of antibiotics is an option for selected children with uncomplicated AOM based on diagnostic certainty, age (2 years), illness severity, and assurance of follow-up either by phone or office visit.

Table 6-6. Antibiotics for Acute Otitis Media

Drug/Brand Name	Adult Dosage	Pediatric Dosage
Amoxicillin (Amoxil, Trimox, Wymox)	500 mg tid: 3.5 g/day	40–90 mg/kg in 2–3 divided doses
Amoxicillin-clavulanate (Augmentin) AugmentinXR Augmentin ES suspension	875 mg q12h (based on amoxicillin component) 2 tabs bid Child >3 mos & <40 kg give 90mg/kg in 2 divided doses	40–90 mg/kg of amoxicillin component in 2 divided doses; to avoid larger doses of clavulanate, some authors recommend providing Augmentin at 40 mg/kg and amoxicillin at 40 mg/kg; newer Augmentin formulations provide clavulanate titrated to the higher amoxicillin dose
Azithromycin (Zithromax)	250 mg (2) to start, then 1 qd x 4 days	10 mg/kg day 1, then 5 mg/kg days 2–5
Cefaclor (Ceclor)	250–500 mg q8h	40 mg/kg in 3 divided doses
Cefdinir (Omnicef)	300 mg q12h (for 5 days in adults)	14 mg/kg in 1 dose or 2 divided doses (for 5 days in children >2 years old)
Cefixime (Suprax)	400 mg qd	8 mg/kg once a day
Cefpodoxime (Vantin)	200 mg q12h for 5 days	10 mg/kg in 2 divided doses for 5 days
Cefprozil (Cefzil)	250–500 mg q12h	30 mg/kg in 2 divided doses
Ceftibuten (Cedax)	400 mg qd	9 mg/kg once a day
Ceftriaxone (Rocephin)	1 gm q12h IM or IV	50 mg/kg IM x 3 days
Cefuroxime axetil (Ceftin)	250–500 mg bid	30 mg/kg in 2 divided doses
Clarithromycin (Biaxin)	500 mg q12h	15 mg/kg in 2 divided doses
Erythromycin-sulfisoxazole (Pediazole)	Not indicated	50 mg/kg in 3 or 4 divided doses (based on erythromycin component)
Loracarbef (Lorabid)	200 mg q12h	30 mg/kg in 2 divided doses
Trimethoprim-sulfamethoxazole (Septra, Bactrim)	1 double-strength tablet q12h (160 mg trim. + 800 mg sulfa)	8 mg/kg trim + 40 mg/kg sulfa in 2 divided doses x 10 days
Trimethoprim (Trimpex, Proloprim)	Not indicated	10 mg/kg in 2 divided doses

When to Consult, Refer, Hospitalize
- Refer to ENT specialist for recurrent acute otitis media
  - 3–4 episodes in 6 months or 4–6 in 12 months
  - Complications of severe infection such as mastoiditis or cholesteatoma
- Refer to ENT specialist for chronic middle ear effusion
  - 3 months or greater in both ears
  - 6 months or greater in one ear
- Refer to ENT specialist for perforation of the TM, nonresponsive to treatment within 48–72 hours, a hearing loss of 20 dB or more post treatment

Follow-Up
EXPECTED COURSE
- Simple cases are resolved in 10 days for AOM and should be reevaluated after treatment completed
- Middle ear effusion commonly persists after course of treatment for acute otitis media
- Effusion is present in 60% of cases at 2 weeks, 40% at 4 weeks, 20% at 2 months, 10% at 3 months
- Recheck can be made in 2–8 weeks depending on reliability of patient/parent

COMPLICATIONS
- Hearing loss
- Perforation of tympanic membrane
- Cholesteatoma
- Advanced infection (acute mastoiditis, meningitis, epidural abscess)

PROBLEMS OF NOSE/SINUSES

Rhinitis

Description
- Hyperfunction and tissue inflammation of the nasal mucosa categorized by the three common causes: Infectious, allergic, and nonallergic (also known as vasomotor rhinitis)

Etiology
- *Allergic rhinitis* is an IgE-mediated hypersensitivity reaction, most commonly related to inhaled seasonal pollen allergens (tree, grass, hay fever) and perennial allergens of dust mites, pet dander, cockroaches, molds, indoor pollutants, and cigarette smoke.
- *Infectious rhinitis* (*common cold*) is most commonly due to the rhinovirus, as well as coronavirus, influenza, parainfluenza, and adenoviruses, or, less commonly, bacteria.
- *Nonallergic* or *vasomotor rhinitis* etiologies are not well understood; thought to be an autonomic response that results in vascular dilatation of the nasal submucosal vessels. Influencing or triggering factors include temperature/humidity change, odors, selected drugs, emotional response, and body positions such as lying down.

- *Other causes*: Perennial form of nonallergic rhinitis is associated with atrophy of the nasal bones and nasal lining in the geriatric population; nasal polyps, benign overgrowths of the nasal mucous membrane, and connective tissue disorders; abuse of nasal decongestants oxymetazoline (Afrin) with rebound edema of the nose after continuous use; and transient rhinitis associated with pregnancy due to hormonal influences in women or foreign body in children

Incidence and Demographics
- Allergic: Affects 8%–20% of children and 15%–30% of adolescents; estimated that up to 75% of children with asthma also have allergic rhinitis
- Infectious: Common in all ages, especially children

Risk Factors
- Exposure to known allergens in susceptible individuals; aging

Prevention and Screening
- Frequent handwashing to reduce risk of infection
- Avoidance of known allergens and use of environmental control measures indoors such as frequent vacuuming with particulate filters, air cleaners (HEPA filters), mattress and pillow encasements, removal of carpeting, air conditioner, keeping indoor humidity <50%

Assessment (See Table 6–7)

Table 6–7. Comparison of Rhinitis Presentations

	Allergic Rhinitis	Infectious Rhinitis (cold)	Vasomotor Rhinitis	Atrophic Rhinitis
Onset	Age 5–20	Anytime	Adulthood	Geriatrics
Common Primary Symptoms	Nasal congestion, sneezing, itchy nose, clear drainage	Congestion, obstruction, sneezing, scratchy sore throat, nasal crusting, cloudy or colored drainage	Abrupt onset congestion and pronounced watery postnasal drip, sneezing	Nasal congestion, thick postnasal drip, repeated clearing of throat, bad smell in nose
Associated Symptoms	Cough, sore throat, itching and puffy eyes	Cough, malaise, headache, fever >100°F, may c/o facial or sinus tenderness	Watery eyes	None

Table 6–7. Comparison of Rhinitis Presentations (cont.)

	Allergic Rhinitis	Infectious Rhinitis (cold)	Vasomotor Rhinitis	Atrophic Rhinitis
Physical Exam Findings	Nasal mucosa pale & boggy Enlarged turbinates Clear watery discharge "Allergic shiners" Nasal salute Mouth-breathing	Edema and hyperemia of mucous membranes, throat erythema without edema, postnasal drainage, lungs clear, cervical lymph nodes tender and enlarged	Turbinates pale and edematous No other findings	Nasal mucosa dry, nonedematous, airway patent No other findings

Differential Diagnosis
- URI
- Foreign body
- Hormonal: Oral contraceptives or pregnancy
- Sinusitis
- Nasal polyps or overgrowths
- Adenoid hypertrophy
- Otitis media
- Endocrine disease (hypothyroidism)

Management
NONPHARMACOLOGIC TREATMENT
- General measures for all types: Hydration, humidification (except for allergic), intranasal irrigation with saline solutions
- Avoidance of known triggers

PHARMACOLOGIC TREATMENT
- Topical antihistamine azelastine HCL 0.1% (Astelin)
- Oral antihistamines: 1st generation products such as diphenhydramine (Benadryl) cause sedation and can impair performance; use with caution
- 2nd generation nonsedating: Fexofenadine (Allegra), loratadine (Claritin), and less sedating Cetirizine (Zyrtec) are preferred for regular use
- Oral decongestants cause vasoconstriction, decrease blood supply to the nasal mucosa, and decreased mucosal edema; can be used with antihistamines; numerous preparations available
- Topical steroids: Not fully effective until several days after initiation of therapy
  - Beclomethasone, fluticasone, triamcinolone preparations all available
  - Refer to packaging for age-usage and dosage
- Immunotherapy: Recommended for patients who have not responded to pharmacologic therapy

        – Series of injections with specific allergens, once or twice weekly
        – Should only be initiated by a trained specialist
- Specific recommendations for each disorder as follows
  – Allergic rhinitis: Intranasal steroids first; oral antihistamines may be added, also topical antihistamine (Astelin) and mast cell stabilizes (NasalCrom); if patient has concomitant allergic eye symptoms, treat also with ocular antihistamine and/or mast cell stabilizer
  – Infectious rhinitis: Acetaminophen or NSAIDs for pain or fever, decongestants (avoid antihistamines as they may over-dry and reduce ability to clear secretions)
  – Rhinitis medicamentosa (drug-induced): Rebound nasal vasomotor rhinitis associated with long-term topical decongestant use that may lead to nasal atony. Discontinue decongestants; use saline solution nasal spray, some relief with intranasal anticholinergic such as ipratropium (Atrovent)
  – Atrophic rhinitis: Guaifenesin (Naldecon Senior EX syrup) for stimulation of mucus, or intranasal saline solution spray

LENGTH OF TREATMENT
- Infectious rhinitis: Treatment for symptom relief only
- Allergic rhinitis usually treated daily throughout allergy season
- Nonallergic rhinitis may be treated daily to prevent symptoms

Special Considerations
- Use medication with caution in geriatric population; medications commonly produce adverse reactions or may interact with other medications they take routinely.
- Use OTC decongestants with caution in patients with diabetes, hypertension, or glaucoma.

When to Consult, Refer, Hospitalize
- Referral to an allergist for allergen immunotherapy for allergic rhinitis that is not easily managed by medications or avoidance of known allergens
- Referral to ENT for those with complications, nasal polyps or growths, or symptoms unmanageable with above-described treatments

Follow-Up
- Routine follow-up is generally 2–4 weeks after initiation of treatment for allergic and nonallergic rhinitis
- Follow up if infectious rhinitis has not resolved in 10 days

EXPECTED COURSE
- Viral rhinitis usually resolves within 7–10 days
- Allergic, vasomotor, and atrophic rhinitis are ongoing problems managed, not cured

COMPLICATIONS
- Rhinitis medicamentosa
- Worsening of related pulmonary conditions (e.g., COPD, asthma)
- Spread of infection: Otitis media, acute sinusitis, pneumonia, bronchitis

Epistaxis

Description
- Hemorrhage from the nostrils, nasopharynx, or nasal cavity (anterior or posterior)
- May be a symptom of an underlying problem

Etiology
- Primarily idiopathic, but may have many other causes; <10% are related to neoplasm or coagulopathy
- Traumatic such as nose-picking, foreign body, sinus fracture or tumor, abuse of inhaled recreational drugs (cocaine)
- Localized irritation secondary to acute or chronic rhinitis, colds, sinusitis, URI
- Vascular abnormalities such as aging sclerotic vessels, arterial venous malformations
- Septal deviation or perforation
- Hypertension (bleeding worsened by but not caused by hypertension)
- Coagulation problems from disease such as von Willebrand disease, leukemias, blood dyscrasias, platelet dysfunction; or medications such as warfarin (Coumadin), NSAIDs, or aspirin, usually secondary to trauma

Incidence and Demographics
- One significant nosebleed is experienced by approximately 10% of the population
- Typically occurs in the young (<10 yrs) and in the older adult (>50 yrs)

Risk Factors
- All of the concomitant or precipitating problems listed under Etiology above

Prevention and Screening
- Adequate moisturizing of the mucous membranes: humidifier, saline nasal spray, along with keeping nails clipped short and away from nose
- Petroleum jelly or antibiotic ointment applied to the anterior nasal septum
- Control of underlying nasal and systemic problems
- Protective athletic equipment, safety precautions to prevent trauma

Assessment
HISTORY
- Patients may present with actively bleeding nose, or may consult for episodes that were resolved with self-care
- Ascertain precipitating events; from which nostril blood first appeared; associated symptoms including nausea and vomiting, URI symptoms
- Inquire about color of blood, coffee-ground emesis, hemoptysis, melena, and medications currently used, particularly aspirin or NSAIDs

PHYSICAL EXAM
- Inspect for site of bleed; note localized or diffuse mucosal irritation, bleeding from 1 or 2 nostrils, venous or arterial source (Table 6–8); obtain vital signs, do complete ENT exam

Table 6-8. Characteristics of Nasal Bleeding Sites

	Anterior Epistaxis	Posterior Epistaxis
Presentation	Typically unilateral	Unilateral or bilateral
Timing	Lasts between a few to 30 min, in isolation or recurrently	Intermittent
Source of Bleed	Typically venous from Kiesselbach's plexus 90% are located here	Typically arterial from posterior nasopharynx More common location in the elderly
Other	Usually less severe, easier to treat More common in young patients	Can result in significant hemorrhage May have nausea or coffee-ground emesis

DIAGNOSTIC STUDIES
- Only recurrent or severe cases warrant extensive evaluation with head radiograph or CT scan
- If significant blood loss is suspected, obtain hemoglobin and hematocrit
- If bleeding disorders are suspected, then obtain a CBC, PT, and PTT

Differential Diagnosis
- Drug-related as an anticoagulant side effect or from abuse (nasal cocaine inhalation)
- Symptom of one of the etiologic agents identified above
- Localized, isolated, benign event

Management
NONPHARMACOLOGIC TREATMENT
- For simple (anterior) nosebleeds, application of direct pinching-type pressure just below the bridge of the nose for 10–15 minutes will stop the bleeding; technique can be taught to the patient for self-care in the event of reoccurrence of a simple nosebleed. Keep the patient in an upright position and apply ice packs over the bridge of the nose.
- If not responsive to above measures, most anterior venous bleeds can be controlled by placing a cotton ball moistened with 1:1000 epinephrine OR vasoconstrictor nose drops (e.g., phenylephrine) just inside the nares and then apply pressure for 5–10 minutes. Some practitioners may also initiate cauterization with silver nitrate sticks or chemical cautery with chromic acid beads to the site of the bleeding.
- For maintenance of nasal hygiene and to avoid recurrence, apply petroleum jelly (Vaseline) to nares routinely for lubrication. Use humidifiers, cut fingernails, and avoid picking.
- For arterial (posterior) bleeds or epistaxis not responding to above acute treatment, immediate referral to an ER or ENT specialist for further treatment procedures, which may include cauterization via silver nitrate stick, bead of chromic acid, or 25% trichloroacetic acid, electrocautery or thermal cautery followed by packing with ribbons of gauze impregnated with petroleum jelly, nasal tampons, or balloon inflation compression.

PHARMACOLOGIC TREATMENT
- Vasoconstrictors and topical anesthetics for bleeding cessation and analgesia
- Examples include cocaine 4%, phenylephrine 0.25% epinephrine 1:1000, lidocaine laryngeal spray, lidocaine jelly 2%, lidocaine solution 4%, viscous lidocaine 2%
- Treatment of underlying disorders

LENGTH OF TREATMENT
- Treatment is episodic for the actual bleeding incident
- Ongoing monitoring and treatment as indicated for the associated underlying disorders

Special Considerations
- None

When to Consult, Refer, Hospitalize
- Immediate referral to an emergency facility or ENT for severe bleeding or bleeding unresponsive to first-line treatment
- Recurrent epistaxis is cause for referral to an ENT specialist

Follow-Up
EXPECTED COURSE
- Excellent prognosis for isolated, idiopathic epistaxis
- Variable outcome depending on underlying cause

COMPLICATIONS
- Nasal obstruction, sinusitis
- Abscess from excessive trauma during packing of nose
- Septal perforation from cauterization therapy
- Vasovagal episode during packing

Sinusitis

Description
- Inflammation or infection of the paranasal sinus cavities, categorized as acute, recurrent, subacute, or chronic
- *Acute sinusitis* is an infection of one or more paranasal sinuses with symptoms lasting 3–4 weeks and that resolve with therapy within 3–4 weeks. It is considered *recurrent* if there are >3 acute episodes per year.
- *Subacute sinusitis* is ongoing symptoms of purulent nasal discharge and inflammation of the sinuses that is resolved in <3 months.
- *Chronic sinusitis* is prolonged inflammation of the sinuses with or without associated infection with symptoms >3 months' duration. There may be irreversible damage to the mucosa.

Etiology
- Predisposing factors include the various forms of rhinitis, nasal polyps, and immunodeficiency. Allergic and vasomotor rhinitis commonly precede recurrent or chronic sinusitis by causing edema and exudate that blocks sinus ostia and impair normal mucociliary clearance.
- The most common bacterial pathogens in acute sinusitis are *Streptococcus pneumoniae*, *Haemophilus influenzea, Moraxella catarrhalis*.
- Polymicrobial pathogens most commonly seen in chronic or subacute sinusitis include anaerobic bacteria and *Staphylococcus aureus*. Anaerobic bacteria are commonly the cause of sinusitis precipitated by dental infections.
- Other infectious causes include viral (rhinovirus, coronavirus, adenovirus); may also be from fungal source (Aspergillus), especially in the immunocompromised.

Incidence and Demographics
- 31 million Americans are affected each year, losing an average of 4 days from work per year
- Complicates approximately 5%–10% of upper respiratory tract infections.
- Sinusitis affects patients with other disease states. It commonly occurs in those with immunodeficiency, asthma, and cystic fibrosis. Medical and surgical management of sinusitis has a significant impact on the improvement of asthma. Chronic sinusitis is an important source of morbidity in cystic fibrosis.

Risk Factors
- Dental or upper respiratory infections
- Anatomic abnormalities: Hypertrophied tonsils and adenoids, deviated septum, nasal polyps, and cleft palate
- Barotrauma
- Immunodeficiency and HIV

Prevention and Screening
- Appropriate treatment of allergies and viral upper respiratory tract infections
- Avoidance of adverse environmental factors, such as cigarette smoke, pollution, and barotrauma
- Practice daily nasal hygiene through the use of normal saline irrigation/spray
- Improve mucociliary clearance by increasing ambient humidity with a humidifier

Assessment
HISTORY
- URI symptoms not improving after 10 days
- Classic presenting symptoms include nasal congestion, yellow/green rhinorrhea, postnasal drainage, facial or dental pain, headache, altered sense of smell, cough that is worse at night
- Other associated symptoms of fever, malaise, fatigue, sore throat, halitosis, and nausea may be present
- Complaints of orbital pain or vision disturbances are indicators of a more serious problem

PHYSICAL EXAM
- Physical examinations should include a complete HEENT (head, eyes, ears, nose, throat) and pulmonary exam, with typical findings in the case of acute sinusitis as follows:
    - Face/sinuses: Tenderness overlying the involved sinus, fever variable
    - Ears: Frequently find middle ear abnormalities and eustachian tube dysfunction
    - Nose: Erythema of the mucosa and purulent drainage
    - Mouth: Postnasal drip on posterior pharyngeal area, halitosis
    - Chest: Potential for wheezing, congestion associated with asthma or URI
- Chronic sinusitis merits a more detailed examination for underlying risk factors
- NOTE: Important serious findings include external facial swelling, erythema, or cellulitis over an involved sinus (periorbital or forehead); vision changes such as diplopia; difficulty moving eyes (EOMs); proptosis; and any abnormal neurologic signs. **These are all indicative of serious complications requiring urgent referral and treatment.**

DIAGNOSTIC STUDIES
- The diagnosis of sinusitis is based on a combination of clinical history, physical examination, nasal cytology, and/or imaging studies
- Imaging studies may be required when the symptoms are vague, physical findings are equivocal, or there is poor response to the initial management
- Plain films of the sinuses are not recommended
- Computed tomography is the preferred imaging technique for preoperative evaluation of the nose and paranasal sinuses secondary to obstruction of the ostiomeatal complex; simple coronal views may be helpful to evaluate recurrent and chronic sinusitis
- Although magnetic resonance imaging has limitations in the definition of the bony anatomy, it is particularly sensitive for evaluation of the frontal, maxillary, and sphenoid sinuses for fungal sinusitis and tumors, so is used for the differential diagnosis between inflammatory diseases and malignant tumors
- Ultrasonography has limited utility but may be applicable in pregnant women and for determining the amount of retained secretions

Differential Diagnosis
- Nasopharyngeal tumor
- Wegener syndrome
- Immotile cilia syndrome
- Nasal polyps
- Nasal septum deviation
- Trauma, foreign body
- Cystic fibrosis
- Granuloma
- Viral URI

Management
NONPHARMACOLOGIC TREATMENT
- There are several comfort measures that may be helpful: Adequate rest, adequate hydration, analgesics as needed, warm facial packs, steamy showers, using saline nasal sprays, and sleeping with the head of bed elevated

PHARMACOLOGIC TREATMENT
- Several medications are useful in the treatment of sinusitis: Antibiotics, intranasal corticosteroids, oral and nasal decongestants.
- Antibiotics are the mainstay of treatment for bacterial sinusitis. High dose amoxicillin is the first-line recommendation. Alternative antibiotics include quinolones, cephalosporins, or macrolides. See specific dosages in Table 6–6 as for otitis media. Note that macrolides generally either do not provide the necessary antibacterial coverage or are associated with too much resistance among pneumococci in the community when used for treating sinusitis.
- Severe cases may require AugmentinXR or a Quinolone first line.
- Failure to respond to first-line antibiotics within 3–5 days warrants switching to a new antibiotic such as amoxicillin/clavulanate (Augmentin XR), cefuroxime axetil (Ceftin), cefpodoxime (Vantin), or Cefdinir (Omnicef).
- Use of nasal corticosteroids in patients with acute sinusitis is reasonable for those with underlying rhinitis or associated bronchial hyperresponsiveness.
- Those patients with significant anatomic obstruction, invasive nasal polyposis, or who have demonstrated marked mucosal edema radiographically benefit from the short-term use of oral corticosteroids.
- Decongestants will reduce mucosal blood flow, decrease tissue edema and nasal resistance, and may enhance drainage of secretions from the sinus ostia. Suggested types include topical decongestants such as oxymetazoline (Afrin) and phenylephrine (Neo-Synephrine) but no longer than 3 days to avoid rebound, and oral decongestants such as pseudoephedrine (Sudafed).

LENGTH OF TREATMENT
- Recommendations are not consistent; however, a 10–14-day course is typical for acute sinusitis.
- Chronic sinusitis should be treated until the patient is well for 7 days.
- For those with incomplete resolution after the above treatment, the antibiotic is continued for another 10–14 days or another antibiotic is tried.

Special Considerations
- Avoid prolonged use of topical decongestants to prevent rebound congestion and dependence.
- Resist the urge and patient demand to treat viral URIs with antibiotics.

When to Consult, Refer, Hospitalize
- Immediate referral for evaluation by an otolaryngologist is indicated for swelling of the forehead or orbital areas, severe pain, and/or vision disturbance.

- Chronic or complicated sinusitis management includes evaluation by a specialist. Indications for referral to an otolaryngologist, allergist, or immunologist include chronic or recurrent sinusitis associated with otitis media; patients who have undergone prior surgical procedures and continue to experience sinusitis; or for complications such as asthma, bronchitis, bronchiectasis or pneumonia, fungal sinusitis, or multiple antibiotic allergies.
- Underlying risk factors are also a reason for referral, such as allergic and nonallergic rhinitis and structural abnormalities.

Follow-Up

EXPECTED COURSE
- Improvement of symptoms within 72 hours and resolution of sinusitis within 10 days

COMPLICATIONS
- Brain abscess, meningitis, osteomyelitis, orbital cellulitis, venous sinus thrombosis, subdural empyema

PROBLEMS OF THE PHARYNX

Pharyngitis/Tonsillitis

Description
- Inflammation of the pharyngeal and/or tonsillar tissue frequently caused by acute infection. Infection by Group A beta-hemolytic *streptococcus* is of greatest concern due to the potential for sequelae (scarlet fever, rheumatic fever, glomerulonephritis) and the potential to avoid such complications by early detection and treatment.

Etiology
- Spread by person-to-person contact via droplets of oral, respiratory, and nasal secretions
- Viral infection accounts for 90% of pharyngitis
- Virus types include Coxsackie, echovirus, respiratory syncytial virus, influenza A and B, Epstein-Barr, adenovirus, coronavirus, herpes simplex, and HIV
- Bacterial agents most common are *Streptococcus pyogenes*; Group A, C, G *streptococcus*; *Arcanobacterium haemolyticum*
- *Mycoplasma pneumoniae* and *Chlamydia pneumoniae* are other infecting organisms that may be found in pharyngitis, though much less commonly
- Fungal infection of *Candida albicans*
- Gonococcal pharyngitis caused by N. *Gonorrhoeae*
- Peritonsillar abscess, a complication of pharyngitis is most likely caused by anaerobic bacteria, Group A beta hemolytic *streptococcus*, H. *influenzae* or S. *aureus*

Incidence and Demographics
- A commonly occurring illness; approximately 30 million cases per year estimated
- Streptococcal pharyngitis most commonly occurs in those under age 18 with a seasonal prevalence during the late winter and early spring months

- Rheumatic fever incidence approximately 64 cases/100,000 cases of Group A beta-hemolytic *streptococcus* infection

Risk Factors
- Exposure to Group A beta-hemolytic *streptococcus*, virus, or other causative agents
- Communal living (dormitories, barracks)
- Immunosuppression, diabetes mellitus (for fungal infection)
- Recent illness, fatigue, exposure to smoke, or excess alcohol intake

Prevention and Screening
- Frequent hand-washing, especially in situations of contact with infected people
- Avoidance of exposure to those infected

Assessment

HISTORY
- Complaint of throat pain that ranges from mild to severe; associated symptoms are variable depending on the underlying etiology (Table 6–9)

PHYSICAL EXAM
- The history and physical alone are only 50% reliable for diagnosis; similar presentation on exam is seen with multiple potential infectious agents

DIAGNOSTIC STUDIES
- Rapid strep antigen screen: 50%–80% sensitivity; >95% specificity; do not culture if positive
- Throat culture remains the "gold standard" for diagnosis of Group A beta-hemolytic *streptococcus*
- If a negative rapid strep screen is found in a patient with a high probability of streptococcus, culture to confirm
- Mono spot is indicated for suspicion of mononucleosis
- CBC with differential reveals WBC increased if bacterial, decreased if viral (not routinely done)
- If indicated, culture for gonorrhea and/or *Chlamydia* infection
- Potassium hydroxide (KOH) wet mount reveals pseudohyphae and budding spores in Candidiasis

Table 6-9. Characteristics of Pharyngitis by Etiology

	Symptoms	Exam Findings
VIRAL		
Coxsackie and others	Sore throat, malaise, fever, headache	Small oral vesicles, ulcers on posterior pharynx, tonsils, buccal mucus
Epstein-Barr	Above + fatigue	Exudative tonsillitis, palatial petechiae, posterior cervical adenopathy; possible maculopapular rash
Primary HIV	Above + myalgia, photophobia lasts few days to 2 weeks	Posterior cervical lymphadenopathy Similar to Epstein-Barr with rash
GROUP A STREP	Sore throat, fever, odynophagia (primarily) Abdominal pain, vomiting, headache	Fever >101°F Erythema, and white or yellow exudate of tonsils and/or pharynx Anterior cervical lymphadenopathy Absence of other URI symptoms/signs generally but not always
Scarlet Fever	Abrupt onset fever, pharyngitis, headache	Sandpaper-like fine, erythematous rash on trunk and extremities (absent on face) that blanches on pressure Appears within 24–48 hours, lasts 4–10 days
Rheumatic Fever	Symptoms develop 1–6 months after strep infection	Various manifestations: heart murmur, polyarthritis, rash (see Chapter 4)
STD		
Chlamydia or Gonorrhea	Chronic sore throat History of oral sex or sexual abuse	Exudative, erythematous pharynx Anterior cervical lymphadenopathy
MYCOPLASMA	Same as strep	Same as strep
FUNGAL		
Candida albicans	History of antibiotic use, immunosuppression, use of inhaled corticosteroids	Thin, diffuse or patchy white plaques on red base on mucous membranes, pharynx, tongue
PERITONSILLAR ABSCESS	Unilateral throat and ear pain Dysphagia, dysphonia, drooling, trismus (difficulty opening mouth due to pain and inflammation)	Erythema and swelling of soft palate Uvula and soft palate edema such that it may appear the uvula "points" towards side of abscess Exquisitely tender, palpable, fluctuant abscess on tonsil Similarly tender, enlarged anterior cervical lymph nodes

Differential Diagnosis
- Etiologic agents identified above
- Epiglottitis
- Thyroiditis
- Postnasal drip related to rhinitis or sinusitis

Management
- The prime reason to identify and treat Group A beta-hemolytic streptococcal pharyngitis is to decrease the risk of acute rheumatic fever.
  NONPHARMACOLOGIC TREATMENT
  - Symptomatic treatment includes forcing fluids to hydrate, gargle with warm salt water, OTC analgesics (acetaminophen, NSAIDS if no contraindications), throat lozenges, and cool-mist humidifier
  - Rest is advisable with pharyngitis associated with mononucleosis
  - NOTE: Peritonsillar abscess requires urgent referral to otolaryngologist for possible IV antibiotics, incision and drainage; tonsillectomy may be recommended as definitive treatment after acute episode resolves

  PHARMACOLOGIC TREATMENT
  - Penicillin V (Pen-Vee K) 500 mg bid or tid is the drug of choice for streptococcus; children: 25–50 mg/kg/day, divided bid–qid all for 10 days
  - If allergic to penicillin, erythromycin (E-mycin 500 mg bid x 10 days); children: 30–50 mg/kg/day, divided tid–qid
  - Alternative treatments: First-generation cephalosporins, azithromycin (Zithromax), clarithromycin (Biaxin)
  - For those with recurrence, a repeat course of antibiotics with clindamycin or Augmentin is recommended
  - For elimination of streptococcus in those who are carriers: Clindamycin (Cleocin) 20 mg/kg/day in 3 divided doses x 10 days, but with asymptomatic carriage generally no treatment is indicated
  - For chlamydial or mycoplasmal infections, when present usually accompanied by lower respiratory tract symptoms: Children: erythromycin 30–50 mg/kg bid x 10 days; adults: doxycycline 100 mg bid x 10 days or azithromycin 500 mg for 1 day followed by 250 mg for 4 days
  - For gonococcal pharyngitis: Ceftriaxone (Rocephin) 125–250 mg IM (consider treatment for chlamydia as well)
  - For Candidias pharyngitis: Nystatin (Mycostatin) 100,000 U/ml oral suspension 4–6 mL qid

  LENGTH OF TREATMENT
  - Antibiotic and antifungal treatments must be carried out for an entire 10-day period

Special Considerations
- Cultures positive for bacteria other than Group A strep are usually not treated
- Household and close personal contacts of patient with strep only treated if symptomatic
- Children may return to school after afebrile and on antibiotic for at least 24 hours
- Advise those diagnosed with mono to avoid contact sports for 4 weeks to avoid possible splenic rupture

When to Consult, Refer, Hospitalize
- Any patient with peritonsillar or retropharyngeal abscess requires urgent referral
- **Patients with symptoms or edema affecting the ability to breath or swallow (e.g., inability to swallow their own saliva) require immediate transfer to hospital**

Follow-Up
- No follow-up necessary unless not resolving
  EXPECTED COURSE
  - Strep pharyngitis typically lasts for 5–7 days, with fever peaking at second to third day; will spontaneously resolve but early treatment of strep pharyngitis decreases symptomatic period by ½–2 days and decreases risk of rheumatic fever
  - Viral pharyngitis will resolve spontaneously
  - Symptoms of rheumatic complications develop in weeks to months following resolution of the pharyngitis

  COMPLICATIONS
  - Infection spread, epiglottitis, lymphadenitis, otitis media, mastoiditis, septicemia, rhinitis, sinusitis, pneumonia
  - Rheumatic fever

Epiglottitis

Description
- Rapid development of cellulitis of the epiglottis and surrounding tissues that potentially results in acute airway obstruction
- **NOTE: An acute and sudden onset of a potentially life-threatening illness**

Etiology
- Abrupt onset and rapid progression of fever, apprehension, and respiratory distress
- Infectious etiology: *H. influenzae* detected in approximately 26% of cases. Other suspected organisms include Group A beta-hemolytic streptococcus, pneumococci, and staphylococci. Unclear if there are viral etiologies.

Incidence and Demographics
- Typically occur in children age 3–8 years, infrequently in adults, but may occur at any age.

Risk Factors
- Unimmunized children

Prevention and Screening
- Immunization with *H. influenzae type B* vaccine available only for children up to age 5.
- Rifampin 20 mg/kg qd x 4 days (max daily dose 600 mg) for close contacts (may be carriers).

Assessment

HISTORY

- Sudden onset of severe pain with swallowing or already unable to swallow own saliva by time of examination, fever, sore throat, swollen glands
- Usually no precipitating URI
- PMH and current medications should be obtained

PHYSICAL EXAM

- Patients are in respiratory distress and may be in shock with a toxic appearance
- Classic posturing of sitting up and leaning forward, tongue hanging out, often holding something (a cup) to spit their saliva out as they can't swallow it without severe pain
- Voice is soft or muffled; there is soft stridor, and minimal cough
- A later finding is hypoxia
- NOTE: Examination of the pharynx should be carried out ONLY with equipment and personnel in place for emergency intubation or tracheotomy for airway maintenance; insertion of a tongue blade into the oral cavity may precipitate laryngeal spasm and acute airway obstruction

DIAGNOSTIC STUDIES

- Blood and epiglottis cultures (obtained under same conditions as examination described above)
- Blood cultures are positive in 90% of patients
- CBC positive for leukocytosis with left shift
- Chest x-ray for screening of pneumonia (25% occurrence rate) and placement of endotracheal tube
- Lateral neck x-ray consistent with inflammation of epiglottis

Differential Diagnosis

- Peritonsillar abscess
- Retropharyngeal abscess
- Diphtheria in unimmunized patients
- Foreign body aspiration
- Lingual tonsillitis
- Sepsis
- Angioedema

Management

- Immediately arrange for monitoring, IV, and maintenance of airway with appropriate personnel and equipment and transport to an emergency setting or hospital with ICU
- Monitor vital signs, oxygen saturation, and be alert for potential abrupt deterioration
- IV antibiotics

Special Considerations

- Incidence decreasing in children since use of HIB vaccine

When to Consult, Refer, Hospitalize
- Immediate consultation with physician or referral to ENT specialist for all patients suspected of having epiglottitis
- Hospitalization for airway management during treatment

Follow-Up
> EXPECTED COURSE
>> • With prompt and appropriate treatment, morbidity and mortality rates are low
>> • Airway management measures usually discontinued within 24–48 hours of treatment

> COMPLICATIONS
>> • Advanced infections: Pneumonia, meningitis, cervical adenitis, septic arthritis
>> • Death from airway obstruction (asphyxia)

PROBLEMS OF THE MOUTH

Oral Candidiasis (Thrush)

Description
- Fungal infection of the oral mucous membranes

Etiology
- Candida albicans is part of normal flora of the oral cavity that causes overt infection when there is a reduction in the competitive oral microflora

Incidence and Demographics
- Essentially a disease of infants but can occur at any age

Risk Factors
- Most common cause in infants and children is long-term use of broad-spectrum antibiotics
- May also arise in immunosuppressed patients
- Conditions that cause decrease in the host resistance (e.g., stress, diabetes, malnutrition, prematurity)
- Use of inhaled corticosteroids (ICS)
- Denture wear

Prevention and Screening
- Judicious use of antibiotics
- Patients using ICS should rinse mouth with alcohol-based mouthwash after each use
- Elderly patients should clean their dentures carefully and frequently

Assessment
> HISTORY
>> • White coating in the mouth
>> • Decreased sucking or appetite due to discomfort, sore throat

PHYSICAL
- White plaques covering the mucous membrane of the oral cavity, particularly the tongue, buccal mucosa, and hard palate, which easily rubs off leaving an underlying red, raw surface
- Membrane consists of an almost pure colony of fungus
- Lesion is confined to the surface mucosa and is not invasive
- Angular chelitis

Differential Diagnosis
- Exudative pharyngitis
- Leukoplakia (adults)

    DIAGNOSTIC STUDIES
    - KOH preparation for microscopy of plaque can be made but not necessary

Management

NONPHARMACOLOGIC TREATMENT
- Determine and treat underlying cause (e.g., antibiotic use, immune problem)

PHARMACOLOGIC TREATMENT
- Topical nystatin (Mycostatin) oral suspension 100,000 units per mL; infants: 2 mL qid, (1 mL on each side of mouth); adults: 4–6 mL (½ dose on each side of mouth) qid, keep in mouth as long as possible before swallowing; clotrimazole trouches 10 mg 5x day
- Gentian violet 1% aqueous solution (effective but messy)
- If resistant to above (rare), fluconazole (Diflucan) or itroconazole (Sporanox)

LENGTH OF TREATMENT
- 7–10 days
- May need to repeat if problem continues on oral antibiotics

Special Considerations
- If occurring in breastfed infant, check mother's nipple area for infection and treat prn

When to Consult, Refer, Hospitalize
- Consult with physician or infectious disease specialist for immunocompromised patient, esophageal infection, failure to resolve as expected

Follow-Up

EXPECTED COURSE
- Resolves in 1–2 weeks depending on severity and host immune status

COMPLICATIONS
- Feeding problems, weight loss

Gingivostomatitis

Description
- Inflammation of the mucosa of the oral cavity that may involve the gingiva, buccal mucosa, or tongue

Etiology
- Viral:
  - Herpes (cold sores)
    - Herpes simplex virus (HSV); primary infection that is usually subclinical; secondary or recurrent infection is more common (recurrent represents reactivation of a latent infection in an immune host with circulating antibodies)
    - 2 subtypes: HSV-1 and HSV-2; both forms can infect either oral or genital mucosa, but HSV-1 usually associated with oral infection
  - Herpangina: Coxsackie virus A is most common but also Coxsackie virus B, echoviruses
  - Hand, foot, and mouth disease: Coxsackie virus A
- Unknown cause:
  - Vincent's angina (trench mouth)
    - Possible anaerobic microorganisms
    - Periodontal infection due to poor dental hygiene or by malocclusion
    - Precipitating events include emotional stress, systemic disease, and immunosuppression
  - Aphthous ulcers
- Other causes:
  - Smoking
  - Food hypersensitivity (citrus, nuts, coffee, chocolate, potatoes, cheeses, figs, gluten)
  - Allergic or toxic drug reactions
  - Riboflavin deficiency
  - Endocrine factors
  - Emotional stress, trauma

Incidence and Demographics
- Herpes; herpangina; hand, foot, and mouth disease; aphthous ulcers
  - Most commonly presents in young children, but can occur at any age
  - Herpes occurs all year; Coxsackie viruses more prevalent in summer and fall
  - Increased incidence in lower socioeconomic status (due to crowded living conditions)
  - Route of spread is usually by close bodily contact or trauma such as teething or a break in the skin
- Aphthous ulcers: More common in females than males
- Vincent's angina: Most commonly seen in young adults and rarely presents in children

Risk Factors
- Crowded living conditions, day care
- Contact with infected person (e.g., kissing, sharing glasses and utensils, participation in contact sports while infected)
- Triggers for reactivation of herpes include sunlight, trauma, fatigue, fever, or illness

Prevention and Screening
- Avoid contact with infected individuals
- Good oral hygiene, proper handwashing
- Adequate nutrition
- Use of sunscreen prior to sun exposure

Assessment

HISTORY AND PHYSICAL EXAM
- Herpes: Fever and irritability precede development of lesions on the lips, gingiva, and tongue; vesicles then break down and become gray ulcers that bleed easily
- Herpangina: Congestion of the oropharynx and posterior oral cavity with erythema and multiple small vesicles that rupture to form superficial ulcers; gingiva and rest of oral cavity are not involved; 25% children under age 5 will have vomiting with herpangina; older children frequently complain of back pain and headache
- Hand, foot, and mouth disease: Mimics herpangina in every aspect, with the addition of vesiculopapular lesions on the palms of the hands and soles of the feet
- Vincent's angina: Sudden onset of acute inflammation; superficial ulceration covered by a gray pseudomembrane surrounded by marked erythema; if membrane removed, leaves very raw area that bleeds easily; halitosis; exclusively in oropharynx
- Aphthous ulcers: Recurring solitary or multiple lesions occurring on the labial, buccal, and lingual mucosa, as well as on the sublingual, palatal, and gingival mucosa; initial lesions are erythematous and indurated papules that erode rapidly to form sharply circumscribed, necrotic ulcers with a gray fibrinous exudate and erythematous halo

DIAGNOSTIC STUDIES
- Viral cultures and/or scrapings can be done but not usually necessary

Differential Diagnosis
- Etiologies mentioned above
- Pharyngitis/tonsillitis
- Oral trauma
- Syphilis
- Squamous cell carcinoma
- Stevens-Johnson syndrome

Management

NONPHARMACOLOGIC TREATMENT
- Fluids, popsicles may be beneficial; gargle/swish with mild mouthwash or 1:1 hydrogen peroxide and water

PHARMACOLOGIC TREATMENT
- Oral anesthetics, but can be harmful and result in self-injury when children chew on anesthetized lips
- Topical acyclovir or penciclovir is often used in treatment of recurrent oral herpes to decrease the duration of HSV shedding, but has minimal effect on the symptoms

- Consider oral acyclovir 400 mg tid x 5–7 days for primary outbreak if severe
- Consider suppressive therapy with oral antivirals for recurrent herpes labialis (>6 episodes/yr) with acyclovir, valcyclovir or famcyclovir
- Antipyretics and analgesics
- Penicillin is the antibiotic of choice for Vincent's angina
- Coating agents such as diphenhydramine hydrochloride elixir with Kaopectate or Maalox 1:1 for aphthous ulcers
- Possible corticosteroids in severe cases

LENGTH OF TREATMENT
- Continue symptomatic treatment until resolution

Special Considerations
- Dentures may cause or aggravate stomatitis in the elderly

When to Consult, Refer, Hospitalize
- If dehydration due to decreased fluid intake, may require hospitalization for IV fluids
- Dental referral for Vincent's angina

Follow-Up
- Follow-up visit in 3–7 days if severe case
  ### EXPECTED COURSE
  - Most cases are self-limiting and resolve in 7–14 days

  ### COMPLICATIONS
  - Usually none; severe cases may result in scarring

PROBLEMS OF THE NECK

Cervical Adenitis

Description
- Enlargement of a cervical lymph node

Etiology
- Most common site of an enlarged cervical lymph node is submandibular and anterior cervical. The superficial lymph nodes are the gateway to the lymphatic system and respond to local infection with reactive lymphadenopathy.
- Local (dental, URI, otitis media, stomatitis) or systemic infection
  - Most common pathogens: S. aureus, S. pyogenes (Group A Strep), and atypical mycobacteria
  - Less common causes: Herpes simplex virus, Epstein-Barr virus, adenovirus, HIV, Group B streptococcus
- Cat scratch disease
- Rarely due to trauma
- Malignant neoplasms (80% of isolated solitary neck masses in adults >40 yrs of age)

- Manifestation of systemic autoimmune diseases such as lupus, rheumatoid arthritis, and sarcoidosis
- Easily mistaken for goiter or thyroid nodule

Incidence and Demographics
- More commonly found in children than adults, occurs at any age

Risk Factors
- Infection
- Systemic disease
- Tobacco and alcohol use (associated with squamous cell carcinoma and 80% of cervical lymphatic tumors)

Prevention and Screening
- Avoid use of tobacco and abuse of alcohol
- Maintain general health with strategies such as adequate nutrition, exercise, and rest
- Avoid contact with those known to have contagious URI

Assessment
HISTORY
- History of recent or current infection
- Duration of the enlarged lymph node, tenderness, change in size
- The patient with malignancy-related lymphadenitis describes it as being present for an undetermined time (gradual enlargement) and becoming larger, nontender, and firm
- Fever, sore throat, ear pain, toothache, rash, unexplained weight loss, night sweats, irritability, cough, and wheezing
- Exposure to cats (cat scratch disease)

PHYSICAL EXAM
- A thorough examination of the teeth, gingiva, oropharynx, and ears is required, assessing for indicators of infection
- All lymph nodes should be assessed to differentiate between an isolated and localized adenitis vs. generalized lymphadenopathy associated with systemic disease
- Physical findings vary depending upon the etiology
- Infection-related lymphadenitis is typically found in the anterior cervical chain and the submandibular nodes. These are soft, tender, warm, and may reveal erythema of the overlying skin. The size of enlargement is variable (2–6 cm) and is usually bilateral.
- Malignancy-related lymphadenitis is often found in the supraclavicular area with a firm texture that is fixed to the skin and underlying tissue. Exam may reveal one or several enlarged nodes along the anterior cervical chain. Lesions may be found in the oral cavity, nose (e.g., unilateral obstruction), or pharynx.
- Examination should carefully differentiate other structures (thyroid, parotid, or salivary glands)

DIAGNOSTIC STUDIES
- Suspected infectious lymphadenitis may be diagnosed clinically; however if severely ill, may require CBC with differential and culture of the infected area (throat, oropharynx)
- Other studies such as blood cultures, TB test, erythrocyte sedimentation rate, heterophil tests or viral titers (Epstein-Barr, cytomegalovirus, *Toxoplasma*) may be required
- CT, ultrasound, or MRI to differentiate among solid, fluctuant, or cystic mass
- Large fluctuant nodes are aspirated and cultured if unresponsive to therapy or worsening
- Referral to specialist if patient is over age 40
- Biopsy of suspected malignancy

Differential Diagnosis
- Malignancy
- Localized infection
- Thyroid enlargement
- Cat scratch disease
- Parotid or salivary gland inflammation

Management
NONPHARMACOLOGIC TREATMENT
- For localized infection, warm compresses for 15 min qid

PHARMACOLOGIC TREATMENT
- OTC analgesics such as NSAIDs or acetaminophen for fever and/or pain
- If cervical adenitis is primary site of infection (suspect *S. aureus, S. pyogenes*):
  - Erythromycin 10 mg/kg/dose qid
  - Amoxicillin/clavulanate (Augmentin) 10–15 mg/kg/dose tid (500 mg tid for adult)
  - Cephalexin (Keflex) 10–20 mg/kg/dose qid or (500 mg bid for adult)
  - Dicloxacillin (Dynapen) 25 mg/kg/day
  - Clindamycin (Cleocin) 30 mg/kg/day
- If atypical mycobacteria
  - Clarithromycin (Biaxin) 7.5 mg/kg/dose bid
  - Rifampin (Rifadin) 5–10 mg/kg/dose q12–24 hours
- If cat scratch disease—controlled studies have not shown antibiotics to affect the course, but may be used
  - Rifampin 5–10 mg/kg/dose q12–24 hours or
  - TMP-SMX (Bactrim) 5 mg of TMP/kg/dose bid
  - Ciprofloxacin (Cipro) 500 mg bid (not recommended for children under 18)

LENGTH OF TREATMENT
- Antibiotic therapy should be continued for 1–2 weeks

Special Considerations
- Have high index of suspicion for malignancy in patients who abuse alcohol or tobacco, or who present with weight loss and night sweats
- In patients with risk factors, screen for HIV infection

When to Consult, Refer, Hospitalize
- If no resolution in symptoms 48–72 hours after treatment initiated, refer for incision and drainage, IV antibiotics
- Refer immediately to emergency facility if difficulty swallowing or breathing
- Refer to surgeon or ENT specialist for excisional biopsy if suspected malignancy (nodes that are matted, hard, or painless without source of regional infection)

Follow-Up
   EXPECTED COURSE
      - Benign lymphadenitis will resolve over time, some within days of treatment, others over the course of 2–3 weeks with or without treatment; if not resolved after 4 weeks, biopsy by an ENT is indicated

   COMPLICATIONS
      - Localized infection that spreads hematologically with sepsis
      - Malignancy and death
      - Obstruction of airway from extending edema and inflammation

CASE STUDIES

Case 1. A 16-year-old female presents with a "severe cold" x 4–5 days.

HPI: Was previously well. Until last week, she had a cold, which is persisting without much improvement. Patient's mother very concerned that she needs antibiotics; claims they are always used by previous providers to treat her daughter's head colds. Feels feverish, has dry cough, runny nose, mostly clear drainage with some yellow mucus in the mornings, scratchy sore throat, and ears "popping." Tried Advil cold and sinus product with benefit.

PMH: Is in general good health, single, and sexually active with boyfriend x 2 months. Denies food, drug, or environmental allergies, smokes 5 cigarettes per day.

Medications: Oral contraceptive, took amoxicillin 500 mg bid yesterday—left over from prescription she was given 2 months ago for "sinusitis."

1. What additional history do you need?
2. What are the risk factors for possible diagnoses?

Exam: Temp is 99.0°F, thin-appearing Caucasian female, NAD, looks mildly ill. Voice quality "nasal." Posterior oropharynx has mild erythema, no lesions or exudate, tonsils not enlarged, neck supple with no lymphadenopathy, ear canals and TMs clear bilaterally. Nasal turbinates mildly erythematous and edematous, watery discharge. Heart: RRR at 88 BPM, lungs clear.

3. What diagnostic tests would you order?
4. What is your differential diagnosis?
5. What treatment plan will you carry out?

Case 2. 22-year-old female college student presents with sore throat and ear ache.

HPI: Sore throat began 3 days ago, was seen at student health center 2 days ago and treated with Pen V K 250 mg qid. Sore throat worse last night and especially c/o severe right ear pain. Notes fever and chills, but did not take temperature; and overall feels very tired and achy. Hurts to swallow, only drinking liquids. Lives in the dormitory. Denies problems with SOB, chest pain, rash, joint pains, nausea, vomiting, or diarrhea.

PMH: Healthy, denies any preexisting medical problems.

Medications: Pen V K, Advil prn for fever and pain x 3 days, last dose 4 hours ago.

Exam: Young Asian female, looks ill. Temp 102.3°F, sinuses nontender, nasal mucosa clear. Ear canals and TMs negative. Throat 4+ erythema on posterior wall, white-yellow purulent exudate on right tonsillar area. Positive trismus, palatal bulge on the right. Neck positive for anterior cervical lymphadenopathy, tender, soft, and mobile. Chest clear. Heart RRR at 110 BPM.

1. What are the most likely possibilities for a differential diagnosis?
2. What information in the history is the most significant?
3. What physical examination components are especially useful for this presentation?
4. Are the findings from the history and physical adequate to make the diagnosis and what diagnostic studies will rule in or out any of the possibilities?
5. What treatment plan will you carry out?

Case 3. A 6-year-old boy presents with severe right ear pain.

HPI: Child was well until this morning, when he awoke at 6 a.m. crying with right ear pain. Mother noted that he felt very hot, did not take temp. Gave Children's Tylenol and he slept a little. Mother later noted drainage from the ear on his pillow.

PMH: Frequent otitis media as an infant/toddler, which he seemed to "grow out of"; never required long-term antibiotics or ventilation tubes; last otitis media was about 2 years ago.

Exam: Young African-American male, looks moderately ill. Temp 101.2°F orally, right ear canal has whitish crust and is moist, no erythema or edema, tragus nontender with manipulation. TM red and bulging, small perforation present. Oropharynx clear, nose clear, neck supple, no lymphadenopathy, heart RRR 110, respirations 32, lungs clear.

1. What additional history is important?
2. What is the differential diagnosis?
3. What historical and physical exam features support the differential?
4. What are the risk factors for otitis media?
5. How will you treat this child?

REFERENCES

American Academy of Pediatrics. (2004). Managing otitis media with effusion. *Pediatrics, 113*(5), 1412–1429.

American Academy of Pediatrics. (2006). *Red book: 2006 Report of the Committee on Infectious Diseases* (26th ed.). Elk Grove Village: Author.

Behrman, R., & Kliegman, R. (2007). *Nelson's textbook of pediatrics* (17th ed.). Philadelphia: W.B. Saunders.

Domino, F. J. (2008). *The 5 minute clinical consult.* Philadelphia: Lippincott, Williams & Wilkins.

Edmunds, M .W., & Mayhew, M. S. (2004). *Pharmacology for the primary care provider* (2nd ed.). St. Louis, MO: Mosby.

Ferri, F. F. (2008). *Ferri's clinical advisor.* St. Louis, MO: Mosby.

Gilbert, D. N., Moellering, R. C., Eliopoulos, G. M., & Sande, M.A. (2008). *The Sanford guide to antimicrobial therapy* (37th ed.). Hyde Park, VT: Antimicrobial Therapy, Inc.

Goroll, A. H., & Mulley, A. G. (2006). *Primary care medicine* (4th ed.). Philadelphia: Lippincott, Williams & Wilkins.

Hay, W., Levin, M. J., Sondheimer, J. M., & Deterding, R. R. (2006). *Current pediatric diagnosis and treatment* (18th ed.). New York: Lange Medica Book/McGraw Hill.

Kleigman, R. M., Marcdante, K. J., Jensen, H. B., & Behrman, R. E. (2006). *Nelson essentials of pediatrics* (5th ed.) Philadelphia: Saunders.

McPhee, S. J., Papadakis, M. A., & Tierney, L. M. (2008). *Current medical diagnosis and treatment* (44th ed.). Norwalk, CT: Appleton and Lange.

National Guideline Clearinghouse. (2006). *Clinical care guideline: pharyngitis (in adults and children).* Ann Arbor: University of Michigan Health System.

Preferred Practice Patterns Committee Glaucoma Panel. (2005, September). *Primary angle-closure glaucoma.* American Academy of Ophthalmology. San Francisco, CA Sept, 15.

Schwartz, M. W. (2008). *The 5 minute pediatric consult.* Philadelphia: Lippincott, Williams & Wilkins.

Scudder, L. (2004). Pars defects in adolescents. *Journal for Nurse Practitioners 1*(1), 23–27.

Spector, S. L., Bernstein, I. L., Li J. T., Berger, W. E., Kaliner, M. A., Schuller, D. E., et al.. (1998). Parameters for the diagnosis and management of sinusitis. *Journal of Allergy and Clinical Immunology, 102*(6 Pt 2): S107–S144.

Stahl, S. M. (2006). *Essential psychopharmacology: The prescriber's guide.* New York: Cambridge University Press.

Taylor, R. (2007). *Manual of family medicine* (2nd ed.). Philadelphia: Lippincott, Williams & Wilkins.

Tierney, L. M., McPhee, S. J., & Papadakis, A. (2008). *Current medical diagnosis and treatment* (44th ed.). Norwalk, CT: Appleton & Lange.

Uphold, C. R., & Graham, M. V. (2003). *Clinical guidelines in family health* (4th ed.). Gainesville, FL: Barmarrae Books, Inc.

U.S. Preventive Services Task Force. (2007). *Guide to clinical preventive services.* Alexandria, VA: International Medical Publishing, Inc.

Respiratory Disorders

Lisa Neri, MSN, CRNP

GENERAL APPROACH

Note: Some respiratory infections can be found in Chapter 4, Infectious Diseases.
- Through careful history and physical, determine the etiology of the problem: infectious (bacterial, viral, or other), allergic, occupational, environmental, congenital defect.
- Most respiratory infections are viral. Treat empirically with antibiotics only if patient has secondary bacterial infection, underlying respiratory condition, or prolonged symptoms.
- Determine whether symptoms are acute or chronic to guide management.
- For dyspnea, determine patient's position at onset of symptoms, relationship to activity, any factors that improve or exacerbate symptoms.
- Assess rate, depth, rhythm, work of breathing, symmetry of chest movement. Rate is critical indicator of respiratory status, especially in children (see Table 7–1).
- Obtain smoking history, smoking exposure.
- Is cough productive or nonproductive? Note color, amount, and consistency of sputum.
- Note nature of cough: paroxysmal, continuous, staccato.
- Assess exercise tolerance, activity level, ability to take bottle or nurse.
- Antitussives should not be given in conditions in which retention of respiratory secretions may be harmful.
- Encourage patients to stay well-hydrated.
- Assess lung status with pulmonary function testing and spirometry (can usually be obtained beginning at age 5).

- Patients with cardiovascular disease, peripheral vascular disease, hyperthyroidism, diabetes mellitus, urinary retention, prostatic hypertrophy, hypertension, and increased intraocular pressure should avoid decongestants.
- In pediatric patients, assess appetite; fluid intake (hydration status); change in sleep pattern; activity in home, school, and day care environment; and immunization history

Table 7–1. Normal Respiratory Rates (counted for 1 minute at rest)

	Preterm	Term	5 Years	10 Years	15 Years	Adults
Normal rate breaths/minute	40–60	30–40	21–25	17–21	14–20	12–15

Red Flags

- Posttussive emesis and all signs and symptoms of respiratory distress should be quickly evaluated, treated with oxygen and bronchodilators if appropriate, or referred to an emergency department.
- *Community-acquired pneumonia*: Consider hospitalization in:
  - Adult patients over age 50, history of comorbid conditions, altered mental status, leukopenia (<4,000), leukocytosis (>30,000), tachycardia, tachypnea, systolic blood pressure <90 mm HG, and temperature <35°C or > 40°C (<95°F or >104°F)
  - Pediatric patients that look toxic, have immunodeficiencies or cardiac or pulmonary disease, are in respiratory distress or dehydrated
- *Hemoptysis* in older patients, smokers, and those who do not respond to treatment for infection have a high index of suspicion for lung cancer. Obtain chest x-ray and refer for bronchoscopy and further work-up
- *Asthma*: Acute exacerbation may present as diminished breath sounds without audible wheezing, but patient may be in severe respiratory distress. Begin treatment, monitor closely, and be on the alert to transfer to an emergency facility.

ACUTE CONDITIONS

Acute Bronchitis

Description
- Acute inflammation of the lining of the tracheobronchial tree associated with cough and mucus production but no lower airway consolidation

Etiology
- Viruses most common (95% of cases): Rhinovirus, coronavirus, adenovirus, influenza, respiratory syncytial virus (RSV)
- *Bordetella pertussis*: Second leading cause
- *Chlamydia pneumoniae, Mycoplasma pneumoniae*, and *Moraxella catarrhalis* are less common
- Secondary bacterial infections: *Streptococcus pneumoniae* and *Haemophilus influenzae* are more common in smokers and patients with chronic obstructive pulmonary disease (COPD)

- Mucous membranes of the airways become inflamed, edematous with increased bronchial secretions. Bronchial epithelium damaged and mucociliary function is impaired.

Incidence and Demographics
- Affects all ages: Severity and frequency increases with cigarette smoking and pre-existing pulmonary disease

Risk Factors
- Patients with underlying increased bronchial reactivity or untreated chlamydial infection may develop chronic bronchial inflammation, which characterizes asthma
- Smoking

Prevention and Screening
- Avoidance of crowds and infected persons during cold and flu season
- Frequent handwashing, smoking cessation
- Influenza vaccination as recommended

Assessment
HISTORY
- Cough characteristics is classic symptom; initially dry then productive with mucopurulent sputum; worse at night
- Acute bronchitis due to pertussis causes a paroxysmal "whooping" cough
- Afebrile or low-grade temperature present; malaise and fatigue; headache (may worsen with coughing); chest burning, substernal pain, occasional dyspnea, wheezing
- Smoking status of patient or household members; infectious illness of household members; past medical history of respiratory diseases

PHYSICAL EXAM
- Afebrile or low-grade temperature less than 101°F (38°C)
- Purulent nasal secretions, postnasal drainage
- Check for sinus tenderness
- Cervical lymphadenopathy; respiratory wheezes, or rhonchi (often clear with cough); tachycardia
- No physical findings of lower airway congestion; in children, upper airway congestion may be heard in the lungs; to differentiate, listen to breathing then compare to auscultation sounds

DIAGNOSTIC STUDIES
- Diagnosis generally based on clinical presentation
- Chest x-ray to rule out pneumonia for patients with severe respiratory symptoms + temperature >37.8°C (100°F), pulse >100/min, and abnormal lung exam
- CBC and sputum culture: Not generally performed unless uncertain of diagnosis
- PPD if at risk for tuberculosis
- Pulmonary function tests (PFT) if asthma or obstructive disease suspected

Differential Diagnosis
- Pneumonia
- Asthma
- Upper respiratory infection/sinusitis
- Influenza
- Allergies
- Cystic fibrosis
- Tuberculosis
- Chronic bronchitis
- Respiratory tract anomalies
- Gastroesophageal reflux
- Congestive heart failure
- Bronchogenic tumors

Management

NONPHARMACOLOGIC TREATMENT
- Rest, adequate hydration, increase humidification of air, smoking cessation

PHARMACOLOGIC TREATMENT
- Antibiotic treatment not generally recommended; most cases are viral
  - Purulent sputum alone not an indication for antibiotic
  - Exceptions: Secondary bacterial infections and adults with chronic obstructive pulmonary disease with change in amount, color, and consistency of sputum: erythromycin 250–500 mg qid (or other macrolide to decrease GI upset); sulfamethoxazole-trimethoprim (Bactrim DS) bid; doxycycline (Vibramycin) 100 mg bid
  - Treatment with agents effective against chlamydia may prevent development of asthmatic symptoms: >8 years old doxycycline 10 mg bid for 2–3 weeks, <8 years old clarithromycin (Biaxin) 7.5 mg/kg every 12 hours
  - For children with cystic fibrosis and comorbidity of chronic lung disease and a persistent cough (>10 days), consider antibiotic therapy
  - Consider antivirals if influenza suspected (Tamiflu or Relenza); start within 48 hours of symptom onset for demonstrable clinical benefit
- Avoid antihistamines; they dry out secretions
- Analgesics for pain of costochondral area due to coughing/fever
- Cough suppressants for night use if difficulty sleeping due to cough
- Expectorants: Efficacy is questionable
- Bronchodilators may be useful if wheezing or bronchospastic cough; albuterol (Proventil, Ventolin) 2 puffs every 4–6 hours x 7 days

LENGTH OF TREATMENT
- If uncomplicated, generally self-limiting, recovery 7–14 days

Special Considerations
- Geriatrics: Monitor closely for complications such as pneumonia
- Other: Symptoms and duration may be worse in smokers
- Adults with pertusis may transmit it to unimmunized children

When to Consult, Refer, Hospitalize
- Refer to pulmonologist or asthma specialist for further evaluation if no improvement in 4–6 weeks or if more severe symptoms

Follow-Up
- If no improvement or symptoms worsen after 72 hours:
  EXPECTED COURSE
  - Generally symptoms resolve in 7–14 days, but cough may persist for 3–4 weeks

  COMPLICATIONS
  - Secondary bacterial infection, pneumonia

Bronchiolitis

Description
- Acute inflammation of the bronchioles resulting in obstruction of the small airways; usually the first episode of wheezing in a child <2 years of age who has physical findings of a viral respiratory infection and has no other explanation for the wheezing, such as pneumonia or atopy

Etiology
- 50%–75% caused by respiratory syncytial virus (RSV); less often by parainfluenza virus or adenovirus
- Small airways become obstructed causing paroxysmal cough, dyspnea, hyperinflation

Incidence and Demographics
- Occurs in 20% of all infants; 1%–2% require hospital admission
- Peak incidence is 3–6 months of age
- Seen in all geographic areas; yearly epidemics occur in winter and early spring

Risk Factors
- Crowded conditions; low socioeconomic status
- Older siblings in the home; day care attendance
- Exposure to secondhand smoke
- Bottle-feeding verses breastfeeding
- More serious obstruction the younger the infant (especially <6 months of age)

Prevention and Screening
- Palivizumab (Synagis) is available for RSV prophylaxis and should be considered for infants and children <2 years old with chronic lung disease, children with hemodynamically significant heart disease, those born at 32 weeks gestation or earlier, or born between 32 and 35 weeks with additional risk factors.
- Influenza vaccine for children 6–59 months of age and their household contacts

Assessment
HISTORY
- Exposure to upper respiratory infection
- Upper respiratory symptoms with nasal discharge and sneezing
- Diminished appetite

- Afebrile or low-grade temperature present
- Gradual development of respiratory distress with wheezing and deep cough, dyspnea, poor feeding, and irritability
- Apnea or cyanosis (apnea may be the only symptom in very young infants)

PHYSICAL EXAM
- Afebrile or low-grade fever
- Nasal congestion with thick, purulent secretions; nasal flaring; retractions
- Cough; tachypnea
- Hyperresonance
- Wheezing; prolonged expiratory phase; fine crackles (wheezing may not be audible if airways are profoundly narrowed)
- Tachycardia and/or mild hypoxemia
- Signs of dehydration: Depressed fontanels, tacky mucous membranes, crying without tears
- Cyanosis of oral mucosa and nail beds
- Hepatosplenomegaly (due to hyperinflated lungs)

DIAGNOSTIC STUDIES
- Usually diagnosed by clinical presentation
- Chest radiography
- CBC with differential
- Pulse oximetry to monitor respiratory status
- Urine specific gravity to monitor hydration
- Nasopharyngeal washings for RSV enzyme immunoassay (rapid results) and culture

Differential Diagnosis
- Pneumonia
- Foreign body
- Exposure to noxious agent
- Asthma
- Croup
- Gastroesophageal reflux (GERD)
- Cystic fibrosis
- Pertussis
- Heart failure

Management
NONPHARMACOLOGIC TREATMENT
- In uncomplicated cases, frequent offerings of clear fluids or diluted milk; frequent suctioning of secretions, with saline and a bulb syringe
- Cool, humidified oxygen if hypoxemic

PHARMACOLOGIC TREATMENT
- Trial of beta 2-adrenergics to see if there is any relief of symptoms: albuterol 5 mg/5 mL solution 0.1–0.15 mg/kg in 2 cc of saline every 20 minutes for 1 hour with continual reevaluation; refer if no response or respiratory distress apparent after treatments
- Racemic epinephrine may reduce wheezing and reduce tachypnea

LENGTH OF TREATMENT
- Inhaled bronchodilators should be continued only if there is a documented clinical response and then given q 4–6 hours; discontinue once signs and symptoms of respiratory distress improve
- Most infants show marked improvement in 3–5 days

Special Considerations
- Glucocorticoids are not routinely recommended in the treatment of previously healthy infants hospitalized with the first episode of bronchiolitis, but may be beneficial to those with chronic lung diseases and those with recurrent episodes of wheezing suggestive of asthma.

When to Consult, Refer, Hospitalize
- Consult with physician or consider an urgent emergency department referral for infants <2–3 months old, marked respiratory distress, hypoxemia on room air, difficulty feeding, dehydration, history of apnea, lethargy, underlying cardiopulmonary disorder

Follow-Up
EXPECTED COURSE
- Vast majority of infants develop a mild infection and are treated as outpatients
- Nonhospitalized infants may continue to cough for 1–2 weeks
- Expect reduction in symptoms in 3–5 days

COMPLICATIONS
- Approximately half of infants go on to develop subsequent wheezing episodes (asthma) or respiratory problems later in life
- Highest risk of complications seen with bronchopulmonary dysplasia (BPD), congenital heart disease, chronic lung disease, prematurity, immunodeficiency
- Infants with cardiopulmonary disease or immunodeficiency are at greater risk for serious sequelae

Croup (Laryngotracheobronchitis)

Description
- Acute inflammatory disease of larynx and subglottic airway, with characteristic "barking" cough, inspiratory stridor, and hoarseness

Etiology
- Parainfluenza is the most common organism in all age groups
- Respiratory syncytial virus (infants)
- M. pneumoniae and influenza virus (children over 5 years)
- Viral infection causes inflammation and edema of subglottic space

Incidence and Demographics
- Most prevalent in late fall and winter
- Most common in children 3 months to 5 years of age, with peak at 2 years
- Male to female ratio is 3:2

Risk Factors
- Exposure in the late fall and winter

Prevention and Screening
- No specific prevention measures except proper handwashing and other preventive measures aimed at decreasing the transmission of respiratory viruses

Assessment

HISTORY
- Length of symptoms; often insidious with a viral URI prodrome
- Inspiratory stridor and "barking" cough often begins at night and is worse at night
- Changes in activity level, alertness, fluid intake, or voiding patterns
- Inquire about *H. influenzae* immunization status

PHYSICAL EXAM (TABLE 7–2)
- Signs and symptoms are variable dependent upon age, degree of airway obstruction, hydration status, and level of fatigue
- Level of consciousness, irritability, lethargy
- Work of breathing: Respiratory rate, nasal flaring, retractions, prolonged expiratory phase
- Inspiratory stridor or stridor at rest; wheezing
- Breath sounds may be diminished from airway narrowing, crackles, rhonchi
- "Barking" cough is characteristic in croup
- Tympanic membranes, throat, sinus may be involved
- Tachycardia caused by fever, respiratory distress, hypovolemia

DIAGNOSTIC STUDIES
- Usually diagnosis of croup is made on clinical presentation without testing
- Pulse oximetry
- Anteroposterior and lateral x-ray of the neck to rule out epiglottitis

Differential Diagnosis
- Foreign body aspiration
- Tumor
- Asthma
- Anaphylaxis
- Peritonsillar abscess
- Spasmodic croup

INFECTIONS
- Epiglottitis
- Bacterial tracheitis
- Diphtheria (uncommon in U.S.)
- Measles (where prevalent)

CONGENITAL
- Tracheo-esophageal fistula
- Laryngomalacia
- Tracheomalacia
- Vocal cord paralysis

Table 7-2. Differentiating Croup From Other Illnesses

	Laryngo-tracheits	Spasmodic Croup	Epiglottitis	Foreign body	Bacterial tracheitis
Age	6 mo–3 yr	3 mo–3 yr	2–6 yr	6 mo–2 or 3 yr	Any age
Etiology	Parainfluenza, RSV, mycoplasma, adenovirus	May be postviral, allergic, GERD, psychogenic	*H. influenzae* type B, other bacteria	Small objects, food, toys	*S. aureus, M. catarrhalis, H. influenzae*
Onset	Insidious	Sudden, at night	Sudden	Sudden	Slow onset, rapid deterioration
Retractions	Yes	Uncommon	Yes	Variable	Yes
Voice	Hoarse	Hoarse	Muffled	Variable	Yes
Position	Normal	Normal	Tripod-sitting, leaning forward	Variable	Variable, usually normal
Barking cough	Yes	Yes	No	Possible	Yes
Fever	Yes	No	Yes	No	Yes

Management

NONPHARMACOLOGIC TREATMENT
- Mild cases can be managed at home
- Humidified air delivered by cool mist vaporizer or steam-filled bathroom
- Take outside into cool night air

PHARMACOLOGIC TREATMENT
- Humidified oxygen
- Aerosolized epinephrine or racemic epinephrine is effective but has short duration (30 minutes to 2 hours)
- Dosage of racemic epinephrine (2.25%) is 0.25 to 1.0 mL of solution in 2–3 mL of normal saline delivered by nebulizer; frequency judged by patient response
- Systemic corticosteroids (prednisone, dexamethasone) are beneficial in severe cases and use remains controversial in mild cases: dexamethasone (Decadron) 4 mg/mL, 0.6 mg/kg IM as a single dose; may consider prednisone 2mg/kg per day in 2 divided doses x 2 days
- Nebulized budesonide has recently been used successfully

LENGTH OF TREATMENT
- Length of treatment is based on clinical response
- Concern about a rebound phenomenon from racemic epinephrine exists; patients who are clinically stable can be discharged safely if 4 hours have elapsed since the last dose of racemic epinephrine and systemic corticosteroids have been given

Special Considerations
- Close monitoring of disease progression; stridor, respiratory rate, pulse oximetry, hydration status, and mental status are critical

- Must rule out epiglottitis; watch for preferred sitting position (tripod position with hands extended), drooling, and muffled voice
- When examining, do not place supine or use tongue blade to examine throat until epiglottis ruled out

When to Consult, Refer, Hospitalize
- Admission is indicated for worsening airway obstruction as evidenced by increasing stridor, hypoxemia, retractions, cyanosis, agitation, fatigue, or inadequate oral intake

Follow-Up
EXPECTED COURSE
- Symptoms may worsen over the first 3 days, so parents/guardian should be advised to return to clinic for increasing stridor or respiratory distress
- For children with moderately severe croup who are discharged, phone contact or clinic follow-up is warranted in 8–24 hours

COMPLICATIONS
- In most cases, croup is a self-limiting illness lasting 3–5 days

Persistent Cough

Description
- Productive or nonproductive cough for greater than 3 weeks
- Chronic cough affects respiration, sleep, and social function

Etiology
- Cough is a physiologic mechanism of expulsion of air from the lungs
- Helps to defend against pathogens and clear the tracheobronchial tree of foreign particles, noxious aerosols, mucus
- Etiology of persistent cough may not be readily apparent due to the wide variety of infectious, mechanical, and physiologic causes (see Table 7–3)

Incidence and Demographics
- Common and frequent presenting complaint in all age groups

Risk Factors
- Cigarette smoking or exposure
- Occupational exposure
- Allergens
- Prevalence is greater in women

Prevention and Screening
- Smoking cessation
- Remove respiratory irritants
- Therapeutic lifestyle changes for GERD

Table 7-3. Most Common Etiology of Chronic Cough by Age

Infants	Toddler/Preschool	School-Age/ Adolescent	Adults
Infection	**Infection**	**Infections**	Smoking, passive
Viral (RSV,	Viral (RSV,	Viral	smoke
adenovirus, influenza,	adenovirus, influenza,	M. *pneumoniae*	Postnasal drip from
parainfluenza)	parainfluenza)	M. *tuberculosis*	sinusitis, allergic
Bordetella pertussis	B. *pertussis*		rhinitis
Chlamydia trachomatis	M. *pneumoniae*	**Other**	GERD
M. *tuberculosis*	M. *tuberculosis*	Asthma	Asthma
		Sinusitis, postnasal drip	Reactive airway
Congenital anomalies	**Other**	Irritants, smoking	disease
Cleft palate	Foreign body	Allergic rhinitis	Chronic bronchitis
Tracheo-esophageal	Asthma	Cystic fibrosis	Bronchiectasis
fistula	Cystic fibrosis	Ciliary dyskinesia	Pneumonia
Vascular ring	Irritants, passive smoke	Psychogenic (habit)	Drug-induced (ACE
	Immunodeficiency		inhibitors)
Other	Ciliary dyskinesia		Irritants
Cystic fibrosis	GERD		Foreign body
Irritants, passive smoke	Sinusitis, postnasal drip		Tuberculosis
Asthma	Immunodeficiency		Lung malignancy
Foreign body			Psychogenic factors
Neurologic impairment			Congestive heart
GERD			failure (CHF)
Immunodeficiency			Interstitial lung disease
			B. *Pertussis*
			Nonasthmatic
			eosinophilic
			bronchitis

Assessment

HISTORY

- Characteristics and timing of cough: Onset and duration
    - Cough at night suggests sinusitis with postnasal drainage, asthma, CHF
    - Paroxysmal coughing >14 days: Pertussis, cystic fibrosis
    - Cough at school, not on weekend: Psychogenic, consider allergy (e.g., mold in building)
- Productive or nonproductive cough (presence or absence of sputum production not used as sole basis for treatment)
- Productive: Bronchitis, cystic fibrosis, tuberculosis, infection (mucopurulent), pneumococcal pneumonia (rust-colored), asthma (thick, tenacious, clear)
- Frequent respiratory infections: Cystic fibrosis
- In children, poor weight gain, delayed milestones: Cystic fibrosis, immunodeficiency
- Foul-smelling, steatorrheic bowel movements: Cystic fibrosis
- Family history of cystic fibrosis (genetic disorder, primarily in Caucasian children)

- Exercise-induced cough associated with asthma, bronchiectasis, or cardiac disease
- Associated symptoms: Fatigue, weight loss, night sweats, fever, indigestion, rhinitis, epistaxis, hemoptysis (consider cancer, tuberculosis, foreign body obstruction, cystic fibrosis, HIV, sinusitis, GERD)
- Precipitating factors: Exercise, cold temperatures, laughing; seasonal may indicate asthma
- Past medical history may be significant for bronchitis, pneumonia, asthma, allergy; choking episodes or heartburn: Gastroesophageal reflux
- Family members ill: Infection; family history of atopy/asthma
- Smokers: Lung tumor, emphysema, chronic bronchitis
- Medication history: ACE inhibitors or beta-blockers

PHYSICAL EXAM
- Appearance/nutritional status
- Nasal discharge, throat clearing, and mucus or mucopurulent drainage in posterior pharynx: Postnasal drip rhinitis, sinusitis
- Respiratory rate, evidence of distress, wheezing, adventitious sounds: Asthma, cystic fibrosis, foreign body, bronchitis, pneumonia, tuberculosis
- Tracheal shift suggest mediastinal mass or foreign body
- Observe for clubbing: Lung malignancy, cardiac source, COPD
- In children, evaluate height and weight and plot on growth curve

DIAGNOSTIC STUDIES
- Tuberculosis skin testing: PPD
- Chest x-ray for cough in smokers, cough >8 weeks in nonsmokers, patients with hemoptysis, and in children and those over 40 years
- Sinus imaging for suspected acute or chronic sinusitis (paranasal sinuses only in children 18 months to 6 years)
- Pulmonary function testing for asthma
- Methacholine bronchoprovocation testing may be positive in absence of clinical findings of asthma
- Barium swallow/esophageal pH monitoring for suspected GERD
- CBC with differential; if infection, mass is suspected
- Wright and gram stains, culture of sputum for productive cough
- Bronchoscopy/endoscopy (particularly useful in children birth to 18 months)
- Sweat test for suspected cystic fibrosis

Differential Diagnosis
- See Table 7–3.

Management
- Important to determine the underlying disorder causing the cough and treat accordingly. While determining cause, consider the following to manage
  ### NONPHARMACOLOGIC TREATMENT
  - Eliminate irritant exposure (smoke, occupational agents); discontinue ACE inhibitors or beta-blockers; increase humidification
  - Therapeutic lifestyle changes for GERD (e.g., smoking cessation, avoiding reflux-inducing foods, small frequent meals, avoid eating 2–3 hours before lying down, elevate the head of bed)

PHARMACOLOGIC TREATMENT
- Antitussives (codeine or dextromethorphan): Use with caution; should not be given in conditions in which retention of respiratory secretions may be harmful; may reserve for nighttime use only
- Codeine phosphate elixir: Adults: 10 mg/5 mL (maximum of 120 mg/day), or 5–10 mL q 4–6 hr prn; children 2–6 years old: 1–1.5 mg/kg/day divided q 4–6 hr; ages 6–12 years: 10 mg q 4–6 hr; may reserve for nighttime use only
- Dextromethorphan HBr (Robitussin DM): Adults: 5 to 10 mL q 4–6 hr prn; children 6–11 months: 1.25 mL q 6–8 hr; ages 12–23 months: 2.5 mL q 6–8 hr; ages 2–6 years: 2.5 mL q 4 hr; ages 6–12 years: 5 mL q 4 hr

LENGTH OF TREATMENT
- For duration of cough or illness

Special Considerations
- Geriatrics: Use decreased dose of antihistamines in allergy, caution with first-generation antihistamine due to increased sedation.
- Pediatrics: A number of nonprescription cough and cold products containing antitussives, decongestants, and antihistamines were voluntarily taken off the market due to many reports of accidental overdose, mostly in children under 2 years. Encourage parents to first check with their healthcare provider before using any cough/cold preparation.

When to Consult, Refer, Hospitalize
- Refer undiagnosed patients with risk factors to specialist
- Consult with physician or pulmonologist for signs of respiratory distress or unresponsive to treatment

Follow-Up
EXPECTED COURSE
- Depending on patient status; patients with negative work-up; follow up every 1–3 months if cough continues

COMPLICATIONS
- Anxiety, exhaustion, self-consciousness, insomnia, lifestyle change, musculoskeletal pain, hoarseness, excessive perspiration, urinary incontinence

Hemoptysis

Description
- Expectoration of blood originating from the lower respiratory tract
  - Hemoptysis is a symptom of underlying disease or pulmonary injury
  - Classifications: Trivial, mild, massive (200–600 mL in 24 hours)

Etiology
- Inflammation of the tracheobronchial mucosa, due to minor erosion from URI or bronchitis, bronchiectasis, tuberculosis, sarcoidosis, Wegner's granulomatosis, lupus pneumonitis

- Bronchovascular fistula
- Bronchogenic carcinoma
- Injury to pulmonary vasculature due to lung abscess, necrotizing pneumonias, aspergillomas, or pulmonary emboli causing pulmonary infarction; trauma; foreign body
- Increase pulmonary capillary pressure due to pulmonary edema, mitral stenosis, AV malformations, or granuloma formation
- Bleeding disorders or anticoagulant therapy
- Nonpulmonary sources: Nose or gastrointestinal tract
- Cryptogenic hemoptysis: Negative work-up, 30%–40% of patients with hemoptysis are due to unknown etiology, 90% resolve in 6 months

Risk Factors
- Most common cause: Acute and chronic bronchitis, followed by bronchogenic carcinoma, then tuberculosis (TB), pneumonia, and bronchiectasis
- Crack cocaine inhalation

Prevention and Screening
- None

Assessment
HISTORY
- Identify patients at risk for conditions noted above
- Smoking history, presence of respiratory infection
- Onset and duration of symptoms; amount and characteristics of sputum
- Determine if nonpulmonary source of bleeding: Vomiting, expectoration from nasopharynx, anticoagulant drug use, substance use, chest trauma
- Associated symptoms: Weight loss, night sweats, dyspnea, fatigue, bruising, hematuria
- TB exposure, dates of last TB test and chest x-ray
- Past cardiac, pulmonary, hematological, or immunological history
- Environmental exposure, asbestos
- Family history of respiratory, cardiac, or hematologic disease

PHYSICAL EXAM
- Fever and tachypnea
- Nail clubbing indicates severe disorder such as lung abscess, tumor, bronchiectasis
- Ears, nasal, pharyngeal exam to determine bleeding source
- Jugular venous distention and ankle edema—heart failure
- Chest exam for pulmonary and cardiac findings
- Lymphadenopathy: TB, carcinoma, sarcoidosis

DIAGNOSTIC STUDIES
- Tuberculin skin test (PPD)
- Chest x-ray
- CBC with differential and platelets
- Gram stain of sputum: infection; acid-fast stain: TB
- Sputum cytologic exam: malignancy

- Renal function, urinalysis
- Coagulation studies: PT, PTT, bleeding time if bleeding present in more than one site
- Bronchoscopy for patients at risk of cancer, TB
- Chest CT: Complementary to bronchoscopy (test of choice for suspected small peripheral malignancies)
- Ventilation-perfusion scan/angiography: Pulmonary embolism

Differential Diagnosis
- See *Etiology* above.

Management
NONPHARMACOLOGIC TREATMENT
- Surgical interventions: Flexible bronchoscopy; angiography for embolization

PHARMACOLOGIC TREATMENT
- Treat underlying illness or infection; refer to specific conditions in text
- Mild cough suppressant but encourage patient to continue expectorating

Special Considerations
- In older adult smoker, think lung cancer until proven otherwise.

When to Consult, Refer, Hospitalize
- Refer patients at high risk for malignancy or if bronchoscopy is indicated to pulmonologist
- Refer if blood persists more than 2–3 days after treatment initiated for respiratory infection
- Hospitalization for patient expectorating large amounts (25–50 mL) in 24 hours

Follow-Up
EXPECTED COURSE
- Mild streaking due to infection should resolve in 2–3 days; with true hemoptysis, patient should follow-up in 12–48 hours

COMPLICATIONS
- Massive hemoptysis is life-threatening

Community-Acquired Pneumonia

Description
- An acute pulmonary infection of the parenchyma of lung involving the alveoli and the interstitial tissue spaces and producing lung field consolidation. Described as "typical" pneumonia when caused by bacteria; "atypical" when caused by *Chlamydia*, *Mycoplasma*, or viruses.
- Community-acquired pneumonia begins outside of the hospital or within 48 hours of hospital admission in a patient who has resided <14 days in a long-term-care facility before symptom onset.

Etiology
PEDIATRICS
- 0–5 months: *Chlamydia pneumoniae*, Group B strep, RSV, respiratory viruses
- 5 months–5 years old: RSV, parainfluenza viruses, *H. influenzae*, *Streptococcus pneumoniae*
- >5 years old: *Mycoplasma pneumoniae*, *S. pneumoniae*, *C. pneumoniae*, and viruses

ADULTS
- <60 without comorbidity: *S. pneumoniae*, *H. influenzae*, *M. pneumoniae*, *C. pneumoniae*, Group A Streptococcus, respiratory viruses
- >60 or with comorbidity: *S. pneumoniae*, respiratory viruses, *H. influenzae*, aerobic Gram-negative bacilli, *Staphylococcus aureus*, community-acquired methicillin-resistant *Staphylococcus aureus* (CA-MRSA)
- Other possible causes: *Neisseria meningitidis*, *Moraxella catarrhalis*, *Klebsiella pneumoniae*, *Pneumocystis carinii*, *Legionella species*, psittacosis, Q fever, tularemia, endemic fungi, *M. tuberculosis*
- While bacterial causes are the most common, viral, fungal, and chemical aspiration all contribute

Incidence and Demographics
- Most deadly infectious disease, sixth leading overall cause of death
- 3–4 million cases each year in U.S.
- Highest incidence in children <5 years old and the elderly

Risk Factors
- Elderly and nursing home residents
- Crowded living conditions
- Seasonal (winter)
- Recent URI, influenza
- Alcoholism, drug abuse
- Existing medical condition (comorbid medical conditions)
- COPD, structural lung disease, smoking
- Airway obstruction or aspiration
- Exposure to bats, birds, soil with bird droppings, rabbits, farm animals, parturient cats

Prevention and Screening
- Influenza, polyvalent pneumococcal, and pertussis vaccines
- RSV prophylaxis in high-risk children <2 years
- Good handwashing

Assessment
HISTORY (SEE TABLE 7–4)
- Onset either abrupt or insidious
- Recent or concurrent URI, fever, cough (productive or nonproductive), dyspnea,

chills, sweats, rigors, fatigue, myalgias, chest discomfort, headache, anorexia, abdominal pain, confusion in the elderly; pleuritic chest pain; patients generally feel unwell
- In pediatrics and the elderly, the presenting complaint may be abdominal pain

PHYSICAL EXAM
- Patient appears ill, particularly with bacterial pneumonia
- Hypothermia or fever, tachypnea, tachycardia
- **Red flag**: Respirations in 2–6-months old >50; 7–35 months old >40; 36+ months old >35
- Dyspnea, use of accessory muscles, nasal flaring, abnormal breath sounds, absent breath sounds, effusion present
- Lung consolidation: Fremitus, egophony, dullness to percussion, rhonchi or rales in lung fields
- Cardiac exam is normal unless underlying disease
- Signs of dehydration
- Assess mental status; may be altered if hypoxic

DIAGNOSTIC STUDIES
- Chest x-ray: Infiltrates confirmed
- Sputum Gram stain if atypical or reportable organism suspected or patient unresponsive to treatment
- Nasopharyngeal washings for RSV enzyme immunoassay (children)
- CBC, blood cultures (usually reserved for hospitalized patients), cold agglutinins, ESR
- WBC elevated (may be low in elderly or immunocompromised patient)

Table 7-4. How to Differentiate Typical and Atypical Pneumonia

Characteristic	"Typical" Pneumonia	"Atypical" Pneumonia
Onset	Often sudden	Usually gradual
Myalgias/ headaches	Not prominent	Often prominent
Fever/shaking chills	Common	Rare
Appearance	Quite ill	Mild to moderately ill
Cough	Productive	Nonproductive paroxysms
Pleuritic pain	Common	Rare
Lung Exam	Dullness, with signs of consolidation	Often minimal abnormal findings
Chest x-ray (CXR)	Localized findings correlate with exam	Involvement in excess of exam findings
Leukocyte count	>15,000/mm³	<15,000/mm³

Differential Diagnosis
- Upper respiratory tract infections
- Asthma
- Bronchitis
- Bronchiolitis
- Croup
- Tuberculosis
- Lung cancer
- Congestive heart failure
- Pulmonary vasculitis
- Atelectasis
- Pulmonary thromboembolic disease

Management

NONPHARMACOLOGIC TREATMENT
- Hydration, high humidity
- Monitor respiratory status, rest
- Smoking cessation, avoidance of secondhand smoke
- Chest physiotherapy for bacterial pneumonia

PHARMACOLOGIC TREATMENT
- Viral pneumonia:
  - Bronchodilator if wheezing present
  - Consider amantadine (Symmetrel) or rimantadine (Flumadine) 100 mg po bid for influenza A
- Typical and atypical pneumonia:
  - Refer to American Thoracic Society's (2007) practice guidelines for treatment based on specific pathogen, and inpatient treatment
  - Empiric treatment often necessary because often not able to identify pathogen
  - Usually use fluoroquinolones, second-generation cephalosporins, amoxicillin/clavulanate (Augmentin), and doxycycline (Vibramycin) for typical pneumonia
  - Usually use macrolides and doxycycline for atypical pneumonia
- Modifying factors for selected patients:
  - Comorbidities and/or suspected penicillin-resistant S. *pneumoniae*: Respiratory fluoroquinolones or betalactam plus a macrolide
  - Suspected aspiration pneumonia: Amoxicillin/clavulanate
  - Young adult (ages 17–40) with no comorbidities: Azithromycin, clarithromycin, or doxycycline

CHOICE OF ANTIBIOTICS
- Macrolides
  - Azithromycin (Zithromax): >12 years old: 500 mg (2 250 mg tablets) initially then 250 mg (1 tablet) qd x 4 days; 6 months old: 10 mg/kg initially then 5 mg/kg qd x 4 days, max of 500 mg initially and 250 mg thereafter
  - Clarithromycin (Biaxin): >2 years old: 500 mg (1 tablet) bid; >6 months: 7.5 mg/kg q 12 h, max of 500 mg bid

– Erythromycin (Erythrocin): >2 years old, 250–500 mg, q 6 h (not generally used due to side effects); peds: 30–50 mg/kg/d in divided doses, max 1 gram per day
- Fluoroquinolones
  – Levofloxacin (Levaquin): 18 and older: 500 mg qd for 7–14 days or 750 mg qd for 5 days
  – Moxifloxacin (Avelox): 18 and older: 400 mg qd for 7–14 days
  – Gemifloxin (Factive): 18 and older: 320 mg qd for 5–7 days
- Doxycycline (Vibramycin): Young adult (18–40): 100 mg bid for 7–10 days

ALTERNATIVES
- Amoxicillin/clavulanate (Augmentin): >40 kg: 875 mg/125 mg bid; <12 weeks old: 30 mg/kg/d q 12 hs, based on amoxicillin component; >12 weeks old: 45 mg/kg/d q 12 h, based on amoxicillin component; adults: 2 gm bid for a minimum of 5 days
- Second-generation cephalosporins (used for typical pneumonia only), all for a minimum of 5 days
  – Cefaclor extended release (Ceclor CD): >12 years old: 500 mg q 12 h; 6 months–12 years: 15 mg/kg q12 h
  – Cefprozil (Cefzil): >12 years old: 250–500 mg q 12 h; 6 months–12 years: 15 mg/kg q 12 h
  – Cefuroxime axetil (Ceftin): >12 years old: 500 mg q 12 h; 3 months– 12 years: 20 mg/kg/d bid
  – Loracarbef (Lorabid): >12 years old: 400 mg q 12 h; 6 months–12 years: 15–30 mg/kg/d bid
- Antitussives
  – Generally cough should not be suppressed and antitussives should be avoided; however, in patients with severe chest discomfort and persistent cough, may consider use of nonnarcotic or low-dose narcotic antitussive for night use only; see section on *Persistent Cough*

LENGTH OF TREATMENT
- Treat uncomplicated bacterial infections for 10 days. Treat *C. pneumoniae*, *M. pneumoniae* for 2 weeks and *Legionella* infections for 3 weeks

Special Considerations
- Elderly residing in nursing homes and young infants at greater risk for morbidity and mortality.
- Drug resistance: Suspect drug-resistant *S. pneumonia* in communities with increased prevalence. Risk factors include age <2 years or >65 years, betalactam or macrolide treatment within the past 3–6 months, alcoholism, medical comorbidities, immunosuppression, exposure to day care.

When to Consult, Refer, Hospitalize
- Consider hospitalization for adult patients over age 65, history of comorbid conditions, altered mental status, leukopenia (<4,000), leukocytosis (>30,000), tachycardia, tachypnea, systolic blood pressure <90 mmHg, and temperature <35°C (95°F) or >40°C (104°F).

- Consider hospitalization in pediatric patients that look toxic; have immunodeficiencies, cardiac or pulmonary disease; in respiratory distress; or dehydrated.

Follow-Up
- 24-hour follow-up contact for patients moderately to severely ill, and 72 hours after beginning antimicrobials for reevaluation.
- For patients who are improving, routine follow-up in 2–3 weeks.
- Patients >40 years old and all smokers, follow-up CXR in 4–8 weeks to rule out underlying bronchogenic carcinoma, which may present as pneumonia.
- In children with recurrent pneumonia, repeat CXR in 4–6 weeks.
  - EXPECTED COURSE
    - Dependent upon pathogen, patient response, complications

  - COMPLICATIONS
    - In adults: Heart failure, renal failure, pulmonary embolism, bacteremia, acute myocardial infection, death
    - In children: If recurrent pneumonia, evaluate for underlying disease

Primary Lung Malignancies

Description
- Bronchogenic carcinomas (lung cancers) include two classes:
  - Non–small cell lung cancer (NSCLC), which includes adenocarcinoma, squamous cell carcinoma, and large cell carcinoma
  - Small cell lung cancer (SCLC) also known as oat cell carcinoma

Etiology
- Cigarette smoking, most important cause in both men and women in U.S.
- Other causes: Secondhand smoke, ionizing radiation (radon gas, therapeutic radiation), asbestos exposure, heavy metals (nickel, chromium), industrial carcinogens
- Possible causes: Lung scarring, air pollution, genetic factors
- Carcinogen causes chromosomal damage, abnormal cell growth, leads to malignancy
- SCLC tumors grow bulky, in middle of chest, metastasize early; squamous cell tumors arise centrally; adenocarcinoma and large cell carcinoma grow peripherally; bronchoalveolar carcinoma (a type of adenocarcinoma) can be multifocal
- Besides direct damage to the airways, lung cancers cause complications through direct extension, metastasis, and paraneoplastic syndromes such as syndrome of inappropriate antidiuretic hormone (SIADH)

Incidence and Demographics
- Lung cancer is the leading cause of cancer death for both men and women.
- Approximately 175,000 new cases of lung cancer in the U.S. per year; 160,000 will die of lung cancer.
- More women die of lung cancer than of breast cancer.
- Most cases present between ages 50 and 70.
- Non–small cell carcinoma: 80% of lung cancers; small cell carcinomas: 20%.

Risk Factors
- Smoking, COPD, industrial and chemical exposure

Prevention and Screening
- NOT SMOKING
- Avoid industrial exposures

Assessment

HISTORY
- Initial symptoms: Cough, hemoptysis, dyspnea
- Persistent cough: Lung cancer is not a common cause of chronic cough (0%–2%), very unlikely in patients who have never smoked
- Coughs developing for the first time and lasting for months, or change in character
- Other symptoms: Chest pain, often made worse by deep breathing; hoarseness; weight loss and anorexia; bloody or rust-colored sputum; fever without a known reason; recurring infections such as bronchitis, pneumonia; new onset of wheezing
- Symptoms of metastasis: Bone pain; weakness or numbness of the arms or legs; dizziness; jaundice; skin tumors; lymphadenopathy

PHYSICAL EXAM
- Findings vary with type of cancer, metastases, and coexisting paraneoplastic syndromes, or may be absent
- 20% of patients present with lymphadenopathy, hepatomegaly, and nail clubbing
- Horner syndrome, Pancoast syndrome, laryngeal nerve palsy with voice hoarseness, phrenic nerve palsy with hemidiaphragm paralysis, and skin metastases occur in less than 5% of cases
- Localized dullness to percussion (atelectasis, effusion)

DIAGNOSTIC STUDIES
- Chest radiographs: Most important initial diagnostic test in predicting whether lung cancer is potential cause of chronic cough
- Sputum cytology if cough persists with cessation of smoking for 4 weeks; proceed with sputum cytology and bronchoscopy even when the chest radiograph is normal
- Fiberoptic bronchoscopy when the chest radiograph suggests that a tumor or an inflammatory pulmonary parenchymal process is present
- CT scan for evaluation of lung parenchyma and pleura, and for cancer staging
- MRI for staging the mediastinum
- PET scanning and other imaging for staging and determination of metastasis

Management
- Presurgical evaluation should consider pulmonary and cardiac status, general health, and acceptable functional status.
- Preoperative radiation may be recommended in certain types of lung cancer.

- In nonsurgical patients and in those with residual tumor in spite of surgical resection, radiation and chemotherapy may be considered.
  NONPHARMACOLOGIC TREATMENT
  - Palliative therapy includes general care of the patient with particular attention to pain control, symptom control, maintenance of adequate nutrition, and psychological support
  - Acupuncture has been found effective in the management of chemotherapy-associated nausea and vomiting, and in controlling pain associated with surgery

  PHARMACOLOGIC TREATMENT
  - Multiple anticancer chemotherapeutic agents are used to treat lung cancer
  - For more complete information, see http://cancernet.nci.nih.gov

  LENGTH OF TREATMENT
  - Duration of treatment depends on type and stage of cancer

Special Considerations
- None

When to Consult, Refer, Hospitalize
- Any patient with suspected lung malignancy should be referred to a pulmonologist for evaluation, with subsequent referral to a thoracic surgeon and/or oncologist for treatment.

Follow-Up
  EXPECTED COURSE
  - Overall 5-year survival rate 10%–15%; patients with SCLC rarely live 5 years
  - 5-year survival rate after curative resection of squamous cell carcinoma is 35%–40%; 25% for adenocarcinoma and large cell carcinoma

  COMPLICATIONS
  - Superior vena cava syndrome, pericardial tamponade, phrenic nerve palsy, recurrent laryngeal nerve palsy, spinal cord compression from metastasis, SIADH, Eaton-Lambert syndrome, hypertrophic pulmonary osteoarthropathy, death

Tuberculosis (TB)

Description
- Systemic disease caused by *Mycobacterium tuberculosis*, of which pulmonary disease is the most common presentation; however, 15% are in other organ systems (extrapulmonary) such as skin, kidneys, bones, genitourinary, meninges, peritoneum, and heart
- Classified as active or latent

Etiology
- Inhalation of aerosolized droplets from an infected person may cause local reaction in periphery of lung that is asymptomatic; rarely causes active disease at this stage.

- Reactivation may occur years later and symptoms of active disease appear.
- Structure of the bacterium M. *tuberculosis* makes it relatively resistant to destruction by macrophages and drugs; it multiplies slowly and may lay dormant for a long period of time.

Incidence and Demographics
- Causes more deaths worldwide than any other infectious disease.
- Annually, 8 million people worldwide develop active TB and 3 million die.
- Approximately 10–15 million people in the U.S. have latent TB infections; about 10% of those will develop active TB at some time in their lives.
- In the U.S., the highest rates are in African-Americans, Hispanics, Asians, and Native Americans.

Risk Factors
- HIV infection is most important risk factor
- Close contacts of people with newly diagnosed infectious TB
- Homeless, immigrants
- Low socioeconomic status, urban crowding
- Institutional or correctional facilities
- Malignancy, malnutrition, IV drug users
- Healthcare workers working with high-risk populations

Prevention and Screening
- Identifying and treating infected individuals early; yearly screening for all at risk.
  - Tuberculin skin tests (TST): Mantoux (PPD) is standard test, establishes exposure to TB; see Table 7–5 for PPD interpretation.
  - A whole-blood interferon gamma assay (e.g., QuantiFERON-TB Gold test or QFT-G test) has been approved by the Food and Drug Administration (FDA). The Centers for Disease Control and Prevention (CDC) recommends that the QFT-G test can be used in all circumstances in which the TST is currently used. Compared with the TST, the QFT-G test is less subject to reader bias and error, can be accomplished after a single patient visit, and may not be as likely to be positive following the BCG vaccine.
- Isoniazid (INH) prevents the disease in most close contacts of infected people and most infected individuals who do not have active TB.
- Preventive therapy indicated for patients in certain risk groups (see Table 7–5).
- Bacillus Calmette-Guerin (BCG) vaccine is indicated only when isoniazid cannot be used. Consider use in persons who are repeatedly exposed and cannot receive standard treatment. Frequently used overseas and may have been used by immigrants; may cause persistent positive PPD.

Assessment
HISTORY
  - Often a person with TB infection will be asymptomatic; assess for risk factors
  - Assess for history of TB, exposure to TB, or treatment for active or latent disease
  - A person with TB disease may have any, all, or none of the following: chronic productive cough; fatigue, malaise; weight loss; anorexia; fever; hemoptysis; night sweats; pleuritic chest pain; lymphadenitis

- Children are usually asymptomatic at initial infection; symptoms may occur 1–6 months later
- Extrapulmonary TB symptoms depend on site affected

PHYSICAL EXAM
- Appear chronically ill, weight loss; chest exam normal or reveal apical rales, increased tactile fremitus on palpation; dullness to percussion
- Evaluate for extrapulmonary TB

DIAGNOSTIC STUDIES
- PPD to assess exposure (see Table 7–5)
- Chest x-ray: Infiltrate in middle and lower lobes in primary TB; fibronodular upper lobe infiltrate in reactivation of disease; see small, homogenous infiltrates, cavitation, hilar and paratracheal lymph node enlargement
- Sputum smear (acid-fast, fluorescence), nucleic acid probe testing, and cultures for definitive diagnosis
- CBC with differential and platelets
- Bronchoscopy

Differential Diagnosis
- COPD
- Asthma
- Pneumonia
- Cancer
- Pleurisy
- Histoplasmosis
- Silicosis
- Interstitial lung disease

Management
NONPHARMACOLOGIC TREATMENT
- Education and counseling regarding the importance of adherence; consider use of community resources such as direct observation therapy (DOT) to ensure adherence
- Review transmission of disease and need for good hygiene, handwashing, secretion precautions, and no sharing of utensils, glasses, etc., for active disease

Table 7–5. Guidelines for Determining a Positive TST and Need for Preventive Treatment

Induration >5 mm	Induration >10 mm	Induration >15 mm
HIV-positive persons	Recent arrivals (< 5 years) from high-prevalence countries	All persons with no risk factors for TB
Fibrotic changes on CXR consistent with old TB	IV drug users	
Patients with organ transplants, other immunosuppressed patients (e.g., receiving the equivalent of >15 mg/d of prednisone for >1 month)	Residents and employees* of high-risk congregate settings: prisons, jails, nursing homes and other healthcare facilities, residential facilities for AIDS patients, and homeless shelters	
	Mycobacteriology laboratory personnel	
	Preexisting medical conditions: Weight loss >10% below ideal body weight, diabetes mellitus, gastrectomy, jejuneal bypass, silicosis, chronic renal failure, malignancy	
	Any child <4 years; infants, children, and adolescents exposed to adults in high-risk categories	

*For persons who are at low risk and are tested at entry into employment, a reaction of >15 mm is considered positive.

Adapted from "Diagnostic standards and classification of tuberculosis," by American Thoracic Society, 2000, *American Journal of Respiratory Care and Critical Care Medicine 2000, 161*, p. 1376.

PHARMACOLOGIC TREATMENT
- Latent disease: Patients in need of preventive therapy (see Table 7–5)
- Isoniazid (INH) is first-line therapy for latent TB in all people; standard dose is 300 mg daily for adults; 10 mg/kg daily for children; can be given twice weekly in higher dose instead of daily
  - Length of therapy is 6–9 months, based on the clinical situation
  - Major adverse reactions are hepatotoxicity, peripheral neuropathy (vitamin B6 daily to decrease neuropathy and CNS effects), and interactions with other drugs
- Alternate therapy is with rifampin 600 mg/d for 4 months for adults and 10–20 mg/d for children for 6 months (max 600 mg/d); should be used to treat contacts of INH-resistant TB patients. **Rifampin cannot be taken by HIV-infected persons taking protease inhibitors or certain nonucleoside reverse transcriptase inhibitors.**
- Current recommendations can be obtained from www.thoracic.org and www.cdc.gov

• Treatment of active disease: First-line drugs include a multidrug regimen of isoniazid, rifampin, pyrazinamide, and ethambutol (Myambutol); may be based on sputum culture

Special Considerations
• Geriatrics often have atypical presentation of disease
• Two-step PPD recommended in the geriatric population because of waning immunity, for healthcare workers, and for employees and residents of congregate settings. PPD is given; if negative, it is repeated in 2 weeks to test for booster effect (positive on second test, indicating infection in the past). If second test is negative, person is considered TB-free and any subsequent positive test indicates a new infection.
• Pregnancy: Pyridoxine given along with INH; streptomycin contraindicated
• Lactation: Small doses of antituberculosis drugs are found in breast milk; however, do not discourage breastfeeding
• Pharmacotherapy may cause interactions with other drugs
• HIV-infected patients should be treated for 9 months

When to Consult, Refer, Hospitalize
• All suspected or confirmed cases should be reported to the local and state health departments.
• Refer all patients with active disease to specialist for treatment.
• Hospitalize patients if incapable of self-care, or if patient is likely to expose new susceptible individuals.
• Some states may incarcerate noncompliant patient to ensure medication is taken.

Follow-Up
EXPECTED COURSE
• Baseline monitoring is not routinely indicated. Baseline monitoring of ALT is recommended for those individuals who chronically consume alcohol, take concomitant hepatotoxic drugs, have viral hepatitis or other liver disease, are pregnant or within 3 months postpartum, and HIV-infected persons. Some experts recommend monitoring for those older than 35 years. Treatment should be interrupted and generally modified for those with ALT 3x the upper limit of normal (ULN) in the presence of hepatitis symptoms and/or jaundice, or 5x ULN in the absence of symptoms.

COMPLICATIONS
• Drug-induced hepatitis, particularly in patients >35 years, frequent monitoring of liver function indicated; drug-induced neuropathy
• Treatment failure most often due to noncompliance
• The death rate for untreated TB patients is 40%–60%
• Drug-resistant TB found in 15% of tuberculosis patients in the U.S.
• Outbreaks of multidrug resistant tuberculosis have been associated with high mortality rates (70%–90%), and median survival rates of 4–16 weeks

CHRONIC CONDITIONS

Asthma

Description
- Chronic inflammatory pulmonary disorder of the airways characterized by episodic and at least partially reversible symptoms of airflow obstruction and hyperreactivity of the airways

  MAJOR GOALS OF ASTHMA THERAPY
  - Reduce impairment
    - Prevent chronic and troublesome symptoms
    - Require infrequent use of inhaled short-acting beta-2 agonists (SABA)
    - Maintain near-normal pulmonary function
    - Maintain normal activity levels
    - Meet patient and family expectations of satisfaction with asthma care
  - Reduce risk
    - Prevent recurrent exacerbations and minimize ED visits
    - Prevent loss of lung function or reduced lung growth in children
    - Provide optimal pharmacotherapy with minimal or no adverse effects of therapy

  FOUR COMPONENTS OF CARE
  - Assessment and monitoring
  - Education
  - Control environmental factors and comorbid conditions
  - Medications

Etiology
- Inflammation and bronchospasm caused by allergic and nonallergic triggers
- Allergy triggers:
  - Seasonal or environmental allergens: Pollens, feathers, warm-blooded pet epithelia, dust mite and cockroach excrement, molds, food additives/preservatives such as sulfites (rare)
- Nonallergic triggers:
  - Exercise-induced asthma, occurring 5–10 minutes following the onset of strenuous activity; related to bronchial heat or water loss
  - Occupational asthma: Triggers in workplace such as fumes, dyes, and chemicals
  - Diseases or infections such as bronchitis, gastroesophageal reflux, rhinitis/sinusitis, viral respiratory infections (especially RSV infections during infancy, rhinovirus <2 years of age)
  - Drug induced: Aspirin, NSAIDs, indomethacin, beta blockers
  - Smoke and pollutants

Incidence and Demographics
- Seventh-ranking chronic condition in the U.S.; African-American males suffer highest mortality rate
- Incidence rising; affects 22 million Americans (6 million children); onset at any age; 12.9 million office visits and 1.7 million ED visits annually
- More common in boys than in girls up to 10 years old, then equal incidence
- Commonly under-diagnosed in pediatrics and geriatrics
- High prevalence in urban and underserved communities

Risk Factors
- Secondhand smoke exposure
- Allergies; atopy in patient or family members
- Genetic predisposition (especially if mother has asthma)

Prevention and Screening
- Avoid allergens, tobacco smoke, foods containing sulfites, aspirin and NSAIDs if sensitive
- Avoid exercise in cold temperatures and during high-pollution levels
- Reduce exposure to triggers by use of air filters and air conditioners; removal of rugs, stuffed animals, pets, etc.
- Treat upper respiratory infections, rhinitis, and gastroesophageal reflux when present
- Recommend influenza vaccination annually

Assessment
HISTORY
- Characteristic symptoms: Episodic wheezing (absent in severe exacerbation), chest tightness, dyspnea, chronic dry or spasmodic cough; symptoms worse at night, with exercise, exposure to cold temperatures, smoke, allergens
- Symptoms of emotional stress, upper respiratory infection, rhinitis/sinusitis, eczema/atopic dermatitis, nasal polyps
- Family history of asthma, allergies, or atopy
- Severity of symptoms (see Table 7–6)

PHYSICAL EXAM
- Findings vary with the severity of the attack; wheezing may not be present, as in cough-variant asthma
- Vital signs, with particular attention to respiratory rate
- Include assessment of the skin, chest, upper respiratory tract
- Signs of atopic dermatitis/eczema, dehydration, nasal discharge, sinus tenderness, mucosal edema and erythema, nasal polyps, postnasal drainage, allergic shiners, allergic salute may be present
- In acute exacerbation, tachypnea, tachycardia, prolonged expiration, audible wheezing (may be absent in severe attacks due to decreased breath sounds), use of accessory respiratory muscles, intercostal retraction, nasal flaring, diaphoresis, distant or diminished breath sounds, hyperresonance, cyanosis, decreased responsiveness
- In severe exacerbation, cyanosis, diaphoresis, diminished breath sounds, pulsus paradoxus (>12 mmHg fall in blood pressure during inspiration)

DIAGNOSTIC STUDIES
- Initial pulmonary function studies are essential for diagnosis, then periodic monitoring (see Table 7–7)
- Peak expiratory flow (PEF) used for monitoring lung status, not to confirm diagnosis. Values vary with height, age, gender. Patient determines "personal best" or average of three readings on optimal day's PEF; <200 mL indicates severe obstruction.
- 80%–100% of patient's "personal best": good control, maintain treatment; 50%–79%: acute exacerbation, adjust treatment; <50%: severe asthma exacerbation, emergency treatment
- Pulse oximetry; pulmonary function tests (PFT; see Table 7–8)/spirometry reveal obstructive dysfunction
- Airflow obstruction indicated by reduced FEV1/FVC ratio (<75%). Partial reversibility; improvement in FVC or FEV1 of at least 15% or improvement in FEF of at least 25% often noted after bronchodilator treatment
- Chest x-ray: Obtain at initial diagnosis in children; shows hyperinflation in uncomplicated episodes
- Skin testing (usually epicutaneous, possibly intradermal) to determine allergic causes
- Bronchial provocation testing confirms diagnosis
- Methacholine, histamine, or exercise challenge test induces symptoms
- CBC if signs of infection and to exclude severe anemia as cause for dyspnea; slight increase of white blood cells during acute attack with eosinophilia related to allergic attack
- Mild arterial hypoxia and hypocapnia indicate fatigue of accessory muscles

Differential Diagnosis

ALL AGES
- Foreign body aspiration
- Acute infections, viral, pneumonia, bronchitis, TB
- GERD
- Aspiration
- AIDS
- Psychogenic cough
- Neuromuscular weakness
- Vocal cord dysfunction (adolescents and young adults)

ADULTS
- COPD
- CHF
- Pulmonary embolism
- Bronchogenic carcinoma
- Cough secondary to ACE inhibitors
- Alpha antitrypsin deficiency

CHILDREN
- Bronchiolitis (RSV)
- Laryngotracheobronchitis (Croup)
- Cystic fibrosis
- Bronchopulmonary dysplasia
- Tracheoesophageal fistula
- Congenital heart disease

Classification of Asthma Severity

- Classification of asthma is based on age and severity of symptoms (impairment and risk)
- Classified as either intermittent or persistent
- Classifying asthma is always a dynamic process; changes can occur frequently
  - Intermittent: Step 1
  - Persistent
    - Mild: Step 2
    - Moderate: Step 3 or Step 4
    - Severe: Step 5 or Step 6

Management

NONPHARMACOLOGIC TREATMENT
- Identify and avoid factors that trigger asthma; control environmental triggers
- Allergy skin testing to determine allergens
- Maintain hydration; increase fluids during exacerbation
- Address family, school, day care issues; provide education, support, and counseling
- Establish a patient/provider partnership with a detailed asthma action plan
- No smoking

PHARMACOLOGIC TREATMENT
- National Heart, Lung, and Blood Institute of the National Institutes of Health has developed general guidelines for the treatment of asthma (see Tables 7–7, 7–9, 7–10)
- Medications are divided into two main groups: quick relief and long-term control. Multiple drug choices, delivery systems, and dosages exist, so check manufacturer information before using.

QUICK RELIEF MEDICATIONS ("RESCUE")
- Short-acting beta-2 agonists (SABA; drugs of choice in acute exacerbation)
  - Albuterol HFA (Proventil HFA, Ventolin HFA), pirbuterol (Maxair), metaproterenol (Alupent)—generally 2 inhalations or 1 nebulization q4h in adults and children
  - Levalbuterol (Xopenex HFA): Children >4 yrs and adults: 2 inh every 4-6 hrs prn
  - Or in adults and children >4 yrs: Levalbuterol (Xopenex) 0.63 or 1.25 mg 1 nebulized solution q6–8h

– Or especially in young children: Albuterol syrup (Proventil, Ventolin) 2 mg/5 mL; children 2–6 years: 0.1–0.2 mg/kg tid max 2gm/day; 6–14 years: 5 mL tid to qid
- Anticholinergic: Ipratropium (Atrovent) 1–2 inh or 1–2 unit dose neb q6h prn (adults only)

LONG-TERM CONTROL MEDICATIONS ("CONTROLLER")
- Systemic corticosteroids may be used qd or qod for severe persistent asthma as well as acute exacerbation; taper is required if treating longer than 7 days
- Inhaled corticosteroids:
    – Beclomethasone dipropionate (Beclovent, Vanceril): Adults: 2 inh of 42 mcg/inh or 1–2 inh of 84 mcg/inh tid–qid; children: 2–4 inh of 42 mcg/inh bid or 1–2 inh of 84 mcg/inh bid
    – Triamcinolone acetate (Azmacort): Adults: 2 inh tid–qid or 4 inh bid; children: 1–2 inh tid–qid or 2–4 inh bid
- Inhaled long-acting beta2 agonists (LABA):
    – Salmeterol (Serevent): 21 mcg/inh, adults: 1 inh q 12 hrs; children >4 yrs: (Serevent discus) 1 inh q 12 hrs
    – Formoterol (Foradil): 12 mcg/inh, adults and children (>5 yrs): 1inh q 12 hrs
- Oral long-acting beta agonists: Albuterol extended release tabs (Volmax, Proventil Repetabs). Adults: 4–8 mg q 12 hrs; children >12 yrs: 4 mg q 12 hrs, ages 6–11: 2mg q12 hrs
- Anti-inflammatory (non-corticosteroid): Adults and children >5 yrs: Cromolyn sodium (Intal) 2 inh of metered dose inhaler (MDI) 0.8 mg/inh qid; neb sol 20 mg/2 mL qid; nedocromil (Tilade) 2 inh qid (children >6 yrs only)
- Leukotriene receptor antagonists:
    – Zafirlukast (Accolate): Adults (12 yrs and older): 20 mg bid; children age 5–11 years: 10 mg bid; take on empty stomach
    – Montelukast (Singulair). Adults: 10 mg qd; age 1–5: 4 mg qd; age 6–14: 5mg qd
- Methylxanthines: Theophylline dose dependent on preparation; maintain serum levels of 12–15 mcg/L

LENGTH OF TREATMENT
- Dependent on the severity of the attacks; goal of treatment is to gain control as quickly as possible and decrease treatment gradually to the least amount of medication needed to maintain control

Special Considerations
- Patients with exercise-induced asthma should be instructed to use prophylactic treatment 5–10 minutes prior to exercise with either SABA or LABA; leukotrienes are an alternative
- Death rate three times greater among African Americans and Hispanics than among Caucasians in U.S.

- Asthma medications should be used with caution in elderly patients as they often do not tolerate side effects. Some have difficulty using inhalers; consider using a spacer.
- Be aware of coexisting heart disease, osteoporosis, liver and kidney disease, which can be aggravated by asthma medications
- For postmenopausal women using inhaled corticosteroids, consider calcium supplements (1,000 to 1,500 mg a day) and vitamin D (800 units a day); consider hormone replacement therapy
- Bone mineral density testing if on long-term inhaled or oral corticosteroids to monitor osteoporosis
- Periodic ophthalmology exam if on oral corticosteroids
- With pregnant/lactating women, use as little medication as possible. If necessary, use inhaled medications first and frequently monitor for toxicity and side effects; however, asthma control is essential for good fetal outcome.
- Most medications are secreted in breast milk
- Pregnancy Category C: Beta adrenergic agonists, theophylline, inhaled and systemic corticosteroids
- Pregnancy Category B: Ipratropium, cromolyn, leukotrienes, ipratropium, and inhaled terbutaline
- Avoid ipratropium in patients with allergy to peanuts or soy; it contains soya lecithin and may precipate an allergic reaction
- In children, monitor growth if using steroids to manage asthma
- Withhold varicella vaccine if child receiving >2 mg/kg or 20 mg/day of oral prednisone

When to Consult, Refer, Hospitalize
- Adults: Severe asthma exacerbation or severe persistent asthma, requiring Step 4 care
- Children: All patients with moderate or severe persistent asthma; consider referral in children <3 years old with mild persistent asthma
- Patient not meeting goals of treatment after 3–6 months of therapy
- Consider referral for other conditions complicating asthma (infections, poorly controlled allergies, GERD, COPD)
- Additional diagnostic testing indicated by clinical presentation
- Immunotherapy is a treatment consideration
- Continuous use of oral corticosteroid therapy or high-dose inhaled corticosteroids, or required 2 bursts of oral corticosteroids in 1 year
- For confirmation of history that suggests an occupational or environmental inhalant or ingested substance is aggravating asthma

Table 7–6a. Classifying Asthma Severity and Initiating Treatment in Children 0–4 Years of Age

Components of Severity		Classification of Asthma Severity (0–4 Years of Age)			
				Persistent	
		Intermittent	Mild	Moderate	Severe
Impairment	Symptoms	<2 days/week	>2 days/week but not daily	Daily	Throughout the day
	Nighttime awakenings	0	1–2x/month	3–4x/month	>1x/week
	Short-acting beta2 agonist use for symptom control (not prevention of exercise-induced bronchospasm [EIB])	<2 days/week	>2 days/week but not daily	Daily	Several times per day
	Interference with normal activity	None	Minor limitation	Some limitation	Extremely limited
Risk	Exacerbations requiring oral systemic corticosteroids	0–1/year	>2 exacerbations in 6 months requiring oral systemic corticosteroids, or >4 wheezing episodes in 1 year lasting >1 day AND risk factors for persistent asthma		
		Consider severity and interval since last exacerbation			
		Frequency and severity may fluctuate over time			
		Exacerbations of any severity may occur in patients in any severity category			
Recommended step for initiating treatment		Step 1	Step 2	Step 3 and consider short course of oral systemic corticosteroids	
		In 2–6 weeks, depending on severity, evaluate level of asthma control achieved. If no clear benefit is observed in 4–6 weeks, consider adjusting therapy or alternative diagnoses.			

Table 7-6b. Classifying Asthma Severity and Initiating Treatment in Children 5–11 Years of Age

Components of Severity		Classification of Asthma Severity (5–11 Years of Age)			
		Intermittent	Persistent		
			Mild	Moderate	Severe
Impairment	Symptoms	<2 days/week	>2 days/week but not daily	Daily	Throughout the day
	Nighttime awakenings	<2x/month	3–4x/month	>1x/week but not nightly	Often 7x/week
	Short-acting beta2 agonist use for symptom control (not prevention of EIB)	<2 days/week	>2 days/week but not daily	Daily	Several times per day
	Interference with normal activity	None	Minor limitation	Some limitation	Extremely limited
	Lung function	• Normal FEV1 between exacerbations • FEV1 >80% predicted • FEV1/FVC >85%	• FEV1 = >80% predicted	• FEV1 = 60%–80% predicted • FEV1/FVC = 75%–80%	• FEV1 <60% predicted • FEV1/FVC <75%
Risk	Exacerbations requiring oral systemic corticosteroids	0–1/year	>2/year		
		Consider severity and interval since last exacerbation			
		Frequency and severity may fluctuate over time for patients in any severity category			
		Relative annual risk of exacerbations may be related to FEV1			
Recommended step for initiating treatment		Step 1	Step 2	Step 3, medium dose ICS option	Step 3, medium dose ICS option, or Step 4
				And consider short course of oral systemic corticosteroids	
		In 2–6 weeks, evaluate level of asthma control achieved and adjust therapy accordingly.			

Reprinted from *National Heart, Blood, and Lung Institute Expert Panel Report 3 (EPR 3): Guidelines for the Diagnosis and Management of Asthma* (NIH Publication No. 08-4051) by National Institutes of Health, 2007, Bethesda, MD: Author.

Table 7–7. Stepwise Approach for Managing Asthma in Children 5–11 Years of Age

Intermittent asthma	Persistent asthma: daily medication Consult with asthma specialist if step 4 care or higher is required. Consider consultation at step 3.					

Step 1

Preferred:

SABA PRN

Step 2

Preferred:

Low-dose ICS

Alternative:

Cromolyn, LTRA, Nedocromil, or Theophylline

Step 3

Preferred:

EITHER:

Low-dose ICS + either LABA, LTRA, or Theophylline

OR

Medium-dose ICS

Step 4

Preferred:

Medium-dose ICS + LABA

Alternative:

Medium-dose ICS + either LTRA or Theophylline

Step 5

Preferred:

High-dose ICS + LABA

Alternative:

High-dose ICS + either LTRA or Theophylline

Step 6

Preferred:

High-dose ICS + LABA + oral systemic corticosteroid

Alternative:

High-dose ICS + either LTRA or Theophylline + oral systemic corticosteroid

Step up if needed

(first, check adherence, inhaler technique, environmental control, and comorbid conditions)

Assess control

Step down if possible

(and asthma is well controlled at least 3 months)

Each step: patient education, environmental control, and management of comorbidities.
Steps 2-4: consider subcutaneous allergen immunotherapy for patients who have allergic asthma (see footnotes).

Quick-relief medication for all patients

- SABA as needed for symptoms. Intensity of treatment depends on severity of symptoms: up to 3 treatments at 20-minute intervals as needed. Short course of oral systemic corticosteroids may be needed.
- Caution: Increasing use of SABA or use >2 days a week for symptom relief (not prevention of EIB) generally indicates inadequate control and the need to step up treatment.

Reprinted from *National Heart, Blood, and Lung Institute Expert Panel Report 3 (EPR 3): Guidelines for the Diagnosis and Management of Asthma* (NIH Publication No. 08-4051) by National Institutes of Health, 2007, Bethesda, MD: Author.

Table 7-8. Definitions of Pulmonary Function Tests

Test	Definition
Spirometry	
FVC	Forced vital capacity: Volume of gas that can be forcefully expelled from the lungs after maximal inspiration
FEV1	Forced expiratory volume in 1 second: Volume of gas expelled in the first second of the FVC (most commonly used to determine asthma status)
FEF25-75	Forced expiratory flow from 25%–75% of the FVC maximal airflow rate
PEFR	Peak expiratory flow rate: Maximal airflow rate achieved in the FVC maneuver
MVV	Maximum voluntary ventilation: Maximum volume of gas that can be breathed in 1 minute (measured in 15 seconds and multiplied by 4)
Lung Volumes	
TLC	Total lung capacity: Volume of gas in the lungs after a maximal inspiration
RV	Residual volume: Volume of gas remaining in the lungs after maximal expiration
ERV	Expiratory reserve volume: Volume of gas representing the difference between functional residual capacity and residual volume
FRC	Functional residual capacity: Volume of gas in the lungs at the end of a normal tidal expiration
SVC	Slowed vital capacity: Volume of gas that can be slowly exhaled after maximal inspiration

Adapted from *Current medical diagnosis and treatment* (44th ed., p. 269), by L. M. Tierney, S. J. McPhee, & A. Papadakis, 2008, Norwalk, CT: Appleton & Lange.

Follow-Up

EXPECTED COURSE
- Requires regular monitoring and evaluation.
- Patients should monitor peak flow rates twice daily to establish baseline and then regularly.
- For acute exacerbation, follow up in 24 hours, then 3–5 days. Follow up weekly until symptoms are controlled and peak flow consistently 80% of predicted, then monthly.
- Once stabilized, follow up every 6 months for a possible reduction in treatment.
- Monitor theophylline levels 2 weeks after initiation of therapy, then every 4 months.

COMPLICATIONS
- Include exhaustion, dehydration, cor pulmonale, airway infection, tussive syncope, rib fracture
- Pneumothorax rare, hypercapnia and hypoxic respiratory failure in severe disease

Table 7–9. Classifying Asthma Severity and Initiating Treatment in Youths 12 Years of Age or Older and Adults

Components of Severity		Classification of Asthma Severity (>12 Years of Age)			
		Intermittent	Persistent		
			Mild	Moderate	Severe
Impairment	Symptoms	<2 days/week	>2 days/week but not daily	Daily	Throughout the day
Normal FEV1/ FVC:	Nighttime awakenings	<2x/month	3–4x/month	>1x/week but not nightly	Often 7x/ week
8–19 yrs 85%	Short-acting beta2 agonist use for symptom control (not prevention of EIB)	<2 days/week	> 2 days/week but not daily, and not more than 1x on any day	Daily	Several times per day
20–39 yrs 80%					
40–59 yrs 75%					
60–80 yrs 70%	Interference with normal activity	None	Minor limitation	Some limitation	Extremely limited
	Lung function	• Normal FEV1 between exacerbations • FEV1 >80% predicted • FEV1/FVC normal	• FEV1 >80% predicted • FEV1/FVC normal	• FEV1 >60% but <80% predicted • FEV1/FVC reduced 5%	• FEV1 <60% predicted • FEV1/ FVC reduced >5%
Risk	Exacerbations requiring oral systemic corticosteroids	0–1/year	>2/year		
		Consider severity and interval since last exacerbation			
		Frequency and severity may fluctuate over time for patients in any severity category			
		Relative annual risk of exacerbations may be related to FEV1			
Recommended step for initiating treatment		Step 1	Step 2	Step 3	Step 4 or 5
				And consider short course of oral systemic corticosteroids	
		In 2-6 weeks, evaluate level of asthma control that is achieved and adjust therapy accordingly.			

Reprinted from *National Heart, Blood, and Lung Institute Expert Panel Report 3 (EPR 3): Guidelines for the Diagnosis and Management of Asthma* (NIH Publication No. 08-4051) by National Institutes of Health, 2007, Bethesda, MD: Author.

Table 7–10. Stepwise Approach for Managing Asthma in Youths 12 Years of Age or Older and Adults

Intermittent asthma	Persistent asthma: daily medication Consult with asthma specialist if step 4 care or higher is required. Consider consultation at step 3.

Step 6
Preferred:
High-dose ICS + LABA + oral corticosteroid
AND
Consider Omalizumab for patients who have allergies

Step 5
Preferred:
High-dose ICS + LABA
AND
Consider Omalizumab for patients who have allergies

Step 4
Preferred:
Medium-dose ICS + LABA
Alternative:
Medium-dose ICS + either LTRA, Theophylline, or Zileuton

Step 3
Preferred:
Low-dose ICS + LABA
OR
Medium-dose ICS
Alternative:
Low-dose ICS + either LTRA, Theophylline, or Zileuton

Step 2
Preferred:
Low-dose ICS
Alternative:
Cromolyn, LTRA, Nedocromil, or Theophylline

Step 1
Preferred:
SABA PRN

Step up if needed
(first, check adherence, environmental control, and comorbid conditions)

Assess control

Step down if possible
(and asthma is well controlled at least 3 months)

Each step: patient education, environmental control, and management of comorbidities.
Steps 2-4: consider subcutaneous allergen immunotherapy for patients who have allergic asthma (see footnotes).

Quick-relief medication for all patients

- SABA as needed for symptoms. Intensity of treatment depends on severity of symptoms: up to 3 treatments at 20-minute intervals as needed. Short course of oral systemic corticosteroids may be needed.
- Use of SABA >2 days a week for symptom relief (not prevention of EIB) generally indicates inadequate control and the need to step up treatment.

Reprinted from *National Heart, Blood, and Lung Institute Expert Panel Report 3 (EPR 3): Guidelines for the Diagnosis and Management of Asthma* (NIH Publication No. 08-4051) by National Institutes of Health, 2007, Bethesda, MD: Author.

Chronic Obstructive Pulmonary Disease (COPD)

Description
- Chronic disease characterized by history of exposure to dust, pollen, and textiles and presence of airflow limitation that is not fully reversible, with or without the presence of symptoms
- Chronic bronchitis defined by history of the presence of a mucus-producing cough most days of the month, 3 months of a year, for 2 consecutive years without other underlying disease to explain the cough
- Chronic bronchitis may precede or accompany pulmonary emphysema: Abnormal permanent enlargement of air spaces within the terminal bronchiole, with wall destruction in absence of fibrosis

- Patients with asthma whose airflow obstruction is not completely reversible are considered to have COPD. The etiology and pathogenesis of the COPD in these patients may vary from those who have chronic bronchitis or emphysema.

Etiology
- Cigarette smoking and environmental tobacco smoke exposure is the most common cause—80% of patients have a history of exposure to tobacco smoke, indoor or outdoor pollution, or industrial dusts and chemicals.
- Bacterial or viral infection, air pollution, and occupational exposures may initially irritate the bronchial tree of patients with COPD.
- Rare genetic cause of emphysema is alpha-1 antitrypsin deficiency.
- Excess mucus in the bronchial tree in chronic bronchitis and enlargement of the distal airspaces in emphysema lead to fixed expiratory flow abnormality.

Incidence and Demographics
- COPD affects more than 10 million people in the U.S.
- Nearly equal prevalence in men and women
- Affects all ages, but is more common in people over age 45
- COPD with asthma is fourth leading cause of death in the U.S.

Risk Factors
- Smokers most likely to develop chronic bronchitis
- Occupations involving high concentrations of dust and fumes are also at high risk: coal miners, metal molders, grain handlers

Prevention and Screening
- Eliminate sources of irritation and infection in the upper and lower respiratory tract
- Encourage smoking cessation and reduction of exposure to secondhand smoke
- Avoid outdoor activities when air pollutant concentrations are high

Assessment
HISTORY
- Duration and characteristics of cough, dyspnea, sputum production
- Exercise/activity tolerance, dyspnea on exertion or at rest
- Chills/fever; weight gain/loss, edema, fatigue, angina
- Tobacco exposure (current smoking, pack year history, environmental tobacco exposure)
- Occupational exposures
- Sleep habits (number of pillows used)
- Increase in sputum production or purulence along with dyspnea signals exacerbation
- Family history of COPD
- Other upper and lower respiratory disease, cardiac disease
- Impact on quality of life, activities of daily living, socioeconomic status

PHYSICAL EXAM
- Clinical findings often absent in early disease. More severe disease typically presents as two distinct patterns as chronic bronchitis progresses to COPD, although many patients have evidence of both disorders

- Ages 30–40 years: Chronic productive cough for mucopurulent sputum, frequent exacerbation, mild dyspnea, overweight, cyanosis, peripheral edema, rhonchi and wheezes common, AP diameter normal
- Age 50 years and older: Dyspnea, rare cough, recent weight loss, use accessory respiratory muscles with breathing, increased anteroposterior (AP) diameter of chest, no abnormal breath sounds
- Disease classifications

Table 7–11. Global Initiative for Chronic Obstructive Lung Disease (GOLD) Classification

Classification	Characteristics
At Risk	Chronic symptoms; exposure to risk; normal spirometry
Mild Disease	FEV1/FVC <70%; FEV1 >80%; w/wo symptoms
Moderate Disease	FEV1/FVC <70%; 50% < FEV1 <80%; w/wo symptoms
Severe	FEV1/FVC <70%; 30% < FEV1 <50%; w/wo symptoms
Very Severe	FEV1/FVC <70%; FEV1 <30% or FEV1 <50% with chronic respiratory failure symptoms

Reprinted from *Global strategy for the diagnosis, management, and prevention of chronic obstructive pulmonary disease* by Global Initiative for Chronic Obstructive Disease (GOLD), World Health Organization, and National Heart, Lung, and Blood Institute, 2006, retrieved March 1, 2008, from www.goldcopd.com.

DIAGNOSTIC STUDIES
- PFT: Reduced FVC, reduced FEV1, reduced ratio of FEV1 to FVC (<70%), increased RV, and increased TLC
- Chest radiographs in emphysema: Hyperinflation, subpleural blebs, parenchymal bullae, flattened diaphragm; in chronic bronchitis: nonspecific peribronchial and perivascular markings at bases ("dirty lungs")
- Consider pulse oximetry during acute exacerbations or in those patients who may be considered for long-term oxygen therapy
- Arterial blood gases (ABGs) unnecessary unless FEV1 <40% of predicted, hypoxia, or hypercapnia suspected; no abnormalities in early COPD; hypoxemia in advanced chronic bronchitis; compensated respiratory acidosis with chronic respiratory failure in chronic bronchitis
- ECG may show sinus tachycardia; abnormalities typical of cor pulmonale in advanced disease with pulmonary hypertension; supraventricular arrhythmia, ventricular irritability, right ventricular hypertrophy
- Alpha 1 antitrypsin level to look for deficiency if COPD occurs before 45 years of age
- Increased hematocrit may be present with chronic bronchitis but not with emphysema

Differential Diagnosis
- Bronchial asthma
- Bronchiectasis
- Bronchopulmonary mycosis
- Congestive heart failure
- Tuberculosis
- Central airway obstruction

Management
- Refer to American Thoracic Society Guidelines for the diagnosis and care of patients with chronic obstructive pulmonary disease (see Tables 7–12 and 7–13)

  NONPHARMACOLOGIC TREATMENT
  - Initiate and support smoking cessation
  - Maintain ideal body weight, well-balanced diet, regular daily exercise
  - Influenza and pneumococcal vaccines
  - Avoid exposure to colds and influenza
  - Avoid respiratory irritants (secondhand smoke, dust, other air pollutants)
  - Increase fluids and humidification
  - Chest physiotherapy in presence of sputum production
  - Breathing exercises; effective cough techniques
  - Supplemental oxygen for patients with resting hypoxemia: 1–3 L/min via nasal cannula 15 hours/day
  - Controversial lung volume reduction surgery and bullectomy (removal of bullae from distal airways, reducing dead space in lung); effective where appropriate

Table 7–12. Stepwise Pharmacologic Therapy for COPD

Stage	Treatment Guideline Recommendations
At Risk	Avoid risk factors; influenza immunization yearly
Mild Disease	Add short-acting bronchodilator when needed
Moderate Disease	Add one or more long-acting bronchodilator(s); pulmonary rehabilitation
Severe	Add inhaled glucocorticosteroids if significant symptoms and noted response in lung function, or if repeated exacerbations
Very Severe	Add long-term oxygen; consider surgical treatments

PHARMACOLOGIC TREATMENT
- Mucolytics and expectorants; questionable effectiveness
- Guaifenesin (Humibid LA): 600 mg tablets, 1–2 tablets bid prn
- Corticosteroids: 2-week therapy of oral steroid for acute exacerbation; inhaled daily therapy if spirometry improves after 6-week to 3-month trial of inhaled steroid
- Bronchodilators: Short- and long-acting beta agonists and anticholinergics, possibly methylxanthine
- Antibiotics for acute exacerbation of COPD
  - Many exacerbations due to bacterial infection: *H. influenzae*, *S. pneumoniae*, *M. catarrhalis*; may be due to viral infection, pneumonia
  - Trimethoprim-sulfamethoxazole (Bactrim DS): 160/800 mg q 12 h

– Amoxicillin-clavulanate (Augmentin): 875/125 mg q 12 h or 500 /125 mg tid
– Doxycycline (Vibramycin): 100 mg bid
– Also may use a fluoroquinolone such as levofloxacin (Levaquin), moxifloxacin (Avelox); azithromycin, cephalosporins
– Antibiotics not indicated in younger patients with mild symptoms and infrequent exacerbation
– Consider use in patients under 60 years old with mild–moderate impairment of lung function (FEV1 >50% predicted value with fewer than 4 exacerbations per year), or elderly patients with moderate or severe impairments and frequent exacerbation
– Long-term oxygen therapy

LENGTH OF TREATMENT
• Chronic condition requiring ongoing therapeutic treatments and monitoring
• Treat exacerbation for 10 days

Table 7–13. Indications for Long-Term Oxygen Therapy

General	In Presence of Right-Sided Heart Failure	Specific Circumstances
$PaO_2 \leq 55$ mmHg or $SaO_2 \leq 88\%$	$PaO_2 \leq 59$ mmHg or $SaO_2 \leq 89\%$	$PaO_2 \geq 60$ or $SaO_2 \geq 90\%$ with lung disease complicated by sleep apnea with nocturnal desaturations not corrected by C-PAP
	EKG evidence of cor pulmonale	If the patient meets criteria at rest, O_2 should also be prescribed during sleep and exercise with appropriate titration
	HCT >55%	If the patient has normal SaO_2 at rest, evaluate for desaturation during exercise or sleep; if $SaO_2 \leq 88\%$, O_2 should be prescribed for those situations
	Clinical evidence of right-sided heart failure	

Special Considerations
- Caution with beta blockers, cough suppressants, antihistamines, sedatives
- Discuss advance directives and end-of-life decisions

When to Consult, Refer, Hospitalize
- Consult with pulmonologist warranted for GOLD stages moderate, severe, and very severe
- Emergency room for signs and symptoms of respiratory failure, severe exacerbation, cor pulmonale
- Refer to pulmonary rehabilitation program if poor exercise tolerance

Follow-Up
> EXPECTED COURSE
>> • Degree of pulmonary dysfunction at initial visit is most important predictor of survival
>> • Poor prognosis especially for severe disease and emphysematous form, median survival approximately 4 years

> COMPLICATIONS
>> • Pulmonary hypertension, cor pulmonale, chronic respiratory failure, spontaneous pneumothorax, left ventricular heart failure

CASE STUDIES

Case 1. A 15-month-old female is brought in by her mother with a cough, runny nose, and low-grade fever. Her mother states she seems to have a cold all the time.
HPI: This current episode started two days ago and the mother is concerned about the frequency of colds. The rhinorrhea is yellow-green, appetite decreased, no symptoms of otitis media but she does have a history.

   1. What additional history would you like?

Exam: Temp 100.6°F, pulse 110, resp 32. Alert and quiet in mother's lap. Nose has moderate amount of thick yellow discharge; cough is wet, deep, and seems barky. Lungs with scattered wheezing and rhonchi in all fields, mild intercostal retractions, no nasal flaring. Rest of exam normal.

   2. What are the possible diagnoses?
   3. What diagnostic tests would you order initially?
   4. Your working diagnosis is bronchiolitis. What is your treatment plan?
   5. On follow-up, your patient is doing much better, but the results of the sweat test have returned positive. What is your course of action now?

Case 2. A 76-year-old male resident of an assisted living facility presents to your office complaining of recent weight loss (10–15 pounds in the last 2 months) and shortness of breath on exertion. Denies any fevers, diaphoresis, chest pain. Has had a nagging cough for the last 3 months, mostly nonproductive.
PMH: Hypertension, hypercholesterolemia.
Medications: Cardizem 180 mg qd, atorvastatin (Lipitor) 20 mg qd. Former smoker, 1 ppd x 30 years.

   1. What additional history would you like to obtain?

Exam: Temp 97.4°F, pulse 80, resp 20, BP 150/90; alert, cooperative male in no apparent distress. Nose: mild edema; chest: slight increase in AP diameter, no retractions, hyperresonance on percussion, no abnormal breath sounds.

   2. What are the most likely differential diagnoses?
   3. What diagnostic tests would you order?
   4. If the PPD is negative, would you do anything further?
   5. What would you do for this patient on this visit?

Case 3. A 35-year-old married Hispanic female presents with a chief complaint of cough for 7 days. She is the mother of three and works in a hardware store. The cough is productive of yellow phlegm and gets worse at night. She also notes some shortness of breath on exertion. She has felt warm off and on for the last 2 days, has had some yellowish rhinorrhea, denies earaches, sore throat.
PMH: Nonsmoker. No past history of asthma, bronchitis, pneumonia. Her children have had colds but currently well. She moved to the U.S. about 6 months ago from Guatemala. No other significant PMH.
Medications: Has tried OTC cold preparations with some relief.

Exam: Temp 100°F, pulse 82, resp 18, BP 128/86. Nose: erythema and edema; throat mild erythema; neck: shotty anterior cervical nodes; lungs: scattered adventitious breath sounds with partial clearing post cough; rest of PE normal.

1. What is your working differential diagnosis?
2. What diagnostic tests would you order?
3. What would you do for this patient at this visit?
4. On return visit, the PPD is positive at 10 mm and she tells you her symptoms are not improved and her fever has been 101°F, but responds well to Tylenol. What is your differential diagnosis now?
5. What diagnostic tests would you order?
6. What would you do regarding the other family members?
7. The CBC with differential results are WBC 12,000, segmented 50%, lymphs 48%; CXR shows increased hilar markings. Would you order an antibiotic? If so, which and why?

REFERENCES

American Academy of Pediatrics. (1999). Screening for tuberculosis in children. *Policy reference guide.* Elk Grove Village, IL: Author.

American Academy of Pediatrics. (2006). *Red book* (26th ed.). Elk Grove Village, IL: Author.

American Thoracic Society. (2000). Treatment of tuberculosis and tuberculosis infection in adults and children. *American Journal of Respiratory and Critical Care Medicine, 161,* S234.

American Thoracic Society. (2007). Guidelines for the initial management of adults with community-acquired pneumonia: Diagnosis, assessment of severity, antimicrobial therapy, and prevention. *American Journal of Respiratory and Critical Care Medicine, 163,* 1730–1754.

American Thoracic Society. (2008). *ATS-CDC-IDSA tuberculosis treatment guidelines for PDA.* Retrieved March 1, 2008, from http://www.thoracic.org/sections/education/palm-programs/pages/ats-cdc-idsa-tuberculosis-treatment-guidelines-for-pda.html

Centers for Disease Control and Prevention. (2008). Summary of notifiable diseases. *MMWR: Morbidity and Mortality Weekly Report 57*(07), 179–183. Retrieved February 25, 2008, from http://www.cdc.gov/mmwr/preview/mmwrhtml/mm5707a4.htm

Crawford-Faucher, A. (2008). Levofloxacin appears safe and effective for CAP in children. *American Family Physician, 77*(6), 838–840.

Dosanjh, D. P., Hinks, T. S., Innes, J. A., Deeks, J. J., Pasvol, G., Hackforth, S., et al. (2008). Improved diagnostic evaluation of suspected tuberculosis. *Annals of Internal Medicine, 148*(5), 325–336.

Edmunds, M. W., & Mayhew, M. S. (2004). *Pharmacology for the primary care provider* (2nd ed.). St. Louis, MO: Mosby.

Garau, J., & Calbo, E. (2008). Community-acquired pneumonia. *Lancet, 371*(9611), 455–458.

Gilbert, D. N., Moellering, R. C. Jr., Eliopoulos, G. M., Sande, M. A., & Chambers, H. F. (2008). *Sanford guide to antimicrobial therapy.* Vienna, VA: Antimicrobial Therapy, Inc.

Goroll, A. H., & Mulley, A. G. (2006). *Primary care medicine* (4th ed.). Philadelphia: Lippincott, Williams & Wilkins.

Graber, M. A., Dachs, R., & Darby-Stewart, A. (2008). Fluticasone or salmeterol alone vs. combination therapy for COPD. *American Family Physician, 77*(5), 587–588.

Khan, K., Wang, J., Hu, W., Bierman, A., & Gardam, M. (2007). Tuberculosis infection in the United States: National trends over three decades. *American Journal of Respiratory and Critical Care Medicine, 177*(4), 455–460.

Kleigman, R. M., Marcdante, K. J., Jensen, H. B., & Behrman, R. E. (2006). *Nelson essentials of pediatrics* (5th ed.). Philadelphia: Saunders.

Mandell, G. L. (Ed.). (2004). *Mandell, Douglas, and Bennett's principles and practice of infectious diseases* (5th ed.). London: Churchill Livingstone.

McPhee, S. J., Papadakis, M. A., & Tierney, L. M. (Eds.) (2008). *Current medical diagnosis and treatment* (47th ed.). New York: Lange Medical Books/McGraw-Hill.

National Cancer Institute. (2007). *Non–small cell lung cancer (PDQ) treatment—Health professionals.* Retrieved February 2008 from http://canernet.nci.nih.gov/index.html

National Heart, Lung, and Blood Institute. (2007). *Expert panel report 3 (EPR 3): Guidelines for the diagnosis and management of asthma* (NIH Publication No. 08-4051). Washington, DC: U.S. Government Printing Office.

Pauwels, R. A., Buist, A. S., Calverley, P. M., Jenkins, C. R., Hurd, S. S., for the GOLD Scientific Committee. (2001). Global strategy for the diagnosis, management, and prevention of chronic obstructive pulmonary disease. NHLBI/WHO Global Initiative for Chronic Obstructive Lung Disease Workshop summary. *American Journal of Respiratory Care Medicine, 163,* 1256–1276.

Rakel, R. E., & Bope, E. T. (2006). *Conn' s current therapy* (pp. 49–226). Philadelphia: Saunders Elsevier.

Rosen, P. (Ed.). (2006). *Emergency medicine: Concepts and clinical practice* (6th ed.). St. Louis, MO: Mosby.

Schwartz, W. (Ed.). (2008). *The 5 minute pediatric consult.* Philadelphia: Lippincott.

Siberry, G. K., & Iannone, R. (Eds.). (2005). *Harriet Lane handbook* (17th ed.). St. Louis, MO: Mosby.

Small, P. M., & Fujiwara, P. I. (2001). Management of tuberculosis in the United States. *New England Journal of Medicine, 345*, 189–200.

Taylor, R. B. (Ed.). (2002). *Family medicine principles and practice* (6th ed.). New York: Springer.

Tierney, L. M., McPhee, S. J., & Papadakis, A. (2008). *Current medical diagnosis and treatment* (44th ed.). Norwalk, CT: Appleton & Lange.

Cardiovascular Disorders

Shirlee Drayton-Brooks, PhD, FNP-BC, APRN-BC

GENERAL APPROACH

- Heart disease and stroke continue to be the leading cause of death in the United States.
- Systolic blood pressure greater than 140 mmHg is a more important risk factor than elevated diastolic blood pressure in persons over 50 years of age.
- Primary and secondary prevention strategies are essential to reduce the risk of heart disease and stroke. Identification of high-risk patients through screening is critical to provide preventive education, early treatment, and appropriate referral.
- Evidence-based national guidelines such as *The Seventh Report of the Joint National Committee on Prevention, Detection, Evaluation, and Treatment of High Blood Pressure* (JNC 7 Express; National Heart, Lung, and Blood Institute, 2003); *The Third Report of the National Cholesterol Education Program Expert Panel on Detection, Evaluation, and Treatment of High Blood Cholesterol in Adults* (National Cholesterol Education Program, 2001); and *Update to ATP III—Implications of Recent Clinical Trials for the National Cholesterol Education Program Adult Treatment Panel III Guidelines* (National Heart, Lung, and Blood Institute, 2004) have been developed to guide treatment decisions.
- Patients should be assessed according to risk stratification and treated to obtain optimal control with individualized drug therapy guided by the patient's clinical profile.
- Problems related to myocardial infarction are one of the four leading causes of malpractice lawsuits.
- The clinician must assess each patient with chest pain and determine whether the condition is life-threatening or safe to manage on an outpatient basis.

- Nonpharmacologic measures are often effective; educate patients to modify lifestyle risk factors.
- Compliance can be a major problem due to health beliefs, cost of medications, side effects, dosing regimens, and difficult lifestyle changes; individualize and simplify treatment and continue to reeducate and support.
- It is important to maintain knowledge of drugs from each class to reduce the potential for medication errors and complications.
- The need for individuals to understand health practices and adhere to therapeutic regimes is critical to reduce health disparities and reduce risk of heart disease.
- Fifty million Americans over 18 years old have metabolic syndrome (American Heart Association, 2008), a constellation of life-threatening health risk factors that increases the likelihood of heart disease, stroke, and death.

Red Flags

- *Chest pain* should be triaged and evaluated promptly to rule out any life-threatening conditions. An immediate brief history will include the age of patient; past medical history focused on cardiac and pulmonary problems; and onset, location, radiation, quality, intensity, and duration of pain. Determine associated symptoms, relieving and aggravating factors, pattern of pain, risk factors for cardiac disease, and family history of hypertension or cardiac disease. Assess vital signs, lung and heart sounds, obtain ECG and pulse oximetry, and integrate assessment findings and risk factors to determine the best management plan. Myocardial infarction (MI) patients may present with severe ischemic pain, which lasts more that 20–30 minutes; is not relieved with nitroglycerin; and may be accompanied by nausea, vomiting, anxiety, diaphoresis, and dyspnea. (MI patients also may have an atypical presentation with pain in arm, jaw, neck, or back without chest pain. Atypical presentation in women includes fatigue without pain.) If acute episode of chest pain, administer oxygen and nitroglycerin, and transport to emergency facility. For non-acute episodes, consult with a physician, refer to cardiologist, or pursue work-up based on history and physical.
- Sudden, spontaneous tachycardia of 140–220 beats per minute is known as *paroxysmal atrial tachycardia* (PAT) and may occur in healthy individuals, older adults, those with chronic obstructive pulmonary disease (COPD), and as a sign of digitalis toxicity. Patient reports that it starts and ends abruptly, lasts minutes to several hours, and may be accompanied by anxiety, dizziness, mild chest pain, and shortness of breath. Rhythm is regular and ECG shows P waves characteristically different than before it started. If asymptomatic and nonrecurrent in healthy individuals, does not need treatment; but if long duration and symptomatic, patient should be referred to emergency department (ED) for treatment. If recurrent, refer to cardiologist.
- Signs and symptoms associated with *pneumothorax* or *pulmonary emboli* include sudden onset of chest pain, hypotension, syncope, dyspnea, tachypnea, and tachycardia. If patient has risk for thrombophlebitis (recent surgery, immobility, oral contraceptive use) or recent fracture, consider pulmonary emboli. Some patients with pulmonary emboli may be asymptomatic. Acute presentation requires transfer to emergency facility.

- Hypertensive patients with sudden onset of knife-like or tearing pain in chest or upper abdomen may have a *dissecting aneurysm*. Initiate emergency transport system immediately.
- Be alert for signs and symptoms of rhabdomyolysis (muscle pain or weakness) that can lead to renal failure when using statin medications and fibric acids.
- Metabolic syndrome, with its constellation of hypertension, diabetes mellitus, hyperlipidemia, and truncal obesity, is associated with increased risk for heart disease and stroke.

Heart Sounds

- Evaluation of heart sounds is an important part of the assessment of any patient with a cardiovascular problem.
- S1 = Closure of the tricuspid and mitral valves; heard best at the 5th left interspace medial to the midclavicular line at the left lower sternal border (LLSB)
- S2 = Closure of the aortic and pulmonary valves; best heard at the second left interspace close to the sternal border
  - Normal splitting of S2 during inspiration is due to greater negative pressure in thoracic cavity = increased systemic venous return = increased blood volume in the right ventricle (RV) = delayed closure of the pulmonary valve
  - Abnormal splitting of S2 (wide splitting, narrow splitting, or single S2) is seen in conditions where the RV ejection time is prolonged (atrial septal defect), the pulmonary valve closes early (pulmonary hypertension), or only one semilunar valve is present (pulmonary atresia, aortic atresia, truncus arteriosus)
- S3 = Low-frequency sound heard early in diastole; related to the rapid filling of the ventricles
  - Heard best at apex or LLSB
  - With tachycardia, forms a "Kentucky" gallop
  - May be normal in children and during pregnancy, except a loud S3 is abnormal (usually audible in conditions with dilated ventricles and decreased compliance)
- S4 = Low-frequency sound heard late in diastole
  - Rare in infants and children
  - Always pathological; seen in conditions with decrease ventricular compliance
  - With tachycardia forms a "Tennessee" gallop
- Gallop = Rapid triple rhythm
  - Results from the combination of a loud S3, with or without S4, and tachycardia

COMMON CARDIOVASCULAR DISORDERS

Hypertension

Description

- Hypertension (HTN) is defined as a persistent elevation of blood pressure measured on three separate occasions with a systolic blood pressure (SBP) >140 mmHg and/or diastolic blood pressure (DBP) >90 (see Table 8–1). It is further classified as either primary (essential, about 95% of cases) or secondary.

- In children, defined as a systolic and/or diastolic blood pressure greater than 95th percentile for gender and age on at least three separate occasions (see Table 8–2).

Etiology
- Hypertension is due to an increase in peripheral arterial resistance.
- Theories of causation include impaired renin-angiotensin cascade, sympathetic nervous system hyperactivity, defect in natriuresis (sodium excretion), and elevated intracellular calcium (excess arterial constriction).
- Essential hypertension is usually idiopathic or may be due to renal retention of salt and water and/or increased endogenous pressure activity. Essential hypertension accounts for the majority of high blood pressure (HBP).
- Secondary hypertension is caused by renovascular disease, vascular problems such as aortic coarctation or renal artery stenosis, endocrine dysfunction such as Cushing syndrome and pheochromocytoma, neurologic disorders, and certain medications (oral contraceptives, corticosteroids, sympathomimetics).

Table 8–1. Classification of Blood Pressure for Adults Aged 18 Years and Older

Blood Pressure in mmHg

Category	Systolic	Diastolic
Normal	<120 and	<80
Prehypertension	120–139 or	80–89
Stage 1 Hypertension	140–159 or	90–99
Stage 2 Hypertension	>160 or	>100

Adapted from "Seventh report of the joint national committee on prevention, detection, evaluation, and treatment of high blood pressure" by A. V. Chobanian, and colleagues, 2003, *Hypertension*, 42(6), pp. 1206–1252.

Table 8–2. Percentile Blood Pressure Readings for Children by Age, Height, and Gender in mmHg

Age (Years)	Girls			Boys		
	5th Percentile	50th Percentile	95th Percentile	5th Percentile	50th Percentile	95th Percentile
1	101/57	104/58	107/60	98/55	102/53	106/59
6	108/71	111/73	114/75	109/72	114/74	117/76
12	120/79	123/80	126/82	119/79	123/81	127/83
17	126/83	129/84	132/86	132/85	136/87	140/89

Adapted from "Hypertension," by V. F. Norwood, 2002, *Pediatrics in Review*, 23(6), pp. 197–208; and "Update on the report of 1987 task force on high blood pressure in children and adolescents," 1996, *Pediatrics*, 79(1), pp. 1–25.

Incidence and Demographics
- In U.S. population: 10%–15% Caucasian, 20%–30% African American
- In pediatric population: 1.2%–13%
- The younger the child and the higher the blood pressure, the more likely to be secondary HTN
- Secondary hypertension generally develops before age 35 or after age 55
- More than ⅓ of patients with hypertension remain undiagnosed even though they may have seen a healthcare provider; at least ⅓ of patients who are diagnosed are not treated to goal BP

Risk Factors
- Major risk factors:
  - >60 years of age; men and postmenopausal women
  - Family history of cardiovascular disease in women under age 65 or men under age 55
  - Hyperlipidemia, diabetes mellitus (DM), smoking
- Other risk factors: Obesity, stress, excessive intake of sodium, high alcohol intake, pregnancy, renal disease, African-American descent, coronary artery disease, left ventricular hypertrophy, cerebrovascular disease, sleep apnea, some medications (oral contraceptives, corticosteroids, NSAIDs, sympathomimetics)

Prevention and Screening
- Patient education for prevention of risk factors (see Box 8–1)
- Blood pressure screening and monitoring using proper technique and equipment (see Table 8–4)

Assessment
HISTORY
- Usually asymptomatic in essential HTN, "silent killer"
- May be occipital headaches upon awakening with severe HTN, dizziness, rarely epistaxis
- Somnolence, confusion, visual disturbances, nausea, vomiting (hypertensive encephalopathy)
- Personal history for risk factors; family history for hypertension
- Past medical history for comorbid conditions such as gout or sexual dysfunction, or effects on target organs

PHYSICAL EXAM
- Elevated blood pressure (usually only sign)
- Body mass index (BMI) may be over 30; children may be obese, or thin with failure to thrive
- Abdominal obesity: Waist circumference >40 inches in men and >35 inches in women

- S4 gallop, possible displaced point of maximal intensity (PMI) due to ventricular hypertrophy
- Renal artery bruit, carotid bruit, hepatosplenomegaly, edema, decreased peripheral pulses, funduscopic changes (AV nicking, etc.) with secondary HTN; or target organ damage—angina/MI, transient ischemic attack (TIA), stroke, peripheral arterial disease

DIAGNOSTIC STUDIES
- Laboratory tests: Urinalysis, urine microalbumin, CBC, blood urea nitrogen, creatinine, calcium, uric acid, lipid profile, serum electrolytes, glucose
- For secondary HTN: Chest x-ray; echocardiogram; renal ultrasound; intravenous pyelogram (IVP); 24-hour urine for aldosterone, free cortisol, catecholamines, and creatinine; dexamethasone challenge test; thyroid profile; renal function tests (BUN/CR); screening panels for various endocrine disorders (thyroid-stimulating hormone [TSH], urine catecholamines, and vanillylmandelic acid [VMA])

Differential Diagnosis
Essential vs. secondary causes of hypertension:
- Pregnancy
- Renal artery stenosis
- Renal failure
- Renal parenchymal disease (polycystic or dysplastic kidneys)
- Coarctation of aorta
- Patent ductus arteriosus
- Aortic insufficiency
- Pheochromocytoma
- Cushing's disease
- Hyperaldosteronism
- Hyperthyroidism
- Neuroblastoma
- Increased intracranial pressure
- Hypervolemia
- Bronchopulmonary dysplasia
- Stevens-Johnson syndrome

Management

NONPHARMACOLOGIC TREATMENT

- Lifestyle modification as in Box 8–1; avoidance of oral contraceptives in at-risk individuals
- Use DASH Diet: Dietary Approaches to Stop Hypertension
- Monitor for target organ damage (TOD); target blood pressure according to risk group

Box 8-1. Lifestyle Modifications for Prevention and Management of Hypertension

Smoking cessation

Lose weight if overweight, and reduce intake of dietary saturated fat and cholesterol

Limit alcohol intake to no more than 1 oz (30 mL) ethanol (e.g., 24 oz [720 mL] beer, 10 oz [300 mL] wine, or 2 oz [60 mL] 100-proof whiskey) per day; 0.5 oz (15 mL) ethanol per day for women and lighter-weight people

Increase aerobic physical activity (30–45 minutes most days of the week)

Reduce sodium intake to no more than 100 mmol per day (2.4 g sodium, 6g sodium chloride, or 1 teaspoon of salt)

Maintain adequate intake of dietary potassium (approximately 90 mmol or 2 g per day), calcium (approximately 1000 mg , and 300mg magnesium daily

Adapted from "Seventh report of the Joint National Committee on Prevention, Detection, Evaluation, and Treatment of High Blood Pressure" by A. V. Chobanian, and colleagues, 2003, *Hypertension*, 42(6), pp. 1206–1252.

Table 8-3. Treatment for Hypertension

BP Classification	Without Compelling Indication	With Compelling Indication
Prehypertension 130–139/85–89	Lifestyle modification	Drugs for compelling indication
Stage 1 140–159/90–99	Diuretic for most; may consider ACEI, ARB, BB, CCB,* or combination	Drug(s) for the compelling indications; other antihypertensive drugs (diuretics, ACEI, ARB, BB, CCB as needed)
Stage 2 160+/100+	Two-drug combination for most (usually diuretic and ACEI, ARB, BB, or CCB)	

*ACEI = ACE inhibitor, ARB = angiotensin II receptor blockers, BB = beta blocker, CCB = calcium channel blocker.
Adapted from "Seventh report of the Joint National Committee on Prevention, Detection, Evaluation, and Treatment of High Blood Pressure" by A. V. Chobanian, and colleagues, 2003, *Hypertension*, 42(6), pp. 1206–1252.

Figure 8-1. Algorithm for the Treatment of Hypertension in Adults

Begin or Continue Lifestyle Modifications

Not at Goal Blood Pressure (<140/90 mmHg)
Lower goals for patients with diabetes or renal disease

Initial Drug Choices
Start with a low dose of a long-acting, once-daily drug, and titrate dose
Low-dose combinations may be appropriate

Uncomplicated Hypertension	Compelling Indications

• Diuretics
• Beta blockers
Specific Indications for Specific Drugs
• ACE inhibitors
• Angiotensin II receptor blockers
• Alpha blockers
• Alpha-beta blockers
• Calcium antagonists
	Diabetes mellitus (type 1) with proteinuria
	  • ACE inhibitors
	Heart failure
	  • ACE inhibitors
	  • Diuretics
	Isolated systolic hypertension in elderly
	  • Diuretics preferred
	  • Long-acting dihydropyridine calcium antagonists
	Myocardial infarction
	  • Beta blockers (non-ISA)
	  • ACE inhibitors (with systolic dysfunction)

Not at Goal Blood Pressure
No response or troublesome side effects
Inadequate response but well-tolerated

Substitute another drug from a different class
Add a second agent from a different class (diuretic if not already used)

Not at Goal Blood Pressure

Continue adding agents from other classes
Consider referral to a hypertension specialist

Adapted from *Sixth report of the Joint National Committee on Prevention, Detection, Evaluation, and Treatment of High Blood Pressure (JNC 6)* (NIH Publication No. 5233), by the National Heart, Lung, and Blood Institute, 1997, Bethesda, MD: National Institutes of Health, p. 32.

PHARMACOLOGIC TREATMENT
- See Tables 8–3 and 8–5 and Figure 8–1
- Compelling indications for treating with medications
  - Heart failure
  - Post–myocardial infarction
  - High coronary disease risk
  - Recurrent stroke prevention
- Children (refer for treatment)
  - Antihypertensive therapy is indicated for HTN treatment in children when the following reasons apply
    » Family history of early complications of hypertension
    » Presence of coronary artery risk factors
    » Dangerously high blood pressure (>12 mmHg over the 99th percentile diastolic or >25 mmHg over the 99th percentile systolic) or presence of end-organ damage (ocular, central nervous system [CNS], cardiac, or renal)
  - Medical management is begun with a single-drug regimen in combination with nonpharmacologic measures; additional drug therapies are initiated as needed
  - Diuretics (contraindicated in patients with renal failure)
    » Furosemide (Lasix): 1–8 mg/kg/day divided q 4–12 h
    » Spironolactone (Aldactone): 1–3 mg/kg/day divided q 6–12 h
    » Hydrochlorothiazide (HCTZ): 1–3 mg/kg/day divided q 12 h
  - Vasodilators (use with adrenergic inhibitor to decrease flushing, headache, tachycardia, salt retention)
    » Hydralazine (Apresoline): 0.75–7.5 mg/kg/day divided q6h
  - Angiotensin-converting enzyme (ACE) inhibitors (should be used with diuretics to enhance effectiveness; avoid in patients with bilateral renal artery stenosis or transplanted kidney)
    » Captopril (Catapres): 1–3 mg/kg/day divided q 8–24 h
    » Enalapril (Vasotec): 0.1–0.5 mg/kg/day divided q 12–24 h
  - Calcium antagonists have limited use in the pediatric population
    » Nifedipine (Procardia): 0.25–3 mg/kg/day divided q 4–6 h
  - Adrenergic inhibitors (propanolol is contraindicated in patients with asthma)
    » Propranolol (Inderal): 1–8 mg/kg/day divided q 6–12 h
    » Atenolol (Tenormin): 1–8 mg/kg/day divided q 12–24 h
- Adults
  - Diuretics: First-line therapy; avoid with history of gout, DM, dyslipidemia
    » Target groups: Congestive heart failure (CHF), osteoporosis, older patients, African Americans, smokers
  - Beta blockers: First-line therapy; avoid with asthma, older Caucasians, conduction disorders, bradycardia
    » Target groups: Young Whites, post-MI, angina, migraine, arrhythmias, tremor, hyperthyroid, preoperative; with CHF use carvedilol (Coreg); with liver disease use labetalol (Labetalol); use with caution in diabetes mellitus, depression

– ACE inhibitors
» Target groups: DM, CHF, post-MI, Whites
» Avoid use in African-American patients, renal stenosis, elevated creatinine
– Angiotensin II receptor blockers (ARB); avoid in renovascular disease)
» Target groups: Identical to ACE with inability to tolerate ACE due to cough
– Calcium channel blockers (CCB); contraindicated in conduction disorders
» Target groups: Angina, coronary artery disease (CAD), African Americans, migraine, isolated systolic HTN in elderly, arrhythmia (nondihydropyridine CCB)
» Avoid grapefruit, cimetidine, ranitidine
» Avoid beta blocker and calcium channel blocker combined (nondihydropyridine)
» Short-acting nifedipine increases cardiac morbidity
– Alpha I adrenergic blockers: Second-line therapy
» Target groups: Benign prostatic hypertrophy, dyslipidemia
» First-dose syncope: Administer q hs; combination with NSAID may decrease effectiveness
– Central alpha 2 agonists; may cause rebound hypertension on withdrawal
» Target groups; monotherapy failure
– Peripheral alpha 2 agonists; limited use

LENGTH OF TREATMENT
• Usually lifelong

Table 8-4. Screening Tests for Causes of Hypertension

Suspected Hypertension Cause	Test
Chronic kidney disease	Estimated glomerular filtration rate (GFR)
Coarctation of the aorta	CT angiography
Cushing syndrome and other glucocorticoid	History; dexamethasone suppression test, excess states including chronic steroid therapy
Drug-induced or drug-related	History, drug screening
Pheochromocytoma	24-hour urinary metanephrine and normetanephrine
Primary aldosteronism and other mineralocorticoid	24-hour urinary aldosterone level or excess states—specific measurements of other mineralocorticoids
Renovascular hypertension	Doppler flow study; magnetic resonance angiography
Sleep apnea	Sleep study with O_2 saturation
Thyroid/parathyroid disease	TSH; serum parathyroid hormone (PTH)

From *Sixth report of the Joint National Committee on Prevention, Detection, Evaluation, and Treatment of High Blood Pressure (JNC 6)* (NIH Publication No. 5233), by the National Heart, Lung, and Blood Institute, 1997, Bethesda, MD: National Institutes of Health.

Table 8-5. Examples of Recommended Drug Therapy for Adults with Hypertension

Drug	Total Daily Dosage	Side Effects
Diuretics Hydrochlorothiazide (HCTZ) Furosemide (Lasix)	12.5–25 mg (once/day) 20–80 mg (2–3x/day)	Anorexia, nausea, vomiting, cramping due to potassium and possibly sodium depletion; increased glucose, uric acid levels
Beta-Adrenergic Blockers Metoprolol (Lopressor) Atenolol (Tenormin)	50–300 mg (1–2x/day) 25–100 mg (1–2x/day)	Bradycardia, depression, fatigue, exercise intolerance, asthma
ACE Inhibitors Lisinopril (Prinivil, Zestril) Captopril (Capoten)	10–40 mg (1–2x/day) 25–150 mg (2–3x/day)	15% have cough, hyperkalemia, ankle swelling, angioedema, leukopenia
Angiotensin Receptor Blockers Losartan (Cozaar) Valsartan (Diovan)	25–100 mg (1–2x/day) 80–320 mg (once/day)	Rare side effects (angioedema, hyperkalemia)
Calcium Channel Blockers Amlodipine (Norvasc) Verapamil (Calan)	2.5–10 mg (once/day) 120–480 mg (1-2x/day)	Peripheral edema, nausea, headache, constipation
Alpha 1 Adrenergic Blockers Prazosin (Minipress) Doxazosin (Cardura)	2–30 mg (2–3x/day) 1–16 mg (once/day)	Dizziness, headache, fatigue, impotence, postural hypotension
Central Alpha 2 Agonists Clonidine (Catapres)	0.2-1.2 mg (2–3x/day)	Dry mouth, syncope, drowsiness, constipation
Peripheral Agents Reserpine	0.05–0.25 mg(1x/day)	Depression, impotence

Special Considerations
- Start with low doses for geriatric patients to avoid serious side effects.
- Pregnancy: Can continue drug used before pregnancy, except ACE inhibitors and ARBs; beta blockers may cause growth retardation in early pregnancy; if HTN develops during pregnancy, use methyldopa (Aldomet) 500 mg to 3 gm qd in divided doses (see Table 8–6).

When to Consult, Refer, Hospitalize
- Consult with physician or specialist when initiating drug treatment for a child with HTN.
- Refer as needed for evaluation and treatment of secondary causes of hypertension.
- Refer to a specialist (nephrologist, cardiologist, ophthalmologist) for end-organ damage.
- Consult physician when no response to first-line therapy, escalating HTN, or HTN emergencies (hypertensive encephalopathy, severe preeclampsia/eclampsia, cerebral hemorrhage, dissecting aortic aneurysm, unstable angina, MI, pulmonary embolism, severe heart failure); hospitalization may be necessary.

Table 8–6. Treatment of Chronic Hypertension in Pregnancy

Drug	Safety Indications
Methyldopa	Preferred based on long-term follow-up studies supporting safety
BBs	Reports of intrauterine growth retardation (atenolol) Generally safe
Labetalol	Increasingly preferred to methyldopa due to reduced side effects
Clonidine	Limited data
Calcium antagonists	Limited data No increase in major teratogenicity with exposure
Diuretics	Not first-line agents Probably safe
ACEIs, angiotensin II receptor antagonists	Contraindicated Reported fetal toxicity and death

ACEIs = angiotensin converting enzyme inhibitors; BBs = beta blockers
From *Sixth report of the Joint National Committee on Prevention, Detection, Evaluation, and Treatment of High Blood Pressure (JNC 6)* (NIH Publication No. 5233), by the National Heart, Lung, and Blood Institute, 1997, Bethesda, MD: National Institutes of Health.

Follow-Up
- Frequent initial follow up until normotensive; then routine visits every 3–6 months depending on patient clinical situation; BP >180 systolic or 110 diastolic, follow up in 48–72 hours.
- Improve adherence by keeping treatment simple and inexpensive, educate patient and family about hypertension, encourage lifestyle modification along with drug treatment.
  EXPECTED COURSE
  - Usually requires lifelong treatment; progression depends on ability to control the disease

  COMPLICATIONS
  - Target organ damage includes stroke, coronary heart disease, left ventricular hypertrophy, congestive heart failure, kidney failure, aortic dissection, retinopathy

Dyslipidemia

Description
- General term used to describe a variety of lipid abnormalities including low-density lipoproteins (LDL), high-density lipoproteins (HDL), and triglycerides (TGL) that deviate from normal ranges and increase the risk of cardiovascular disease. Elevation in blood lipids is often due to abnormal lipid metabolism (see Tables 8–7 and 8–8).

Table 8-7. Classification of Lipoproteins

Low-Density Lipoprotein Cholesterol (mg/dL)	
<100	Optimal
100–129	Near optimal/above optimal
130–159	Borderline high
160–189	High
>190	Very high
Total Cholesterol (mg/dL)	
<200	Desirable
200–239	Borderline high
>240	High
High-Density Lipoprotein Cholesterol (mg/dL)	
<40	Low
>60	High
Triglycerides (mg/dL)	
>150	Increased CHD risk

Adapted from *Third report of the Expert Panel on Detection, Evaluation, and Treatment of High Blood Cholesterol in Adults* (Adult Treatment Panel III) (NIH Pub. No, 01-3670) by the National Cholesterol Education Program, 2001, Bethesda, MD: Author.

Table 8-8. Normal Cholesterol and Triglyceride Levels in Children

Age	Cholesterol	LDL	HDL	Triglycerides
0–4 years M	117–209	—	—	30–102
F	115–206	—	—	35–115
5–9 years M	125–209	65–133	39–76	31–104
F	130–211	70–144	37–75	33–108
10–14 years M	123–208	66–136	38–76	33–129
F	128–207	70–140	38–72	38–135
15–19 years M	116–188	64–134	31–65	38–152
F	124–209	61–141	36–76	40–136

Adapted from *Pediatric cardiology for practitioners* (4th ed.) by M. Park, 2002, St. Louis, MO: Mosby.

Etiology
- Hyperlipidemias (also called dyslipidemia) are either primary (some genetic forms) or secondary (related to fat, calorie, and alcohol intake; medication use; or caused by metabolic diseases such as hypothyroidism, diabetes mellitus, liver disease, obesity, and nephrosis).
- Familial or genetic syndromes include familial hypercholesterolemia, polygenic hypercholesterolemia, familial defective apolipoprotein B-100, familial hypertriglyceridemia, familial combined hyperlipidemia, familial hyperchylomicronemia with marked increase in triglycerides.
- Total cholesterol is influenced by four major classes of lipoproteins: chylomicrons, very low-density lipoproteins (VLDL), LDL, and HDL.
- HDL carries fat away from blood vessels and prevents or delays atherosclerosis.

- LDL facilitates forming of cholesterol deposits in the blood vessels.
- Isolated elevated LDL may be seen in familial hypercholesterolemia (FH).
- Other causes: Thyroid disease, Cushing's disease, hepatic disease, malignancy, pancreatitis.

Incidence and Demographics
- 105 million people have high total cholesterol ($\geq$200 mg/dL).
- Familial combined hyperlipidemia: 1/300 persons.
- Familial hypercholesterolemia: 1/500 persons.
- The prevalence of cholesterol screening during the preceding 5 years increased from 67.3% in 1991 to 70.8% in 1999.

Risk Factors
- Obesity, high saturated fat diet, sedentary lifestyle, cigarette smoking, excess alcohol use
- More common in males
- Elevated plasma fibrinogen, elevated homocysteine
- Lipoprotein (a): Predictor of premature atherosclerosis
- Syndrome X: Metabolic syndrome that can involve glucose intolerance, central obesity, hyperlipidemia, and hypertension; at high risk for coronary artery disease
- Low HDL is a major risk factor for CAD; high HDL (>60) is protective

Prevention and Screening
- Screen for above risk factors
- Interventions for smoking cessation, hypertension, weight management, increasing physical activity, and lipid management
- Treat comorbid conditions
- Measure blood pressure in all adults at least every 2.5 years
- Assess dietary intake with routine evaluations
- Measure lipid profile in adults 20 years of age and older at least every 5 years
- Promote American Heart Association diet for all persons

Assessment
HISTORY
- Obtain history for other CHD risk factors, family history of hyperlipidemia, dietary and alcohol intake, exercise
- Rarely produces symptoms unless there are symptoms of related diseases, reactions to medications
- Symptoms predisposing disease: Weight gain, cold intolerance, constipation, edema, central obesity, purple striae, fat wasting, hepatomegaly, xanthomas, corneal arcus, ear lobe crease, plaques on funduscopic exam, poor wound healing, recurring rashes/pruritus, hypertension
- Medications such as thiazide diuretics, treatment for acute pancreatitis, hepatitis, renal disease

PHYSICAL EXAM
- Xanthomas: In familial hypercholesterolemia; papules, plaques, or nodules in the tendons, eyelids, buttocks, knees, and skin folds
- Corneal arcus prior to age 50–60 years, young Whites

- Milky white serum (hypertriglyceridemia)
- Obesity

DIAGNOSTIC STUDIES
- Fasting fractionated lipid profile to include total cholesterol, triglycerides, HDL, LDL, VLDL, apolipoprotein
- Comprehensive metabolic panel to detect other metabolic abnormalities
- Urinalysis to detect kidney disease
- Thyroid screening: TSH, FT4
- Liver function tests to rule out liver disease and prior to starting medication
- Baseline ECG

Differential Diagnosis

Primary versus secondary causes:
- Nephrotic syndrome
- Chronic renal failure
- Diabetes mellitus
- Hypothyroidism
- Cushing's syndrome
- Chronic liver disease
- Excessive alcohol intake
- Pancreatitis
- Obesity
- Hyperuricemia
- Medications
- Pregnancy

Management

NONPHARMACOLOGIC TREATMENT
- Lifestyle modifications: Smoking cessation, increased physical activity, moderation of alcohol intake, increased use of soy products, diet changes
- LDL is the primary indicator for treatment
- All patients with hyperlipidemia should be started on American Heart Association (AHA) Step 2 diet; AHA recommends a well-balanced diet of lean meat, poultry, fish, vegetables, fruits, breads, and low-fat dairy products and limiting eggs, fat, sweets, and high-fat desserts for all adults
  - Step 1 diet reduces serum cholesterol by 3%–14% (maintenance for general public)
  - Step 2 diet confers additional 3%–7% benefit compared Step 1 (therapeutic for lipid-lowering)
- Guidelines from the National Cholesterol Education Program known as Adult Treatment Panel (ATP) III recommend daily intake of less than 7% of calories from saturated fat, less than 35% of calories from total fat provided most is from unsaturated fat, less than 200 mg of dietary cholesterol; use of foods rich in soluble fiber; weight control; and physical activity that improves HDL
- See Table 8–9 for LDL goals and initiation of treatment
- If 3–6 months of diet therapy not effective in reaching LDL goal, start medications
  - Saturated fat <10% of total calories
  - Total fat <30% of total calories

- Dietary cholesterol <300 mg/day
- Carbohydrates approximately 55% of calories
- Protein 15%–20% of calories
- Increase dietary fiber: Oatmeal, oat bran, raw fruits and vegetables
- Exercise; weight loss in overweight patients

Table 8-9. LDL Goals and Initiation of Treatment

Risk Category	LDL Goal	Level To Start TLC**	Level To Consider Drug Therapy
CHD or CHD risk equivalents* (10-year risk >20%)	<100 mg/dL	>100 mg/dL	>130 mg/dL 100–129: Consider initiating therapy, treat other risk factors, or use nicotinic acid or fibrate if high TG or low HDL
2+ risk factors (10-year risk 10%–20%)	<130 mg/dL	>130 mg/dL	>130 mg/dL
2+ risk factors (10-year risk <10%)	<130 mg/dL	>130 mg/dL	>160 mg/dL
0–1 risk factor (10-year risk assessment not necessary)	<160 mg/dL	>160 mg/dL	>190 mg/dL 160–189 mg/dL: Drug therapy optional; consider if single severe risk factor, multiple life-habit or emerging risk factors, or 10-year risk nearly 10%

*CHD risk equivalents: Clinical CHD, symptomatic carotid artery disease, peripheral arterial disease, abdominal aortic aneurysm
**TLC: Therapeutic lifestyle change
†10-year risk based on clinical conditions such as diabetes, multiple risk factors, age, sex, total cholesterol, HDL, blood pressure and its treatment

Adapted from *Third report of the Expert Panel on Detection, Evaluation, and Treatment of High Blood Cholesterol in Adults* (Adult Treatment Panel III) (NIH Pub. No, 01-3670) by the National Cholesterol Education Program, 2001, Bethesda, MD: Author.

PHARMACOLOGIC TREATMENT (SEE TABLE 8-10)
- HMG CoA reductase inhibitors ("statins"):
  - Drug of choice for all patients with diagnosed CAD
  - Lowers LDL; increases HDL
  - Evening dosing
  - Atorvastatin (Lipitor), lovastatin (Mevacor), simvastatin (Zocor): Metabolized by cytochrome P-450 (CYP)3A4

- Drug/food interactions: Cyclosporine, erythromycin, itraconazole, ketoconazole, fibric acid, diltiazem, verapamil, fluoxetine, nefazodone
- Contraindicated in liver disease, pregnancy, lactation
- Rhabdomyolysis may develop if fibrate used in patient with renal dysfunction
- Monitor liver function tests
- Bile acid sequestrants:
  - May safely be used in combination with other lipid-lowering medications
  - Used to lower LDL
  - Use with caution if triglycerides >300 (may increase triglycerides 20%–30%)
  - Interference with other drugs (1 hr before med or 4 hrs after) and fat-soluble vitamins
  - Side effects: Constipation, flatulence, nausea
  - Cholestyramine (Questran) maintenance dose 2–4 packs a day
  - Colestipol (Colestid) maintenance dose 5 g given qd or bid
- Nicotinic acid:
  - Lowers total cholesterol and triglycerides, increases HDL
  - Caution in DM and gout; monitor liver toxicity
  - Liver function tests, blood glucose, uric acid prior to initiation
  - Low dose, titrate slowly to avoid flushing, pretreat with aspirin ½ hr prior to dose
  - Initiate 500 mg qd, increase by 500 mg q 4 weeks
  - Side effects: flushing, hypotension, nausea
- Fibric acids:
  - Lower triglycerides, increase HDL
  - Rhabdomyolysis and renal failure may develop in patients also using statins
  - Monitor liver function tests
  - Generally well-tolerated
  - Side effects: Dizziness, dyspepsia, diarrhea, blurred vision
  - Gemfibrozil (Lopid) bid dosing
- Children: Drug therapy recommended for children 10 years old and older after an adequate diet trial of 6 months
- Criteria for treatment:
  - LDL remains >190 mg/100 mL
  - LDL remains >160 mg/100 mL and a positive family history of coronary artery disease and two or more cardiovascular disease risk factors
  - Only bile acid sequestrants (cholestyramine or colestipol) are recommended (see Table 8–11)

Table 8-10. Recommended Drug Therapy for Hyperlipidemia

Drug	Daily Dosage Range	Class
Atorvastatin (Lipitor)	10–80 mg	HMG CoA
Fluvastatin (Lescol)	20–80 mg	HMG CoA
Lovastatin (Mevacor)	20–80 mg	HMG CoA
Pravastatin (Pravachol)	10–40 mg	HMG CoA
Simvastatin (Zocor)	5–80 mg	HMG CoA
Cholestyramine (Questran)	8–24 g	Bile acid sequestrant
Colestipol (Colestid)	5–30 g	Bile acid sequestrant
Gemfibrozil (Lopid)	1200 mg	Fibrate
Fenofibrate (Tricor)	67 mg–200 mg	Fibrate
Niacin	1.5–3.0 g	Nicotinic acid
Nicotinic Acid (Niaspan)	1–3.0 g	Niacin extended release

Table 8-11. Recommended Bile Acid Sequestrant Therapy for Children with Hyperlipidemia

Daily Doses of Cholestryamine	TC and LDL Levels (mg/100mL)
1	TC <245, LDL <195
2	TC 245–30, LDL 195–235
3	TC 301–345, LDL 236–280
4	TC 345

(1 dose = 9-gram packet of cholestyramine or 5-gram packet of colestipol)

Adapted from *Pediatric cardiology for practitioners* (4th ed.) by M. Park, 2002, St. Louis, MO: Mosby.

LENGTH OF TREATMENT
• Usually lifelong

Special Considerations
• Females using conjugated estrogens reduces LDL approximately 15% and increases HDL approximately 15%; use as adjunct, not as replacement to cholesterol-lowering agents
• Total cholesterol and LDL levels are not measured before 2 years old and no treatment is recommended before that age
• Pregnancy and lactation: Levels are normally elevated, usually do not test
• Elderly: Treatment is controversial, insufficient studies

When to Consult, Refer, Hospitalize
• Refer all pediatric and adult patients who are not controlled with therapy to a cardiologist and endocrinologist
• Refer if pregnant, comorbid conditions
• Refer to dietitian, especially if poor dietary compliance
• Immediate treatment for triglycerides >1,000; may need to be hospitalized

Follow-Up
- Every 1–2 years with lipid profile for patients not requiring drug therapy
- Visits for patients requiring drug therapy should include tolerance to medication (myalgias), diet assessment, compliance with exercise routine, 24-hour recall of diet, and appropriate lab tests
- Inquire about new medications; many medications affect lipid parameters
- Monitor lipids and liver function test every 6 weeks on drug therapy until goal reached
- Visits every 4–8 weeks initially, until lipid control achieved, then every 6 months; with comorbid conditions, every 3–4 months
    EXPECTED COURSE
    - Dependent on etiology, CAD
    - 1% decrease in cholesterol will decrease risk of CAD by 2%

    COMPLICATIONS
    - CAD progression, stroke
    - Peripheral vascular disease
    - Rhabdomyolysis, liver dysfunction secondary to drug treatment
    - Pancreatitis (with triglycerides over 1,000)

Coronary Artery Disease (CAD)/Ischemic Heart Disease (IHD) Angina Pectoris

Description
- Coronary artery disease may develop over years as a result of atherosclerotic lesions that decrease the arterial lumen. Over time, blood flow may be reduced to the heart, producing cardiac ischemic disease.
- Angina is a clinical manifestation of ischemic heart disease when blood flow to an artery is compromised sufficiently to decrease myocardial oxygen and produce subsequent chest discomfort (angina).
    - Classic: Substernal pressure or heaviness associated with exertion or anxiety, resolving with rest
    - Women under 50 with angina frequently awaken from sleep with chest pain
    - Types include:
        - Stable: Pain duration less than 15 minutes; no change in frequency, severity, or duration of anginal symptoms during the preceding 6 weeks
        - Unstable: Recent change in characteristic angina symptoms and may occur at rest
        - Variant (Prinzmetal): Transient ST-segment elevation, at rest, with angina symptoms related to coronary spasm usually involving right coronary artery

Etiology
- Plaques formed on the intimal lining of artery are composed of lipoproteins, cellular components, and extracellular matrix molecules. These cause the inner lining of the blood vessels to thicken and the blood vessels to lose elasticity.
- Atherosclerosis first appears as a fatty streak, which progresses for about 30 years.
- Foam cells form and plaque begins to form, then develops into multilayered plaque with stabilizing fibrous cap.

- As early as the fourth decade the plaque becomes unstable and the foam cells necrose and rupture underneath the fibrous cap.
- With progression, the fibrous cap tears and bleeds to produce a thrombus, which occludes the blood vessel either completely or partially and causes decreased blood flow and ischemia or necrosis (myocardial infarction).
- The process of atherosclerosis is accelerated by HTN, DM, hyperlipidemia, genetics, coronary artery vasospasm, aortic stenosis, and aortic insufficiency.

Incidence and Demographics
- Male prevalence through majority of life span until women reach menopause, where occurrence rises; equal gender incidence after age 70.
- Highest incidence occurring fifth through seventh decade.

Risk Factors
- Male, HTN, hyperlipidemia, DM, tobacco use, familial history of premature cardiac death (prior to age 55); menopausal women without estrogen replacement
- Cocaine
- Advancing age
- Obesity

Prevention and Screening
- Modifiable lifestyle changes associated with coronary risk factors
- Treatment comorbid conditions: CAD, HTN, DM, hyperlipidemia
- Low-fat and low-sodium diet
- Regular aerobic exercise
- Avoid excessive alcohol intake; smoking cessation

Assessment
HISTORY
- Classic presentation of substernal pressure or heaviness associated with exertion or anxiety and relieved with rest or nitroglycerin
- Each patient has typical pattern: subjective description of tightness, squeezing, burning, pressure, heaviness
- A change in the patient's typical pattern is indicative of unstable angina

PHYSICAL EXAM
- Vital signs: Elevation in BP, pulse, and respirations
- Holosystolic murmur may be present
- Transient S3 or S4
- Mitral valve prolapse, intermitted claudication may be present
- Sparse hair growth on distal extremities with associated peripheral vascular disease

DIAGNOSTIC STUDIES
- ECG at the time of the pain may show changes; between episodes, ECG may be normal
- ECG normal in 25%–50% patients during angina episode; may find evidence of prior MI (Q waves)

- ECG unreliable in patients with bundle branch block, Wolf-Parkinson-White syndrome
- Chest x-ray: Assess heart size, look for pulmonary edema, pleural effusions, and aortic aneurysm
- Exercise stress test: S-T segment depression (less accurate in women)
- Exercise thallium imaging: Hypoperfusion found in areas with diminished uptake
- Used for clarification with ECG abnormalities, often in women, digoxin and beta blocker usage
- CBC, electrolytes, cardiac enzymes, pulse oximetry as indicated
- Radionuclide ventriculography: Left ventricle imaging to differentiate infarction from ischemia
- Technetium: Tagged RBC, highly sensitive for CAD (nonspecific)
- Coronary angiography: Definitive for diagnosis of CAD
- Rapid sequence MRI: Calcified coronary arteries (not sensitive to coronary lesions)
- CT scan not recommended

Differential Diagnosis

CARDIAC
- Pericarditis
- Aortic dissection
- MI
- CHF

GASTROINTESTINAL
- Gastroesophageal reflux (GERD)
- Cholecystitis
- Esophageal spasm
- Peptic ulcer

RESPIRATORY
- Costochondral pain
- Pneumothorax
- Pneumonia
- Pleurisy
- Asthma
- Pulmonary emboli

MUSCULOSKELETAL
- Chest wall syndrome
- Shoulder arthropathy

PSYCHOLOGICAL
- Anxiety
- Panic disorders
- Depression

Management

NONPHARMACOLOGIC TREATMENT

- Modification of risk factors: Weight, smoking, stress, aerobic activity, diet low in saturated fat and sodium
- Cardiac rehabilitation as indicated

PHARMACOLOGIC TREATMENT

- Optimal management of comorbid conditions: Hyperlipidemia, diabetes, CHF, hypertension, arrhythmias
- New guidelines suggest treatment in patients with symptomatic chronic stable angina to prevent MI or death and to reduce symptoms
    - Aspirin or clopidogrel when aspirin is absolutely contraindicated
    - Beta blockers
    - Low-density lipoprotein (LDL) cholesterol-lowering therapy with a statin
    - Angiotensin-converting enzyme (ACE) inhibitor
- Agents that should be used in patients with symptomatic chronic stable angina to reduce symptoms only are sublingual nitroglycerin or nitroglycerin spray for immediate relief of angina
- Calcium antagonists (long-acting) or long-acting nitrates when beta blockers are clearly contraindicated
- Calcium antagonists (long-acting) or long-acting nitrates combined with beta blockers when beta blockers alone are unsuccessful

DRUG-SPECIFIC

- Nitroglycerin: 0.3 to 0.6 mg SL 5 minutes before any activity likely to produce angina
- Nitrates (long-acting): Used to promote coronary vasodilatation
    - Patient education regarding storage and use of nitroglycerin so it will remain effective, when and how to take it, when to go for medical help
    - Monitor for hypotension with nitroglycerin use
    - Drug tolerance develops rapidly in patients taking nitroglycerin; patient should have a planned drug-free interval of 10–14 hours on a scheduled basis
    - Isosorbide dinitrate: 5–40 mg tid
    - Isosorbide mononitrate: 10–40 mg po bid or sustained release 60–120 mg qd
    - Nitro-Dur skin patch 0.2–0.8 mg/hr, on for 12 hours then off for 12 hours
- Aspirin: 81–325 mg qd
- Hyperlipidemic medication: Lower LDL to 100 or lower; see section on hyperlipidemia above
- Beta blockers: Decrease heart rate, contractility, and oxygen requirements
    - Monitor bradycardia, fatigue, depression, CHF, asthma
    - Metoprolol (Lopressor) 25–200 mg bid, atenolol (Tenormin) 25–200 mg qd
- Calcium channel blockers: Coronary vasodilatation with reduction myocardial oxygen
    - Best drug for vasospasm
    - Monitor headache, pedal edema, constipation
    - Avoid verapamil and diltiazem in patients with arrhythmias

      – Coronary spasm: Nifedipine XL (Procardia) 30–120 mg qd; verapamil (Calan) 120–320 mg qd; diltiazem (Cardizem) 120–480 mg qd
      – Avoid short-acting calcium channel blockers

LENGTH OF TREATMENT
- Depends on etiology
- Often until revascularization

Special Considerations
- Women often have atypical symptoms and limited interpretation of diagnostic tests
- Geriatric patients: Low therapeutic doses to avoid side effects, monitor closely
- Pregnancy: Exclude other diagnoses, cardiologist to follow

When to Consult, Refer, Hospitalize
- Consult with a physician for new and uncontrolled cases
- Refer to cardiologist for invasive procedures; coronary revascularization, intolerable symptoms and medication failure, stenosis of left main artery >50% with or without angina, left ventricular dysfunction and three vessel damage, unstable angina with ischemia on exercise stress test, post infarction continuing angina or ischemia
- Transfer to nearest ED and hospitalize for acute angina unrelieved with pharmacologic therapy; crush 325 mg aspirin and swallow en route to medical facility

Follow-Up
- Individualize follow-up dependent on symptoms and condition; minimum every 3 months
- Patient education regarding storage and use of nitroglycerin so it will remain effective, when and how to take it, when to go for medical help
  ### COMPLICATIONS
  - MI, cardiac arrest, CHF, death

Myocardial Infarction

Description
- Myocardial tissue death (necrosis); results from myocardial oxygen demand severely compromised by thrombus formation leading to subsequent reduction in coronary blood flow with total coronary occlusion (Q-wave transmural infarction) or nonocclusion (Non–Q-wave nontransmural infarction—patent but highly narrowed artery)

Etiology
- CAD: Coronary thrombosis secondary to ruptured atherosclerotic plaque
- Coronary spasm

Incidence and Demographics
- Global incidence with mortality 30%–40%
- Male preponderance fourth through sixth decade, equal by age 70

Risk Factors
- See CAD risk factors above

Prevention and Screening

- 81 mg aspirin a day
- Evaluate the presence and control status of major risk factors for coronary heart disease (CHD) for all patients approximately every 3–5 years
- Calculate 10-year risk (National Cholesterol Education Program global risk) of developing symptomatic CHD for all patients with two or more major risk factors to assess the need for primary prevention strategies
- Patients with established CHD should be identified for secondary prevention efforts, and patients with a CHD risk equivalent (e.g., atherosclerosis in other vascular beds, diabetes mellitus, chronic kidney disease, or 10-year risk greater than 20% as calculated by Framingham equations) should receive equally intensive risk factor intervention as those with clinically apparent CHD

History

- Often presents as nonspecific presentation of illness in elderly
- Women may have nonstandard presentation; frequently awakened at night with pain
- Elderly patient may have no symptoms—"silent MI"
- Shortness of breath, CHF
- Pain radiation at rest or minimal activity
- Classic: Oppressive retrosternal chest pain, not relieved by nitroglycerin; nausea or vomiting; diaphoresis
    PHYSICAL EXAM
    - High incidence of mortality within first hour following cardiac event
    - May have obvious pain; usually reduced sensitivity to pain in elders— "silent MI"
    - Nonspecific presentation, delirium, syncope, weakness
    - Vital signs: Hypotension, tachycardia, dyspnea
    - General appearance: Apprehensive, appears ill, ashen color
    - Respiratory: Shortness of breath, rales
    - Heart: S3, S4, new mitral regurgitation murmur, arrhythmia

    DIAGNOSTIC STUDIES
    - ECG diagnostic in 85% of cases with ST segment elevation, "Q" waves, inverted T waves
        - Subendocardial infarction: Note ST segment depression (may be only finding)
    - Cardiac enzymes (see Table 8–12)
        - Creatine kinase (CK): CK-MB2 to CK-MB2 ratio >1.5, infarction is suggested (more sensitive early marker prior to elevation of CK-MB)
        - Troponin T and troponin I (not found in muscle or blood of healthy person) are more specific than CK-MB; become positive 4–12 hours after onset of MI
        - LDH: LDH1 exceeds LDH2 levels in pathology; less specific than cardiac enzymes
        - Troponin T and troponin 1 confers greater sensitivity

Table 8-12. Cardiac Enzymes in the Diagnosis of MI

Lab	Onset	Comment
CK: MB 1 & 2	3–4 hours	Sensitive, not specific
Troponin I & T	3.5 hours	Highly specific
LDH 1 & 2	24 hours	Sensitive, not specific

Differential Diagnosis
- Unstable angina
- Aortic dissection
- Pericarditis
- Pulmonary embolism
- Esophageal spasm
- Biliary tract disease
- Gastroesophageal reflux disease
- Pancreatitis
- Chest wall muscle spasm

Management

NONPHARMACOLOGIC TREATMENT
- Acute: Immediate emergency room care for evaluation and stabilization
- Post-MI: Diet low in saturated fat and sodium; caloric restriction if appropriate
- Post-MI: Treat underlying risk factors (hypertension, hyperlipidemia)

PHARMACOLOGIC TREATMENT
- Acute:
  - Nitroglycerin SL 0.3–0.6 mg every 5 minutes, total three doses
  - Chest pain unrelieved—transport to nearest emergency room or chest pain center
  - Aspirin 160–325 mg, preferably chewable
  - O2 via nasal cannula at 2 liters, if available
  - Thrombolytic therapy may confer benefit if initiated within 3–12 hours after onset of pain
- Post-infarction:
  - Treatment of hyperlipidemia
  - Smoking cessation
  - Antiplatelet agent
    » Aspirin 81–325 mg qd unless contraindicated
    » Clopidogrel (Plavix) 75 mg po qd if unable to tolerate aspirin
  - Beta blockers improve survival rates:
    » With the exception of marked CHF or bronchospasm, improve mortality
    » Monitor bradycardia, fatigue, depression
    » Metoprolol (Lopressor) 25–200 mg bid
    » Atenolol (Tenormin) 25–200 mg qd
  - Calcium channel blockers are not effective and are indicated for secondary prevention

- ACE inhibitors should be considered for all patients:
  » In patients with left ventricular dysfunction, improves morbidity
  » HOPE study showed reduction of mortality in patients without CHF
  » Most effective for patients with diabetes, hypertension
  » Monitor cough and renal function, including hyperkalemia
  » Rare: Life-threatening angioedema caused by drug
  » Lisinopril 2.5–10 mg QD; start with small dose, titrate up
  » PEACE study suggests ACE inhibitors do not lower mortality in stable patients with normal heart function
- Glycosides: Consider use in CHF
- Nitrates:
  » Effective for residual ischemia and coronary atherosclerosis
  » Monitor hypotension

Special Considerations
- None

When to Consult, Refer, Hospitalize
- Acute: Immediate referral to emergency department by ambulance, not by family or friends
- Patients with symptoms that may represent acute coronary syndrome (ACS) should not be evaluated solely over the telephone but should be referred to a facility that allows evaluation by a physician and the recording of a 12-lead electrocardiogram (ECG) and biomarker determination (e.g., an emergency department or other acute-care facility)
- Patients with symptoms of ACS (chest discomfort with or without radiation to the arm[s], back, neck, jaw, or epigastrium; shortness of breath; weakness; diaphoresis; nausea; lightheadedness) should be instructed to call 9-1-1 and be transported to the hospital by ambulance rather than by friends or relatives
- Initial post MI care and evaluation by cardiologist

Follow-Up
- Long-term management; see at least every 3 months
  EXPECTED COURSE
  - Two variables dictate course: status of vessel disease and ventricular damage
    - Main left CAD: 20% mortality first year; single vessel damage has 2% mortality; double vessel damage has 3%–4% mortality; triple vessel damage has 5–8% mortality
    - Left ventricular dysfunction: Ejection fraction (EF) <40% doubles annual mortality rate
  - Overall mortality rate 10% in hospital phase, 10% mortality during first year
  - 60% of deaths occur in the first hour

  COMPLICATIONS
  - Death
  - Chronic heart failure
  - Ventricular tachycardia or ventricular fibrillation in first 24 hours
  - Atrial fibrillation and flutter, bradycardia, heart block
  - Deep vein thrombosis

- Pulmonary embolism
- Mitral regurgitation
- Cardiogenic shock

Chronic Heart Failure/Congestive Heart Failure (CHF)

Description
- A clinical syndrome characterized by insufficient cardiac output to meet the metabolic demands of the body, due to either decreased contractility (systolic failure) or decreased ventricular filling (diastolic failure). It is classified as left heart failure (acute) or right heart failure (chronic) and may present as acute, pure left-sided failure; chronic, pure right-sided failure; or as an acute exacerbation of chronic failure.
- Formerly called congestive heart failure; the nomenclature has switched to chronic heart failure over the past few years.

Etiology
- Most common cause in children is congenital heart disease with volume or pressure overload.
- Acquired causes are metabolic abnormalities, severe hypoxia, acidosis, viral infection, myocarditis, acute rheumatic carditis, rheumatic valvular heart disease, cardiomyopathy, prolonged SVT, complete heart block, severe anemia, acute hypertension, and bronchopulmonary dysplasia.
- Left-sided failure: An acute process causes abrupt decrease in the output of a previously healthy heart. This might include acute MI, acute papillary muscle rupture, acute dysrhythmia, acute valvular regurgitation, or drug toxicity.
- Right-sided failure: Chronic strain on compensatory mechanisms finally produces a hypertrophied heart that cannot keep up with metabolic demands. Chronic strain may be caused by chronic hypertension; hypertrophic or restrictive cardiomyopathy; chronic, subclinical sympathetic nervous system stimulation; chronic valvular stenosis/regurgitation causing higher pressure; and drug toxicity.

Incidence and Demographics
- Occurs in infants through old age
- Male preponderance until age 75, then equal occurrence
- Most frequent hospital admitting diagnosis

Risk Factors
- Factors precipitating CHF in patients with underlying heart disease include:
  - Patient noncompliance with medications
  - Excess salt intake, stress, obesity, pulmonary infection
  - Uncontrolled hypertension
  - Inadequate therapy
  - Progression or complications of underlying disorder such as arrhythmias and cardiac muscle damage
  - Increased or decreased volume, anemia, electrolyte imbalance
  - Drugs such as NSAIDs, acetaminophen, beta blockers, steroids, digitalis toxicity, alcohol

Prevention and Screening

- Control of underlying disorder
- Monitor for and treatment of risk factors

Assessment

HISTORY (SEE TABLE 8-13 FOR CHF CLASSIFICATION)
- Dyspnea on exertion, diminished exercise capacity, weakness
- Nocturia, orthopnea, paroxysmal nocturnal dyspnea, nocturnal cough
- Edema
- Anorexia
- Infants present with poor feeding, poor weight gain, tachypnea that worsens during feeding, and cold sweat
- Older children may c/o shortness of breath (especially with activity), puffy eyelids, swollen feet, or exercise intolerance

Table 8-13. NY Heart Association Functional Classification of Chronic Heart Failure

Class	Activities That Are Tolerated
Functional Class 1	Ordinary physical exertion does not limit activity
Functional Class 2	Ordinary physical activity presents slight limitations
	Patient experiences fatigue, dyspnea, angina, palpitations
Functional Class 3	Comfortable at rest; physical activity presents marked limitations
Functional Class 4	Symptoms at rest; any physical activity presents marked limitations

PHYSICAL EXAM
- Overall appearance, noting whether short of breath on walking or sitting
- Basilar rales, wheezes, S3 gallop rhythm, displaced PMI
- Cool extremities, cyanosis, color
- Change in mental status
- Ascites, hepatomegaly
- Hypotension, pulsus alternans, tachycardia, tachypnea
- Frothy pink sputum
- Edema, rapid weight gain
- Jugular venous distention
- While elements of both left- and right-sided failure often exist in a patient, it is often possible to identify the etiology of the problem by sorting symptoms into these two categories:
  - **Left-sided failure** produces signs and symptoms of acute low cardiac output and high pulmonary pressures: dyspnea at rest, anxiety, chest discomfort/heaviness, pale skin, murmur of mitral regurgitation, S3 gallop, crackles through most of the lung field bilaterally, frothy cough

– **Right-sided failure** produces symptoms of compensated chronic fluid retention/overload: dyspnea with exertion, easily fatigued, paroxysmal nocturnal dyspnea, orthopnea, anorexia, basilar rales, abdominal fullness, jugular venous distention, lower-extremity edema, hepatosplenomegaly, hepatic/splenic hum, pulsatile chest wall heave, displaced point of maximal impulse, single or multiple murmurs of stenosis or regurgitation

DIAGNOSTIC STUDIES
- CHF is a clinical diagnosis and diagnostic tests are only used to assist in identifying the cause and to determine severity and identify complications
- Chest x-ray: Pleural effusions, pulmonary edema, cardiomegaly, and to rule out pneumonia
- Electrocardiogram: Identify arrhythmias, type of heart disease, possible left ventricular strain
- Echocardiogram: Ejection fraction (EF) determines severity; assists in determining the cause of CHF (type of heart defect, enlarged chambers, decreased left ventricular function)
- Electrolytes, BUN, creatinine, cardiac enzymes, urinalysis, arterial blood gases, pulse oximetry
- Cardiac catheterization: Not routine (important for primary etiology)
- Endomyocardial biopsy: Only useful for myocarditis or infiltrative disease

Differential Diagnosis
- Renal disease
- Failure to thrive
- Chronic obstructive pulmonary disease
- Nephrotic syndrome
- Cirrhosis
- Pulmonary emboli
- Acute MI
- Pneumonia
- Asthma
- Bacterial endocarditis
- Chronic venous insufficiency

Management
- The severity of the CHF dictates the course of medical/surgical management; goal is to improve quality of life by reducing symptoms.
    NONPHARMACOLOGIC TREATMENT
    - Identify and treat underlying disease and control precipitating factors
    - Control leg edema with elastic pressure stockings and elevation of legs
    - Sodium and fluid restriction, daily weight assessment
    - Patient education, cardiac rehabilitation: Goal is to balance activity with metabolic restriction
    - Oxygen
    - Other options: Surgical—valve replacement and cardiac transplant

Table 8-14. Drug Treatment for Adults with Chronic Heart Failure

Drugs	Treatment Regimen	Common Side Effects
Cardiac Glycosides		
Digoxin (Lanoxin)	Loading dose 1.0 mg po over 24 hours, starting 0.5 mg rather than 0.25 mg q 12 x 2 Maintenance 0.25 mg qd, or 0.125 mg qd if risk of toxicity	GI—anorexia, nausea CNS—apathy, weakness, headache Cardiac—arrhythmia Not indicated for acute MI Monitor toxicity
Diuretics		
Furosemide (Lasix)	Initial dose 20–80 mg qd Dose dependent on acute vs. chronic management	Electrolyte disturbances, orthostatic hypotension, Dizziness, weakness, GI upset Ototoxicity if rapid IV
Hydrochlorothiazide (HCTZ)	Mild symptoms—25–50 mg qd	Anorexia, nausea, vomiting, cramping
Metolazone (Zaroxolyn)	2.5–5 mg 1 hour prior to furosemide Generally, once or twice a week	Marked electrolyte imbalance, CNS effects
Spirolactone (Aldactone)	25–50 mg qd or in divided doses	Hyperkalemia
Angiotensin-Converting Enzyme (ACE) Inhibitors		
Captopril (Capoten)	6.25–12.25 mg tid	Angioedema, hypotension Cough—may be significant Hyperkalemia—use with caution in renal impairment
Enalapril (Vasotec)	2.5 mg bid, titrate to 10 mg bid	Same as above
Lisinopril (Zestril)	20 mg qd	Same as above
Quinapril (Accupril)	10 mg qd	Same as above
Beta Blockers		
Carvedilol (Coreg)	3.25 po bid, titrate *slowly* to 25 mg bid or tid	Bradycardia, depression, fatigue
Metoprolol (Lopressor)	5 mg bid, titrate to 100 mg bid	Same as above
Vasodilators		
Hydralazine (Apresoline)	10 mg qid; target dose 300 mg daily Requires 8–12 hour nitrate-free period before starting	GI side effects, hypotension, headaches, tachycardia
Isosorbide dinitrate (Isordil)	5–10 mg tid; target dose 160 mg daily	Same as above

PHARMACOLOGIC TREATMENT (SEE TABLE 8-14)
- Pediatric patients requiring medications should be managed by cardiologist
- Patients frequently need a 3–4 drug regimen to control symptoms based on cardiac impairment
- Diuretics reduce preload and left ventricular filling

- ACE inhibitors are cornerstone of therapy; prevents progression of left ventricular dysfunction
- Beta blockers improve ventricular function and reduce post-infarction mortality
- Glycoside improves contractility in systolic failure
- Vasodilators reduce after-load
- Anticoagulants prevent thrombus formation; generally used when EF < 20%

LENGTH OF TREATMENT
- Acute episodes: Until resolution and stabilization of symptoms
- Chronic condition: Indefinite

Special Considerations
- Geriatric patients: Special attention to dosage requirements
- Lactation: Multiple drug regimen is of concern

When to Consult, Refer, Hospitalize
- Consult with a physician for initial diagnosis with management plan
- Refer all pediatric patients, pregnant and lactating women with CHF to a cardiologist for treatment
- Refer if complications or exacerbation is not responsive to treatment

Follow-Up
- Follow up every 3 months if stable
- Provide patient education about diet, activity, medication, self-monitoring, and what symptoms to report

EXPECTED COURSE
- Chronic: Poor prognosis if ejection fraction less than 20% or steady decline after diagnosis
- Acute: Generally responsive to initial treatment

COMPLICATIONS
- Electrolyte disturbances, arrhythmias, digitalis toxicity

Syncope

Description
- A temporary loss of consciousness, accompanied by fainting; loss of muscle tone; and possibly brief tonic contractions of the face, extremities, and trunk

Etiology
- Systemic hypotension leads to brief cerebral ischemia, causing loss of function
- Simple syncope usually is a vasovagal event, triggered by fear, pain, excitement, or extended periods of standing still, especially in warm environments
- Cough syncope is seen predominantly in asthmatic children
- Long QT syndrome is usually characterized by a loss of consciousness during exercise or emotional stress and is accompanied by cardiac rhythm abnormalities
- Vasomotor due to impaired vasoconstriction resulting in hypotension with decreased cerebral perfusion; includes vasovagal and carotid sinus syncope

- Postural (orthostatic) hypotension: Dehydration, autonomic insufficiency, medication
- Cardiogenic syncope: Disturbances of rhythm, conduction, or hemodynamics
- Psychiatric disorders: Anxiety, depression, conversion disorder
- Neurologic disorders (rare): Vertebrobasilar TIAs or migraines
- Pathophysiology related to reflex-mediated vasomotor instability; decreased cardiac output or blood flow obstruction; metabolic disruptions (hypoglycemia, hypoxia, hyperventilation); neurologic events (seizures, cerebrovascular diseases)

Incidence and Demographics
- 30% of adults will experience at least one episode of syncope
- 3% of all ED visits
- Vasodepressor syncope or "fainting" is common in young women, associated with stress or pain
- A diagnosis can be made in 45%–50% of cases
- Syncopal events occur in 10%–15% of all adolescents
- Simple syncope is uncommon before age 10–12 and occurs more frequently in girls

Risk Factors
- Cardiac disease, diabetes
- Vasodilators, diuretics, adrenergic blocking agents
- Age, family history of sudden death
- Prolonged QT syndromes
- Asthma and cough

Prevention and Screening
- Adequate hydration

Assessment
HISTORY
- Detailed history including symptoms before and after event (position changes, prolonged standing, exposure to warm environment)
- Lightheadedness, diaphoresis, nausea, visual changes before event
- Length of loss of consciousness, seizure activity, height of fall, any injuries including to tongue
- Confusion or drowsiness after event
- Associated cardiac or neurological symptoms: Chest pain, diaphoresis, palpitations, headache, diplopia, aphasia, unilateral motor weakness, paresthesia
- Incontinence of bladder or bowel
- Past medical history: Cardiac, neurologic; family history of heart disease, seizures
- Medications: Vasodilators, beta blockers, diuretics, anticholinergics
- Recent drug or medication use
- Interview family member or witness

PHYSICAL EXAM
- Vital signs including orthostatic changes
- Cardiovascular: Arrhythmia, murmurs, displaced PMI (cardiomegaly), bruits, difference in blood pressure between arms including orthostatic pressures
- Neurologic exam for focal deficits

DIAGNOSTIC STUDIES
- ECG for arrhythmia and other cardiac disease
- Chest x-ray (CXR) if associated coughing
- CBC and electrolytes to rule out anemia, metabolic abnormalities
- Fasting blood glucose, thyroid function tests
- Pregnancy testing in women of child-bearing age
- Echocardiography to rule out valvular disease, particularly if murmur
- Stress testing if exertional syncope to rule out ischemia
- Holter or event monitoring to rule out arrhythmia
- Tilt table to evaluate autonomic dysfunction
- Electrophysiologic studies if recurrent event and still no known etiology
- Electroencephalography if seizure history or seizures suspected
- Brain imaging if focal neuro signs (CT or MRI)
- Carotid or transcranial Doppler studies if bruits or to rule out vertebrobasilar insufficiency

Differential Diagnosis
- Vasomotor syncope
- Orthostatic hypotension
- Acute myocardial infarction
- Sick sinus syndrome
- Drug reaction
- Cough or micturition
- Conduction disorders (AV block)
- Arrhythmias
- Aortic stenosis
- Pulmonary stenosis or hypertension
- Congenital anomalies with right-left shunting
- Seizure
- Vertebrobasilar TIA
- Psychogenic cause (hyperventilation)
- Metabolic abnormality

Management
NONPHARMACOLOGIC TREATMENT
- In cases of benign syncope (vasomotor), explain etiology to patient and advise to lie down when prodromal symptoms occur
- Simple syncope can be managed by avoiding triggers, pushing fluids, and salt-loading during hot weather
- Also the patient can be taught to contract the calf muscles repeatedly while sitting or standing still
- Long QT syndrome can sometimes be managed by the implantation of a cardiac pacemaker
- Occasionally, left cervicothoracic sympathectomy is necessary

PHARMACOLOGIC TREATMENT
- Medical management depends on etiology
- Use smallest doses of antihypertensive medications, eliminate any unnecessary drugs

- Beta adrenergic blocking agents for recurrent episodes of simple syncope or prolonged QT syndrome
- Improved management of asthma episodes

Special Considerations
- Further evaluation is necessary in presence of known heart disease, arrhythmias, pathological murmurs, and exertional syncope
- With geriatric patients, increased risk secondary to comorbidities, polypharmacy, autonomic neuropathy, and dehydration due to decreased fluid intake
- Syncope common in third trimester of pregnancy due to aortocaval compression by the enlarged uterus in the supine position; try left side lying position

When to Consult, Refer, Hospitalize
- Hospitalize for ventricular tachycardia, sustained supraventricular tachycardia, suspected myocardial infarction, medication that can cause malignant arrhythmias (torsades de pointes with quinidine), or any other high risk for cardiac syncope
- Hospitalize for acute focal neuro signs
- Hospitalize older people who cannot be safely managed in their present living environment
- Refer to cardiology if prolonged QT syndrome is suspected or simple syncope is hard to control
- Neurology referral for new-onset seizures
- Mental health evaluation if psychogenic origin suspected

Follow-Up
EXPECTED COURSE
- Depends on etiology; patient may outgrow simple syncope by young adulthood

COMPLICATIONS
- Depends on etiology
- Increased risk of complications with heart disease, advanced age, and polypharmacy

Murmurs

Description
- Murmurs are sounds created when there is turbulent forward blood flow due to partial obstruction of a stenotic heart valve or turbulent backward flow through an incompetent valve due to faulty valve closure (regurgitation) that produces an abnormal sound distinguishable from other heart sounds.
- Innocent (functional, physiologic, benign) murmurs: Turbulent flow as blood is ejected from a chamber or due to increased or vigorous flow across a valve; associated with no structural abnormality.

Etiology
- Organic: Congenital or acquired (atherosclerosis)
- Functional: Resulting from another medical condition such as anemia, fever, thyrotoxicosis, pregnancy
- Innocent murmurs: No evidence of cardiac pathology
- Rheumatic fever is a potential contributor to all murmurs
- Infective endocarditis: Regurgitation murmurs
- Other contributing factors include:
  - Aortic stenosis: Congenital and senile calcifications
  - Aortic regurgitation: High blood pressure, aortic dissection, syphilis, collagen vascular disease
  - Mitral regurgitation: Ruptured chordae tendineae, CAD, mitral valve prolapse
  - Tricuspid regurgitation: Right ventricular failure, right ventricular infarction

Incidence and Demographics
- Murmurs are common and may occur in all ages.
- 80% of children have innocent murmurs sometime during childhood, usually beginning at age 3.
- An innocent murmur is a frequent finding in the third trimester of pregnancy.
- The elderly often have a II/VI systolic ejection murmur due to decreased compliance of heart.

Risk Factors
- Age: Children and elderly have the most murmurs
- Physiologic states of increased metabolic demand: Fever, anemia, pregnancy, hyperthyroidism
- Heart disease

Prevention and Screening
- Prevention through treatment of streptococcal pharyngitis to prevent rheumatic fever
- Screening through periodic routine examinations

Assessment
HISTORY
- Symptoms such as shortness of breath, syncope, chest pain, palpitations, exercise intolerance indicate pathologic murmur
- Family history of heart disease; prenatal and perinatal history
- Signs or history of infections and illness
- Activity level and endurance; feeding; crying; cyanosis

PHYSICAL EXAM
- Skin color and moisture; nail clubbing
- Vital signs; pulses; posture
- Neck for distended veins, bruits, and thyromegaly
- Lungs for adventitious sounds

- Chest for asymmetry, precordial bulge, thrill, heave, and point of maximal impulse
- Abdomen for organomegaly
- Extremities for edema
- Assessment of murmurs:
    - Grading of intensity (see Table 8–15)
    - Location: Area with greatest intensity
    - Radiation: Heard in direction of blood flow
    - Pitch: High, medium, low
    - Quality: Soft, harsh, rumbling
- Timing: Within the cardiac cycle (systolic between S1/S2; diastolic between S2/S1)
    - Once auscultated, a murmur must be identified as systolic or diastolic
    - S1 is mitral and tricuspid valve closure
    - S2 is aortic and pulmonic valve closure
    - The period between S1 and S2 is systole
    - The period between S2 and S1 is diastole

Table 8-15. Grading of Murmurs

Grade	Characteristics
I/VI	Very faint, and may not be heard in all positions
II/VI	Quiet but heard immediately upon placing the stethoscope on the chest
III/VI	Moderately loud
IV/VI	Loud accompanied by palpable thrill
V/VI	Very loud, heard with a stethoscope partly off the chest; accompanied by palpable thrill
VI/VI	Heard with the stethoscope entirely off the chest and accompanied by palpable thrill

Table 8-16. Heart Sounds and Related Heart Values Positions

Diastole	Systole	Diastole	Systole
S2	S1	S2	S1
A/P close	M/T close	A/P close	M/T close
M/T open	A/P close	M/T open	A/P close

Figure 8-2. Standard Chest Auscultatory Points

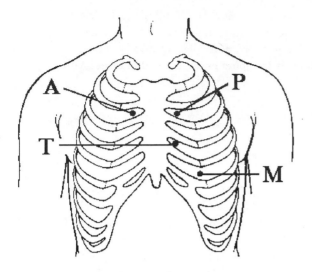

- Murmurs that occur after S1 and before S2 are systolic murmurs
  » Mitral and tricuspid regurgitation (backflow through an incompetent valve)
  » Aortic and pulmonic stenosis (turbulent flow through a tight opening)
- Murmurs that occur after S2 and before S1 are diastolic murmurs
  » Aortic and pulmonic regurgitation (backflow through an incompetent valve)
  » Mitral and tricuspid stenosis (turbulent flow through a tight opening)
• Placement of murmurs:
  - Once murmurs are identified as systolic or diastolic, the likely valve of origin must be identified by location
  - Murmurs loudest at the second intercostal space, right sternal border, are likely aortic murmurs
  - Murmurs loudest at the second intercostal space, left sternal border, are likely pulmonic murmurs
  - Murmurs loudest at the fourth intercostal space, left sternal border, are likely tricuspid murmurs
  - Murmurs loudest at the fifth intercostal space, midclavicular line, are likely mitral murmurs
• Systolic regurgitant murmur: Murmur begins with S1 and usually lasts throughout systole (pansystolic or holosystolic); caused by blood flow from a chamber that is at a higher pressure throughout systole than the receiving chamber (ONLY associated with ventricular septal defect [VSD], mitral and tricuspid regurgitation [MR and TR])
• Diastolic: Early diastolic (caused by the incompetence of the aortic or pulmonary valve); middiastolic (caused by turbulence of the tricuspid or mitral valve); or presystolic (caused by flow through the atrioventricular valves during ventricular diastole—tricuspid or mitral stenosis [TS or MS])

- Continuous murmur: S1 through S2; conditions such as patent ductus arteriosus (PDA)
- Innocent heart murmurs (functional, physiologic, benign); see Table 8–17
  - Left sternal border (LSB), second through fourth left interspaces and apex
  - Grade I–II/VI; low pitch; soft, short, nonradiating, midsystolic
  - Variable loudness; heard best in supine position and diminishes with upright position

Table 8–17. Types of Murmurs

Type of Murmur	Characteristics of the Murmur
Systolic murmur	Occurs between S1 and S2
	Systolic ejection murmur: Interval between S1 and the onset of the murmur (also referred to as crescendo-decrescendo); caused by blood flow through stenotic or deformed semilunar valves or by increased blood flow through normal semilunar valves
	Systolic regurgitant murmur: Murmur begins with S1 and usually lasts throughout systole (pansystolic or holosystolic); caused by blood flow from a chamber that is at a higher pressure throughout systole than the receiving chamber (ONLY associated with VSD, MR, and TR)
Diastolic murmur	Occurs between S2 and S1
	Classified as early diastolic and caused by the incompetence of the aortic or pulmonary valve, atrial and pulmonic regurgitation (AR, PR); middiastolic, caused by turbulence of the tricuspid or mitral valve; or presystolic, caused by flow through the atrioventricular valves during ventricular diastole (tricuspid or mitral stenosis [TS, MS])
Continuous murmur	Occurs with S1 and continues through the S2 into diastole
	Seen with conditions such as patent ductus arteriosus (PDA), pulmonary artery (PA) stenosis, Blalock-Taussig shunt
Innocent heart murmurs (functional murmur) See Table 8–18	Murmurs that arise from cardiovascular structures in absence of anatomic abnormalities (80% of children have innocent murmurs sometime during childhood, usually beginning at 3 years old); also referred to as functional, benign, or physiological murmurs

- Interpretation of murmurs
  - Once timing and placement are identified, the valvular disorder is evident
  - A systolic murmur at the second intercostal space, right sternal border, is an aortic murmur occurring when the aortic valve is open—aortic stenosis
  - A diastolic murmur at the second intercostal space, right sternal border, is an aortic murmur occurring when the aortic valve is closed—aortic regurgitation
  - A systolic murmur at the fifth intercostal space, midclavicular line, is a mitral murmur occurring when the mitral valve is closed—mitral regurgitation
  - A diastolic murmur occurring at the fifth intercostal space, midclavicular line, is a mitral murmur occurring when the mitral valve is open—mitral stenosis

Systolic Murmurs

AORTIC STENOSIS

- Second intercostal space (IC) right of sternum, with patient sitting and leaning forward
- Valve is open when stenotic murmur occurs and is caused by forward flow through stenotic valve
- Begins after S1 and is a crescendo-decrescendo or diamond-shaped ejection murmur
- Radiation into neck from aortic area
- Medium pitch with variable intensity
- Harsh, loudest at base; musical at apex
- Midsystolic
- Systolic thrill may be present
- Seen frequently in the elderly and associated with a diminished S2

TRICUSPID REGURGITATION

- Lower LSB
- Begins with S1; high-pitched, smooth, blowing quality
- Pansystolic regurgitant murmur, increases in intensity with inspiration
- Right ventricular lift
- Always associated with pathology, usually diseased right ventricle from rheumatic heart disease

VENTRICULAR SEPTAL DEFECT

- LSB (3rd to 5th ICS)
- Radiation wide over precordium but not into axilla
- Loud (particularly base), harsh, pansystolic regurgitant murmur with thrill

Table 8-18. Classification of Innocent Murmurs in Children

Vibratory murmur (Still's murmur)	Usually detected at 3–6 years old; uncommon before 2 years old
	Described as a musical, buzzing, "twanging string," or vibratory sound
	Heard best at the middle left sternal border (MLSB) or between the left lower sternal border (LLSB) and apex when the patient is in the supine position; diminishes when the patient is upright or does the Valsalva
	Midsystolic and grade II–III/VI in intensity; not accompanied by a thrill
	Intensity may increase with anemia, fever, or exercise; ECG and CXR normal
Pulmonary ejection murmur	Usually detected at 8–14 years old; heard best at the upper left sternal border (ULSB)
	Early to midsystolic; grade I–III/VI in intensity; not accompanied by a thrill; soft and blowing
	EKG and CXR are normal

Table 8–18. Classification of Innocent Murmurs in Children (cont.)

Pulmonary flow murmur of the newborn	Blood flow through the sharply angulated right and left pulmonary arteries at birth; usually detected in newborns, especially those with low birthweights, and disappears by 3–6 months of age
	Heard best at the ULSB
	Midsystolic and grade I–II/VI in intensity; not accompanied by a thrill
	Transmits well to the right and left chest, back, and both axillae
	Normal EKG and CXR
Venous hum	Originates from turbulence in the jugular venous system
	Usually detected at 3–6 years old
	Heard best at the infraclavicular and supraclavicular areas (disappears when the patient is supine or when the neck veins are gently occluded)
	Continuous humming murmur
	Normal EKG and CXR
Carotid bruit	Originates from turbulence in the carotid arteries; detected at any age
	Systolic ejection murmur; grade II–III/VI in intensity
	Rarely, a thrill is palpable over the carotid artery
	Normal EKG and CXR

HYPERTROPHIC OBSTRUCTIVE CARDIOMYOPATHY
- LSB
- No radiation
- Murmur increases with Valsalva maneuver, decreases with patient squatting
- Midsystolic

PULMONIC STENOSIS
- LSB 2nd or 3rd ICS, pulmonary area
- Generally no radiation unless loud, then toward left neck
- Variable intensity, medium pitch
- Midsystolic: Begins after S1 with crescendo-decrescendo contour
- Associated with thrill if significant pathology; usually congenital cause

MITRAL REGURGITATION
- Location: Apex; frequently radiates to wide area of chest and to left axilla
- Intensity variable, often loud; does not increase with inspiration
- Pitch is high with a blowing quality
- S3 usually also heard
- Pansystolic regurgitant murmur frequently accompanied with thrill
- Begins with S1 (which may be decreased)
- Valve is closed when the murmur occurs; noise caused from backflow through incompetent valve
- Always pathologic

Diastolic Murmurs
− Always indicative of heart disease
− Often heard best with bell of the stethoscope

MITRAL STENOSIS
- Listen with patient in left lateral decubitus position; also with exercise
- Diastolic rumbling murmur that begins after a short period of silence after S2
- Low in pitch, heard best with bell of stethoscope in light skin contact
- No radiation
- Loudest at apex; best heard after mild exercise

AORTIC REGURGITATION
- Heard at LSB with patient leaning forward and listening with diaphragm pressed firmly on the chest
- Early diastolic murmur that begins immediately after S2 and diminishes in intensity
- Blowing, high-pitched, decrescendo
- Heard with rheumatic heart disease or syphilis

PULMONARY VALVE INSUFFICIENCY
- LSB 2nd ICS
- Radiates mid-right sternal border
- High-pitched, loudest base, decrescendo murmur

Continuous Murmurs (quality often varies when patient changes position)
− Patent ductus arteriosus
− Coarctation of the aorta
− Peripheral pulmonary stenosis

DIAGNOSTIC STUDIES
- ECG to detect underlying heart disease
- CBC to look for signs of infection, anemia
- Chest x-ray to evaluate heart failure, size of heart
- Echocardiography: Valve pathology and systolic/diastolic function
- Angiography for more thorough evaluation
- Fluoroscopy demonstrates calcified aortic valve

Differential Diagnosis
• See descriptions of systolic and diastolic murmurs above.

Management
NONPHARMACOLOGIC TREATMENT
- Patient education on disease entity and lifestyle modifications for underlying disorder
- Valvular surgical repair

PHARMACOLOGIC TREATMENT
- Stabilize hemodynamic deficiencies
- Antibiotics for endocarditis prophylaxis as indicated

LENGTH OF TREATMENT
• Often a chronic condition

Special Considerations
• Geriatric patients: Aortic stenosis common
• Pregnancy: Monitor murmurs throughout pregnancy with intervention and cardiac consultation for any change in objective findings

When to Consult, Refer, Hospitalize
• Consult or refer if symptomatic (signs of heart failure, growth failure, syncope, cyanosis); diastolic murmur; systolic murmur that is loud (grade III/IV or with a thrill), long in duration, and transmits well to other parts of the body; abnormally strong or weak pulses; abnormal cardiac size or silhouette or pulmonary vasculature on CXR
• Refer to pediatric cardiologist for murmur in conjunction with chromosomal abnormalities (especially Trisomy 13, Trisomy 18, and Trisomy 21)
• If abnormal ECG and symptomatic, hospitalization may be necessary

Follow-Up
• Asymptomatic patients should be assessed at least annually and at every visit
• Innocent murmurs: No follow-up necessary
• Monitor murmurs associated with pregnancy; if worsen, refer to cardiology
  COMPLICATIONS
    • Chronic heart failure
    • Poor activity tolerance; growth and development problems
    • Progression of mitral stenosis has potential for thrombus formation and hypoxia
    • Progression of mitral regurgitation is associated with dyspnea and orthopnea
    • Atrial fibrillation with mitral stenosis and mitral regurgitation
    • Stroke and/or TIA
    • Bacterial endocarditis

Mitral Valve Prolapse (MVP)

Description
• A condition characterized by decreased ventricular load resulting in prolapse of the valve leaflets during systole
• Produces a mid systolic click and late systolic murmur

Etiology
• Strong familial pattern, associated with connective tissue disorder such as Marfan syndrome and Ehlers-Danlos syndrome (nearly all patients with Marfan syndrome have MVP); systemic lupus erythematosus (SLE)
• One-third of patients with MVP have congenital heart disease (atrial septum defect, ventricular septum defect, or Ebstein's anomaly)
• May be caused by rheumatic endocarditis or ruptured chordae tendineae post MI
• May be idiopathic; 50% of cases in children are idiopathic

- Pathology involves abnormal valvular collagen leading to degeneration. Excessive tissue increases orifice size. Function of the papillary muscle and chordae apparatus is abnormal. MVP is the most common cause of mitral regurgitation.

Incidence and Demographics
- Adolescents and young adults; more common in females and thin patients; may be comorbid with minor chest wall deformities
- 3% of general population; 5% of pediatric population; 75% without morbidity/mortality

Risk Factors
- Familial history
- Connective tissue disorders
- Mitral regurgitation

Prevention and Screening
- Proper dental care and prophylaxis to prevent endocarditis
- Anticoagulation to prevent thrombus/embolus for patients with risk factors
- Screening through periodic routine exams

Assessment
HISTORY
- Frequently asymptomatic
- Palpitations, lightheadedness, dyspnea, fatigue, syncope
- Anxiety, panic attacks
- Possible chest pain, usually mild

PHYSICAL EXAM
- Murmur and clinical findings may vary from visit to visit
- Late systolic murmur: Begins in mid or late systole and can continue through S2
- Mid and late systolic clicks may be audible
- Positional murmur changes: When standing or with Valsalva, click is closer to the first heart sound (S1); with squatting, click farther from first heart sound (S1)
- Body build: Thin, tall in some cases
- Autonomic abnormalities: Orthostatic hypotension
- Mitral regurgitation (MR): Holosystolic murmur, radiation to axilla, frequent thrill
- A high incidence of thoracic skeletal anomalies (80%) are seen in association with MVP:
    - Pectus excavatum (50%)
    - Straight back (20%)
    - Scoliosis (10%)

DIAGNOSTIC STUDIES
- Echocardiogram: Diagnostic and should be repeated with significant change in murmur or accompanying clinical findings; will detect and quantify MR
- ECG: Usually normal; possible atrial or ventricular arrhythmias; left atrial/ventricular enlargement
- CXR: Normal

- Tilt table test to identify autonomic dysfunction
- Holter monitor to identify arrhythmia

Differential Diagnosis
- Stenotic mitral or tricuspid valve
- Pericarditis
- Tricuspid valve prolapse
- Papillary muscle dysfunction
- Hypertrophic cardiomyopathy

Management
NONPHARMACOLOGIC TREATMENT
- No treatment or activity restrictions in patients with asymptomatic MVP (about 75%)
- Patients who are symptomatic (palpitations, lightheadedness, syncope) or have arrhythmias should undergo treadmill exercise testing and/or ambulatory ECG monitoring
- Surgery: Mitral valve replacement

PHARMACOLOGIC TREATMENT
- Prophylactic antibiotics with invasive procedure and dental cleaning if there is MR, to prevent endocarditis
- Beta blockers such as atenolol (Tenormin) 25–50 mg if patient has exercise-induced arrhythmias, palpitations, and panic attacks
- Digoxin used with inotropic deficit
- Anticoagulation for atrial fibrillation and MR: Warfarin (Coumadin) maintain INR (International Normalized Ration) 2.0–3.0
- Sodium chloride tablets for low baseline intravascular volume, abnormal renin-aldosterone response, and abnormal compensatory response

LENGTH OF TREATMENT
- Lifelong monitoring and treatment unless surgical valve replacement

Special Considerations
- Males older than 50 have higher incidence of complications
- Pregnancy may improve symptoms of MVP

When to Consult, Refer, Hospitalize
- Referral to a cardiologist for initial diagnosis, symptomatic patients, arrhythmias, and complications.

Follow-Up
- Monitor for MR q year with echocardiogram for problems; q 2–3 years for mild/moderate murmur with regurgitation; q 5 years for click only
  #### EXPECTED COURSE
  - 25% function with little problem for several decades; however, with increased decline in valve function, may progress rapidly to demonstrating greater symptoms
  - 75% stable lifetime function

COMPLICATIONS
- Uncommon, usually relate to underlying heart disease
- Stroke and/or TIA from embolus
- Progression to or worsening MR
- CHF, arrhythmia
- Infective endocarditis
- Sudden death

Atrial Fibrillation

Description
- Common arrhythmia, acute or chronic, characterized by nonsynchronized irregular atrial and ventricular activity
- Untreated rates vary from atrial 200–600/minute with ventricular rate 80–180/minute
- Difference between apical rate and pulse rate is pulse deficit
- Non–life-threatening by itself; however, has major risk of embolism

Etiology
- Extra-cardiac causes include pulmonary embolus, surgery, alcohol intoxication and withdrawal, hyperthyroidism
- May be preceded by premature atrial contraction
- May be idiopathic or due to a variety of cardiac causes including rheumatic heart disease, cardiomyopathy, atrial septal defect, mitral valve prolapse, sick sinus syndrome, acute myocardial infarction, heart failure, and pericarditis
- Chaotic electrical activity within the atria; AV node is continuously stimulated by atrial impulses, therefore, the ventricular rate is irregular and usually rapid
- Ineffective atrial emptying results in hemodynamic instability, poor cardiac output, and stasis of blood

Incidence and Demographics
- Increases with aging
- High reccurrence of episodes
- 2%–4% of adult population

Risk Factors
- Conditions leading to the above etiologies

Prevention and Screening
- Avoid excessive alcohol, caffeine, and nicotine
- Treat comorbid conditions
- Assess and aggressively respond to triggers that comprise hemodynamic stability: acute MI, chronic heart failure, or pulmonary embolus

Assessment
HISTORY
- Variable symptoms from asymptomatic to severe
- Initial presentation may be with paroxysmal rhythm
- Palpitations, angina, fatigue, decline in activity level, marked dyspnea, dizziness, syncope

- Review of systems (ROS) for symptoms of hyperthyroidism, underlying cardiac disease, alcohol use

PHYSICAL EXAM
- Tachycardia, irregular pulse—marked deficit between apical rate and radial pulse
- Pallor, orthostatic blood pressure changes
- Peripheral edema, jugular venous distension
- Tachypnea
- CNS disturbance: Decreased mental acuity

DIAGNOSTIC STUDIES
- ECG: Confirmatory with absent P waves, irregular ventricular rate, and rhythm 100–160 beats
- Cardiac event monitor
- Echocardiogram or transesophageal echo (TEE) to assess underlying cardiac dysfunction
- Thyroid function tests
- Ventilation perfusion scan if pulmonary embolus suspected (shortness of breath, chest pain)

Differential Diagnosis
- Hyperthyroidism
- Hypertension
- Pulmonary embolus
- Atrial flutter
- Sinus tachycardia
- Alcoholism

Management

NONPHARMACOLOGIC TREATMENT
- Treat underlying disorders
- Invasive therapy for refractory cases: cardioversion; radiofrequency catheter ablation of AV node
- Pacemaker implantation

PHARMACOLOGIC TREATMENT
- Acute:
  - Managed in hospital setting under care of cardiologist for cardioversion and possible anticoagulation
  - IV digoxin (Lanoxin), ibutilide (Corvert), beta blockers, and calcium channel blockers administered to break arrhythmia (pharmacologic cardioversion)
- Chronic (rate control):
  - Digoxin: Loading dose 0.25 mg bid x 2 days or start at maintenance dose; maintenance 0.125–0.25 mg qd
    » Check drug levels 6–8 hours after last dose or prior to dose
    » Monitor toxicity: Fatigue, anorexia, weakness, and nausea
    » Digoxin ventricular response control less effective with activity

» Active individuals consider beta blocker or calcium channel blocker
- Beta blockers: Metoprolol (Lopressor) 50–100 mg qd; atenolol (Tenormin) 25–100 mg qd (side effects: bradycardia, fatigue, depression, impotence)
- Calcium channel blockers: Verapamil (Calan) 120–480 mg qd; diltiazem (Cardizem) 90–360 mg qd (side effects: constipation, dizziness, headaches)
- Use caution with medication; some have depressing effect on the AV node
- Antithrombotic therapy: Warfarin (Coumadin) is drug of choice for chronic atrial fibrillation
    » Aspirin 325 mg qd in patients with contraindication to warfarin
    » Arrhythmia >48 hrs: Anticoagulation therapy maintained 3–4 weeks prior to cardioversion
- Profile for those most at risk of stroke secondary to atrial fibrillation includes age over 65 years; previous TIA or stroke; high blood pressure; heart failure; thyrotoxicosis; clinical coronary disease; mitral stenosis; prosthetic heart valve; diabetes

LENGTH OF TREATMENT
- Anticoagulation therapy is indefinite unless situations arise that would contraindicate therapy

Special Considerations
- Geriatric patients: Prevalent problem
- Pregnancy (rare): Digoxin safe; cardioversion does not affect fetus; anticoagulation may result in spontaneous abortion although heparin does not cross placenta
  - Recommendations for IV heparin during first trimester, oral warfarin second and third trimester

When to Consult, Refer, Hospitalize
- Initially, refer all patients to cardiologist for evaluation and management plan; refer pregnant women for management; and refer patients who are not controlled back to cardiologist for evaluation

Follow-Up
- At least monthly follow up for INR if on warfarin (target 2.5)
    EXPECTED COURSE
    - Prognosis dependent on underlying cause
    - Exercise and activity levels may be limited due to hemodynamic instability

    COMPLICATIONS
    - Heart failure
    - Stroke, peripheral arterial embolism
    - Bradycardia, torsades de pointes with drug treatment; bleeding with anticoagulants

CONGENITAL HEART DEFECTS

Patent Ductus Arteriosus (PDA)

Description
- The ductus arteriosus is a normal fetal structure between the left pulmonary artery and the descending aorta.
- Functional closure of the ductus arteriosus usually occurs within 48 hours after birth. Anatomic closure is completed by 2–3 weeks of age.
- PDA becomes clinically significant if it persists past neonatal period; unlikely to close spontaneously after that time and may produce signs and symptoms of pulmonary overcirculation.

Etiology
- Idiopathic
- High altitude
- Maternal exposure to rubella during the first trimester
- Genetic or familial

Incidence and Demographics
- Full term infants: 0.5/1,000 live births; at high altitudes (>4,500 feet), 15/1,000 live births
- Premature infants: 8/1,000 live births; prevalence in infants with birthweight <1,750 grams is 45%; <1,200 grams birthweight, 80%

Risk Factors
- Genetic predisposition with environmental triggers such as viruses and drugs
- Prematurity

Assessment
HISTORY
- Symptoms dependent on volume of pulmonary blood flow; patients are usually asymptomatic with a small PDA
- A moderate to large shunt PDA may cause symptoms of chronic heart failure (tachypnea, sweating, poor feeding/poor weight gain), irritability, and lower respiratory tract infections

PHYSICAL EXAM
- Classic finding is a "machinery" murmur with continuous systolic and diastolic components, heard best at upper left sternal border (ULSB) and left infraclavicular area; no murmur may be heard with severe left ventricular failure
- Patients with a small PDA usually have normal physical growth and normal pulses/pulse pressure
- Tachycardia, tachypnea, crackles in cases of pulmonary over-circulation
- Hyperdynamic precordium

DIAGNOSTIC STUDIES
- ECG: Normal or left ventricular, atrial hypertrophy depending on amount of the shunt
- Chest x-ray: Normal with a small PDA. Varying degrees of cardiomegaly with enlargement of left atrium (LA), left ventricle and ascending aorta. Increased pulmonary vascular markings proportionate to the amount of left-to-right shunting.
- Echocardiography: Doppler studies can provide functional information. Dimensions of left atrium and ventricle can indirectly assess the amount of left-to-right shunting; greater the dilation of these chambers, the larger the shunt.
- Cardiac catheterization: Not necessary for diagnostic evaluation

Differential Diagnosis

- Atriovenous malformations (systemic, pulmonary or coronary)
- Venous hum
- Ventricular septal defect with aortic regurgitation
- Pulmonary atresia
- Persistent truncus arteriosus
- Aortopulmonary septal defect (AP window)
- Peripheral pulmonary stenosis
- Total anomalous venous connection
- Collaterals in coarctation of the aorta in Tetralogy of Fallot/pulmonary atresia
- Anomalous origin of the left coronary artery from the pulmonary artery
- Ruptured sinus of Valsalva aneurysm

Management

PHARMACOLOGIC TREATMENT
- Indomethacin (prostaglandin synthetase inhibitor) during the neonatal period
- 0.2 mg/kg intravenously q 12 h for up to three doses
- Contraindications to the use of indomethacin include blood urea nitrogen >25 mg/dL or creatinine >1.8 mg/dL, platelet count <80,000/mm3, necrotizing enterocolitis, hyperbilirubinemia, and bleeding tendency (including intracranial hemorrhage)

SURGICAL
- Premature infants
    - If medical therapy is unsuccessful or indomethacin is contraindicated after 2–3 attempts, surgical repair indicated
    - Percutaneous coil embolization is performed in the cardiac catheterization laboratory; percutaneous closure not currently available for very small or preterm infants; new devices under study which may make it feasible to close even large PDAs or PDAs in small infants
    - Surgical ligations performed via thorascopy with minimal surgical incision is the currently used procedure
        » The existence of a PDA, regardless of size, is an indication for surgery
        » A PDA ligation is performed between 6 months and 2 years of age; asymptomatic infants may be closed electively at time chosen by family and surgeon

» Surgical mortality is less than 1%
» Complications are rare and include injury to the laryngeal nerve (hoarseness), the left phrenic nerve (left hemidiaphragm paralysis), or the thoracic duct (chylothorax)

Special Considerations
None

When to Consult, Refer, Hospitalize
• Refer all patients with a PDA type murmur to a cardiologist

Follow-Up
• No activity restrictions unless pulmonary hypertension is present
• Infective endocarditis prophylaxis for 6 months after surgery/coil embolization
• Controversial whether children with silent PDAs detected by ultrasound but not clinically significant should be repaired at all
    COMPLICATIONS
        • Complications post-surgery are unusual; may include infective endocarditis, CHF, recurrent pneumonia, pulmonary vascular obstructive disease (PVOD), pulmonary hypertension, pulmonary or systemic emboli
        • Rarely, aneurysm of the PDA may occur

Atrial Septal Defect (ASD)

Description
• A defect (opening) in the atrial septum
• Four types of atrial defects: Primum defect (30%), secundum defect (50%–70%), sinus venosus defect (<10%), coronary sinus septal defect (<10%)

Etiology
• No known genetic cause and most ASDs are sporadic. Primum ASDs are associated with trisomy 21.

Incidence and Demographics
• Isolated cases (those not associated with other cyanotic heart lesions) occur in 0.5–1/1,000 live births (5%–10% of all CHD cases)
• ASDs account for <10% of congenital heart disease in infants, but >30% of cases diagnosed in adults as findings may be subtle and not detected

Risk Factors
• Genetic predisposition with environmental triggers such as viruses and drugs
• Prematurity

Assessment
    HISTORY
        • Even with moderate to large ASDs, infants and children are usually asymptomatic
        • Children with significant defects may be small, but true failure to thrive is rare

- Physiologic impact of the left-to-right shunt increases with age, initially manifests as exercise intolerance and can lead to overt CHF
- Progressive increase in symptoms in 2nd and 3rd decade of life

PHYSICAL EXAM
- In large defects, height and weight may be slightly below normal
- Heart rate usually normal, may have mild tachycardia; blood pressure is normal
- May be prominent precordial bulge or right ventricular heave
- Classic finding is wide, split S2; may have split S1 with loud second component
- II–III/VI medium-pitched systolic ejection murmur heard best at ULSB or LMSB secondary to pulmonary valve stenosis
- Middiastolic rumble at the LLSB due to increased flow across the tricuspid valve may be heard with large left-to-right shunts

DIAGNOSTIC STUDIES
- ECG: Usually normal sinus rhythm; right axis deviation (RAD) and mild right ventricular hypertrophy (RVH) or right bundle branch block may be seen
- Chest x-ray: May be normal or may show cardiomegaly with right atrial enlargement (RAE) or right ventricular enlargement (RVE), prominent main pulmonary artery (MPA), increased pulmonary vascular markings (PVMs). Large pulmonary artery best seen on lateral view
- Echocardiography: Transthoracic or transesophageal technique, can identify location of ASD, able to demonstrate pulmonary venous return
- Cardiac catheterization: Not necessary for diagnostic evaluation; performed if defect can be closed using an atrial occluder device

Differential Diagnosis
- Pulmonary stenosis
- Innocent murmur
- Physiologic "flow" murmur (e.g., anemia, fever)
- Tricuspid stenosis

Management
- Patients with isolated defect 3–8 mm in size have a spontaneous closure rate of 80% by 18 months of age.
- Patients with an isolated defect <3 mm in size diagnosed by 3 months of age have a spontaneous closure rate of 100% by 18 months of age.
- ASDs >8 mm in size rarely close spontaneously.
- Infective endocarditis does not occur in patients with an isolated ASD
  NONPHARMACOLOGIC TREATMENT
  - Exercise restriction unnecessary

  PHARMACOLOGIC TREATMENT
  - If signs, symptoms of CHF develop, treatment with digoxin and diuretics is indicated
  - Infective endocarditis prophylaxis unnecessary unless there are associated cardiac lesions

SURGICAL
- High pulmonary vascular resistance (PVR) is a contraindication for surgery
- Surgery postponed until 3–4 years of age because of high incidence of spontaneous closure; surgery performed during infancy, however, if CHF develops and does not respond to medical management
- Surgical closure of the ASD
- Direct closure of the defect with a patch or stitch closure
- Incision is made through a median sternotomy
- Performed under cardiopulmonary bypass through an atrial approach
- Surgical mortality is less than 1%. The mortality rate is higher during infancy and in patients with a high PVR
- Complications include postoperative arrhythmias (7%–20%) and cerebrovascular accident
- Placement of an atrial occluder ("clamshell" device) to close the ASD (done in the cardiac catheterization laboratory) may be possible for secundum defects

Special Considerations
- None

When to Consult, Refer, Hospitalize
- Refer all patients with an ASD-type murmur to a cardiologist

Follow-Up
- Patients without chronic heart failure are managed conservatively. If after the first year of life, patient is asymptomatic with small ASD, see every 1–2 years to monitor for spontaneous closure of the ASD.
    POSTOPERATIVE FOLLOW-UP
    - Cardiology visit periodically
    - No activity restrictions unless complications from surgery have occurred
    - No infective endocarditis prophylaxis for an isolated ASD
    - Long-term follow-up required for patients with postoperative arrhythmias

    COMPLICATIONS
    - Chronic heart failure and pulmonary hypertension (in the third to fourth decade of life)
    - Atrial arrhythmias (flutter/fibrillation)
    - Holt-Oren Syndrome: Tricuspid or mitral insufficiency
    - Rarely, cerebrovascular accident

Ventricular Septal Defect (VSD)

Description
- A defect (opening) in the ventricular septum
- VSDs are classified as membranous or muscular, depending on the location of the defect
- Defects vary in size ranging from tiny openings with no hemodynamic compromise to large openings with accompanying pulmonary hypertension and chronic heart failure

Etiology
- Unknown

Incidence and Demographics
- VSD is the most common form of congenital heart disease (CHD), usually detected by a murmur heard between 2 and 6 weeks.
- Isolated cases (those not associated with other cyanotic heart lesions) occur in 1.5-2/1,000 live births (15%–20% of all CHD cases); VSDs are the most common lesion in chromosomal syndromes, however, >95% of children with a VSD have normal chromosomes.
- 3 % of children with VSDs have a parent with a VSD.
- 30%–50% close in first 2 years.

Risk Factors
- Genetic predisposition with environmental triggers such as viruses and drugs
- Prematurity

Prevention and Screening
- Early referral

Assessment
HISTORY
- Patients with small VSDs are usually asymptomatic with normal growth and development.
- Symptoms vary with size of the VSD and degree of left-to-right shunting. Patients with moderate to large shunt VSDs show delayed growth and development, increased incidence of respiratory infections, decreased exercise tolerance, and signs and symptoms of chronic heart failure (CHF). CHF usually does not occur until 6–8 weeks of life, after the fall in pulmonary vascular resistance and pulmonary artery pressure.
- Infants may have severe dyspnea, feeding difficulties, profuse perspiration, and duskiness with crying or infection.

PHYSICAL EXAM
- Small VSD:
  - Patients are acyanotic and well-developed
  - Precordial activity is normal, thrill is typically not palpable
  - Normal physiologic splitting of S2
  - II–VI/VI harsh systolic regurgitant murmur heard best at the LLSB
- Moderate-to-large VSD:
  - Infants may be failure-to-thrive and show signs of chronic heart failure (usually by 2 months of age)
  - Hepatomegaly may be present
  - Tachycardia
  - Increased intensity of the precordial impulse
  - S2 is narrowly split
  - II–VI/VI harsh holosystolic murmur heard best at the LLSB, may obscure 1st and 2nd heart sounds
  - Apical diastolic rumble

DIAGNOSTIC STUDIES
- ECG: Normal with a small VSD. Left ventricular hypertrophy (LVH) and occasional left atrial enlargement may be seen with moderate VSDs. Combined ventricular hypertrophy (CVH) with or without left atrial enlargement with large VSDs. Monitor for possible pulmonary hypertension or pulmonic stenosis, which results in right ventricular hypertrophy (RVH).
- Chest x-ray: Normal with a small VSD; with moderate to large shunt VSDs, cardiomegaly of varying degrees that involves the LA, LV, and sometimes the RV. Pulmonary vascular markings (PVMs) increased. The degree of cardiomegaly and increased PVMs is directly proportionate to the amount of left-to-right shunting.
- Echocardiography: Two-dimensional echo can determine the anatomical location, size and number of VSDs. Doppler studies can provide visualization of the shunt. Used to screen for development of left ventricular outflow tract disease and spontaneous closure.
- Cardiac catheterization: Strongly recommended for critically ill children prior to surgery. Provides detailed information about the anatomic location of the VSD, quantitative measurements of shunting, and level of pulmonary vascular resistance.
- Selective left ventriculography: Shows "gooseneck" deformity of left ventricular outflow tract.

Differential Diagnosis
- Tricuspid regurgitation
- Mitral regurgitation
- Patent ductus arteriosus
- Atrial septal defect
- Subaortic membrane

Management
- Small defects spontaneously close up to 75% of the time; moderate defects close 30%–50%; large defects will decrease in size as the patient grows but have a low spontaneous closure rate. Muscular defects have a higher spontaneous closure rate than membranous defects.

  NONPHARMACOLOGIC TREATMENT
  - Observation only for small-to-moderate VSDs
  - Frequent feedings of high-caloric formula, orally or through a nasogastric tube, may help growth failure in children with moderate to large VSD

  PHARMACOLOGIC TREATMENT
  - Infective endocarditis prophylaxis as long as VSD present and until 6 months after surgical correction
  - If signs and symptoms of CHF develop, treatment includes digoxin and diuretics
  - Anemia should be corrected by oral iron therapy

SURGICAL
- If growth failure cannot be improved with medical management, VSD should be closed surgically within first 6 months of life; surgery should be postponed for infants who respond to medical therapy to allow time for spontaneous closure
- Surgical closure of a VSD
- Direct closure of the defect with a patch or stitch closure through a median sternotomy
- Surgical mortality is 2%–5% after 6 months of age; higher in patients less than 2 months of age and those with multiple VSDs or associated defects
- Complications include a residual VSD shunt (20% of patients), right bundle branch block (10% of patients), complete heart block (<5% of patients) and rarely cerebrovascular accident

Special Considerations
- None

When to Consult, Refer, Hospitalize
- Refer all patients with a VSD-type murmur to a cardiologist

Follow-Up
- Patients without chronic heart failure or pulmonary hypertension managed conservatively, with close monitoring of growth. 78%–80% of children with small VSDs will have spontaneous closure during the first 2 years of life.
- Patients <6 months with CHF and growth failure should be seen monthly.
  POSTOPERATIVE FOLLOW-UP
  - Cardiology follow-up as directed by surgery
  - No activity restrictions unless complications from surgery have occurred
  - Infective endocarditis prophylaxis may be discontinued 6 months after surgery; however, if there is a residual VSD, continue infective endocarditis prophylaxis indefinitely
  - Long-term follow-up is required for patients who had transient heart block postoperatively, whether a pacemaker was placed or not

  COMPLICATIONS
  - Subacute bacterial endocarditis
  - Pulmonary overcirculation/pulmonary hypertension
  - Left ventricular volume overload
  - Aortic insufficiency
  - Eisenmenger syndrome
  - Acquired left ventricular outflow tract obstruction
  - Aneurysm of the interventricular septum
  - Mitral regurgitation leading to valve replacement
  - Heart block requiring pacemaker placement

Coarctation of the Aorta (CoA)

Description
- Discrete narrowing of the aorta, just opposite the site of insertion of the ductus arteriosus (juxtaductal position)
- Two distinct presentations:
  - Neonatal period: Coarctation is usually severe, associated with closing of the ductus arteriosus, presents at 4–10 days of life
  - Infancy, childhood: Typically no symptoms, coarctation is less severe, may have good collateral flow to the descending aorta

Etiology
- Cause is unknown

Incidence and Demographics
- Occurs in 0.8–1/1,000 live births (8% of all CHD cases)

Risk Factors
- Other cardiac defects such as aortic hypoplasia, bicuspid aortic valve (85%), PDA (60%), ventricular septal defect (50%), mitral valve abnormalities, and Shone syndrome (multiple left-sided obstruction lesions including mitral stenosis, subaortic membrane, valvular aortic stenosis) are often associated with CoA
- Turner syndrome (XO): 30%–35% have CoA

Prevention and Screening
- Early referral

Assessment
HISTORY
- Symptomatic infants:
  - Poor feeding and weight gain
  - Dyspnea
  - Signs of chronic heart failure
  - Circulatory shock
  - Normal newborn discharge examination (if the PDA had not closed and was supplying blood flow to the descending aorta)
- Asymptomatic children:
  - Majority of children are asymptomatic until late childhood
  - Occasionally, complaints of pain and/or weakness in the legs following exercise, headache secondary to hypertension

PHYSICAL EXAM
- Symptomatic infants:
  - Hallmark is absent or weak femoral pulses
  - Pale, varying degrees of respiratory distress
  - Oliguria or anuria
  - General circulatory shock with severe acidosis
  - Differential cyanosis (lower part of body appears cyanotic due to right-to-left ductal shunting)

– Decreased or absent lower-extremity pulses; qualitative difference between brachial and femoral pulse
– Blood pressure discrepancy between the upper and lower extremities (higher in the arms)
– Loud single S2; a gallop is usually present
– Nonspecific systolic ejection murmur, although 50% of sick infants do not have a murmur
- Asymptomatic children:
  – Normal growth and development
  – Decreased or absent lower extremity pulses
  – Hypertension in upper extremities (normally thigh or calf systolic pressure higher than arm)
  – Systolic thrill may be present in the suprasternal notch
  – Accentuated A2, normally split S2
  – II–IV/VI systolic ejection murmur heard best at the URSB, MLSB, or LLSB that radiates to the left interscapular region posteriorly
  – Frequently an ejection click is audible

DIAGNOSTIC STUDIES
- ECG: Usually normal. RVH or right bundle branch block (RBBB) may be present in infants; LVH can be seen in older children with long-standing CoA.
- Chest x-ray: Marked pulmonary edema and cardiomegaly in symptomatic infants. In older children, the heart size is normal or slightly enlarged. A "3 sign" on an overpenetrated CXR (due to a double aortic curve/abnormal contour of the arch) or an E-shaped indentation on a barium-filled esophagus may be seen. Rib notching between the fourth and eighth ribs may be present in older children but is rare before the age of 5 years. Rib notching is erosion of the ribs caused by dilated intercostal collateral vessels.
- Echocardiography: Two-dimensional echo and color flow Doppler studies can show the site and extent of coarctation as well as provide information about left ventricular function and other left-sided lesions.
- Cardiac catheterization allows measurement of pressure above and below coarctation.
- MRI may be used to further define the location and severity of the CoA and provide data about collateral vessels.

Differential Diagnosis
- Aortic stenosis
- Pulmonary stenosis
- Patent ductus arteriosus

Management
NONPHARMACOLOGIC TREATMENT
- Symptomatic infants:
  – Oxygen
  – Surgical intervention to follow
- Asymptomatic children:
  – Patients with mild CoA should be followed closely for the development of hypertension or systolic pressure differences between the arms and legs

PHARMACOLOGIC TREATMENT
- Symptomatic infants:
    - Prostaglandin E1 infusion to reopen the ductus arteriosus (0.5 mcg/kg/min)
    - Correction of acidosis and metabolic disturbances
    - Inotropic agents (dopamine or dobutamine)
    - Diuretics
- Asymptomatic children:
    - Patients with mild CoA should be followed closely for the development of hypertension or systolic pressure differences between the arms and legs; occasionally these children will require chronic antihypertensive therapy, usually with beta blockers or ACE inhibitors, most commonly if repair done <5 years old

SURGICAL
- Symptomatic infants:
    - Surgery to repair the CoA should be performed urgently on infants with CHF
    - Surgical correction of CoA
    - Surgery is performed without bypass through a left posterolateral thoracotomy
    - Types of repair include:
        » End-to-end anastomosis (area of coarctation resected, distal and proximal aorta anastomosed end-to-end)
        » Patch aortoplasty (area of coarctation incised, elliptical Dacron patch sutured in place to widen diameter)
        » Subclavian flap aortoplasty (distal subclavian artery divided, flap of proximal portion of vessel used to expand the coarcted area)
    - Ductus is always ligated with these surgical techniques
    - Surgical mortality is less than 5%
    - Complications include residual obstruction and/or recoarctation (6%–33%) and postoperative renal failure
    - Balloon angioplasty may be performed if recoarctation occurs
- Asymptomatic children:
    - Upper extremity hypertension or a systolic gradient of >20 mmHg between upper and lower extremities is an indication for elective repair of a CoA in children 2–4 years old; mortality is less than 1%
    - Older children should be operated on as soon as the diagnosis of CoA is made
    - Surgical correction of CoA
    - Surgery performed without bypass through a left posterolateral thoracotomy
    - Types of repair are the same as in symptomatic infants
    - End-to-end is the repair of choice for discrete CoA in older children
    - Complications include spinal cord paralysis producing paraplegia due to limited collateral circulation during cross-clamping of the aorta (0.4%), postoperative rebound hypertension, and post-coarctectomy (reperfusion) syndrome
    - Balloon angioplasty of a native (unoperated) CoA is controversial; may be performed if recoarctation

Special Considerations
- None

When to Consult, Refer, Hospitalize
- Refer all patients with a CoA-type murmur to a cardiologist
- Refer patients with hypertension to a cardiologist if other causes have been ruled out

Follow-Up
- Symptomatic infants should be followed every 6–12 months to evaluate for recoarctation
- Asymptomatic children can be seen annually to assess for persistent hypertension, recoarctation, subaortic stenosis, and persistent myocardial dysfunction
- Infective endocarditis prophylaxis indefinitely due to associated bicuspid aortic valve and recoarctation

CYANOTIC CONGENITAL HEART DEFECTS

Tetralogy of Fallot (TOF)

Description
- A syndrome of congenital heart defects. The four components of TOF are:
  1. Large VSD located in the membranous region of the ventricular septum
  2. Pulmonary stenosis
  3. Overriding aorta
  4. Obstructive right ventricular hypertrophy

Etiology
- Cause is unknown

Incidence and Demographics
- Occurs in 0.2–0.3:1,000 live births (8% of all CHD cases); most common cyanotic CHD beyond 1 week of age
- Associated defects:
  - Right aortic arch (25%)
  - Pulmonary atresia (15%)
  - Abnormal coronary arteries (5%)
  - Pulmonary branch stenosis
  - Systemic collateral arteries that feed into the lungs
  - ASD
  - Microdeletion of chromosome 22q11 (Velocardiofacial syndrome)

Risk Factors
- Genetic predisposition with environmental triggers such as viruses and drugs
- Prematurity

Assessment

HISTORY

- Heart murmur audible in the newborn period
- Most patients are symptomatic with cyanosis present at birth
- History of hypoxic spells, especially with crying or exercise
- Parents may describe child as squatting while walking
- Patients with acyanotic (pink) TOF are asymptomatic
- Hypoxic spells ("Tet" spells)
- Spells usually occur after crying, feeding, or defecation
- Spells usually consist of rapid and deep breathing, irritability and prolonged crying, increased cyanosis, and decrease in intensity of murmur
- Severe hypoxic spell may lead to limpness, convulsion, cerebral vascular accident (CVA), or even death

PHYSICAL EXAM

- Varying degrees of cyanosis, with hypercyanosis occurring later in infancy
- Growth retardation if cyanosis is severe
- Tachypnea
- Clubbing may be present if the cyanosis has been long standing (usually >6 months)
- Normal S1 and single S2 (because the aorta is located more anteriorly than normal)
- Active precordium, grade III–IV/VI systolic ejection murmur heard best at the middle and upper left sternal border (caused by right ventricular outflow tract obstruction); the greater the obstruction, the softer the murmur
- Continuous murmur representing PDA shunt may be audible in patients with TOF and pulmonary atresia

DIAGNOSTIC STUDIES

- ECG: Normal QRS axis with acyanotic TOF and right axis deviation with cyanotic TOF. Right ventricular hypertrophy (RVH) and right atrial hypertrophy are usually present. Combined ventricular hypertrophy (CVH) may be seen in acyanotic TOF.
- Chest x-ray: X-ray findings in patients with acyanotic TOF are the same as in those with a small to moderate VSD. With cyanotic TOF, heart size < normal. PVMs are decreased. Heart may appear "boot-shaped" because of a concave main pulmonary artery with an upturned apex. Right aortic arch (25%) and right atrial enlargement (25%) may be present.
- Echocardiography: Two-dimensional echo can determine the anatomical location, size, and number of VSDs; assess the anatomy of the RVOT, pulmonary valve, and pulmonary arteries; and image the coronary arteries. Doppler studies can provide visualization of the VSD shunt and estimate a pressure gradient across the RVOT obstruction.
- Cardiac catheterization: Recommended prior to surgical repair of TOF.

Differential Diagnosis

- Aortic stenosis

Management

- Treatment of cyanotic spells includes knee-chest positioning, oxygen, intravenous fluid bolus, sodium bicarbonate to treat acidosis, morphine sulfate to calm child, vasoconstrictors (epinephrine or phenylephrine) to increase systemic vascular resistance, beta blockers (Inderal) to cause RVOT relaxation.

   PHARMACOLOGIC TREATMENT
   - Treat iron deficiency anemia since anemic children are more likely to have a CVA
   - Infective endocarditis prophylaxis

   SURGICAL
   - Asymptomatic and acyanotic children are repaired at 6–12 months of age
   - Asymptomatic and minimally cyanotic children are repaired at 3–24 months of age, depending on the amount of pulmonary artery hypoplasia
   - Mildly cyanotic infants who have had a palliative shunt procedure may have a complete repair 1–2 years after the shunt procedure
   - Symptomatic infants with a favorable RVOT and pulmonary arteries are repaired at 3–4 months of age
   - Surgical repair of TOF
   - Patch closure of VSD and reconstruction of the RVOT by resection of the infundibular tissue and placement of a transannular patch
   - Incision is made through a median sternotomy under cardiopulmonary bypass
   - Surgical mortality 2%–5% during the first two years of life, higher in patients <3 months of age and >4 years old and those with severe pulmonary hypoplasia, associated defects
   - Complications include bleeding during the postoperative period, pulmonary valve regurgitation, residual RVOT obstruction, RV dysfunction, residual VSD, right bundle branch block and rarely, complete heart block or ventricular arrhythmias

Special Considerations

- None

When to Consult, Refer, Hospitalize

- Refer all patients with a TOF type murmur to a cardiologist

Follow-Up

- Symptomatic infants should be seen monthly until surgical repair. Asymptomatic children can be seen every 3–6 months until surgical repair.

   POSTOPERATIVE FOLLOW-UP
   - Cardiology follow-up
   - Varying levels of activity restrictions may be necessary
   - Infective endocarditis prophylaxis should be continued indefinitely
   - Long-term follow-up is required for patients who had sinus node dysfunction, surgical heart block, or ventricular arrhythmias postoperatively, whether a pacemaker was placed or not

COMPLICATIONS
- Hypoxic spells ("Tet" spells)
- Right ventricular dysfunction
- Ventricular arrhythmias
- Rarely, brain abscess and cerebrovascular accident
- Infective endocarditis
- Polycythemia

PERIPHERAL VASCULAR DISORDERS

Peripheral Arterial Disease

Description
- Chronic or acute entity consisting of obstruction or narrowing of the major arteries, commonly affecting the lower extremities and most frequently a result of atherosclerosis

Etiology
- Acute thrombus leading to embolus
- Chronic atherosclerotic lesions
- Inflammatory component in thromboangiitis obliterans (Buerger's disease), giant cell (temporal) arteritis
- May also be caused by trauma or entrapment (thoracic, popliteal)

Incidence and Demographics
- Elderly
- Male preponderance

Risk Factors
- Age >40 years
- Tobacco usage
- Hyperlipidemia, hypertension, atherosclerosis
- Diabetes mellitus or fasting serum glucose >110 mg/dL
- Obesity

Prevention and Screening
- Lifestyle modification
- Identification and treatment of comorbid conditions

Assessment
HISTORY
- Acute: Pain, paresthesia, paralysis, pallor, pulselessness
- Chronic: Lower extremity aching, fatigue occurring with activity and relieved by cessation of activity (intermittent claudication); pain develops at rest as disease progresses
- Aorta: Back or abdominal pain; femoral: hip, buttock, calf pain
- See Table 8–19 for classification of peripheral vascular disease

Table 8-19. Fontaine Classification of Peripheral Vascular Disease

Stage	Clinical Feature
1	Silent
2	Intermittent claudication
3	Rest ischemia
4	Ulceration or gangrene

PHYSICAL EXAM
- Pale, cool, diminished, or absent pulses in extremity; bruit of femoral artery possible
- Severity determined by amount of time required for venous filling and return of color
- Absent or decreased hair and nail growth of the lower extremities
- Waxy pallor of the affected extremity, or dependent rubor with hyperemia due to compensatory reflex vasodilation of the microvasculature causing bright red distal extremity

DIAGNOSTIC STUDIES
- Diagnosis is clinical but Doppler ultrasound used to determine severity
- Angiography for acute or surgical candidates

Differential Diagnosis
- Musculoskeletal strains
- Osteoarthritis
- Acute arterial spasm
- Deep vein thrombus (DVT)
- Acute embolic conditions
- Thromboangiitis obliterans (Buerger's disease)

Management
NONPHARMACOLOGIC TREATMENT
- Acute arterial occlusion: Avoid elevating affected extremity; protect extremity and refer for heparin therapy immediately
- Smoking cessation
- Control/treat comorbid diseases: Hyperlipidemia, diabetes mellitus, hypertension
- Initiate prescribed exercise program: Preferably walking to point of pain to develop collateral circulation
- Educate patient about signs and symptoms that require immediate attention
- Stage 3: Diagnostic testing for possible surgery

PHARMACOLOGIC TREATMENT
- Acute: Heparin IV; possible embolectomy
- Chronic: Pentoxifylline (Trental) 400 mg tid; aspirin or cilostazol (Pletal) 100 mg bid decreases platelet aggregation
- ASA 81–324 mg/day for all patients

Special Considerations
- Risk of arterial occlusion increases with age

When to Consult, Refer, Hospitalize
- Refer to vascular surgeon for new onset, severe, Stage 3 or greater symptoms, acute arterial occlusion, arteriosclerosis obliterans (proliferation of the intima leads to occlusion of lumen of the arteries)

Follow-Up
- Follow up every 3 months if stable
- Patient education about medications, care of feet
    - EXPECTED COURSE
        - Chronic: Symptoms differ, with slow progression to rapid deterioration

    - COMPLICATIONS
        - Amputation
        - Gangrene

Superficial and Deep Venous Thrombosis

Description
- Deep venous thrombosis (DVT): Acute blood clot formation in the deep lower extremity or pelvic veins with ambiguous presenting signs or symptoms
- Superficial: Acute inflammation and clot formation with associated redness and tenderness along superficial vein

Etiology
- Thrombosis consist of red blood cells, platelets, and fibrin attached to part of the inflamed vessel wall
    DVT caused by:
    - Immobilization secondary to surgery, prolonged bed rest, prolonged travel by plane or car
    - Venous incompetence, vascular wall injury
    - Chronic heart failure
    - Hypercoagulable states: Inherited coagulation deficits, malignancy, and estrogen usage
    Superficial thrombosis (Saphenous vein frequently involved) caused by:
    - IV therapy, trauma
    - Bacterial infection

Incidence and Demographics
- Common; approximately 1–2 million cases per year
- Female preponderance
- High incidence with total hip replacement

Risk Factors
- DVT
  - Obesity
  - Orthopedic surgery, immobility, trauma
  - Pregnancy, oral contraceptives
  - Malignancy, coagulation defects
  - Venous catheters
  - Rheumatoid disease, lupus
  - High altitude elevations, polycythemia vera
- Superficial
  - Aseptic procedures

Prevention and Screening
- Limit period of immobilization
- Prophylactic anticoagulation for associated risk factors
- Avoidance of estrogen-containing oral contraceptives, or use low dose
- Post-surgical mechanical leg compression

Assessment
HISTORY
- DVT is frequently asymptomatic
- Possible unilateral leg pain or tenderness of calf, swelling, and discoloration
- With superficial thrombosis: Acute episode with definite time frame, local redness, tender cord, swelling, dull pain over inflamed vein, fever

PHYSICAL EXAM
- DVT: Reproducible tenderness with calf compression (Homan's sign), leg circumference greater compared to uninvolved leg due to swelling, cool extremity with weak distal pulses; however, signs often unreliable
- Superficial thrombosis: Isolated induration, redness, and tenderness along vein, but no significant swelling of the extremity

DIAGNOSTIC STUDIES
- Anticoagulation therapy baseline: Platelets, PT, PTT, CBC, LFTs, occult blood; monitor platelets daily with heparin treatment
- B-mode ultrasound combined with Doppler flow detection: Highly sensitive and specific for popliteal and femoral thrombi
- Impedance plethysmography: Accurate compared to duplex ultrasound which is less precise in the detection calf vein thrombi
- Nuclear scanning: Tagged fibrinogen 125 detects active clot formation
- Contrast venography: Most sensitive and specific contrast venography; most effective

Differential Diagnosis
- Cellulitis
- Musculoskeletal strain
- Lymphedema
- Acute arterial occlusion
- Ruptured Baker cyst

Management

NONPHARMACOLOGIC TREATMENT
- DVT:
  - Initially hospitalize with bed rest and leg elevation, anticoagulation
  - After stabilization, prompt mobilization
  - Intermittent pneumatic compression followed by graded pressure stockings
  - Calf DVT can be treated as outpatient
- Superficial:
  - Bed rest with leg (or extremity) elevated, local heat
  - If sepsis, hospitalization often required

PHARMACOLOGIC TREATMENT
- Anticoagulation therapy for DVT acute treatment and prophylaxis
  - Heparin: IV 5,000 units IV titrated to PTT 2–5 seconds above control; Subcautaneous 5,000 units 2–3 times day (stops propagation of thrombus; allows fibrinolysis)
    » Plethysmogram or ultrasound prior to discontinuation to ascertain resolution
    » Heparin and warfarin concurrent with heparin starting day 3; heparin discontinued day 5 or 6
- PT therapeutic International Normalized Ratio 2.5–3.0 with warfarin therapy
  - Thrombolytic agents: Streptokinase and urokinase; aspirin not beneficial
  - Filtering devices: Umbrella in vena cava traps emboli, useful if anticoagulants are contraindicated
  - For superficial thrombosis: NSAIDs; appropriate antibiotic if septic

LENGTH OF TREATMENT
- Treat single-episode DVT for 3 months; longer if recurrent, associated with pulmonary embolus
- Aseptic inflammation of superficial thrombosis subsides in 1–2 weeks

Special Considerations
- Geriatric patients: Common due to predisposing factors, age-related coagulation deficiencies
- Pregnancy: Use heparin because Coumadin is a teratogen
- Lactation: Unknown if heparin and warfarin are secreted in breast milk
- Oncology patients risk hemorrhage with heparin

When to Consult, Refer, Hospitalize
- Consult with physician for evaluation and management, possible hospitalization
- Refer to vascular specialist for recurrences or complications

Follow-Up
- Monitor oral anticoagulation and for signs of recurrence
- Provide patient education about wearing support hose, warfarin complications, symptoms of pulmonary embolism (PE)

EXPECTED COURSE
- Prognosis is good once danger of PE has passed

COMPLICATIONS
- Pulmonary embolism
- Chronic venous insufficiency
- Septic thrombophlebitis, osteomyelitis with superficial thrombosis

Venous Insufficiency

Description
- A chronic condition characterized by noninflammatory incompetence of the venous backflow valves in the veins of the lower extremities. Blood is regurgitated through the valves, resulting in engorgement and secondary edema of the lower leg.

Etiology
- Venous valves become incompetent and are not able to maintain efficient flow of blood back to heart.
- May be caused by leg trauma, prior thrombophlebitis, or conditions that cause abnormally high venous pressure.

Incidence and Demographics
- Female predominance
- Onset late adulthood

Risk Factors
- Trauma, obesity, pregnancy, history of thrombophlebitis
- Prolonged immobility, particularly standing
- Familial tendency, increases with age

Prevention and Screening
- Early aggressive treatment of thrombophlebitis
- Avoidance of prolonged standing and immobility
- Weight loss if appropriate
- Avoidance of restrictive lower-extremity garments

Assessment
HISTORY
- Pain varies from minimal discomfort to marked pain with ulcers
- Lower extremity edema worsens with prolonged standing
- Mild pruritus of lower extremity, scratching
- Recurrent stasis ulcers, weeping, crust formation
- Previous history of thrombophlebitis at site
- Bilateral aching in the lower extremities—typically worse at night
- Bilateral lower extremity edema with prolonged standing; relieved when legs elevated

PHYSICAL EXAM
- Hyperpigmentation of distal extremity; appears brown or reddish, brawny hyperpigmented thick skin
- Wet ulceration may be present distally, often over medial aspect of lower leg

- Edema of lower extremity
- Varicosities may be present
- Check femoral, popliteal, dorsalis pedis, posterior tibial pulses

DIAGNOSTIC STUDIES
- Stasis ulcer: Culture and sensitivity
- Doppler studies: Assess vascular status

Differential Diagnosis
- Cellulitis
- Chronic renal disease
- Lymphedema
- Acute phlebitis
- Fungal infection
- Atopic dermatitis
- Severe contact dermatitis
- Neurodermatitis

Management
NONPHARMACOLOGIC TREATMENT
- Elastic stockings prior to ambulation
- Elevation of foot of bed
- Avoid prolonged positions or inactivity
- Weight reduction for obese patients
- Refer for wound debridement and management
- Treat ulcers with antimicrobial dressing or Unna boot

PHARMACOLOGIC TREATMENT
- Diuretic therapy
- Corticosteroid creams such as hydrocortisone cream, triamcinolone 1% for itching
- Oral antibiotic for positive wound culture
- Broad-spectrum antifungal (clotrimazole)

LENGTH OF TREATMENT
- Chronic condition
- Treat exacerbations until resolution

Special Considerations
- Control edema; venous ulcer will not heal or remain healed with edema

When to Consult, Refer, Hospitalize
- Refer to vascular specialist or wound care center for refractory ulcers

Follow-Up
- Depends on clinical situation; usually every 3 months if stable
- Patient education about use of support hose, weight loss, sitting whenever possible
  EXPECTED COURSE
  - Chronic, recurrent with frequent exacerbation if poor compliance to preventive measures

COMPLICATIONS
- Bacterial infection
- Stasis ulcers
- Thrombus

Varicose Veins

Description
- Superficial, dilated, tortuous veins arising from incompetent valves and high venous pressure in the lower extremities, usually distant and involving the saphenous vein

Etiology
- Congenitally incompetent valves
- Prior thrombophlebitis
- Pregnancy, obesity, ascites
- Idiopathic, may have familial tendencies

Incidence and Demographics
- Female preponderance
- 20% of adult U.S. population

Risk Factors
- Prolonged weight bearing, standing
- Pregnancy, obesity
- Clothing apparel that causes vasoconstriction of lower extremities

Prevention and Screening
- Weight control
- Elevation of lower extremities
- Elastic support when ambulatory
- Avoidance of restrictive clothing

Assessment
HISTORY
- Fatigue, aching, heaviness, cramping primarily of lower extremities
- Menses may be precipitating factor

PHYSICAL EXAM
- Dilated and tortuous veins
- Standing offers gravitational advantage to visualize veins
- Hyperpigmentation of distal leg
- Veins are palpable

Differential Diagnosis
- Chronic venous insufficiency
- Peripheral neuropathy
- Nerve root compression
- Osteoarthritis—hip

- Arterial insufficiency
- Lymphedema
- Postphlebitic syndrome

Management

NONPHARMACOLOGIC TREATMENT
- Elastic compression stockings up to the knee prior to ambulation
- Avoid prolonged weight-bearing and standing; do not cross legs when sitting
- Weight loss; elevate leg when sitting
- Avoid restrictive garments
- Low-sodium diet in salt-sensitive individuals
- Sclerotherapy, laser surgery, or ligation and stripping of saphenous vein for severe, refractory cases

PHARMACOLOGIC TREATMENT
- Hydrochlorothiazide (HCTZ) 12.5mg qd prn with fluid retention

LENGTH OF TREATMENT
- Chronic problem

Special Considerations
- Pregnancy: Frequent problem

When to Consult, Refer, Hospitalize
- Referral to surgeon if severe and refractory

Follow-Up
- If symptomatic

EXPECTED COURSE
- Improvement with surgery
- Usually worsens with dependent positions such as standing

COMPLICATIONS
- Thrombophlebitis, varicose ulcers
- Secondary fungal and bacterial infection
- Eczema
- Neuritis from scarring secondary to stripping surgery

CASE STUDIES

Case 1: Lori is a 44-year-old White female who presents to the clinic for a well-woman exam. She works as a telephone operator in a busy law firm office. Lori voices no complaints today. Diet recall indicates high-fat meals, including junk foods. She states she loves cheese.
PMH: Smokes two packs per day for 15 years; past medical history significant for hypertension; drinks three beers daily.
Medications: Hydrochlorothiazide 50 mg qd

    1. What additional history would you ask regarding her cardiovascular status?

Exam: Vital signs: BP 128/84; Wt: 133 lbs, Ht: 64 inches, eyes: yellow-orange raised lesions on eyelids; remainder of exam is unremarkable.

    2. Would you order any diagnostic test on this patient?
    3. If your suspicions are correct, what actions would be required?
    4. When Lori returns to the clinic 6 months later with total cholesterol 252, HDL 30, and LDL 170, how will you intervene?
    5. What complications can occur with this problem and the treatment regimens?

Case 2: Baby Joe is 1 month old and presents to the clinic because he is not feeding well and his mother states he is losing weight. Baby Joe was delivered vaginally at 36 weeks gestation. His birthweight was 4 lbs 9 oz. The baby is taking 2 oz of formula over a 55-minute period.
Medications: None.

    1. Are there any other history questions you would like to ask?

Exam: Vital Signs: Temp: 98.0°F/ear, Resp: 60, HR: 180, Wt: 5 lbs 2 oz. Crying and irritable, sweating; systolic thrill, II/VI continuous murmur at the upper LSB, rate 180; respiratory rate 60 with bilateral crackles; hepatomegaly noted.

    2. What are your differential diagnoses?
    3. What is your management plan?

Case 3: Mr. Jones is 56 years old and presents to the clinic complaining of decreased appetite, shortness of breath, and swelling in his feet. He is unable to perform normal activities without becoming winded and has a productive cough.
PMH: 6 lb weight gain in the past 7 days. Past medical history significant for hypertension, hyperlipidemia, and MI.
Medications: Lipitor 20 mg/day, Monopril 40 mg/day

    1. What additional history would you ask?

Exam: Vital signs: BP 90/40; Pulse 120; Resp 24; Skin: cyanotic; CV: S3 gallop, jugular distention; Lungs: basilar rales and wheezing; Abdomen: hepatomegaly, ascites; Extremities: 3+ pedal edema bilaterally

2. What diagnostic studies would you order?
3. What is your differential diagnosis?
4. What is your management plan?

REFERENCES

Ahmed, A. (2003). American College of Cardiology/American Heart Association chronic heart failure evaluation and management guidelines: Relevance to the geriatric practice. *Journal of the American Geriatric Society, 51,* 123–126.

ALLHAT Collaborative Research Group. (2002). Major outcomes in high-risk hypertensive patients randomized to angiotensin converting enzyme inhibitor or calcium channel blocker vs diuretic: The antihypertensive and lipid lowering treatment to prevent heart attack trial. *Journal of the American Medical Association, 288,* 2981–2997.

American Academy of Family Physicians. (2004). Risk classification for stroke, death, and atrial fibrillation. *American Family Physician 6*(7), 1739–1740.

American Heart Association. (2008). *Metabolic syndrome.* Retrieved November 16, 2008, from http://www.americanheart.org/presenter.jhtml?identifier=4756

Anderson, J. L., Adams, C. D., Antman, E. M., Bridges, C. R., Califf, R. M., Casey, D. E. Jr., et al. (2007). ACC/AHA 2007 guidelines for the management of patients with unstable angina/non ST-Elevation myocardial infarction. *Circulation, 116*(7): e148–304.

Centers for Disease Control and Prevention. (2003). *A public health action plan to prevent heart disease and stroke.* Retrieved March 1, 2008, from www.cdc.gov/dhdsp/library/action_plan/pdfs/action_plan_3of7.pdf

Centers for Disease Control and Prevention. (2003). State-specific trends in high blood cholesterol awareness among persons screened — United States, 1991–1999. *MMWR: Morbidity and Mortality Weekly Report, 50*(35), 754–758.

Chobanian, A. V., Bakris, G. L., Black, H. R., Cushman, W. C., Green, L. A., Izzo, J. L., Jr., et al. (2003). Seventh report of the Joint National Committee on Prevention, Detection, Evaluation, and Treatment of High Blood Pressure. *Hypertension, 42*(6), 1206–1252.

Dickerson, L. M., & Gibson, M. V. (2005). Management of hypertension in older persons. *American Family Physician, 17*(3), 469-476.

Expert Panel on Detection, Evaluation and Treatment of High Blood Cholesterol. (2001). Executive summary of the third report of the NCEP expert panel in adults. *Journal of the American Medical Association, 285*(10), 2486. Retrieved November 19, 2008, from www.nhlbi.nih.gov

Gibbons, R. J., Abrams, J., Chatterjee, K., Daley, J., Deedwania, P. C., Douglas, J. S., et al. (2002). ACC/AHA 2002 guideline update for the management of patients with chronic stable angina: A report of the American College of Cardiology/American Heart Association Task Force of Practice Guidelines (Committee on the Management of Patients With Chronic Stable Angina). *Journal of the American College of Cardiology, 41,* 159–168. Retrieved November 19, 2008, from www.acc.org

Massie, B. M., & Amidon, T. A. (2003). Heart. In L. M. Tierney, Jr., S. J. McPhee, & M. A. Papadakis (Eds.), *Current medical diagnosis and treatment* (42nd ed., pp. 312–408). New York: Lange Medical Books/McGraw-Hill.

National Cholesterol Education Program. (2001). *Third report of the expert panel on detection, evaluation, and treatment of high blood cholesterol in adults* (Adult Treatment Panel III; NIH Pub. No, 01-3670). Bethesda, MD: Author.

National Heart, Lung, and Blood Institute. (1997). *Sixth report of the Joint National Committee on prevention, detection, evaluation, and treatment of high blood pressure* (JNC 6) (NIH Publication No. 5233). Bethesda, MD: National Institutes of Health.

National Heart, Lung, and Blood Institute. (2003). *Seventh report of the Joint National Committee on prevention, detection, evaluation, and treatment of high blood pressure (JNC 7 Express).* (NIH Publication No. 5233). Bethesda, MD: National Institutes of Health.

National Heart, Lung, and Blood Institute. (2004). *ATP III update 2004: Implications of recent clinical trials for the ATP III guidelines.* Retrieved March 12, 2008, from http://www.nhlbi.nih.gov/guidelines/cholesterol/atp3upd04.htm

Norwood, V. F. (2002). Hypertension. *Pediatrics in Review, 23*(6), 197–208.

Park, M. (2002). *Pediatric cardiology for practitioners* (4th ed.). St. Louis, MO: Mosby.

Snow, V., Barry, P., Gibbons, R. J., Owens, D. K., Williams, S. V., Mottur-Pilson, C., et al. (2004). Primary care management of chronic stable angina and asymptomatic suspected or known coronary artery disease: A clinical practice guideline from the American College of Physicians. *Annals of Internal Medicine, 141*(7), 562–567.

Snow, V., Barry, P., Fihn, S. D., Gibbons, R. J., Owens, D. K., Williams, S. V., et al. (2004). Evaluation of primary care patients with chronic stable angina: Guidelines from the American College of Physicians. *Annals of Internal Medicine, 141*(1), 57–64.

Solenski, N. J. (2004). Transient ischemic attacks: Part I. Diagnosis and evaluation. *American Family Physician, 6*(7), 1665–1681.

Solenski, N. J. (2004). Transient ischemic attacks: Part II. Treatment. *American Family Physician, 6*(7), 1665–1681.

Sontheimer, D. L. (2006). Peripheral vascular disease: Diagnosis and treatment. *American Family Physician, 73*(11), 1971–1976.

Update on the report of 1987 task force on high blood pressure in children and adolescents. (1996). *Pediatrics, 79*(1), 1–25.

U.S. Preventive Services Task Force. (2002). Aspirin for the primary prevention of cardiovascular events: Recommendation and rationale. *Annals of Internal Medicine, 136,* 157–160.

Van Vlaanderen, E. (2001). Revised guidelines for acute MI. *Clinical Advisor, March 2001,* 31–34.

Wing, L. M., Reid, C. M., Ryan, P., Beilin, L. J., Brown, M. A., Jennings, G. L., et al. (2003). A comparison of outcomes with angiotensin converting enzyme inhibitors and diuretics for hypertension in the elderly. *New England Journal of Medicine, 348,* 583–592.

Yusuf, S., Sleight, P., Pogue, J., Bosch, J., Davies, R., & Dagenais, G. (2000). Effects on angiotensin converting enzyme inhibitor, ramipril, on cardiovascular events in high risk patients: The Heart Outcomes Prevention Evaluation (HOPE) Study Investigators. *New England Journal of Medicine, 342,* 145–153.

Gastrointestinal Disorders

Barbara Rideout, MSN, APRN-BC

GENERAL APPROACH

- The elderly are less likely to feel pain with abdominal conditions and do not always present with the classic symptoms or lab findings, are more likely to have vague diffuse pain, and tend to have less acute presentation.
- Iron deficiency anemia in a male, postmenopausal female, or elderly patient always warrants an upper and lower endoscopy to rule out a gastrointestinal source of bleeding or cancer.
- Antidiarrheals should never be given to patients under 5 years old, nor any patient with bloody diarrhea, fever, fecal leukocytes, and abdominal pain due to the possible development of a systemic infection from retained toxins. These patients require prompt evaluation and referral.
- All tender, nonreducible hernias must be referred to a surgeon for prompt evaluation.
- Always repeat abdominal exam before discharging the patient to validate initial results or detect new findings; document assessment.
- Always examine the tender area last to avoid referred pain.

Red Flags
- Patient who presents with fever, chills, leukocytosis (elevated total white blood count [WBC] with increased neutrophils [polys] and bands on the differential) and rebound tenderness warrants rapid assessment and referral to an acute care facility for a surgical consultation
- Abdominal pain lasting >6 hours or pain that wakes the patient at night requires evaluation and possible referral

- *Pyloric stenosis* presents as projectile vomiting in infants between 2 weeks and 5 months of age due to hypertrophy of the pyloric muscle, which causes increasing duodenal obstruction
  - Infant is hungry, willing to eat after vomiting, but becomes progressively dehydrated
  - There may be visible gastric peristaltic waves from left to right across the abdomen
  - Palpable pyloric mass, like an olive, best palpable during feeding or immediately after vomiting
  - The infant should be referred to a pediatric surgeon immediately

GASTROINTESTINAL SIGNS AND SYMPTOMS

Dysphagia

Description
- Difficulty in swallowing (oropharyngeal dysphagia) and having food pass from the mouth down the esophagus to the stomach (esophageal dysphagia)
- Patients describe oropharyngeal dysphagia as a feeling of food getting stuck, indicative of upper esophageal or pharyngeal disease
- Odynophagia is painful swallowing, an alarm symptom that requires immediate evaluation to determine cause and treatment
- May be a structural or neuromuscular problem caused by such conditions as gastroesophageal reflux disease (GERD), esophageal spasm, Barrett's esophagus, benign esophageal or peptic stricture, esophagitis, esophageal rings (also webs and diverticula), carcinoma, goiter, myasthenia gravis, multiple sclerosis, hypothyroidism, Parkinson's disease, achalasia, scleroderma, polymyositis
- May present as difficulty swallowing solids or liquids, described as trouble initiating a swallow; coughing; choking; nasal regurgitation (oropharyngeal dysplasia); sensation of food "sticking" after it is swallowed (esophageal dysphasia)
- May present as chest pain
- It is NOT attributed to normal aging

Etiology
- Structural abnormalities
- Muscular weakness or incoordination of swallow
- Peristalis or emptying of esophagus

Incidence and Demographics
- Exact prevalence unknown; 10 million persons are evaluated each year in U.S.
- May be as high as 22% in persons over age 50 years

Prevention and Screening
- Identify at-risk persons: previous stroke, cervical spinal cord injury

Assessment
- Perform a careful history and physical exam and appropriate studies to determine underlying cause
- Associated symptoms include heartburn, weight loss, hematemesis, coffee ground emesis, anemia, and regurgitation
- May include ENT, cardiac, pulmonary, abdominal, and neuromuscular exam

- Diagnostic work-up may include:
  - CBC and stool for occult blood to evaluate for bleeding (carcinoma)
  - Liver function tests to evaluate for metastatic process
  - BUN, albumin to evaluate nutritional status
  - Thyroid function tests to rule out hypothyroidism
  - ECG and cardiac work-up if chest pain is the presenting symptom
  - Endoscopy: Standard test for the diagnosis and management of esophageal diseases because it allows for biopsy and a definitive tissue diagnosis
  - Barium swallow or upper GI series; often done first to differentiate between mechanical lesions and esophageal motility problems; if a motility problem is suspected, barium swallow should be done first; if a mechanical lesion is suspected, an endoscopy is often done first
  - Esophageal pH recording to evaluate for GERD if difficulty establishing diagnosis
  - Video esophagography–esophageal manometry (not a first line test)

Differential Diagnosis
- Functional dysphagia
- Neurogenic dysphagia
- Psychogenic dysphagia
- Esophageal cancer
- Vascular rings
- Achalasia
- Radiation injury
- Scleroderma

Management
- Outpatient treatment if patient not malnourished and not at high risk for aspiration
- Treat identifiable condition
- Goal is to treat the underlying cause and maintain nutritional status during work-up; consider liquid supplementation
- Elderly may have poor fitting dentures that contribute to problem

Special Considerations
- Use thickened liquids for persons with dysphagia to prevent aspiration

When to Consult, Refer, Hospitalize
- Refer any patient with new symptoms and no obvious treatable cause to a gastroenterologist—particularly the older patient, and those with weight loss, bleeding, iron deficiency anemia, history of chronic GERD, history of heavy alcohol and tobacco use

Abnormal Liver Function Tests (LFTS)

Description
- Serum liver chemistries are useful in evaluating liver function. Alanine and aspartate aminotransferase (ALT is highest in liver disease and AST is less specific; elevated in liver, cardiac, skeletal muscle, kidney, brain, pancreas, or lung disease), evaluate hepatic cellular integrity; bilirubin (direct and indirect), alkaline phosphatase (ALP), and gamma-glutamyl transpeptidase (GGT) assess hepatic excretion; and prothrombin time (PT) and serum albumin evaluate hepatic protein synthesis.

Etiology
- Elevated aminotransferases (ALT and AST) are typically caused by acute hepatocellular injury.
- These enzymes are found in multiple tissues and are released into the plasma in response to cellular injury.
- AST is found predominately in the liver; therefore, it is more specific than ALT for evaluating hepatocellular damage.
- ALT is found in liver, cardiac, skeletal, kidney, and brain tissue and elevated levels alone may indicate tissue damage in any of those organ systems (e.g., myocardial ischemia or musculoskeletal injury).
- ALT and AST do not indicate the severity of liver injury as they may be normal in severe disease.
- The highest levels of ALT and AST (usually >500 units/liter) occur with severe viral hepatitis, drug-induced liver injury (e.g., acetaminophen, phenytoin, rifampin), or ischemic hepatitis. Moderate elevations (usually <300 units/liter) are present in mild acute viral hepatitis, chronic active hepatitis, cirrhosis, and liver metastases. Mild elevation may be present in biliary obstruction, with higher levels suggesting the development of cholangitis (causing hepatic cell necrosis). In alcoholic liver disease, the AST/ALT ratio may be >2. A ratio of AST/ALT >1 may be seen with fatty liver as seen associated with pregnancy.
- An elevated bilirubin (a degradation product of heme) should be fractionated to determine if it is predominantly conjugated (direct, processed by the liver) or unconjugated (indirect, not processed by the liver).
- Elevations in direct bilirubin are usually caused by impaired excretion of bilirubin from the liver due to hepatocellular disease, biliary tract obstruction, drugs, or sepsis.
- Indirect bilirubin elevation is caused by hemolysis or ineffective erythropoiesis (increased bilirubin production); neonatal jaundice, Gilbert's or Crigler-Najjar syndromes (impaired bilirubin conjugation due to enzyme deficiency); or when hepatic bilirubin uptake is decreased due to drugs, heart failure, or portosystemic shunting.
- Alkaline phosphatase is an enzyme found in various tissues including the liver, bone, intestine, and placenta (more than 80% from liver and bone).
- Elevated ALP levels (in the absence of bone disease or pregnancy) usually represent impaired biliary tract function.
- Fractionation of an elevated serum ALP can be done to determine the source; however, elevation of other liver function tests is helpful in establishing a hepatic cause.
- Mild to moderate increases (usually 1–2 times normal) occur with hepatocellular disorders such as hepatitis or cirrhosis.

- High serum elevations (up to 10 times normal or greater) can occur with extrahepatic biliary tract obstruction (usually a gallstone blocking the common bile duct) or intrahepatic cholestasis (bile retention in the liver) as seen with drug-induced cholestasis and biliary cirrhosis.
- The ALP is usually mildly elevated in incomplete biliary tract obstruction and in metastatic and infiltrative liver disease (e.g., leukemia, lymphoma, and sarcoidosis).
- An elevated ALP is also present in nonhepatic disorders, with the most common being bone disease (Paget's disease and bone metastases).
- Elevated GGT, in liver disease, is useful in differentiating the origin of an elevated ALP (hepatic vs. bone), as they both tend to increase in similar hepatic diseases.
- GGT is also a highly sensitive indicator of acute alcohol ingestion and of other agents that stimulate the hepatic microsomal oxidase system, such as barbiturates and phenytoin.
- GGT enzyme is also present in the pancreas, kidney, heart, and brain, and elevations may occur in disorders involving those organ systems.
- A prolonged PT is caused by impaired hepatic synthesis of coagulation factors seen in significant liver disease and/or with vitamin K deficiency that may occur with malnutrition, malabsorption (e.g., cholestasis, steatorrhea, pancreatic insufficiency), and warfarin use. If administration of vitamin K corrects the PT, then a deficiency was present.
- Decreased serum albumin, the primary protein synthesized by the liver, may be caused by chronic liver disease, or by other nonhepatic factors such as malnutrition, hormonal factors, or excessive protein loss (nephrotic syndrome or protein-losing enteropathy).
- Inadequate hepatic protein synthesis may lead to a decreased serum albumin; however, because of its long half-life (14–20 days), albumin stores are often adequate. In liver disease, it is often an indicator of a chronic process.
- Decrease in ALT and AST with increase in plasma bilirubin concentration and a prolonged PT is indicative of a poor prognosis.

Incidence and Demographics
- Unknown

Risk Factors
- Alchohol
- Drugs metabolized by liver
- Genetic predisposition

Prevention and Screening
- Annual evaluation of LFTs in high-risk patients

Assessment
HISTORY
- The most important part of the evaluation
- Many patients are asymptomatic with mild, transient elevations
- Generalized symptoms of fever, anorexia, malaise, weight loss, jaundice, arthralgias, myalgias, rash, and pruritus may be present
- Gastrointestinal symptoms: Anorexia, nausea, vomiting, abdominal pain, dark urine, and pale stools
- Additional history is aimed at identifying potential risk factors: History of

hepatitis exposure, gallstones, transfusions, previous surgery, medications (including vitamins and herbs, OTCs, acetaminophen), alcohol and drug use, sexual practices, occupational exposure, and travel history

PHYSICAL EXAM
- Skin exam: Jaundice (include sclera), spider angiomas, palmar erythema, gynecomastia, caput medusae (annular purple discoloration around umbilicus or ostomy), and ecchymosis
- Abdominal exam: Ascites, tenderness (usually right upper quadrant), enlarged gallbladder, hepatomegaly, and splenomegaly; the liver may be smaller than normal in advanced liver disease
- Extremities: Asterixis, temporal and proximal muscle wasting, and peripheral edema

DIAGNOSTIC STUDIES
- If the patient is asymptomatic, repeat liver function tests first; if normal, repeat testing in 3–6 months is suggested
- If repeat is abnormal, obtain hepatitis serologies to exclude viral hepatitis A, B, and C (see section on viral hepatitis)
- If the patient is symptomatic, further tests are guided by history and physical exam (see Table 9–1); consider:
  - Mono spot and CMV IgG, IgM titers
  - Abdominal ultrasound: Best screening test to evaluate for gallstones; it can also detect biliary tree dilation, biliary obstruction, cholecystitis, fatty liver, and liver parenchymal disease
  - Computed tomography (CT) scan (with IV contrast): Best test to evaluate liver parenchymal disease and space-occupying lesions (tumor or abscess); also can assess biliary tree dilation and identify obstructing lesion
  - Magnetic resonance imaging (MRI): Similar to CT scan but can better visualize vessels without the use of IV contrast
  - Endoscopic retrograde cholangiopancreatography (ERCP) and percutaneous transhepatic cholangiography (PTC): Usually done after screening with ultrasound, CT, or MRI to further assess cause, location, and extent of biliary tree abnormalities
  - Liver biopsy: Definitive study to determine the cause and extent of hepatocellular and infiltrative liver disease; biopsy may be guided using ultrasound or CT

Management
- Aimed at correcting underlying cause
  NONPHARMACOLOGIC TREATMENT
  - Avoid drugs and other agents that are hepatotoxic
  - Management will vary depending on etiology

Table 9-1. Interpreting Liver Function Tests

Liver Function Test	Enzyme Found In	Cause of Elevation	Seen in the Following Conditions	Comments
Bilirubin: Direct (conjugated, processed by liver)	Liver, blood, urine	Impaired excretion of bilirubin from the liver	Hepatocellular disease, biliary tract obstruction, drugs	
Bilirubin: Indirect (unconjugated, not processed by the liver)	Liver, blood, urine	Hepatic bilirubin uptake is decreased	Hemolysis, drugs, heart failure	
Alkaline Phosphatase	Bone, liver	Impaired biliary tract function (cholestasis) or infiltrative liver disease hepatic excretion	**Mild:** hepatitis, cirrhosis, early cancer **High:** biliary tract obstruction, cholestasis	Increases with age, women > men Also elevated in bone disease
GGT	Liver, pancreas, kidney, heart brain	Hepatic excretion	Sensitive for acute alcohol ingestion	Differentiates the origin of an elevated ALP between bone and liver
Transaminases	Many tissues	Acute hepatocellular injury—from necrosis or inflammation	**Mild:** biliary obstruction, mild viral chronic or active and alcoholic hepatitis, wcirrhosis, and liver metastases **High:** viral hepatitis, drug-induced liver injury	Do not indicate severity of liver injury; most common cause of elevation is alcoholic hepatitis
ALT	Predominantly liver, more specific test	Celiac disease		
AST	Liver, cardiac, skeletal, kidney, brain			AST twice as high as ALT typical of alcoholic liver injury
Prothrombin Time	Blood	Impaired hepatic synthesis of coagulation factors	Significant liver disease	
Albumin	Blood serum	Impaired hepatic protein synthesis, excess protein loss	Chronic liver disease, malnutrition	May decrease with age

Special Considerations
- Geriatric patients: Higher incidence of neoplasm in this age group
- Pregnancy: Elevated ALP common since present in placental tissue; CT scans are contraindicated

When to Consult, Refer, Hospitalize
- Consult with or refer to a physician or specialist when significantly abnormal liver function tests persist without an identifiable cause, or for symptomatic patients in need of specialized diagnostic tests and management

Follow-Up
- Recheck studies every 3–6 months

Constipation/Encopresis

Description
- Constipation is a symptom as well as a diagnosis where there is decrease in the frequency of stools, excessive difficulty passing stools, and straining with defecation.
- Encopresis is fecal soiling or staining underwear after 4 years of age either due to constipation (retentive) or other factors such as resistance to toilet training or reluctance to leave activities to use toilet.

Etiology
- Stool remains in the colon for a prolonged period of time
- Most common cause is functional etiologies which include poor dietary intake of fiber and fluids, behavioral habits such as change in environment with travel or schedule, sedentary lifestyle. Occurs in children most often when cereal is first introduced to diet, during toilet training, or entry to school
- Psychogenic; chronic constipation can begin in the first year of life
- Neurologic dysfunction causing a change in colonic motility; often seen in the elderly; people with diabetes, spinal cord injury, or neurological diseases such as multiple sclerosis or Parkinson's disease
- Metabolic disorders such as hypothyroidism, hyperparathyroidism, hypokalemia, hypercalcemia, and uremia
- Obstruction; anorectal pain from fissures, hemorrhoids, abscesses or proctitis, mechanical
- Medications: Opiate analgesics, calcium channel blockers, anticholinergics, diuretics, aluminum-based antacids, calcium and iron supplements, NSAIDs, antihistamines, antipsychotics, antiparkinson agents, congenital disorders, and laxative abuse

Incidence and Demographics
- 2.5 million healthcare visits/year for constipation; increased incidence in elderly
- 4% of all pediatric visits are for constipation; in pediatrics the peak age is 2–4 years and males > females

Risk Factors

- Aging, chronic disease, medications, poor dietary fiber in diet and decreased fluid intake, immobility
- Children with inappropriate expectations from parents regarding GI physiology; pregnancy; breastfed infant (due to iron supplementation in mother)

Prevention and Screening

- Exercise, increase daily fiber and fluid intake
- If possible, establish time each day to defecate and do not ignore the urge to defecate
- Anticipatory guidance regarding toilet training techniques

Assessment

HISTORY

- Determine patient's/family's definition of constipation
- Stool history (constipation since birth may indicate Hirschsprung's): Decreased frequency to <2 times weekly; excessive straining/difficulty defecating, bloated feeling, rectal fullness, persistent sense of need to evacuate
- Current pattern, character, consistency, color, straining, blood, soiling of underwear
- Use of laxatives, manual extraction, fecal or urinary incontinence
- Medications, diet, fluid intake, anorexia, abdominal or rectal pain, and weight loss
- Family history: Colon cancer, Hirschsprung's disease, other bowel diseases
- In children, also inquire about toilet training history, abuse, trauma, history of behavioral problems

PHYSICAL EXAM

- Vital signs, including weight, growth parameters
- Distention, abdominal tenderness, palpable stool in the colon, and decreased bowel sounds may be present
- Rectal exam: Sphincter tone, fissures, size of rectal vault, rectal prolapse, presence of stool and consistency, masses
- In frail elderly, evaluate systemic signs of fever, delirium, urinary retention, arrhythmias, and tachypnea

DIAGNOSTIC STUDIES

- Stool for occult blood; rarely, CBC to check for leukocytosis and anemia (indication of colorectal cancer)
- Electrolytes, calcium, BUN, creatinine, and glucose to rule out hyperparathyroidism, hypokalemia, hypercalcemia, and uremia; thyroid function tests to rule out hypothyroidism
- Flat plate and upright abdominal films to evaluate for obstruction
- Colonoscopy or barium enema if patient is anemic to evaluate for colorectal cancer; consider in any adult with new onset after age 40

Differential Diagnosis
- All ages:
  - Partial obstruction
  - Irritable bowel syndrome
  - Spinal cord lesions/trauma
  - Hypothyroidism
  - Rectal prolapse
  - Rectocele
  - Neurological myopathies
  - Rectal fissures
- Adults:
  - Colon cancer
  - Hemorrhoids
  - Irritable bowel syndrome
- Children:
  - Hirschsprung's disease
  - Cerebral palsy
  - Breastfeeding
  - Cystic fibrosis
  - Down syndrome

Management
NONPHARMACOLOGIC TREATMENT
- Infants <6 months old:
  - If exclusively on formula or breast milk, continue with same; review formula preparation and fluid intake of breastfeeding mother
- Infants 6–12 months old:
  - Continue present formula or breastfeeding
  - Offer water between feedings
  - Add high-fiber food such as prunes, apricots, plums, peas and beans
  - May add apple juice or Karo syrup to diet
- Toddlers and preschoolers:
  - Increase water intake and decrease juice intake
  - Offer whole fruits instead of juice
  - Increase fiber in diet so child is receiving child's age plus 5 = the grams of fiber per day required
- All over 5 years of age:
  - Increase fiber; age 3–15: Age + 5 = g of fiber/day; adults: 20–35 g/day
  - Increase fiber gradually, over a 2-week period
  - Increase fluid intake, particularly water; for adults, 1.5–2 liters/day
  - Physical exercise; bowel training program/behavior modification
- Nonretentive encopresis:
  - Increase child's responsibility, provide incentives
  - Counsel parents to stop any pressures on child regarding defecation, accidents
  - No punishment for defecating in pants

PHARMACOLOGIC TREATMENT
- If after a month the nonpharmacological methods are not effective:
- Children:
  - Lactulose, sorbital and Miralax are generally well-tolerated in children.
  - Mineral oil orally 1–3 mL/kg/day (should not be used under a year of age because of risk of aspiration); this needs to be disguised to get children to swallow it; is usually second line.
  - Initiation phase: Home colonic clean out (goal: yellow liquid stools) often achieved using high doses of MiraLax (2–3 capfuls for 2 or more days with dosing more dependent on findings on physical exam than age and weight dosing) or using repeated doses of magnesium citrate (use age and weight dosing and repeat bid to tid for 2 or more days); fleet enemas often needed in this phase; because this is more invasive and often difficult for parents and child, this decision needs to be made in the context of physical examination
  - Surfactants—used to soften stools; docusate sodium (Colace) for children 3–6 years, 20–60 mg/day; 6–12 years, 40–150 mg/day; used short-term up to 2 weeks; may be used longer and do not induce dependency
- Adults:
  - Hydrophilic colloids or bulk-forming agents: Psyllium (Metamucil, Fiberall) 3.4 grams 1–3 times daily; methylcellulose (Citrucel) 2 grams 1–3 times daily; polycarbophil (FiberCon) 1 gram 1–4 times daily; can be used on a long-term basis
  - Surfactants: Used to soften stools; docusate sodium (Colace) 50–200 mg daily; used short-term up to 2 weeks; may be used longer and does not induce dependency
  - Osmotic laxatives: Used for acute constipation and should not be used long-term; should result in a bowel movement in 0.5–3 hours, or longer; magnesium hydroxide suspension (Milk of Magnesia) 30–60 mL x one dose (should not be given to patients with renal insufficiency); magnesium citrate 240 mL bottle x one dose; sodium phosphate (Fleet enema) x one
  - Stimulants: Stimulate fluid secretion, colonic contraction; may cause cramping; use infrequently
  - Lubiprostone (Amitiza) 24 mcg bid is approved for chronic constipation in adults as well as irritable bowel syndrome, constipation type
- Management for constipation with fecal impaction:
  - First removal of impaction by use of sodium phosphate enemas; 2–3 enemas over a 2-day period
  - Once impaction removed, begin long-term therapy
    » Mineral oil: Adults 60 mL/dose, max 2 doses/day; children 1 mL/kg/dose bid, max 90 mL /day OR
    » Lactulose: Adults 15 mL bid; children 0.5 mL/kg/dose bid
    » Treat for 3–6 months along with nonpharmacological treatments

LENGTH OF TREATMENT
- Varies depending on agent used; see specific agents

Special Consideration
- Evaluate diet, fluid intake, medications, activity in older adult

When to Consult, Refer, Hospitalize

- Refer to a gastroenterologist if patient fails to respond to treatment; stool positive for occult blood, weight loss is present, and over the age of 50 with sudden, unexplained change in bowel pattern
- In children, refer to gastroenterologist if child has failed at initial attempts to disimpact or to surgeon if symptoms of obstruction

Follow-Up

- Patient education should be provided regarding food, diet, exercise, and medications
  EXPECTED COURSE
  - With treatment, constipation should resolve in several days if there is no significant underlying problem such as bowel obstruction
  - With exercise, a daily bowel regimen, and an increase in fiber and fluids, constipation should, for the most part, resolve permanently
  - In cases of fecal impaction, follow up every 2 months after impaction removed for 6 months to evaluate progress

  COMPLICATIONS
  - Bowel obstruction, socialization, enuresis, decreased appetite

Diarrhea

Description

- Increased frequency, looseness, and volume of stools; may be either acute or chronic condition; infants 6–24 months are at highest risk of morbidity and mortality

Etiology

- Diarrhea is produced by one or more of the following: abnormal intestinal motility, decreased water absorption, and/or increased fluid secretion
- *Acute diarrhea*: Most commonly caused by infectious agents, bacterial toxins, or drug (see Table 9–2)
- *Chronic diarrhea*: Can be due to many causes but often from hardy agents spread by fecal-oral route

Incidence and Demographics

- Common worldwide; accounts for about 12% of hospitalizations for children <4 years old

Risk Factors

- Day care setting
- Travel to area with water and soil contamination
- Improper cooking and preparation methods, especially street vendors where constancy of temperature is an issue
- Recent antibiotic use

Prevention and Screening

- Handwashing, particularly after using bathroom
- Avoid water supply while traveling to endemic areas
- Proper food preparation and cooking

Assessment

HISTORY
- Determine if symptoms were sudden in onset or chronic
- Obtain medication history, including any recent courses of antibiotics plus laxative or antacid use
- Inquire about sexual practices and risk for HIV infection
- Obtain description of bowel pattern, contributing factors such as certain foods or stress, family history, and stool characteristics (bloody, watery, with mucous, fatty, foul-smelling)
- Weight loss, ecchymosis, peripheral neuropathy, joint pains
- Travel history: Incubation period is 2–4 days for many viruses
- Surgical history; history of exposure to others with similar illness
- Symptoms of hyperthyroidism

PHYSICAL EXAM
- There may be signs of dehydration: Tachycardia, confusion, orthostatic hypotension, poor skin turgor, dry mucous membranes, depressed fontanelle, eyes sunken, crying without tears, listless, decreased urine output; fever is variable and ranges from afebrile to significant elevations
- Make sure to weigh patient, particularly infants
- Abdominal exam may reveal hyperactive bowel sounds and generalized tenderness
- Signs of peritonitis (rebound tenderness) may be seen with severe inflammatory diarrhea
- Particularly in children, look for other possible causes of diarrhea such as otitis media and urinary tract infection (UTI)

DIAGNOSTIC STUDIES
- Based on presentation, severity, and duration; test if symptoms severe or diarrhea lasts >7 days
- Stool cultures, ova and parasites, *Clostridium difficile* toxin, occult blood
- Stool for fecal leukocytes; with noninflammatory diarrhea, tissue invasion does not occur so fecal leukocytes are not found; with inflammatory diarrhea, fecal leukocytes are generally present; ELISA assay, latex agglutinations, or PCR for rotavirus
- CBC to look for anemia, leukocytosis, and eosinophilia (often seen in parasitic infections and inflammatory bowel diseases)
- Electrolytes; evaluate for hypokalemia, hyponatremia
- BUN and creatinine; elevations may be indicative of dehydration
- Blood cultures if systemic infection is suspected—high fever, chills, leukocytosis
- In patients with diarrhea lasting >3 weeks:
  – Sigmoidoscopy or colonoscopy to diagnose colitis
    » Evaluate for malabsorption: Vitamin B12, folate, vitamin D, albumin, cholesterol, iron, iron binding capacity, prothrombin time, D-xylose absorption test, 24-hour fecal fat collection to diagnose steatorrhea

Table 9–2. Common Causes of Acute Diarrhea

Organism	Transmission	Incubation	Signs and Symptoms	Type of Stools	Lab Data	Special Notations
Viral Rota and Norwalk	Fecal-oral	24–72 hours	Nausea, vomiting, cramps Fever	Watery	No WBCs in stool	Most common causes: Rotavirus in children (6–24 months) More common in winter Norwalk in all others Vomiting most prominent symptom in children Diarrhea most prominent symptoms in adults
Bacterial *Staphylo-coccus* *aureus*	Food: Ham, poultry, creams, mayonnaise	30 min–6 hours	Nausea, vomiting, cramps	Soft, not watery	No WBCs in stool	Onset abrupt, others with symptoms, look for common source
Clostridium *perfringens*	Food: Beef, ham, Mexican cuisine	8–12 hours	Nausea, vomiting, epigastric pain	Watery	No WBCs in stool	Onset not as abrupt as with *S.* *aureus*
Campylobacter *jejuni*	Food: Chicken Water Fecal material	1–7 days	Nausea, vomiting, abdominal pain, malaise, fever	Watery, gross and occult blood	WBCs in stool Positive culture	Abdominal pain can mimic appendicitis
Salmonella	Food: Poultry, red meat, eggs, unpasteurized milk Water Contact with infected pets (turtles, reptiles) Fecal-oral	6–72 hours	Nausea, vomiting, abdominal cramps, fever	Watery, gross and occult blood	WBCs in stool Positive culture	Common in children <5 and adults >70 years

Table 9-2. Common Causes of Acute Diarrhea (cont.)

Organism	Transmission	Incubation	Signs and Symptoms	Type of Stools	Lab Data	Special Notations
Shigella	Food Water Fecal-oral	1–7 days	Abdominal pain Fever	Watery, Occult blood, No gross blood	WBCs in stool Positive culture	Most common in 1–4-year-olds, common in child care centers
Escherichia coli	Food, water contaminated with feces "Traveler's diarrhea"	10 hours–6 days	Abdominal cramps	Watery	Usually no WBCs Positive culture	History of recent travel
Protozoal Giardia lamblia	Fecal-oral Water	1–4 weeks	Abdominal pain, flatulence, distention, Anorexia	Soft, pale, watery foul-smelling	Stool positive for ova and parasites (O&P)	An acute presentation of chronic or recurrent diarrhea

Adapted from *Clinical guidelines in family practice* (4th ed.), by C. R. Uphold & M. V. Graham, 2003, Gainesville, FL: Barmarrae Books, Inc.

Differential Diagnosis
- Appendicitis
- Volvulus
- Cystic fibrosis
- Intussusception
- Inflammatory bowel syndrome
- Irritable bowel syndrome
- Meningitis
- Pancreatitis
- Pneumonia
- Lactose intolerance
- Colon cancer

Management
NONPHARMACOLOGIC TREATMENT
- Adequate hydration with fluids containing electrolytes and carbohydrates
- In infants without signs of dehydration, continue with formula or breast milk but increase amount. May change to soy-based formula for diarrhea (Isomil/DF, Enfamil, Prosobee or Lactofree) while ill
- Normal diet when patient able to tolerate; no longer recommending BRAT diet (bananas, rice, applesauce, toast) because not calorie-dense and not enough fat and protein

- In children with signs of mild dehydration, give 50 mL/kg of oral replacement therapy (ORT) such as Pedialyte, plus 10 mL/kg for each stool over a 4-hour period; sports drinks may be used in children >3 years old
- If vomiting present, start with small volumes: 5 mL q 2–3 minutes and increase gradually if vomiting subsides; also increase ORT by estimated volume loss with emesis

PHARMACOLOGIC TREATMENT

- Antidiarrheal agents: If no contraindications (fever, bloody stools), may consider using:
    - Loperamide (Imodium): Adults: 4 mg initially followed by 2 mg after each loose stool for a maximum of 16 mg in 24 hours; NOT recommended in children
    - Bismuth subsalicylate (Pepto-Bismol): Adults: 2 tablets or 30 mL q 30–60 minutes, max 8 doses/day; children 6–9 years: 10 mL q 30–60-minutes; 9–12 years: 15 mL q 30–60 minutes, max 8 doses/day
- In adults, empirical antibiotic treatment while awaiting stool culture results for patients with moderate to severe fever, bloody stools, tenesmus, or the presence of fecal leukocytes
    - Fluoroquinolones: Drugs of choice as they provide good coverage for most invasive bacterial pathogens
    - Ciprofloxacin (Cipro) 500 mg bid OR levofloxacin (Levaquin) 500 mg daily
    Alternative agents
    - Trimethoprim-sulfamethoxazole 160/800 (Bactrim DS) bid OR erythromycin 250–500 mg qid
- If *Giardia* or *C. difficile* is suspected:
    - Metronidazole (Flagyl) 250 mg tid for 7 days (avoid alcohol use during and for 48 hours after); for C.Difficile, 500 mg tid for 10–14 days
    - Option for C. Difficile, oral vancomycin
- Generally antibiotics are not used to treat children until the causative organism is known and then only:
    - *Campylobacter*: Erythromycin 20–50 mg/kg/day divided into 4 doses for 5–7 days
    - *Shigella*: Bactrim 1mL/kg/day divided into 2 doses for 5 days
    - *E. coli*: Bactrim 1 mL/kg/day divided into 2 doses for 3 days
    - *Giardia*: Furazolidone 6 mg/kg/day divided into 4 doses for 7–10 days (Furox-one 5mg/kg/day in 4 divided doses
    - Alinia: New product for *Giardia*; may be given orally; do not use in children younger than 12 months; suspension for ages 1–11 yrs; tablets only; tablets only for 12 years and older

LENGTH OF TREATMENT

- Depends on underlying cause; for acute diarrhea due to an infection, generally treat 5–7 days

Special Considerations
- For chronic diarrhea, treatment may vary according to underlying cause
- Geriatric patients at greater risk for dehydration and complications
- Neonates are at greater risk for severe infection and should be immediately referred
- Pregnancy and lactation: If antimicrobials are required, check safety profile for use during pregnancy and lactation
- Other: Immunocompromised patients are a greater risk for chronic diarrhea from an infectious process such as cryptosporidium (a common, self-limiting infection that people with an intact immune system are able to clear in a few days without treatment)

When to Consult, Refer, Hospitalize
- Consult with physician for any child with significant signs and symptoms of dehydration (>10% increased pulse rate, poor skin turgor, depressed fontanelle, delayed capillary refill, <1 mg/kg/hour urine output)
- Consult for possible hospitalization for infants <3 months with bacterial diarrhea
- Any patient with bloody diarrhea, fever, acute abdominal pain, and leukocytosis should be referred and evaluated immediately in an acute-care setting
- Anyone who has not had resolution of diarrhea within 3 weeks needs to be referred to a gastroenterologist for evaluation

Follow-Up
- Depends on cause and severity; none may be necessary if hydration maintained
    EXPECTED COURSE
    - Acute diarrhea should resolve in 24–48 hours

    COMPLICATIONS
    - Will vary depending on underlying cause: Dehydration, electrolyte imbalance, sepsis, shock, malnutrition, anal fissures, and hemorrhoids

Pyloric Stenosis

Description
- Hypertrophy of the pyloric muscle, causing increasing duodenal obstruction resulting in projectile vomiting in infants 2–4 weeks of age

Etiology
- Cause unknown; genetic predisposition and environmental factors include neonatal hypergastrenemia and gastric hyperactivity, increased vascularity, post-macrolide antibiotic (erythromycin) exposure, or treatment of pertussis in first 2 weeks of life

Incidence and Demographics
- 1:500 live births
- Males are affected 3–4 times more often than females
- Caucasians (2–4:1,000) have higher incidence than Hispanics (1.8:1,000) and African Americans (0.7:1,000)
- Slight familial incidence

Risk Factors
- Firstborn males
- History of hyperbilirubinemia

Prevention and Screening
- Close monitoring of vomiting in first 4 weeks of life

Assessment

HISTORY
- Vomiting begins at 2–8 weeks of age, rapidly progressing to projectile; peaks at 3–5 weeks
- Presentation may be later in premature infants; evolves more slowly and is less projectile
- Infant is hungry
- Fretfulness
- Eventual dehydration, weight loss, lethargy are late findings

PHYSICAL EXAM
- Visible gastric peristaltic waves from left to right across the abdomen
- Palpable pyloric olive in the right upper quadrant (RUQ)
- Note hydration status
Diagnostic studies:
- Hypochloremic alkalosis with potassium depletion
- Abdominal ultrasonography demonstrates hypoechoic ring and increased measurement of the pylorus: >4 mm thickness or <16 mm length
- Upper GI demonstrates delayed gastric emptying with narrowing and elongation of the pyloric channel

Differential Diagnosis
- Overfeeding
- Improper handling
- Protein or lactose intolerance
- GERD
- Gastroenteritis
- Metabolic disorders
- Infections, including sepsis, UTI
- CNS disorders (e.g., bleed, hydrocephalus)

Management
- Referral to pediatric surgery for pyloromyotomy

When to Consult, Refer, Hospitalize
- Surgical consultation and admission to the hospital

Follow-Up
EXPECTED COURSE
- Following surgery, nothing by mouth for 12–24 hours, then advance to full feeds by 36–48 hours
- Discharge when tolerating full-strength feeds
- Surgery is considered curative

COMPLICATIONS
- Gastric spasms cause continued spitting of feeds after surgery; encourage parents to feed small volumes slowly and frequently reassure the family
- Overfeeding a ravenous baby can lead to regurgitation

Cystic Fibrosis (CF)

Description
- Most common lethal genetic disease in the U.S., caused by defect on chromosome 7, autosomal recessive inheritance pattern
- Classic diagnostic triad is elevated sweat chloride concentration; production of abnormally tenacious mucus secretion in the gut, pancreas, and hepatobiliary system, resulting in obstruction and chronic pulmonary disease
- CF should be considered in any infant with chronic diarrhea and failure to thrive. There is a possible association between GERD and CF; although CF affects GI system, long-term progressive pulmonary disease leads to mortality

Etiology
- CF gene is located on the long arm of chromosome 7

Incidence and Demographics
- 1:2,500 White births
- Median survival rate is 30 years

Risk Factors
- Autosomal recessive inheritance
  - Parents are carriers and are clinically normal
  - Males and females equally affected
  - Inheritance horizontal, siblings affected but parents are not
  - The recurrence risk is 1:4 for each pregnancy
  - 1 in 22 persons is a carrier

Prevention and Screening
- Prenatal screening of future pregnancies
- Artificial insemination

Assessment
HISTORY
- Newborn period
  - Meconium ileus
  - Prolonged jaundice

- Infancy/childhood
  - Failure to thrive
  - Parents may report that child's tears or skin are salty-tasting
  - GI discomfort with increased flatulence
  - Constipation and/or bulky, greasy stools
  - Fat-soluble vitamin deficiency
  - Recurrent or persistent pneumonia
  - Heat prostration
  - Intussusception of the appendix
- Late childhood/early adulthood
  - Pancreatitis
  - Cirrhosis
  - Gallstones

PHYSICAL EXAM
- Poor growth
- Wheezing, dyspnea, cough
- Digital clubbing, cyanosis
- Abdominal distention, pain
- Increased flatulence secondary to pancreatic insufficiency and malabsorption, foul-smelling stools
- Hypoalbuminemia, edema, hepatomegaly
- Higher incidence of rectal prolapse, nasal polyps

DIAGNOSTIC STUDIES
- Positive sweat test: Sweat chloride >60 mmol/L; may be unreliable in infants <1 month old
- Genetic confirmation

Differential Diagnosis
- Failure to thrive
- Celiac disease
- Chronic sinusitis
- Reactive airway disease
- Bronchiectasis

Management
NONPHARMACOLOGIC TREATMENT
- High-caloric nutritional support, 100–150 Kcal/day
- Multidisciplinary team approach
- Nighttime nasogastric/gastrostomy/jejunostomy supplementation as necessary
- Chest physiotherapy before meals

PHARMACOLOGIC TREATMENT
- Pancreatic enzyme supplementation (lipase) <2,500 units/kg/meal
- Vitamin replacement: Particularly A, E, D, K, as these are poorly absorbed secondary to steatorrhea

• If GERD coexists, administer sucrafate 2 hours before and 1 hour after oral medications
• Ensure appropriate immunizations, including annual influenza vaccine
• Early treatment with antibiotics for respiratory infections, especially antipseudomonal agents
• May need aerosolized bronchodilator therapy

LENGTH OF TREATMENT
• Lifelong; therapy centers on optimal growth and nutrition and management of respiratory infections and symptoms

When to Consult, Refer, Hospitalize
• Hospitalization frequently necessary to treat infection and for pulmonary symptom management

Follow-Up
EXPECTED COURSE
• The average life span is 30 years; with current improved treatment regimens, life expectancy is increasing, challenging the adult providers who need to co-manage with pediatric consultants

COMPLICATIONS
• Continued failure to thrive
• Progression of respiratory insufficiency to obstructive airway disease
• 95% of males with CF are infertile secondary to failure of development of structures of the Wolffian tract (vas deferens)
• Decreased female fertility
• Death

Acute Abdominal Pain

Description
• New onset of pain in the abdominal area

Etiology
• Abdominal pain can be caused by obstruction of hollow viscus, altered bowel motility, capsular distention, peritoneal irritation, mucosal ulceration, vascular insufficiency, nerve injury, abdominal wall injury, or pain referred from an extra-abdominal site
• Common etiologies in various age groups are:
  – All ages: Gastroenteritis, viral most common
  – <2 years old: Trauma, intussusception, incarcerated hernia, UTI, and intestinal malrotation
  – 2–5 years old: Sickle cell anemia, right lower lobe pneumonia, UTI
  – >5 years: Appendicitis
  – Adolescent: Dysmenorrhea, ectopic pregnancy, tubo-ovarian pathology
  – Adults: Pancreatitis, cholecystitis, renal stones, peptic ulcer disease (PUD)

Assessment

HISTORY

- Determine the onset, progression, migration, character and intensity, and localization
- Onset: *Sudden, rapid, or gradual*
  - Sudden: Patient is able to relate time of onset to a precise moment
    » Most often associated with perforation of the gastrointestinal tract that may be caused by a duodenal or gastric ulcer, diverticulum, or a foreign body
    » Other causes: Ruptured ectopic pregnancy, ruptured aortic aneurysm, mesenteric infarction, or an embolism of the abdominal muscle
  - Rapid: Begins within a few seconds and increases in severity in a short period of time
    » Often associated with intestinal obstruction, ureteral stone, cholecystitis, pancreatitis, diverticulitis, appendicitis, and penetrating duodenal or gastric ulcer
  - Gradual: Pain that slowly becomes more severe over a course of hours or days
    » History of onset is vague
    » Often associated with a chronic inflammatory process, neoplasm, or a large bowel obstruction
- Progression:
  - Perforated bowel often presents as a sudden onset of pain that dramatically abates if the perforation seals off and there is no further leakage of bowel content or blood into the peritoneum
  - A small bowel obstruction may present as intermittent attacks of pain that progress into a steady constant pain suggestive of vascular compromise
- Migration:
  - Pain that changes from the original site of onset to another location
  - Acute appendicitis may begin as periumbilical or epigastric pain and then localize to the right lower quadrant
  - A perforated duodenal ulcer causes pain initially in the epigastrium (due to leakage of gastric contents); can migrate to the lower quadrants where the gastric material localizes in the abdominal cavity
  - Cholecystitis often causes irritation of the phrenic nerve resulting in diaphragmatic pain that can radiate to the right shoulder, right scapula, or between the shoulder blades (Kehr's sign)
- Character and intensity:
  - Cramping, dull, or aching and is either constant or intermittent
  - Cramping (or colicky) abdominal pain increases in intensity in short waves, with intermittent periods of complete absence of pain; often is associated with mechanical small bowel obstruction; short pain-free intervals may indicate a more proximal bowel obstruction, whereas, longer pain-free intervals may indicate a more distal obstruction
  - Dull or aching abdominal pain that is constant is often caused by distention or edema of the abdominal wall, bowel wall, or from the inflammation of an abdominal organ (such as the capsule of the liver or spleen)

- Localization:
  - Visceral pain due to distension of a hollow viscus is often localized poorly and often perceived in the midline; epigastric, midabdominal, or lower abdominal area
  - Patients with visceral pain frequently change positions in an attempt to alleviate the pain
  - Somatic pain is due to peritoneal inflammation and is usually sharper and more localized to the diseased area
  - Patients with peritonitis often lie still on one side with their knees and hips flexed
  - Pain from peritonitis is intensified by jarring motions (bumping into the bed)
  - In children, the closer the pain is to the umbilicus, less likely it is to be organic
- Additional information:
  - Have the patient rate his/her pain on a scale of 1–10
  - Determine if pain interferes with sleep; factors that precipitate or relieve the pain; relationship of pain to meals, specific foods, menstrual cycle, urination, defecation, exertion, and inspiration
  - Fever, chills, nausea, vomiting, diarrhea, constipation, or urogenital symptoms may be present
  - Blood in the stool, urine, or emesis may be present
  - Social history including alcohol and intravenous drug use
  - Gynecological history: Evaluate for possible pregnancy or sexually transmitted disease (STD)
  - In children, include questions regarding irritability, ability to console, fussiness with feedings, when crying does infant clench fists or draw feet up

PHYSICAL EXAM

- Assess for fever, tachycardia, orthostatic hypotension, pallor, jaundice, perspiration, restlessness, and body positioning
- Abdominal exam: Perform with knees flexed if in severe pain
- Observe for any surgical scars, distention
- Bowel sounds: High-pitched tinkling sounds suggest a dilated bowel with air and fluid under tension; rushes of high-pitched sounds indicate intestinal obstruction; absent bowel sounds indicate an ileus or peritonitis
- Inspect and palpate for hernias: Abdominal, inguinal, umbilical
- Palpate for localized tenderness, rigidity, guarding, and rebound tenderness (an indication of peritonitis); check for CVA tenderness (with pyelonephritis or urolithiasis)
- Evaluate for hepatosplenomegaly and fluid wave (ascites from liver disease)
- Assess for Rovsing's sign, psoas sign, obturator sign (see appendicitis), and Murphy's sign (see cholecystitis)
- Rectal exam: rectal wall pain can be an indication of appendicitis or abscess
- Pelvic exam: for all women with abdominal pain
- In children assess growth parameters
- Other systems for possible origin because of possibility of referred pain, based on history

DIAGNOSTIC STUDIES
- CBC with differential; may show leukocytosis or anemia
- Serum electrolytes, glucose, BUN, and creatinine
- LFTs may be abnormal with liver involvement (AST, ALT, Alk phos, bilirubin, PT, PTT)
- Amylase and lipase may be elevated in pancreatic disease
- Beta HCG: Always obtain in women of childbearing age
- STD testing if appropriate
- Urinalysis to rule out infection and hematuria (children with appendicitis may have some RBCs and WBCs in urine)
- Check stool for blood
- Abdominal ultrasound or transvaginal ultrasound for possible tubo-ovarian pathology
- CT scan for possible appendicitis, abscess, diverticular disease, and enlarged pancreas
- Consider if diagnosis unclear:
    - ECG: Rule out referred pain from cardiac etiology
    - Chest x-ray to evaluate for heart, lung, and mediastinal disease
    - Flat plate and upright abdominal film
    - Abdominal MRI
    - Upper and lower GI barium studies
    - Endoscopy, colonoscopy, sigmoidoscopy
    - ERCP
    - Hydroxy-iminodiacetic acid (HIDA) gallbladder scan

Differential Diagnosis
- Diffuse pain
    - Generalized peritonitis
    - Metabolic disturbances
    - Psychogenic illness
    - Gastroenteritis
- Right upper quadrant
    - Cholecystitis
    - Cholelithiasis
    - Hepatitis
    - Hepatic abscess
    - Right lower lobe pneumonia
    - Subphrenic abscess
- Right lower quadrant
    - Appendicitis
    - Cecal diverticulitis
    - Ectopic pregnancy
    - Ovarian cyst/torsion

- Endometriosis
- Pelvic inflammatory disease
- Ureteral calculi
- Mittelschmerz (colicky pain associated with ovulation)
- Left upper quadrant
  - Splenic enlargement/hematoma
  - Left lower lobe pneumonia
  - Cardiac disease
  - Pancreatitis
- Left lower quadrant
  - Diverticulitis
  - Ectopic pregnancy
  - Ovarian cyst/torsion
  - Endometriosis
  - Mittelschmerz
  - Ureteral calculi
  - Pelvic inflammatory disease
- Epigastric or midline
  - Gastritis
  - Cardiac disease
  - Peptic ulcer disease
  - Pancreatitis
  - Abdominal aortic aneurysm

Management
- Varies depending on the underlying cause of the abdominal pain (see specific gastrointestinal problems discussed in this chapter)

Special Considerations
- Geriatric patients: Presentation may be subtle, without classic symptoms

When to Consult, Refer, Hospitalize
- Refer for immediate surgical evaluation in cases of acute abdominal pain associated with high fever with leukocytosis, clinical findings suggestive of peritonitis, evidence of bleeding
- Consult with a physician or refer to specialist if diagnosis is unclear or patient is unstable

Follow-Up
- Varies by etiology

COMMON GASTROINTESTINAL CONDITIONS

Acute Gastroenteritis (AGE)

Description
- General term used to describe symptoms of nausea, vomiting, and/or diarrhea caused by inflammation from infection of the stomach and intestinal mucosa. Symptoms may be caused by cholinergic hyperactivity or by the gut as it attempts to rid itself of irritating contents.

Etiology
- The visceral afferent nerves of the GI tract and the chemoreceptors are stimulated and send messages to the cerebral cortex that induce vomiting
- Diarrhea is produced from the increased fluid secretion caused by inflammation of the bowel lining, or by damage to bowel mucosa or abnormal intestinal motility
- Most commonly caused by a viral, bacterial, or protozoal/parasitic infection
- Also can occur from an allergic or chemical reaction, from swallowed inorganic materials, or emotional stress
- Gastric distress is one of the most common adverse reactions to medication

Incidence and Demographics
- Very common worldwide

Risk Factors
- Foreign travel, ingesting contaminated food or water
- Exposure to others who have an infectious gastroenteritis
- Day care or institutional living
- Medication adverse effects
- Recent course of antibiotics
- Lactose intolerance

Prevention and Screening
- Careful food preparation, good handwashing, properly cleaning fresh fruits and vegetables prior to eating; drink bottled water and cooked foods when traveling to foreign countries. Use bottled water for ice in drinks and tooth brushing.

Assessment
HISTORY
- Acute onset of nausea, vomiting, and/or diarrhea; usually multiple episodes; symptoms may vary from mild to severe
- Fever, abdominal pain, anorexia, malaise, myalgia, and headache may be present
- Characteristics of diarrhea: watery, soft, with mucus or blood

PHYSICAL EXAM
- With severe AGE, may see symptoms of dehydration and electrolyte imbalance including dry, flushed skin; dry mucous membranes; poor skin turgor; decreased urine output; rapid pulse; and orthostatic blood pressure
- Bowel sounds may be hyperactive

- There may be diffuse abdominal tenderness and distention or abdominal exam may be unremarkable
- Significant localized rebound tenderness is unusual; if present, especially with a fever and an elevated WBC, suspect other cause

DIAGNOSTIC STUDIES
- Obtain laboratory work if no spontaneous resolution of symptoms within 72 hours
- Stool for culture and ova and parasites to identify a causative organism if present: *Shigella, Salmonella, E. coli* O157:Y7
- Stool for C. *difficile*, especially if recent course of antibiotic
- Stool for leukocyte and occult blood to rule out bacterial infection
- CBC with differential to evaluate for leukocytosis and eosinophilia (increased number of eosinophils commonly seen in parasitic infections)
- Electrolytes to evaluate for dehydration and electrolyte abnormalities

Differential Diagnosis
- Acute appendicitis
- Cholecystitis
- Fecal impaction
- Ileus
- Inflammatory bowel disease
- Irritable bowel syndrome
- Bowel obstruction
- Pelvic inflammatory disease
- Diverticulitis

Management
NONPHARMACOLOGIC TREATMENT
- Often initial treatment is supportive: bed rest, fluid replacement, and advancing the diet as tolerated
- Clear liquid diet advance as tolerated using BRATY diet: bananas, rice, applesauce, toast, yogurt
- Children age 5 years to adults: No solid foods; give clear liquids in small amounts (15 mL q 10 min) and gradually increase if no vomiting occurs; if no vomiting for 4 hours and tolerating 8 oz/hour, may begin small amount of regular foods as tolerated; if vomiting reoccurs at any point, let stomach rest (approximately one hour) then restart small amounts of clear liquids
- In younger children >1 month and <5 years, give ORT at 50 mL/kg over 4 hours; start with sips and gradually increase; may continue formula or regular diet if able to tolerate

PHARMACOLOGIC TREATMENT
- Antidiarrheal agents are controversial in acute gastroenteritis because the causative pathogen needs to be eliminated from the body; in mild to moderate diarrheal illness, antidiarrheals can be used with caution (but not if fever and blood in stool)
- If vomiting continues despite slow intake of fluids, consider use of antiemetic

- Chemoreceptor trigger zone suppressors will suppress vomiting; antihistamines more effective for nausea than for acute vomiting; antimotility agents to suppress diarrhea prolong absorption time of water in the gut but also may cause retention of organism/toxin
- Antibiotics are used only when an organism is isolated and symptoms are not resolved; when leukocytes or dysentery are present, for treatment of *Shigella*, when there are 8–10 stools per day, if patient is immunocompromised; consider metronidazole, trimethoprim-sulfamethoxazole, fluoroquinolones

Special Considerations
- Geriatric and pediatric patients are at higher risk for dehydration
- Pregnancy and lactation: If antimicrobials are required, check safety profile before use

When to Consult, Refer, Hospitalize
- Hospitalization required with severe dehydration, electrolyte imbalance, and/or metabolic acidosis; in the elderly or immunocompromised; and for severe abdominal pain, rebound tenderness, or neurological symptoms

Follow-Up
- None may be necessary if patient remains hydrated
    - EXPECTED COURSE
        - Usually self-limiting with vomiting limited to 24–48 hours, diarrhea may last 3–5 days; inflammation of the bowel due to a drug reaction may last for several weeks

    - COMPLICATIONS
        - Severe dehydration, electrolyte imbalance, and metabolic acidosis

Gastroesophageal Reflux Disease (GERD)

Description
- Symptomatic condition characterized by reflux or retrograde passage of low pH gastric contents into the esophagus causing pain, irritability, or vomiting; in children—poor weight gain, respiratory disorders
- In infants, it is the regurgitation of some of a feeding; 47% of all infants <2 months of age display normal physiologic gastroesophageal reflux without associated symptoms at least 2 times daily and outgrow this by 10 months to 1 year
- Reflux disease may cause damage to the esophageal mucosa with or without failure to thrive, occult blood loss, anemia, and possibly aspiration pneumonia with or without wheezing

Etiology
- Inappropriate lower esophageal sphincter (LES) relaxation allows for gastric contents to be refluxed into esophagus. The turgor of the lower esophageal sphincter is influenced by age, intra-abdominal pressure, length of esophagus below diaphragm, hormones, food, and neurologic interventions.
- Esophageal peristalsis impairment allowing for slow clearance of refluxed contents
- Delayed gastric emptying: Gastroparesis (common in people with diabetes)

- Sliding hiatal hernia (protrusion of the stomach wall through the diaphragm) may predispose patients to GERD
- Frequent, excessive, or chronic reflux will decrease the esophageal mucosal resistance to acid, causing esophageal inflammation
- In children, dysfunction of sphincter tone, esophageal motility, and gastric emptying may be caused by delayed maturation of one or all of these barriers
- Pathological verses physiological reflux differs in both frequency and volume

Incidence and Demographics
- Affects up to 40% of the U.S. adult population
- 47% of all infants <2 months display physiologic reflux, outgrown by 18 months in 90% of cases

Risk Factors
- Hiatal hernia, abnormal esophageal clearance, gastric outlet obstruction, obesity
- Medications that decrease LES tone: Anticholinergics, meperidine, theophylline, calcium channel blockers, nitrates, nicotine, alcohol, caffeine, mint, chocolate, increased estrogen levels (oral contraceptives), citrus and spicy foods, and foods high in fat and other foods that can decrease LES tone
- Eating large meals or lying down within 3 hours after eating; >16 oz/day of cola consumption
- Wearing tight clothing around the chest or abdomen; obesity; anxiety; cigarette smoking or exposure to secondhand smoke; children with neurological impairment or esophageal atresia; premature infants

Preventon and Screening
- Avoid spicy foods, caffeine, smoking, mints

Assessment
HISTORY
- Typical symptoms: Heartburn (pyrosis) described as a burning retrosternal discomfort radiating upward towards the neck that occurs 30–60 minutes after meals
- Symptoms are exacerbated by lying supine or bending over and improve with sitting up or taking antacids
- Excessive salivation, regurgitation, halitosis, sour or bitter taste into the mouth is common
- In children, inquire about type, amount, and frequency of feedings and regurgitation; choking during feedings; any bile or blood in regurgitation; any fevers, diarrhea; upper respiratory infection (URI) symptoms, history of respiratory illnesses, otitis media; any developmental delays
- Atypical symptoms: Dysphagia, odynophagia (painful swallowing), chest pain, hoarseness, cough, sore throat, nausea, and asthma

PHYSICAL EXAM
- Exam often normal; assess hydration status
- Adults—weight; children—plot height/weight on growth curve
- Respiratory and cardiac exam; abdominal exam to check for tenderness and masses; stool for occult blood

- Mental status, irritability, lethargy
- Assess developmental milestones in infants; neurologic exam if presents as unexplained vomiting

DIAGNOSTIC STUDIES
- Diagnosis can be made without further diagnostic tests in children if typical symptoms of heartburn and regurgitation are present, if history and physical exam are normal, child is developmentally on track, and growing appropriately
- Diagnostic studies are recommended when the diagnosis of GERD is uncertain, when symptoms not resolved with 4 weeks of empiric treatment, or if complications are suspected as indicated by atypical symptoms (listed above); symptoms that indicate a more serious etiology such as a cardiac cause for chest pain; evidence of bleeding (guaiac-positive stools or hematemesis); anemia; weight loss; symptoms that persist despite treatment, or daily symptoms
- Barium swallow/upper GI study: Usually first test ordered but is the least sensitive for diagnosing GERD; main value is to assess anatomy and rule out malrotation and obstruction; useful as a screening test to exclude complications of GERD (mucosal irregularities and ulcer) and to evaluate dysphagia (caused by stricture)
- Fluoroscopy can demonstrate presence of reflux, as well as rule out other causes of vomiting, such as gastric outlet obstruction
- Esophageal pH monitoring can measure the number of acid reflux events as well as the duration of each event in a given period of time; pH probe indicated to tailor medical management but not necessary in those infants who present with pathologic reflux that has caused a life-threatening event
- Esophagogastroduodenoscopy (EGD) aids in the evaluation of the degree of esophagitis from reflux; biopsies are obtained to assess mucosal integrity; evaluation of other disorders such as Crohn's disease, eosinophilic or infectious esophagitis, peptic ulcers, stricture or webs, and bleeding points can also be made
- Stool for occult blood; CBC to rule out anemia

Differential Diagnosis
- Infants:
  - Overfeeding
  - UTI
  - Pyloric stenosis
  - Partial upper intestinal obstruction
  - Otitis media
  - Pneumonia
- Older ages:
  - Cardiac spasm or MI
  - Peptic ulcer disease
  - Esophageal tumor/stricture
  - Esophagitis
  - Esophageal motility disorders
  - Esophageal structural disorders
  - Hiatal hernia

- All ages:
  - Gastroenteritis
  - Milk/soy intolerance
  - Celiac disease
  - Infections
  - Hepatitis
  - Drug-induced
- Drugs affecting the lower esophageal sphincter:
  - Nitrates
  - Nicotine
  - Narcotics
  - Theophylline
  - Anticholinergics
  - Estrogen
  - Somatostatin
  - Prostaglandins

Management
- Goals are to relieve symptoms, heal esophagitis, and prevent complications

  ### NONPHARMACOLOGIC TREATMENT
  - Lifestyle modification is step 1 therapy and the key component to management
  - In adults, elevate head of bed on 6-inch blocks or use wedge under mattress
  - Avoid eating 2–3 hrs before lying down and eat smaller, more frequent meals
  - In infants, hold infant upright for 15–30 minutes after feeding; prop upright in infant seat/car seat
  - In infants also recommend smaller and more frequent feedings
  - Lose weight if overweight; avoid tight-fitting clothing
  - Avoid substances that cause symptoms, including foods high in fat, citrus and spicy foods, mint, chocolate, caffeine, and alcohol; patients with GERD and breastfeeding mothers of infants with GERD should stop smoking
  - If taking medications that decrease LES tone, seek appropriate alternatives

  ### PHARMACOLOGIC TREATMENT
  - Pharmacological treatment in children under the age of 2 years is discouraged
  - Acid-neutralizing drugs may be initiated if nonpharmacologic treatment is not effective (see Table 9–3)
  - In mild symptoms, use over-the-counter antacids
  - Liquid more effective than tablet form
  - Antacids can decrease absorption of other medications (e.g., fluoroquinolones, tetracycline, ferrous sulfate); separate dosing by 2 hours
  - Aluminum or magnesium hydroxide—adults: 10–30 cc po qid; children: 0.5–2 mL/kg/dose 3–6 times/day
  - Step 2 therapy involves adding histamine-2 (H2) receptor antagonists if symptoms not relieved by lifestyle modification or antacids within 2–3 weeks
  - H2 receptor antagonists suppresses gastric acid secretion; symptomatic improvement occurs in approximately 80% within 6 weeks
  - Cimetidine (Tagamet): Adults: 400 mg bid, maximum 800 mg bid; children: 10 mg/kg/dose qid

- Potential drug interactions with theophylline, warfarin, nifedipine, propranolol, and phenytoin
- Ranitidine (Zantac): 150 mg bid, maximum 300 mg bid; famotidine (Pepcid) 20 mg bid, maximum 40 mg bid; nizatidine (Axid) 150 mg bid
- Reevaluate 2 weeks after starting therapy with H2 antagonists.; if effective, continue for 8–12 weeks
- If symptoms do not resolve go to step 3 therapy: Add a prokinetic agent; use higher dose H2 antagonist (see maximum dosages above) for an additional 8–12 weeks; or change from H2 antagonist to a proton pump inhibitor for 4–8 weeks
- Prokinetic agents increase LES tone and promote gastric emptying; used for mild–moderate symptoms, typically in combination with H2 receptor antagonists or proton pump inhibitors
- Metoclopramide (Reglan): Adults: 5–10 mg qid; children: 0.1 mg/kg/dose 20–30 min ac and hs
- Used less frequently because of its potential for central nervous system side effects such as drowsiness, confusion, depression, and extrapyramidal reactions
- Proton pump inhibitors suppress gastric acid secretion to a greater degree than H2 blockers; the initial treatment in patients with erosive esophagitis confirmed by endoscopy; take 1 hour before meal
- Omeprazole (Prilosec): Adults: 20–40 mg q am; children: 0.7–3.3 mg/kg/day in 1–2 doses
- Lansoprazole (Prevacid): 15–30 mg qd; esomeprazole (Nexium) or rabeprazole (Aciphex) 20 mg qd (1–11 yrs., <30 kg, 15 mg daily; >30 kg, 30 mg daily)

Table 9-3. Drugs Commonly Used for GERD

Drug	Dose
Acid Neutralization	0.6–2 mL/kg/dose 3-6 times/day
Aluminum or magnesium hydroxide	1–4 tablets/day in divided doses
Calcium carbonate	
Acid Suppression	40 mg/kg/day divided tid or qid
H2 blockers	5–10 mg/kg/day divided bid, tid, or even qid
Cimetidine (Tagamet)	1 mg/kg/day divided bid
Ranitidine (Zantac)	10 mg/kg/day divided bid
Famotidine (Pepcid)	
Nizatidine (Axid)	
Proton Pump Inhibitors*	0.7–3.3 mg/kg/day in 1–2 doses
Omeprazole (Prilosec)	1.4 mg/kg/day
Lansoprazole (Prevacid)	
Prokinetic Agent	0.1–0.2 mg/kg/dose up to qid
Metoclopramide (Reglan)	1–3 mg/kg tid
Erythromycin	
Cholinergic Agent	0.1–0.2 mg/kg/dose up to qid
Bethanechol	

*PPIs ideally should be administered 15–30 minutes before the first meal of the day

LENGTH OF TREATMENT
- Reconsider diagnosis if no response to proton pump inhibitors after 8 weeks
- Treat erosive esophagitis with proton pump inhibitors for 12 weeks
- 85% of infants with GERD improve with age as they become more erect and advance to more solid diet
- If patient has a good response to therapy, gradually withdraw medication while continuing lifestyle modifications
- Maintenance therapy with H2 blockers (continue usual treatment dosage) or proton pump inhibitors (omeprazole 20 mg or lansoprazole 15 mg daily) should be considered to prevent relapse that occurs in 80% within 6 months (see dosages under peptic ulcer disease); lifestyle modification should continue throughout treatment and indefinitely to prevent relapse

Special Considerations
- Pregnancy: Predisposition due to elevated hormone levels and increased intra-abdominal pressure from pregnant uterus; antacids generally safe in pregnancy
- Lactation: Antacids generally safe

When to Consult, Refer, Hospitalize
- Consult with or refer to a physician or gastroenterologist when the patient does not respond to treatment or has symptoms of dysphagia, evidence of blood loss, iron deficiency anemia, or significant weight loss; or for pediatric patients with anatomic abnormalities suspected or if there is poor weight gain or developmental delay
- Referral for surgery (gastric fundoplication; step 4 therapy) when all other approaches have failed

Follow-Up
- 2-week intervals until improvement noted, then monthly
  EXPECTED COURSE
  - In infants, 85% will have resolution when they are able to sit/stand and have begun eating solids
  - Often a chronic, relapsing condition in adults; however, the majority of patients with GERD respond well to medical therapy without developing complications or requiring surgery
  - Annual endoscopy with biopsy indicated in patients with Barrett's esophagus

  COMPLICATIONS
  - Hemorrhage (3%), peptic stricture (10%–15%), Barrett's esophagus (10%), adenocarcinoma with Barrett's esophagus

Peptic Ulcer Disease (PUD)

Description
- Ulceration in the gastric or duodenal mucosa caused when the normal protective coating of the stomach is penetrated and irritated by acid secretion, causing pain

Etiology
- Nonsteroidal anti-inflammatory drugs (NSAIDs)

- *H. pylori* infection associated with 95% of duodenal ulcers
- Acid hypersecretory states (e.g., Zollinger-Ellison syndrome, caused by a gastrin-secreting tumor)
- Ulceration extends through the muscularis mucosa and is usually 5 mm or greater in diameter

Incidence and Demographics
- In the U.S., approximately 500,000 new cases and 4 million occurrences per year
- Duodenal ulcers are 5 times more common than gastric ulcers; more than 95% occur in the duodenal bulb or pyloric channel; occur more often between the ages of 30 and 55
- Benign gastric ulcers commonly occur in the antrum (60%) and at the junction of the antrum and body on the lesser curvature (25%); occur more often between the ages of 55 and 70
- Geriatric patients: Increased mortality with initial attack >60 years old

Risk Factors
- Aging (decrease in gastric mucosal protective mechanisms)
- Corticosteroid use, stress; aspirin (ASA) and chronic NSAID use increase risk of gastric ulcers
- Smoking, alcohol use do not appear to cause peptic ulcer disease

Prevention and Screening
- Consider using COX2 inhibitor type of NSAIDs (e.g., celecoxib [Celebrex]) to reduce the incidence of ulcer, spare gastric mucosal prostaglandin synthesis
- Misoprostol (prostaglandin analog) 100–200 mcg tid–qid, or a proton pump inhibitor bid, given prophylactically in combination with NSAIDs to prevent NSAID-induced ulcers, for increased risk with age >70, use of anticoagulants or corticosteroids, and previous history of peptic ulcer and/or complications
- Stop smoking; stress management
- Take NSAIDs with food and only when needed; avoid chronic use

Assessment

HISTORY (DIAGNOSIS OFTEN MADE BY CLINICAL PRESENTATION)
- Classic symptom is epigastric pain (dyspepsia) described as a gnawing or dull ache that fluctuates throughout the day
- With duodenal ulcer, discomfort occurs 1–3 hours after meals and may awaken patient at night; pain is relieved by eating, antacids, or vomiting
- With gastric ulcers, symptoms are more variable; food may increase or decrease symptoms; and anorexia, nausea, vomiting, and weight loss are more common
- Melanotic stools: In elderly and NSAID-induced ulcers there may be no symptoms until bleeding or perforation occur

PHYSICAL EXAM
- Abdominal exam may reveal mild, localized epigastric tenderness to deep palpation
- Stool may be positive for occult blood

DIAGNOSTIC STUDIES
- *H. pylori* detection by serum antibodies or endoscopic biopsy (see below) should be evaluated in all patients with diagnosed peptic ulcer disease
- CBC to exclude anemia from GI blood loss and leukocytosis due to ulcer perforation; stool occult blood
- Amylase in patients with significant epigastric pain to exclude pancreatic disease
- Fasting serum gastrin level to screen for Zollinger-Ellison syndrome; consider in patients with multiple recurrent ulcers, and in those with ulcer and no *H. pylori* or NSAID use (hold H2 receptor antagonists for 24 hrs. and proton pump inhibitors for 1 week because they may falsely elevate levels)
- Upper endoscopy: Best test to diagnose peptic ulcer disease; allows for biopsy to detect malignancy (>5% of gastric ulcers are malignant at time of presentation) and *H. pylori* infection (through rapid urease test or histology); recommended in patients who test positive for *H. pylori* infection (serum antibody) under age 45 and for all patients over age 45
- Barium upper GI series: May be used to screen uncomplicated symptoms of dyspepsia; however, cannot distinguish between benign and malignant gastric ulcers
- Urea breath test (*H. pylori* generates urease): Diagnoses active *H. pylori* infection; useful in evaluating symptomatic patients who have been previously treated for *H. pylori* (if breath test positive, indicates unsuccessful eradication); the serum *H. pylori* antibody may persist for up to 18 months after treatment, even in those patients who have been successfully treated; proton pump inhibitors should be held for 7 days prior to test to avoid a false-negative result

Differential Diagnosis
- Gastroesophageal reflux
- Cholecystitis
- Pancreatitis
- Diverticulitis
- Biliary tract disease
- Gastric carcinoma
- Cardiovascular disease
- Angina/MI

Management
- Goal: Eradicate bacteria, provide environment for ulcer healing
  NONPHARMACOLOGIC TREATMENT
    - Stop NSAIDs
    - Maintain well-balanced diet
    - Smoking should be discouraged as it slows ulcer healing and increases risk for reoccurrence
    - Stress management
    - Surgery for refractory ulcers rarely is performed

PHARMACOLOGIC TREATMENT
- In patients who do not need an endoscopy, have normal CBC and test negative for *H. pylori*:
  - Proton pump inhibitors (omeprazole and lansoprazole): Suppress gastric acid secretion to a greater degree than H2 receptor antagonists; give 1 hour before meals (see Table 9–4)
  - H2 receptor antagonists: Suppress basal and nocturnal gastric acid secretion; less effective inhibition of meal-stimulated acid production
    » Cimetidine (Tagamet), ranitidine (Zantac), famotidine (Pepcid), or nizatidine (Axid)
    » Cimetidine has potential drug interactions with theophylline, warfarin, nifedipine, propranolol, and phenytoin
  - Sucralfate (Carafate): Enhances mucosal defenses; efficacy is equal to H2 receptor antagonists in treating duodenal ulcers; inhibits the absorption of certain medications (i.e., digoxin) and dosing should be separated by 2 hours and taken 1 hour before meals

NSAID-induced ulcer disease
- Antibiotic therapy not necessary
- Discontinue NSAID if possible
- Substitute COX2 inhibitor when possible
- Once daily proton pump inhibitor
- Prostaglandin analog (misoprostol) used if NSAID is continued
- Proton pump inhibitor for acute ulcer for 4–8 weeks, or indefinitely for prophylaxis
- Antacids: No longer used as first-line treatment due to newer agents; commonly used to provide symptom relief in addition to other therapies on an as-needed basis

H. pylori ulcer disease
- Use antibiotic combinations including amoxicillin combined with tetracycline, metronidazole, or clarithromycin; bismuth subsalicylate may be used as a third agent
- Either proton pump inhibitor or a histamine 2 receptor antagonist is required to provide an environment for healing of existing ulcer
- In patients with complicated ulcer (bleeding, nausea, and significant pain), initiate treatment with proton pump inhibitor first to relieve symptoms, followed by treatment regimen for *H. pylori* if test is positive

Table 9–4. Treatment of Active Peptic Ulcer Disease

Drug	Duodenal Ulcer	Gastric Ulcer
Omeprazole (Prilosec)	20 mg qd	20 mg bid
Lansoprazole (Prevacid)	15 mg qd	30 mg qd
Cimetidine (Tagamet)	800 mg q hs	400 mg bid
Ranitidine (Zantac)	300 mg q hs	150 mg bid
Nizatidine (Axid)	300 mg q hs	150 mg bid
Famotidine (Pepcid)	40 mg q hs	20 mg bid
Sucralfate (Carafate)	1 g qid	Not indicated

LENGTH OF TREATMENT
  • Active peptic ulcer: Reevaluate in 2 weeks; if symptoms improving
    continue treatment
  • With proton pump inhibitors, treat uncomplicated duodenal ulcer for 4 weeks,
    gastric or complicated ulcer for 6–8 weeks
  • With H2 antagonists, treat uncomplicated duodenal ulcer for 6 weeks, gastric
    ulcer for 8–12 weeks
  • With H. pylori, give medications for 10–14 days minimum; may require
    retreatment if symptoms recur

Special Considerations
• Pregnancy: Misoprostol may cause uterine contractions resulting in abortion

When to Consult, Refer, Hospitalize
• Refer to a gastroenterologist for endoscopic evaluation in patients with symptoms of GI
  bleeding (iron deficiency anemia, hematemesis, or melena), persistent vomiting, and
  weight loss; severe epigastric pain that may suggest ulcer penetration or perforation;
  patients over the age of 50 with new onset of dyspepsia; persistent symptoms after
  several weeks of treatment or for recurrent symptoms after finishing treatment; all
  gastric ulcers

Follow-Up
• Evaluate effectiveness of therapy 2 weeks after initiation and again after completion
  (4–12 weeks)
• Using a urea breath test, confirm eradication of H. *pylori* in patients that continue to
  have symptoms or relapse (may require retreatment with different antibiotic regimen)
• Successful H. *pylori* eradication decreases peptic ulcer recurrence to 20% per year
• All gastric ulcers should be reevaluated by endoscopy with cytology after treatment to
  document resolution and exclude malignancy

COMPLICATIONS
  • Hemorrhage, ulcer perforation or penetration, gastric outlet obstruction

Irritable Bowel Syndrome (IBS)

Description
• The American Gastroenterology Association defines irritable bowel syndrome (IBS) as
  a combination of chronic and recurrent GI symptoms not explained by structural
  or biochemical abnormalities.
• Symptoms may be constant or intermittent but must be present for 3 months.
• Symptoms include recurrent abdominal pain and distension, improved after bowel
  movement. Onset associated with a change in frequency or appearance of stool;
  subtypes include constipation predominant, diarrhea predominant, and variable
  stool pattern.

Etiology
• Pathophysiology is unknown but may be related to an increase in 5-HT, a neurotransmitter controlling intestinal motility and visceral afferent responses. This increase
  maybe caused by normal or noxious stimuli.

- Specific food intolerance (lactose; high fat; citrus or spicy foods; dietetic sweeteners; and gas-producing foods such as beans, cabbage, and raw onions)
- Malabsorption of bile acids
- Heightened visceral pain perception

Incidence and Demographics
- Common, occurs in 15%–30% of the population, median age 35; also occurs in children and the elderly
- 2:1 females: males; one-third have history of illness from childhood; no known genetic factors

Risk Factors
- Familial history
- Presence of other functional disorders
- Emotional and physical stress (e.g., anxiety, excessive worry, major loss, improper diet, overwork, decreased sleep, and poor physical fitness) can exacerbate symptoms

Prevention and Screening
- Stress reduction
- Maintain healthy lifestyle by eating a well-balanced, high-fiber, low-fat diet; regular exercise; and adequate sleep
- Avoid foods or other substances that exacerbate symptoms (see specific foods listed above)
- Avoid caffeine, tobacco, and alcohol

Box 9–1. Diagnostic Criteria for Irritable Bowel Syndrome

Continuous or recurrent symptoms for at least 3 months, including:
- Abdominal pain or discomfort relieved with defecation
- Associated with a change in frequency of bowel movements or
- Associated with a change in consistency of bowel movements

Two or more of the following at least 25% of the time:
- >3 stools/day or <3 stools/week
- Altered stool passage (straining, urgency, feeling of incomplete evacuation)
- Altered stool form (lumpy/hard or watery/loose)
- Passage of mucus from rectum
- Bloating or feeling distension of abdomen

Adapted from "Medical position statement: Irritable bowel syndrome" by the American Gastroenterological Association, 1997, *Gastroenterology*, *112*, 2118–2119.

Assessment
HISTORY
- Rome III criteria requires that adult or child be old enough to provide an accurate history of the abdominal pain, which can be described as sharp or dull, crampy or burning; usually periumbilical or LLQ; present at least 12 weeks, not necessarily consecutive, in the previous 12-month period, relieved with defecation and associated with a change in stooling form or frequency;

also has increased number of stools, abnormal stool form (hard, lumpy, watery, alternating), abnormal stool passage (straining, urgency, feeling of incomplete evacuation), mucus, bloating, feeling of abdominal distension

- Constipation is described as small, infrequent, hard stools or straining to defecate
- Diarrhea (usually 4–6 stools day) is described as watery, ribbon-like, with clear mucus in the stool
- Blood in stool and waking at night to defecate is more likely inflammatory bowel disease
- Often alternates between both constipation and diarrhea; increased flatulence and bloating may be present; symptoms are exacerbated by meals and stress, and are usually relieved by defecation
- History of increased emotional or physical stress, depression, or preoccupation with bowel habits
- Weight loss—none with IBS
- Diet, eating patterns, medications, treatments tried, family history (colon cancer)
- In women, take menstrual history and any association of symptoms with menstruation
- Abdominal pain relieved by defecation; preoccupation with bowel symptoms

PHYSICAL EXAM
- See Box 9–1
- Usually normal; no weight loss
- Lower abdominal tenderness or distension may be present but not pronounced; a tender cord may be palpated over the sigmoid colon (left lower quadrant), which indicates the presence of stool; abdominal tympany if air trapping is present; mildly hyperactive bowel sounds may be present
- Digital rectal exam is normal, although may have discomfort on exam

DIAGNOSTIC STUDIES
- CBC with differential, erythrocyte sedimentation rate (ESR), and thyroid function tests are normal; stool test for occult blood negative
- In patients with diarrhea, stool studies are negative (culture, ova and parasite, and C. *difficile*, WBCs and fat)
- Flexible sigmoidoscopy, colonoscopy, barium enema when symptoms are severe or prolonged, to exclude inflammatory or malignant disease; indicated for patients older than 40
- Small bowel series to rule out Crohn's disease when diarrhea predominates
- Abdominal plain radiograph during an acute episode of abdominal pain to exclude bowel obstruction

Differential Diagnosis
- Inflammatory bowel disease
- Constipation
- UTI
- Infectious diarrhea
- Esophagitis
- Antibiotic use

- Thyroid disease
- Chronic pancreatitis
- ASA/NSAIDs
- Diverticulitis
- Giardiasis
- Celiac disease
- Endometriosis
- Cystic fibrosis
- Cholecystitis
- Lactose intolerance
- Colon cancer
- Malabsorption

Management

NONPHARMACOLOGIC TREATMENT
- Patients should keep a diary in which foods, symptoms, and daily events are recorded to identify possible exacerbating factors
- Dietary changes: Avoid foods and other agents that worsen symptoms
- All patients should try a lactose-free diet for 2 weeks to exclude lactose intolerance
- A high-fiber diet (20–30 g/day) is recommended; may cause bloating and flatulence initially but usually resolves in few weeks (increase gradually); use 1 teaspoon bran powder 2–3 times/day added to food or in 8 oz liquid
- Management of stress through relaxation techniques and behavior modification, emotional support, address patient fears

PHARMACOLOGIC TREATMENT
- Medications required only in severe cases
  - Bulk-forming agents may be better tolerated than bran, used in mixed IBS
    » Psyllium (Metamucil) 1 tablespoon in 8 oz of fluid up to 3 times day
    » Methylcellulose (Citrucel) 1 tbsp in 8 oz of fluid up to 3 times day
  - Anticholinergic agents: Relieve spasm and abdominal pain
    » Dicyclomine hydrochloride (Bentyl) 10–20 mg qid prn
    » Hyoscyamine sulfate (Levsin) 0.125 mg 1–2 (tabs or tsp) q4h orally or sublingually prn
  - Antidiarrheal agents: Used on an as-needed basis
    » Loperamide hydrochloride (Imodium) 4 mg initially, then 2 mg after each loose stool prn (max 8 mg/day); diphenoxylate with atropine (Lomotil) 1–2 tablets qid prn
  - If constipation primary problem may use lactulose 15–30 mL/dose, max 60 mL/day if increased fiber not effective, or lubiprostone (Amitiza) 8-24 mg bid
  - Treatment for flatulence
    » Simethicone (Phazyme, Gas-X) 125 mg qid prn with meals and q hs
  - Antidepressants are controversial but may be effective for some patients with chronic, unremitting abdominal pain
    » Tricyclic: Amitriptyline (Elavil) 25–50 mg q hs
    » Serotonin reuptake inhibitors: Sertraline (Zoloft) 25–50 mg, initially and increase up to 200 mg daily or fluoxetine (Prozac) 20–40 mg, if depression coexists

LENGTH OF TREATMENT
- • High-fiber diet and avoidance of exacerbating agents should be continued indefinitely
- • Use other agents as needed for symptomatic management

Special Considerations
- • Symptoms usually decrease with age
- • Pregnancy: Check safety profile of all medications

When to Consult, Refer, Hospitalize
- • Refer to or consult with a physician or gastroenterologist for severe symptoms, symptoms of nocturnal diarrhea, hematochezia, fever and weight loss; new onset of symptoms in patients over 40 years old; patients that have persistent symptoms despite treatment with diet, bulking agents, and antispasmodics
- • Refer to a psychologist for counseling and stress management if appropriate

Follow-Up
- • Every 2 weeks until symptoms improve, then every month for six months if continued improvement
    EXPECTED COURSE
    - • Most respond well to treatment during the initial 12-month period; however, irritable bowel syndrome is a chronic relapsing condition that may require prolonged therapy

    COMPLICATIONS
    - • Depression, anxiety disorders, loss of work or school days

Ulcerative Colitis

Description
- • Ulcerative colitis is a chronic, relapsing inflammatory disease of the colon and rectal mucosa
- • Disease may be limited to the rectum (ulcerative proctitis) or involve the entire colon
- • It is characterized by acute exacerbations and remissions

Etiology
- • Etiology unknown but possibly autoimmune or genetic predisposition
- • Inflammatory process causes diffuse friability and erosions that result in bleeding

Incidence and Demographics
- • Usually manifests between the ages of 15–35, with a second smaller peak in the 7th decade of life; can occur as early as 5 years old
- • In U.S., occurs in 5–10 per 100,000; females more common than males
- • Geriatric patients: Increased mortality with initial attack >60 years old

Risk Factors
- • Tenfold increased risk of disease if first-degree relatives affected
- • Jewish descent

Prevention and Screening
- Familial predisposition

Assessment

HISTORY
- Classic symptom is bloody diarrhea; other symptoms include crampy lower abdominal pain (commonly left lower quadrant, relieved by defecation), fecal urgency, tenesmus, nocturnal diarrhea
- More severe cases have fever, anemia, anorexia, and weight loss
- Extra-intestinal manifestations such as oligoarticular arthritis, ankylosing spondylitis, uveitis, oral aphthous ulcers, pyoderma gangrenosum, and erythema nodosum; occur in about 25% of cases as in Crohn's disease
- In children, growth retardation, delayed puberty

PHYSICAL EXAM
- Orthostatic blood pressure and heart rate measurements are done to determine volume status
- Abdominal exam may reveal tenderness or signs of peritonitis; digital rectal exam may reveal red blood and mucus
- Signs of extra-intestinal manifestations such as arthritis, skin rashes, and eye manifestations

DIAGNOSTIC STUDIES
- CBC to evaluate anemia from bleeding; may show leukocytosis
- Erythrocyte sedimentation rate and C-reactive protein are increased in active inflammation
- Albumin may be low
- Stool studies to exclude infection (culture, ova and parasites, C. *difficile* toxin)
- Sigmoidoscopy is diagnostic; mucosa appears friable and inflamed; purulent exudates and ulcers may also be present; biopsy can differentiate ulcerative colitis from specific types of infectious colitis
- Colonoscopy should not be performed in severe active disease because of the risk of perforation; may be performed when symptoms improve on therapy to determine the extent of disease
- Plain abdominal radiographs are obtained in severe colitis to exclude toxic megacolon (colon becomes atonic and dilated more than 6 cm and is associated with symptoms of toxicity)
- Barium enemas are not useful during acute disease and may precipitate toxic megacolon

Differential Diagnosis
- Crohn's disease
- Trauma
- Enterocolitis
- Infectious colitis
- Juvenile polyps
- IBS
- Ischemic colitis

- Appendicitis
- Hemolytic uremic syndrome
- Radiation induced proctitis
- Henoch-Schönlein purpura

Management

NONPHARMACOLOGIC TREATMENT
- Maintain well-balanced, high-fiber diet; avoid caffeine and gas-producing foods
- Surgical intervention: Curative with total colectomy; indications include severe colitis that does not respond to steroid treatment, patients with toxic megacolon that fail to improve after 48–72 hours (before perforation occurs), and in high-grade dysplasia

PHARMACOLOGIC TREATMENT
- Fiber supplements or bulk-forming agents if not achieved through diet
  - Bran powder 1–2 tbsp bid, or psyllium (Metamucil) 1 tbsp in 8 oz of fluid up to 3 times day, or
  - Methylcellulose (Citrucel) 1 tbsp 8 oz of fluid up to 3 times day
- Anti-inflammatory agent in mild to moderate disease, effective in inducing remission
  - Sulfasalazine (Azulfidine) and prednisone tablets or liquid for children >2 years and adults; mesalamine (Rowasa) suppository for rectal involvement, enema for left-sided colitis; hydrocortisone suppository/enema
- Antidiarrheal agents should not be used during the acute phase as may precipitate toxic megacolon, but are safe and beneficial in mild chronic symptoms
  - Loperamide (Imodium) 4 mg initially, then 2 mg after each loose stool prn (max 8 mg/day)
  - Diphenoxylate with atropine (Lomotil) 1–2 tablets qid prn
  - Immunomodulators are used for more severe disease

LENGTH OF TREATMENT
- Treatment is dictated by symptoms; exacerbations treated several weeks to 2–3 months
- Establish good working relationship with patient and gastroenterologist as you manage the primary care problems of the patient

Special Considerations
- Pregnancy: Acute exacerbations typically occur in the first trimester; advised to postpone becoming pregnant until after one year of remission; continue sulfasalazine with folic acid supplementation during pregnancy to maintain remission
- Prednisone is safe in pregnancy; immunosuppressants are unsafe and should be avoided

When to Consult, Refer, Hospitalize
- Refer to a gastroenterologist for initial diagnostic studies and management and when acute exacerbation does not respond to usual therapy
- Refer to a surgeon for surgical intervention if severe disease unresponsive to treatment

- Hospitalization is indicated for patients who present with fulminant colitis with symptoms of high fever, sepsis, profuse bloody diarrhea, abdominal pain, and severe dehydration

Follow-Up
- Colon cancer screening with colonoscopy and biopsy every 1–2 years, beginning 7–8 years after disease onset (colon cancer incidence triple in patients with U.C. for >10 years)

  EXPECTED COURSE
  - Acute exacerbations are usually well-controlled with medication and patients do not require surgery
  - Most never require hospitalization
  - Patients who have more severe disease that is resistant to therapy require surgery (up to 20% of patients), which results in complete cure of the disease

  COMPLICATIONS
  - Toxic megacolon, perforation, strictures, anemia, colorectal cancer

Crohn's Disease

Description
- Crohn's disease (regional enteritis) is a chronic, relapsing disease characterized by patchy inflammation that occurs anywhere in the gastrointestinal tract, but most commonly the terminal ileum and the proximal colon.

Etiology
- Pathogenesis of bowel disease unknown
- Often causes ulcerations, strictures, fistulas, and abscesses because the inflammatory process involves all layers (transmural) of the intestinal wall
- One-third of patients have small bowel involvement only, often of the terminal ileum (ileitis); one-half of patients have small bowel and colon involvement, commonly the terminal ileum and proximal ascending colon (ileocolitis); 20% of patients have only colon involvement
- Possible genetic predisposition
- Possible environmental factors, bacteria, viral, dietary

Incidence and Demographics
- Onset usually occurs at 15–25 years with a second, smaller peak at 55–65
- More common in women than men
- Incidence 20–100/100,000 in the U.S.
- 25% present in childhood with an average age of onset 7.5 years
- More common in Whites and those of Jewish descent

Risk Factors
- First-degree relative has disease
- Anxiety may exacerbate symptoms
- Smoking

Prevention and Screening
- Maintain good nutritional status
- Stress management

Assessment

HISTORY
- Findings variable; depends on location and extent of disease
- Delayed growth and development in children
- Common presentation includes nonbloody diarrhea, abdominal pain (often right lower quadrant or periumbilical), nausea, vomiting, and weight loss; low-grade fever and malaise may be present
- More serious disease may present with bowel obstruction, fistulas complicated by infection, and perianal disease (anal fissure, perianal abscess or fistula)
- Patients may have high fever, dehydration, severe abdominal pain, significant weight loss, malnutrition, post-prandial bloating
- Extra-intestinal manifestations of Crohn's occur in 25% and include oligoarticular arthritis, ankylosing spondylitis, uveitis, oral aphthous ulcers, pyoderma gangrenosum, and erythema nodosum
- If disease is confined to colon, may present with rectal bleeding and diarrhea

PHYSICAL EXAM
- Abdominal exam may reveal a tender mass, which represents thickened or inflamed intestine; commonly found in the right lower quadrant
- Rectal exam to evaluate for perianal disease (fissures, fistulas, abscesses and "blind" sinus tracts)
- Exam for extra-intestinal findings

DIAGNOSTIC STUDIES
- CBC may reflect leukocytosis from inflammation or abscess, iron deficiency anemia due to mucosal blood loss, megaloblastic anemia from B12 deficiency due to terminal ileum disease and malabsorption, or anemia of chronic disease
- Erythrocyte sedimentation rate (ESR) or C-reactive protein elevated during active inflammation
- Decreased albumin levels due to malabsorption, intestinal protein loss, or chronic disease
- Stool culture, ova and parasites, and C. *difficile* toxin to exclude infectious cause for diarrhea
- Upper gastrointestinal series with small bowel follow-through
- Colonoscopy is superior to barium enema in evaluating the colon as it allows for biopsy
- Serologic testing to distinguish between Crohn's disease and ulcerative colitis
  - Antineutrophil cytoplasmic antibodies (pANCA) only present in 5–10% patients with Crohn's disease (much higher in ulcerative colitis)
  - Antibodies to yeast S. *cerevisiae* (ASCA) present in 60%–70% patients with Crohn's disease (much lower in ulcerative colitis)
  - Combination of negative pANCA and positive ASCA is 50% sensitive and 97% specific for Crohn's disease

Differential Diagnosis
- Ulcerative colitis
- Gastroenteritis
- Hemolytic uremic syndrome
- Acute appendicitis
- PUD
- Henoch-Schönlein purpura
- IBS
- Constipation
- Psychosocial problems
- Lactose intolerance
- Infectious diarrhea
- Lymphoma
- Ischemic colitis
- Carcinoma

Management
- Goals are to treat symptoms and control the disease process
    NONPHARMACOLOGIC TREATMENT
    - Maintain a well-balanced diet high in protein and vitamins, particularly B12 and iron
    - Avoid dairy products that contain lactose if they exacerbate symptoms
    - A low-roughage diet (no raw fruits or vegetables, nuts, seeds, etc.) may be beneficial during acute exacerbations
    - Stress management; relaxation techniques
    - Psychosocial support is very important in these patients, given the chronicity of this disease
    - Surgical intervention—not curative; one-half of patients require at least one surgery

    PHARMACOLOGIC TREATMENT
    - Parental vitamin B12 and medium-chain triglyceride supplementation are given if malabsorption results (common in patients with extensive terminal ileum disease or resection)
    - Iron supplements are needed in patients with chronic blood loss
    - Drug of choice: Prednisone for acute exacerbations: 40–60 mg/day for 2–3 weeks; taper 5 mg week to 20 mg/day; taper 2.5 mg per week to a maintenance dose required for some individuals
    - Loperamide (Imodium) as needed
    - Enteral therapy (tube feedings) or total parental nutrition (TPN) are indicated when patients are unable to tolerate an oral diet for 5 days

    LENGTH OF TREATMENT
    - Acute exacerbation: Treatment with sulfasalazine or mesalamine for 3 weeks usually improves symptoms; however, some may require 2–3 months
    - Patients who fail to improve after 3 weeks of mesalamine should have systemic corticoids added
    - Work closely with the specialist while providing primary care to this patient

Special Considerations
- Pregnancy: Sulfasalazine and steroids are safe in pregnancy

When to Consult, Refer, Hospitalize
- Refer to gastroenterologist for treatment of diarrhea with bile acid sequestrants, antidiarrheals, sulfasalazine, corticosteroids, some antibiotics, and immunomodulators
- Refer to or consult with a gastroenterologist for initial diagnostic studies and management and for acute exacerbations
- Hospitalization is required in acute exacerbations when symptoms persist
- Surgical intervention may be required to remove severely affected bowel or to provide bowel rest

Follow-Up
- Provide patient education about disease process, medication, diet; colonoscopy screening after 10 years of disease due to increased incidence of colon cancer
- Follow up according to specialist recommendations and for exacerbation of symptoms
- All patients will require emotional support
  - EXPECTED COURSE
    - Chronic, with acute exacerbations and periods of remission; progression of disease is common with the average patient having surgery every 7 years

  - COMPLICATIONS
    - Toxic megacolon fistula, abscess, perforation, bowel obstruction, perianal disease, malabsorption, and colon cancer (increased risk, but not as high as with ulcerative colitis)
    - Complications from chronic steroid use include aseptic necrosis of the hip, cataracts, osteoporosis, diabetes, and hypertension
    - Depression in 30%–50% of patients with severe disease

Colic

Description
- Excessive crying in an infant who is otherwise well. Crying lasts longer than 3 hours per day, at least 3 days/week, for at least 3 weeks in an infant <3 months old. Symptoms often peak at 6 weeks.

Etiology
- Exact pathophysiology unknown; historically believed to be problem with interaction between infant and environment although many researchers question this assumption
- Several possible etiologies: Normal variant, maternal/child interaction, family tensions, immaturity of GI tract, stimulus sensitivity, infant temperament, food allergy or intolerance
- May be associated with excessive gas, cow's milk, or other food intolerance

Incidence and Demographics
- Occurs in one-third of all infants
- Occurs equally in breastfed and bottle-fed, males and females

Risk Factors
- Inadequate psychosocial support for the mother

Prevention and Screening
- Family predisposition

Assessment

HISTORY
- Obtain crying history: Age of onset, frequency, duration, pattern; inconsolable for short periods
- Feeding history, elimination patterns
- Interventions tried and their effectiveness
- Ask how things are going at other times regarding infant's behavior and activity

PHYSICAL EXAM
- Growth parameters, developmental milestones
- Careful abdominal examination to assess for masses, tenderness
- Observe parent–child interaction
- Tensing of the infant with clenching of fists; fussy during feeding

DIAGNOSTIC STUDIES
- None necessary if adequate weight gain, meeting developmental milestones, and normal exam

Differential Diagnosis
- Normal crying
- Incarcerated inguinal hernia
- Inadequate feeding techniques
- Cow's milk allergy
- Gastroesophageal reflux
- Lactose intolerance
- Breast milk transmission of irritating substances
- Otitis media

Management

NONPHARMACOLOGIC TREATMENT
- Reassure parents that no physical problem is present; educate regarding normal infant crying
- Soothe infant by providing motion (swing, rocker, car seat), papoose carrier, snug bundling
- Ensure adequate burping during feeding
- Encourage and provide support for the mother
- Switching to hypoallergenic formula (casein hydrolysated whey) may be helpful
- Avoiding cow's milk in diet of breastfeeding mothers may also help
- Chamomile tea has been found to decrease the incidence within 7 days

PHARMACOLOGIC TREATMENT
- No drug therapy is indicated, though may consider trial of simethicone (Mylicon) drops 0.3 cc qid after meals and every evening prn; caution parents that this is not a universally effective therapy

LENGTH OF TREATMENT
- Colic is a self-limiting condition, which gradually improves
- Virtually gone by the age of 4 months

Special Considerations
- Frequent telephone contact with caregivers is helpful to provide support

When to Consult, Refer, Hospitalize
- Consult or refer for any signs of infection, obstruction, weight loss, feeding intolerance
- Referral of parents for treatment of psychosocial problems if indicated

Follow-Up
EXPECTED COURSE
- Gradual resolution of symptoms with support and increased age of infant

COMPLICATIONS
- Abuse, overfeeding, maternal anger, poor parental bonding

CONDITIONS THAT MAY WARRANT SURGERY

Appendicitis

Description
- Inflammation of the variform appendix (small, blind pouch projecting from the cecum), causing obstruction of the lumen of the appendix. Early diagnosis key to decrease both morbidity and mortality associated with rupture.

Etiology
- Obstruction is the cause in 30%–40% of cases and is commonly caused by a fecalith (a hard concentration of fecal matter and calcium salts), foreign body, inflammation, or neoplasm.
- Other causes include hypertrophy of the lymphoid tissue associated with a viral infection (e.g., measles), trapped barium after an imaging study, foreign body (e.g., seeds), intestinal worms (e.g., pin worms), tumor, or adhesions that cause obstruction.
- Obstruction leads to a build-up of mucosal secretions that causes the appendix to become inflamed and may lead to gangrene or perforation.

Incidence and Demographics
- Most common in people age 10–30 with peak incidence at 15–24
- In patients >50 years and <5 years, classic symptoms less frequent though perforation is more common, with a higher mortality and morbidity

- A ruptured appendix occurs in one half of children under 6 years of age with appendicitis
- Most common cause of abdominal pain requiring surgery in childhood and adolescence

Risk Factors
- Family history, intra-abdominal tumors, recent gastrointestinal illness especially viral or worm infestation
- Recent radiographic study using barium

Prevention and Screening
- None

Assessment

HISTORY
- Classic presentation:
  - Pain begins gradually; usually starts as vague, colicky, cramping, and poorly localized to the periumbilical or epigastric area, often associated with the urge to defecate or pass flatus which help to reduce the pain; pain can vary depending on location of appendix; migration of periumbilical pain to RLQ is one of the most predictive features of appendicitis
  - Lasts approximately 4–6 hours, followed by increased, steady pain that is more localized generally to the right lower quadrant (although site can vary because appendix is not always located in RLQ)
  - Usually aggravated by motion or coughing; pain during car ride is suspicious of rebound tenderness
  - Anorexia is frequent; nausea and vomiting also can occur
  - May have constipation or diarrhea; fever usually low-grade or absent
- Atypical presentation in children:
  - Initial symptom is vomiting
  - May have GI and genitourinary (GU) complaints
- URI symptoms, fever >101°F:
  - Less likely to exhibit abdominal tenderness, rebound tenderness, anorexia, and altered bowel sounds
- Atypical presentation in elderly:
  - Mental confusion, no fever, less abdominal tenderness

PHYSICAL EXAM
- Normal or mild elevation in temperature; if febrile may also be tachycardic
- Patient may be lying with knees flexed and guarding abdomen
- Abdominal exam: RLQ tenderness with rebound and guarding are usually present at McBurney's point; positive Rovsing's sign (pain referred to the right when direct pressure applied to LLQ), positive psoas sign (pain when raises right leg against resistance), and a positive obturator sign (pain when the right hip and knee are flexed and thigh is rotated inward)
- In neonates, a palpable abdominal mass and abdominal wall cellulitis may be evident
- In children <2 years, fever and diffuse abdominal tenderness are primary presentation

- In children 2–12 years, fever and RLQ tenderness is paramount
- Abdominal tenderness may be absent if appendix located in pelvis or behind cecum
- Involuntary guarding and rebound tenderness are indicative of a ruptured appendix
- May present with tender flank, rectum, or pelvis; therefore, a rectal and pelvic exam plus assessing for CVA tenderness is essential
- Mass from abscess may be palpable if perforation occurred several days prior to exam
- Serial exams are important until diagnosis made or ruled out

DIAGNOSTIC STUDIES
- CBC frequently shows a moderate leukocytosis
- Urinalysis to exclude hematuria and infection
- Urine Beta-HCG (b-HCG) should be performed in post-menarchal females
- Flat plate and upright abdominal x-ray to exclude intestinal obstruction, bowel perforation, or ureteral calculus; identification of a fecalith
- Pelvic ultrasound or abdominal CT preferred over x-ray to detect appendiceal inflammation, free fluid, abscess, or other causes of abdominal pain

Differential Diagnosis
- Life-threatening:
  - Ectopic pregnancy
  - Intestinal obstruction
  - Torsion or perforation of viscus
  - Abdominal aneurysm
  - Atypical presentation of MI
- Other possible differential diagnosis:
  - Acute gastroenteritis
  - Ruptured ovarian cyst or follicle
  - Twisted ovarian cyst and endometriosis
  - Perforated ulcer
  - Acute diverticulitis
  - Pelvic inflammatory disease
  - Acute pancreatitis
  - Cholecystitis
  - Ureteral calculus
  - Pyelonephritis constipation
  - Hemolytic uremic syndrome
  - Henoch-Schönlein purpura
  - Inflammatory bowel disease (IBD)
  - UTI
  - Mesenteric adenitis
  - Meckel's diverticulum
  - Pneumonia
  - Sickle cell
  - Pharmacologic disease
  - Pelvic inflammatory disease
  - Intussusception

Management
NONPHARMACOLOGIC TREATMENT
- Surgery (appendectomy) required
- Avoid use of cathartics or enemas due to risk of perforation
- Push fluids before appendectomy *treatment*
- Antibiotics should not be given if the diagnosis of appendicitis is in question because they can mask the presence or development of perforation
- If perforation or abscess does occur, IV antibiotics are given

Special Considerations
- Pregnancy: May present with atypical pain due to displacement of the appendix by the uterus
- Acute appendicitis may be the first manifestation of Crohn's disease

When to Consult, Refer, Hospitalize
- Immediate referral to a surgeon for appendectomy

Follow-Up
EXPECTED COURSE
- Recovery from an uncomplicated appendectomy is approximately 1 week

COMPLICATIONS
- Abscess and/or perforation of the bowel with subsequent peritonitis; either requires drainage and/or IV antibiotics

Intussusception

Description
- Telescoping of part of the bowel into another; results in decreased blood flow. Ischemia and infarction of intestine may occur if not treated. Ileocolic intussusception is most common, accounting for 80% of cases.

Etiology
- Idiopathic: Most commonly, cause is unknown
- Pathologic: Lead point found, occurs secondary to an abnormality in the bowel such as Meckel's diverticulum, polyps, intestinal duplication, hematoma, intestinal parasites, or, in older children, a malignancy
- Recent history of viral illness postulated to cause an increase in lymph tissue called Peyer's patches, thought to be a lead point for the intussusception

Incidence and Demographics
- Peak incidence is 3–36 months of age; males > females, 2:1
- 2–4 cases/1,000 live births per year; 75% of cases in children >5 years are associated with lead point
- Incidence has seasonal variations; peaks coincide with seasonal viral gastroenteritis

Risk Factors
- Recent history of viral illness postulated to cause an increase in lymph tissue called Peyer's patches, thought to be a lead point for the intussusception
- Patients with cystic fibrosis have an increased risk

Prevention and Screening
- None

Assessment

HISTORY
- Cramping, intermittent colicky pain
- Screaming, pulling legs upward during episode, followed by period of lethargy
- Pallor
- Bloody stool after the onset of symptoms
- "Currant jelly" stool is a late finding

PHYSICAL EXAM
- Pale, lethargic
- Sausage-shaped mass may be palpable across the midline
- Bowel sounds may be normal early, may be hyperactive during painful episodes; absent bowel sounds are a late finding

DIAGNOSTIC STUDIES
- CBC to rule out infection
- Abdominal x-ray reveals staircase pattern due to invagination of intestine
- Ultrasound is diagnostic
- Contrast enema is both diagnostic and therapeutic

Differential Diagnosis
- Gastroenteritis
- Tumor
- Constipation
- Meckel's diverticulum
- Incarcerated inguinal hernia
- Malrotation/volvulus
- Hirschsprung's disease
- Obstruction secondary to volvulus, stricture, fecal impaction, adhesions

Management

NONPHARMACOLOGIC TREATMENT
- Nasogastric decompression
- Contrast enema reduction done by an experienced radiologist
- Surgery indicated if signs of peritonitis, shock, or incomplete radiologic reduction

PHARMACOLOGIC TREATMENT
- None

LENGTH OF TREATMENT
- If reduction complete, restart feedings; discharge from the hospital takes place after the child has tolerated a full liquid diet

Special Considerations
- Radiologic reduction should not be attempted if symptoms present >5 days, in infants <3 months of age, or in any child with peritonitis or shock, in whom perforation is suspected

When to Consult, Refer, Hospitalize
- Immediate referral to pediatric emergency center
- Urgent surgical consultation recommended before radiologic reduction undertaken

Follow-Up
EXPECTED COURSE
- Children are usually discharged from the hospital 24 hours after reduction
- Surgical reduction is required if radiologic reduction is unsuccessful; manual reduction is undertaken; if not successful, resection of the affected bowel is indicated

COMPLICATIONS
- Recurrence: 10%, usually within 24 hours of radiologic reduction; less likely after surgical reduction
- Perforation: 1% occurrence during reduction
- Bowel necrosis, GI bleeding, sepsis, shock

Abdominal Hernias

Description
- A defect in the abdominal wall that allows intra-abdominal contents to protrude from the normal location.
- Hernias also can develop at sites of previous surgical incisions (incisional hernia).
- Clinically, all hernias can be described as reducible (contents can be pushed back into the abdominal cavity), nonreducible (contents cannot be pushed back into the abdominal cavity), incarcerated (a nonreducible hernia in which the flow of intestinal contents is obstructed), or strangulated (an incarcerated hernia in which the blood supply of the hernia contents is compromised)

Etiology
- Congenital or acquired defect in the abdominal wall
- Situations or conditions that raise intra-abdominal pressure increase occurrence (e.g., Valsalva, ascites, pregnancy)
- Incomplete or poor healing of a surgical incision can predispose to the development of an incisional hernia

Incidence and Demographics

- Umbilical: Common in infants; more common in African-American children, higher incidence in low birthweight infants. In adults, occurs in middle-aged multiparous women, patients with ascites, and the elderly.
- Epigastric: Common in men 20–50 years old
- Incisional: Common in peritoneal dialysis patients
- Femoral: Second most common hernia in both men and women, rare in children; incidence increases with age

Risk Factors

- Congenital defect in abdominal wall
- Activities and conditions that increase intra-abdominal pressure such as constipation, straining during micturition, chronic cough, weight-lifting, ascites, pregnancy, obesity
- Postoperative wound infection, dehiscence

Prevention and Screening

- Avoid excessive straining and lose weight if overweight; good body mechanics
- Screen on physical exams

Assessment

HISTORY
- Umbilical hernia: In infants, asymptomatic; adults may have vague, intermittent pain and tenderness
- Epigastric hernias: Present with a small painless mass
- Incisional or ventral hernia: Recent surgery, smoker, post-op wound infection
- Peristomal hernia: Patients with ostomy
- Strangulated hernias present with severe pain, fever, nausea and vomiting, abdominal distension, and constipation

PHYSICAL EXAM
- Inspection and palpation in both the supine and standing positions, while the patient performs a Valsalva maneuver; abdominal exam to evaluate tenderness, masses, hepatomegaly, and ascites; digital rectal exam to exclude enlarged prostate
- Umbilical or ventral: Palpate the umbilical region in the supine position while the patient raises head and performs a Valsalva maneuver
- Epigastric: Usually a small mass located midline between the umbilicus and xiphoid cartilage
- Incisional: Presents as a bulge through a surgical incision

DIAGNOSTIC STUDIES
- Diagnosed by history and physical exam
- CBC may show leukocytosis if strangulation is present
- Ultrasound may be helpful to diagnose a hernia in patients who report symptoms but have no palpable mass; can differentiate an incarcerated hernia from an enlarged lymph node or other cause

Differential Diagnosis

- Muscle strain
- Arthritis
- Lipoma
- Lymphadenopathy
- Diastasis recti

Management

NONPHARMACOLOGIC TREATMENT

- Patients with symptomatic, reducible inguinal hernias, who have relative contraindications to surgery, may wear a truss (keeps hernia reduced); however, this is not always effective
- Elective herniorrhaphy (hernia repair) is indicated for all abdominal hernias before incarceration and strangulation occurs; patients with evidence indicating a strangulated hernia must undergo emergent surgery
- Uncomplicated hernia repair is often done under local or spinal anesthesia on an outpatient basis

PHARMACOLOGIC TREATMENT

- None indicated
- Significant pain, if present, is suggestive of a more serious complication such as incarceration or strangulation, and should not be masked by narcotics

Special Considerations

- Geriatric patients: Inguinal and umbilical more common with increasing age
- Diastasis recti is a separation of the two rectus abdominis muscles, causing a ridge of abdominal contents to bulge slightly; it has no clinical consequence
- Pregnancy: Increases risk for developing a hernia due to increased abdominal pressure

When to Consult, Refer, Hospitalize

- Refer to a surgeon for evaluation

Follow-up

EXPECTED COURSE

- Risk of reccurrence after hernia repair—epigastric up to 10%; nonmesh incisional hernias recur 30%–50%; mesh-repaired hernias recur 20%

COMPLICATIONS

- Ischemic bowel with a strangulated hernia; bowel obstruction

Inguinal Hernia

Description

- Protrusion of abdominal viscus or bowel loop through a weakened opening of the abdominal wall at the inguinal area; may be reducible, nonreducible, incarcerated, or strangulated

Etiology
- Defect in the normal musculofascial integrity allowing bowel to protrude into the inguinal area
- Classified as direct or indirect:
  - Direct: Bowel protrudes directly through inguinal canal and emerges at the external inguinal ring
  - Indirect: Bowel protrudes through the internal abdominal ring, traverse the spermatic cord through inguinal canal and to the external inguinal ring
- Reducible vs. nonreducible: Reducible if contents can be pushed back into the abdominal cavity; nonreducible if they cannot
- Incarcerated inguinal hernia is a nonreducible hernia in which intestinal flow is completely blocked
- Strangulated inguinal hernias are incarcerated with compromised blood supply

Incidence and Demographics
- Of all abdominal hernias 75% are inguinal
- Men > women
- In children with a congenital defect of the processus vaginalis, over 50% of hernias are diagnosed during first year of life
- Indirect Inguinal hernias more common in the young however incidence increases 4–5 times after age 50

Risk Factors
- Congenital defect: Processus vaginalis remains patent (indirect)
- Increase intra-abdominal pressure such as with obesity, liver disease or Valsalva maneuvers (cough, exertion, defecation, constipation)

Prevention and Screening
- Family predisposition

Assessment
HISTORY
- May be asymptomatic, with hernia an incidental finding on examination
- Mild presentation of discomfort, dull aching, or swelling at groin/scrotal area
- Acute distress, acute scrotal pain and colicky pain, nausea and vomiting if incarcerated and/or strangulated
- Explore circumstances and precipitating events to onset of symptoms, whether it is better or worse with exertion or straining, position changes such as standing or supine, and whether the patient can reduce the hernia; this aids in evaluating the acuity of the situation as needing immediate surgery, elective surgical repair, manual reduction, or self-monitoring

PHYSICAL EXAM
- External inguinal area may be unchanged with an indirect hernia
- Inguinal bulging if a direct hernia is present
- Heaviness and palpable mass of the scrotum with an indirect hernia, either upon simple palpation or with invagination of the finger up to the inguinal ring; the hernia may be palpable in this position only with a Valsalva maneuver

- Transillumination of the scrotum is opaque and dull if hernia is present in the scrotum
- Abdominal exam may be normal or reveal abdominal distention, tenderness, and bowel sounds that may be hyperactive, heard in the scrotum, or entirely absent if incarcerated; the severity of the hernia correlates to increasingly abnormal findings

DIAGNOSTIC STUDIES
- None

Differential Diagnosis
- Hydrocele
- Epididymitis
- Lymphadenopathy
- Muscle, ligament, tendon injuries
- Varicocele
- Spermatocele cysts
- Tumor

Management
NONPHARMACOLOGIC TREATMENT
- If mild and asymptomatic, watchful waiting is indicated
- Explain to all patients with a plan of "watchful waiting" the signs of incarceration and strangulation and need for prompt treatment
- If reducible and nontender, elective surgical repair should be considered
- If incarcerated, urgent referral to surgeon for reduction then repair
- If strangulated, urologic emergency requiring immediate surgical referral

LENGTH OF TREATMENT
- Self-monitoring for signs or symptoms of changes (pain, nonreducible) ongoing, with annual examination

Special Considerations
- None

When to Consult, Refer, Hospitalize
- Refer to a surgeon all patients with symptomatic hernia.

Follow-Up
EXPECTED COURSE
- Courses may be variable, depending on precipitants; congenital defects will progress with age; contributing factors of obesity or poor body mechanics with exertion or Valsalva maneuvers may be improved and minimize their effect on recurrence

COMPLICATIONS
- Peritonitis, infarcted bowel
- Recurrence is 0.5%–15%

Cholecystitis

Description
- Acute or chronic inflammation of the gallbladder

Etiology
- More than 90% of cases are due to cystic duct obstruction by an impacted stone.
- Formation of gallstones is from supersaturation of products in bile exceeding their maximum solubilities.
- Gallstones consist predominantly of either cholesterol or calcium.
- Other causes include gallbladder stasis that can occur from prolonged acute illness, fasting and hyperalimentation, gallbladder infection; vasculitis; carcinoma of the gallbladder and/or bile ducts; other tumors that compress the gallbladder and/or bile ducts; infectious agents in clients with AIDS.
- Pain arises from the gallbladder contracting against an obstruction.

Incidence and Demographics
- Occurs in 16–20 million people in the U.S., with 1 million new cases each year.
- Gallstones are less common in African Americans except those who have sickle cell anemia.
- Geriatric patients: atypical presentation; at higher risk for developing complications, most common indication for abdominal surgery.

Risk Factors
- Mnemonic: Fat, fair, forty, flatulent, female
- Increases with age; body habitus, obesity, or rapid weight loss
- Childbearing, pregnancy, being female; family, maternal history of gallstones
- Drugs: Contraceptive hormones, hormone replacement therapy, ceftriaxone
- Ethnicity: Pima Indians, Scandinavians
- Hyperalimentation; ileal and other metabolic diseases such as diabetes mellitus, Crohn's disease

Prevention and Screening
- Low-fat, low-carbohydrate, high-fiber diet and physical activity

Assessment
HISTORY
- Acute:
    - Epigastric or right upper quadrant pain, nausea, vomiting, and fever
    - Pain may radiate to the right shoulder, scapula, or between the shoulder blades if there is irritation of the phrenic nerve (Kehr's sign)
    - Pain is usually precipitated by a large or fatty meal
    - Past medical history of biliary colic
- Chronic:
    - Less severe abdominal pain
    - Episodes shorter in duration (<3 hours) and recurrent

PHYSICAL EXAM
- Jaundice may be present if there is biliary obstruction (15% of acute cases)
- Positive Murphy's sign (sudden intake of breath, inspiratory arrest on palpation of the right upper quadrant due to pain)
- Guarding and rebound tenderness may be present
- Geriatric patients: Localized tenderness may be only presenting symptom, no fever or pain

DIAGNOSTIC STUDIES
- Leukocytosis, an elevated ALT (>300 IU/L), AST, GGT, and alkaline phosphatase usually present
- Elevated bilirubin may be seen with or without obstruction
- Serum amylase may also be elevated, especially if a biliary duct obstruction has occurred at or near the pancreatic duct causing a concomitant pancreatitis
- Ultrasound: 95% sensitivity and specificity for diagnosis of gallstones

Differential Diagnosis
- Pneumonia
- Thoracic disease
- Angina
- Appendicitis
- Bowel obstruction/IBD
- Pancreatitis
- Hepatitis
- Peptic ulcer disease
- GERD
- Cancer of gall bladder or bile ducts
- Right kidney disease

Management
NONPHARMACOLOGIC TREATMENT
- For chronic cholecystitis, decrease fat in diet

PHARMACOLOGIC TREATMENT
- For chronic cholecystitis, consider using ursodiol (Actigall) 8–10 mg/kg/day divided bid or tid
- For acute cholecystitis, referral to surgeon

Special Considerations
- In obese, diabetic, elderly, or immunosuppressed patient, severe inflammation of the gallbladder with gangrene, necrosis may occur without obvious signs and symptoms
- High risk for gallbladder carcinoma: Pima Indians, calcified gallbladder, gallbladder polyps >10 mm, gallstones >2.5 cm, anomalous pancreaticobiliary duct junction

When to Consult, Refer, Hospitalize
- Refer all to surgeon for evaluation; those with acute cholecystitis require hospitalization

Follow-Up
- Provide patient education about diet, medications
  EXPECTED COURSE
    - Uncomplicated cholecystectomy usually followed by complete resolution of symptoms

  COMPLICATIONS
    - Gangrene, necrosis, cholangitis, and other complications of surgery
    - Mortality rate is markedly increased for elderly who have cholecystectomy for acute cholecystitis

Colorectal Cancer

Description
- Malignancy of the large intestine including the rectum

Etiology
- Most colon cancers are adenocarcinomas that begin as adenomatous polyps (benign epithelial growths)

Incidence and Demographics
- Second leading cause of death due to malignancy in U.S., with 55,000 deaths occurring annually
- Increased prevalence in developed countries, urban areas, and advantaged socioeconomic groups
- Higher incidence in people of German, Irish, Czechoslovakian, and French decent

Risk Factors
- Incidence increases after age 40, with 90% of new cases occurring over age 50
- Previous history or family history of adenomatous polyps
- Family history of colorectal cancer, especially in a first-degree relative diagnosed before age 55
- Familial polyposis
- Inflammatory bowel disease
- History of breast or gynecological cancer
- Barrett's esophagus
- Obesity
- Cigarette smoking

Prevention and Screening
- Annual digital rectal examination with annual stool checks for occult blood in all persons over 40
- Colonoscopy is the recommended screening test for colorectal cancer beginning at age 50
- High-risk patients with first-degree relative with colon cancer should have a colonoscopy, recommended beginning at 40 (or 10 years before cancer diagnosis in relative, whichever is earlier). Patients with a negative screening colonoscopy need future screenings every 3–5 years.

- Direct effect of diet remains unproven; however, a diet high in fiber, fruits, and vegetables shows promise in decreasing colorectal cancer. Calcium supplementation and a daily aspirin also have been shown to be beneficial

Assessment

HISTORY
- Often colorectal cancer reaches advanced stages without symptoms
- Symptoms may include rectal bleeding, altered bowel habits (constipation, occasional diarrhea, pencil-thin stools)
- Signs and symptoms of anemia

PHYSICAL EXAM
- A mass may be palpated in the abdomen
- Rectal mass may be palpated on digital exam
- The liver should be evaluated for enlargement suggesting metastatic disease
- Enlarged inguinal lymph nodes

DIAGNOSTIC STUDIES
- Stool for occult blood: False positives can be caused by ingestion of red meat, iron, or aspirin, and from upper GI bleeding; false negatives can occur from vitamin C ingestion and intermittent bleeding
- CBC to evaluate for iron deficiency anemia
- Elevated liver function tests raise concern for possible liver metastasis
- Carcinoembryonic antigen (CEA) has not been shown to be efficacious for colorectal cancer screening; however, useful as a marker for treatment response in patients who have been diagnosed with colorectal cancer; if treatment response occurs, the CEA level should decrease
- Colonoscopy with biopsy confirms diagnosis
- Abdominal CT used to evaluate for metastatic disease in patients with colorectal cancer

Differential Diagnosis
- Rectal polyps
- Hemorrhoids
- Rectal fissures
- Colorectal strictures
- Diverticulosis
- Colorectal infections
- Inflammatory lesions
- Other neoplasms
- Inflammatory bowel disease
- Masses outside bowel wall

Management
- Depends on cancer stage (tumor size and extent of bowel wall invasion, lymph node involvement, presence of metastasis) and type of tumor
- Surgery is the treatment of choice

NONPHARMACOLOGIC TREATMENT
· Referral to surgeon for surgery and/or radiation

PHARMACOLOGIC TREATMENT
· Chemotherapy

Special Considerations
· None

When to Consult, Refer, Hospitalize
· If colon cancer is suspected or diagnosed, refer to a surgeon
· Patients with a family history of colon cancer or a history of adenomatous polyps should be followed regularly by a gastroenterologist

Follow-Up
EXPECTED COURSE
· Depends on the stage of the cancer and type of tumor

COMPLICATIONS
· Complications associated with chemotherapy, radiation, surgery, and/or metastasis

Acute Pancreatitis

Description
· Inflammation of the pancreas causing release of pancreatic enzymes into the surrounding tissue
· With acute pancreatitis, there is usually complete restoration of pancreatic function; when recovery is incomplete, the patient develops chronic pancreatitis

Etiology
· Most cases are related to biliary tract disease from a large gallstone causing a blockage of the pancreatic duct or from excessive alcohol consumption
· This causes the release of pancreatic enzymes that cause local and systemic symptoms
· Other causes include hypercalcemia, hyperlipidemia, viral infections (e.g., mumps), renal failure, certain medications, and abdominal trauma

Incidence and Demographics
· Estimated 15 per 100,000
· Equal distribution between genders
· Acute, no predominant age
· Chronic, usually related to alcohol intake, ages 35–45

Risk Factors
· Alcohol abuse
· Gallstones, hyperlipidemia, hyperparathyroidism, hypercalcemia
· Abdominal trauma, renal failure, certain viral infections

- Certain medications (diuretics, valproic acid, didanosine [ddI], sulfonamides, azathioprine)
- Noncompliance with diabetes and hyperlipidemia treatment

Prevention and Screening
- Decrease alcohol consumption; a low-fat, low-cholesterol diet

Assessment

HISTORY
- Abrupt onset of epigastric or left upper quadrant abdominal pain, often radiating to the back, described as steady and severe
- Pain is worsened by movement or lying supine and improves when sitting or leaning forward
- Nausea and vomiting are generally present
- There may be a history of alcohol intake or a heavy meal prior to the onset of pain

PHYSICAL EXAM
- Low-grade fever, epigastric or left upper abdominal tenderness, and distention are usually present
- Occasionally an upper abdominal mass can be palpated due to pancreatic inflammation or presence of a pseudocyst (a sac of pancreatic enzymes surrounding the pancreas)
- Absent bowel sounds may occur if a paralytic ileus is present
- Mild jaundice, tachycardia, hypotension, pallor, and sweating can be seen

DIAGNOSTIC STUDIES
- Serum amylase and lipase will be significantly elevated
- Urinalysis may show proteinuria, increased osmolality, glycosuria, and casts
- CBC may show leukocytosis (10,000–25,000)
- Alkaline phosphatase and ALT and ALT may be mildly elevated
- Serum calcium may be decreased in severe acute disease
- In chronic disease labs may be normal
- Flat plate and upright abdominal film to rule out perforated ulcer or intestinal obstruction
- Chest x-ray may be needed to rule out chest pathology
- Abdominal CT scan may be used to demonstrate an enlarged pancreas or pseudocyst

Differential Diagnosis
- Acute cholecystitis
- Acute intestinal obstruction
- Perforated duodenal ulcer
- Leaking aortic aneurysm
- Renal stone
- Acute mesenteric ischemia
- Gastroenteritis

Management

NONPHARMACOLOGIC TREATMENT
- Referral for hospitalization and treatment of underlying cause, unless mild case and tolerating fluids

Special Considerations
- Can occur in children secondary to trauma (should increase suspicion of child abuse)

When to Consult, Refer, Hospitalize
- Hospitalization required for IV hydration while NPO, pain management, and monitoring response
- Surgical consultation required in all cases of acute pancreatitis with evidence of abscess formation or infected pancreatic tissue

Follow-Up
- For recurrent episodes of pancreatitis:

EXPECTED COURSE
- Most uncomplicated cases subside in 3–7 days

COMPLICATIONS
- Pancreatic pseudocysts, abscesses, stricture of the common bile duct, diabetes mellitus, chronic pancreatitis, and occasionally pancreatic cancer

Diverticulitis/Diverticulosis

Description
- Diverticulosis is the presence of a diverticulum (herniation of mucosa through muscular wall of the colon)
- Diverticulitis is an inflammation of a diverticulum, usually caused when undigested food and bacteria remain in the diverticular outpouching and serve as an area where localized abscess and peritonitis begin
  - Infection can vary from a small abscess to peritonitis
  - Size of the inflamed diverticula vary from small to large, and the number can be one to several dozen
  - Diverticula are more common in the sigmoid colon (left colon) than in the right colon

Etiology
- Diverticula develop from increased intraluminal pressure that results from insufficient intake of fiber
- Subsequently, infection and inflammation result from mechanical obstruction from retention of undigested food residues and bacteria in the diverticula
- Thought to be a result of poor dietary fiber intake over many years that results in hypertrophy, thickening, and fibrosis of the bowel wall from movement of hard stool under increased intraluminal pressures

Incidence and Demographics
- Common in Western countries; uncommon in developing countries
- More common in women

Risk Factors
- Low-fiber diet, increased age, sedentary lifestyle

Prevention and Screening
- High-fiber diet; avoid foods with small seeds that can become trapped in the diverticula

Assessment

HISTORY
- Complaints vary with severity of the inflammation and infection; diverticulosis is asymptomatic
- Crampy left lower or mid-abdominal pain that may radiate to the back, or acute pain that is localized to the left lower quadrant
- Fever, constipation, loose stool, and/or nausea and vomiting may be present

PHYSICAL EXAM
- There may be left lower quadrant tenderness with a palpable mass and hypoactive bowel sounds
- Rebound tenderness also may be present and may be suggestive of a perforated diverticulum
- Rectal exam may reveal a palpable mass (indicating a pelvic abscess) and heme-positive stool

DIAGNOSTIC STUDIES
- CBC shows a mild to moderate leukocytosis; ESR elevated in diverticulits; CBC may be normal in diverticulosis
- Flat plate and upright abdominal film to look for free air (sign of perforation), ileus, and small or large bowel obstruction
- Abdominal scan with IV and oral contrast to delineate pericolic abscesses
- Barium enema should not be obtained in the acute phase due to risk of perforation; perform after patient has responded to medical management to exclude other problems such as a mass
- If a mass or stricture is seen, a colonoscopy should be performed to rule out malignancy after acute episode resolved

Differential Diagnosis
- Appendicitis
- Ruptured ovarian cyst or follicle
- Twisted ovarian cyst
- Endometriosis
- Ruptured ectopic pregnancy
- Pelvic inflammatory disease
- Crohn's disease
- Colon cancer

- Ischemic bowel
- Intestinal obstruction

Management
NONPHARMACOLOGIC TREATMENT
- Outpatient treatment for majority of cases with only mild abdominal tenderness, tolerating fluids, low-grade fever, and leukocytosis <12,000; initial liquid diet followed by low-residue diet
- Gradually increase dietary fiber after acute phase; avoid eating seeds, nuts, corn
- If condition worsens or lacks improvement in 48–72 hours, hospitalize; or if peritoneal signs or septicemia
- Surgical management required for signs of abscess or perforation

PHARMACOLOGIC TREATMENT
- Mild symptoms: Metronidazole (Flagyl) 250–500 mg po q8h plus either trimethoprim-sulfamethoxazole 160/180 (Bactrim DS) po q 12 h or other antibiotic (Cipro, Augmentin) for 7–10 days
- May treat pain with anitspasmodics, opiates(not meperidine-increases intrluminal pressure)
- Stool softeners until dietary fiber can be increased
- Moderate to severe symptoms require hospitalization, IV antibiotics, and nasogastric intubation

LENGTH OF TREATMENT
- Mild symptoms: 14 days
- Moderate to severe symptoms: Length of treatment may vary

Special Considerations
- Elderly less likely to have classic symptoms; pursue evaluation despite mild presentation
- No alcohol if metronidazole ordered; it will provoke severe vomiting

When to Consult, Refer, Hospitalize
- Hospitalization with surgical consultation should be obtained in all patients with severe diverticulitis (fever, elevated WBC, rebound tenderness, vomiting, rectal pain) and for those who fail to improve after 48–72 hours of medical management
- Hospitalization often required for elderly with acute diverticulitis and multiple medical problems

Follow-Up
- Within 3 days, sooner if worsens; response to antibiotics should occur in 3 days
  ### EXPECTED COURSE
  - Diverticulitis recurs in one-third of patients who receive medical management. Recurrent attacks are an indication for elective surgical resection

  ### COMPLICATIONS
  - Perforation, peritonitis, hemorrhage, and bowel obstruction

CONDITIONS OF THE RECTUM AND ANUS

Hemorrhoids

Description
- Hemorrhoids are varicosities of the hemorrhoidal venous plexus that are classified as either internal (above pectinate line) or external (below pectinate line)
- These varicosities may be dilated, prolapsed, or thrombosed, often causing painful swelling at the anus

Etiology
- Anal cushions become displaced, etiology unknown
- Prolapse of a vascular anal cushion through the anal canal becomes entrapped by the anal sphincter and a hemorrhoid is formed

Incidence and Demographics
- Occurs in 50% of adults over age 50
- Uncommon under age 25 except in pregnancy

Risk Factors
- Constipation, prolonged sitting or standing
- Weight-lifting
- Pregnancy, obesity
- Congestive heart failure, portal hypertension
- Rectal surgery, loss of muscle tone
- Anal intercourse

Prevention and Screening
- High-fiber diet
- Avoid constipation and straining to defecate
- Proper body mechanics when lifting
- Avoid prolonged periods of sitting or standing; change position frequently
- Weight loss if overweight

Assessment
HISTORY
- Rectal bleeding (usually painless and bright red); rectal discomfort, itching, burning
- Inquire about possible risk factors
- Constipation or straining

PHYSICAL EXAM
- External hemorrhoids are a soft and painless mass exterior to the anal verge
- Internal hemorrhoids may be palpated by digital rectal exam or visualized by anoscopy
- If thrombosed, hemorrhoids are bluish in color, firm, and tender to palpation

DIAGNOSTIC STUDIES
- Diagnosed by physical exam; if normal exam but has bleeding, colonoscopy in those over 40
- CBC to rule out anemia

Differential Diagnosis
- Anal skin tags
- Crohn's disease
- Anal fissure
- Prolapse of rectal mucosa (common in elderly)
- Abscess
- Rectal polyps
- Rectal or anal carcinoma

Management
NONPHARMACOLOGIC TREATMENT
- Eliminate risk factors when possible
- Avoid direct pressure on hemorrhoid while sitting
- Warm sitz baths 2–3 times daily for 20 minutes, witch hazel compresses (Tucks) tid-qid prn
- High-fiber diet (20–30 g/day) and increased fluid intake (eight 8 oz glasses/day)

PHARMACOLOGIC TREATMENT
- Bulk-forming laxatives to soften stool and prevent constipation
  – Psyllium (Metamucil) 1 tbsp in 8 oz of fluid up to 3 times day
  – Methylcellulose (Citrucel) 1 tbsp in 8 oz of fluid up to 3 times day
- Stool softeners to reduce straining during defecation
  – Docusate sodium (Colace) 50–200 mg/day
- Topical hydrocortisone preparations to relieve pain, itching, and inflammation; cream, foam, and suppositories are available
  – Anusol-HC, ProctoFoam-HC, Hydrocortisone cream 1%–2.5% prn
- Local analgesic spray, suppository, or cream provides pain relief
  – Benzocaine (Hurricane), pramoxine (Anusol), or dibucaine (Nupercainal) prn

LENGTH OF TREATMENT
- Use topical hydrocortisone preparations for a maximum of 2–3 weeks; stool softeners and bulk-forming laxatives may be used indefinitely to prevent reoccurrence

Special Considerations
- Pregnancy: Common, usually resolve spontaneously after delivery

When to Consult, Refer, Hospitalize
- Refer to a colorectal surgeon when symptoms do not respond to conservative treatment within 3–4 weeks; when patients present with severe pain, thrombosis, strangulation, ulceration, perianal infection, rectal prolapse, or for recurrent symptomatic hemorrhoids

- Refer patients over 40 with rectal bleeding, despite hemorrhoids, to a gastroenterologist for sigmoidoscopy and/or colonoscopy to evaluate for other causes of GI bleeding and to exclude cancer

Follow-Up
EXPECTED COURSE
- Patients should follow up for further evaluation if there is no improvement in symptoms within 2 weeks of initiating treatment, if rectal bleeding is excessive or persists, or if constipation continues

COMPLICATIONS
- Bleeding, thrombosis, strangulation, secondary infection, ulceration, and anemia

Pinworms

Description
- Pinworm infestation characterized by perianal itching, usually at night or early morning, caused by deposit of eggs at anal opening

Etiology
- Enterobius vermicularis infection
- Adult worms invade intestine, migrate to anus, and deposit eggs on the perianal skin at night; larvae develop over 6 hours and are ingested, re-inoculating the host
- Transmission occurs when individual touches anus, then touches hands or belongings of another individual, allowing the second person to come in contact with eggs

Incidence and Demographics
- Affects 6%–15% of children in the U.S.; may affect household contacts of affected children; most frequently occurs in children 5–10 years of age
- Spread by fecal-oral transmission; unrelated to personal hygiene

Risk Factors
- Shared toys, bedding, clothing with infected individual
- Day care attendance

Prevention and Screening
- Good hygiene, handwashing

Assessment
HISTORY
- Nocturnal and early morning anal itching

PHYSICAL EXAM
- Difficult to observe during physical examination
- Small, white, threadlike worm occasionally visible

DIAGNOSTIC STUDIES
- Tape test: Parents use sticky tape, touch the anal opening with the tape to obtain specimen when child first arises in morning; may need up to 3 specimens since worms may not lay eggs every night

Differential Diagnosis
- Other parasitic infestation
- Bacterial vaginitis
- Fungal vaginitis
- Diaper dermatitis
- Chemical dermatitis
- Habit
- Anal fissure

Management
NONPHARMACOLOGIC TREATMENT
- Wash clothing, underclothing, bedding of infected individual in hot water
- Early morning bathing removes most eggs; frequent handwashing, trim fingernails short
- Family members may need to be treated

PHARMACOLOGIC TREATMENT
- Drug of choice: Mmebendazole (Vermox) 100 mg chewable tablet, single dose, may repeat in 3 weeks
- Pyrantel Pamoate (Pin-X) 11mg/kg, not to exceed 1 g
- Albendazole (Albenza) 10 mg/kg
- Doses need to be repeated in 1–2 weeks to ensure cure
- All should be used with caution in children <2 years

LENGTH OF TREATMENT
- Second dose recommended 3 weeks after initial dose to insure eggs that hatched after initial treatment are eradicated

Special Considerations
- Recurrence is common if all contacts are not treated

When to Consult, Refer, Hospitalize
- Referral or hospitalization is not indicated

Follow-Up
EXPECTED COURSE
- Improvement is expected within a few days

COMPLICATIONS
- Recurrence
- Urethritis, vaginitis may occur from migration of the worm from perineum

Anal Fissure

Description
- Anal fissure is a tear in the lining of the anal canal distal to the dentate line
- Most commonly seen in posterior midline (men); anterior midline may occur in women
- Once they occur, become cyclical in nature

Etiology
- Usually associated with the passage of a large hard stool; can occur with anal stenosis
- Trauma to anal wall causing pain and inflammation, but usually no infection due to local defenses

Incidence and Demographics
- Incidence unknown, though very common
- Typically occur in first 3–4 years of life
- Can occur in all age groups

Risk Factors
- Sexual abuse should be considered in a child with any abnormal findings; uncommon in children
- Constipation
- Trauma

Prevention and Screening
- Avoid constipation
- Increase fluids and fiber

Assessment
HISTORY
- Passage of a large or hard, dry stool
- Crying during defecation, severe pain
- Bright red blood evident on the toilet paper
- Streaks of blood around stool

PHYSICAL EXAM
- Fissure often can be seen if careful inspection of the anal area is performed

DIAGNOSTIC STUDIES
- Not indicated unless the source of the bleeding cannot be identified; may require anesthesia

Differential Diagnosis
- Juvenile polyp
- Intussusception
- Inflammatory bowel disease
- Gastroenteritis
- Necrotizing enterocolitis

Management

NONPHARMACOLOGIC TREATMENT
- Anal dilatation is necessary if anal stenosis is present, requires referral
- High-fiber diet or fiber supplements
- Warm sitz baths

PHARMACOLOGIC TREATMENT
- Stool softener to facilitate easy passage and prevent stool withholding
- Topical antibiotic ointment bid
- Hydrocortisone cream bid to tid
- Topical anesthetics
- Topical nitroglycerin increases local blood flow and reduces pressure in anal sphincter to facilitate healing
- Botulinum toxin may be used and has fewer side effects than nitroglycerin therapy

LENGTH OF TREATMENT
- Treat until soft stool is produced and the fissure is healed

Special Considerations
- Suspect sexual abuse when more than one fissure is present or if child

When to Consult, Refer, Hospitalize
- Consult or refer to surgeon or colorectal specialist if symptoms persist after 90 days of treatment
- Need to report to child protective authorities if sexual abuse is suspected

Follow-Up
- 1–2 weeks
  EXPECTED COURSE
  - Uncomplicated; resolves when fissure is healed and constipation resolved

  COMPLICATIONS
  - Recurrence, skin ulceration
  - Fecal incontinence

CONDITIONS OF THE LIVER

Viral Hepatitis

Description
- Inflammation of the liver caused by a viral infection that may be acute (<6 months duration) or chronic (>6 months duration) that produces liver dysfunction with a broad range of severity
- Six types of viral hepatitis have been identified: A, B, C, D, E, and G
- Hepatitis B virus (HBV) and hepatitis C virus (HCV) account for 60%–80% of chronic hepatitis

Etiology
- Hepatitis A virus (HAV): An RNA hepatovirus
- Hepatitis B virus (HBV): A DNA hepadnavirus with an inner core protein and outer surface coat component
- Hepatitis C virus (HCV): An RNA togavirus
- Hepatitis D virus (HDV): A defective RNA virus that only occurs in persons with Hepatitis B infection
- Hepatitis E virus (HEV): An RNA virus similar to calicivirus
- Hepatitis G virus (HGV): Recently identified flavivirus

Incidence and Demographics
- HAV: 125,000–200,000 infections per year; 70% are symptomatic, 33% have serologic evidence for past HAV infection
- HBV: 140,000–320,000 infections per year, 1–1.25 million with chronic infection; more than 500,000 carriers; post-transfusion infection occurs in less than 1%
- HCV: 35,000–180,000 infections per year; chronic infection will develop in >85% of those infected; approximately 4 million HCV carriers; 10% have no known source of infection
- HDV: Occurs in 1% of HBV-infected persons, primarily among intravenous drug users; endemic in some Mediterranean countries, affecting 80% of HBV carriers
- HEV: Outbreaks commonly occur in India, Burma, Afghanistan, Algeria, and Mexico; rare in the U.S.; usually occurs in persons who traveled to endemic areas
- HGV: 900–2,000 infections per year; 0.3% of acute viral hepatitis

Risk Factors
- See Table 9–5

Table 9-5. Comparison of Viral Hepatitis Transmission

Virus	Transmission	Risk Factors	Incubation	Chronicity
Hepatitis A	Fecal-oral	Contaminated food and water Common in overcrowded, poor sanitation areas, also close contacts	15–50 days	No
Hepatitis B	Blood Body fluids	Transfusion Needle-sharing Exposure to infected body fluids Sexual activity Perinatal transmission	45–160 days	Yes

Table 9-5. Comparison of Viral Hepatitis Transmission (cont.)

Virus	Transmission	Risk Factors	Incubation	Chronicity
Hepatitis C	Blood Body fluids	Transfusion Needle-sharing High-risk sexual behavior Cocaine use Low risk of perinatal transmission	14–180 days	Yes
Hepatitis D	Blood Body fluids	Acute or chronic hepatitis B Immigrants from endemic countries Positive sexual contacts	45–160 days	Yes
Hepatitis E and G	Fecal-oral	Third world countries (rare in U.S.)	15–60 days	No

Prevention and Screening
- Healthcare providers need a high index of suspicion
- Universal precautions should be practiced by all healthcare and day care workers when in contact with blood, blood products, or body fluids
- Safe sex practices
- Avoid intravenous drug use and sharing of needles
- Screening of all blood products for HBV and HCV infection
- Proper hygiene and handwashing by food handlers
- Screen all pregnant women for HBV infection
- Vaccination against hepatitis A and B (see Table 9–6)
- Immune globulin to all close personal contacts of those with hepatitis A; traveling to endemic areas; with chronic liver disease or clotting disorders; sewage workers and food handlers, day care workers

Table 9-6. Hepatitis Vaccines

Virus	Vaccine	Target Population	Dosing Regimen	Dose
Hep A	Havrix, Vaqta Twinrix (A and B)	International travelers Children >2 years living in endemic areas Chronic liver disease Men who have sex with men IV drug abusers Occupational risk	*Age 2–18 years:* Havrix, either 2- or 3-dose schedule; Vaqta, 2-dose schedule. *Age >18 years:* 2-dose schedule of Havrix; 3-4 dose schedule of Twinrix Second dose given 6–12 months after the first Havrix	2–18 years: 0.5 mL >18 year: 1 mL IM anterolateral thigh in children, deltoid in adults
Hep B	Recombivax or Engerix-B	All infants All children not previously vaccinated Healthcare workers People with high-risk behaviors	3 doses given at 0, 1, and 6 months	0–19 years: 0.5 mL >19 years: 1.0 mL IM in anterolateral thing for children; deltoid for adults
	Pediarix (combination DPT, HepB, and polio Comvax combination HIB and HepB		Many are given in combination with routine pediatric doses in single injection	
Hep C, D, E, G	None available			

Assessment
- Symptoms of viral hepatitis are similar, however, the severity of symptoms may vary among types, ranging from asymptomatic infection without jaundice to fulminant hepatitis (severe form of acute hepatitis indicated by encephalopathy, hypoglycemia, bleeding, and prolonged prothrombin time)
  HISTORY
  - Symptoms vary according to phase of disease
  - Pre-icteric phase: Fatigue, malaise, anorexia, nausea, vomiting, headache, aversion to smoking and alcohol
  - Icteric phase: Weight loss, pruritus, right upper quadrant pain, clay-colored stool; frequently have pronounced jaundice and may appear mildly toxic to acutely ill (see Table 9–7)

PHYSICAL EXAM
- General toxicity varies with disease severity
- Jaundice of the skin, sclera, and mucous membranes
- Lymphadenopathy usually present in the cervical and epitrochlear areas
- Abdominal exam: Liver tenderness with hepatomegaly present in >50%, splenomegaly present in 15%
- Dark urine or clay-colored stools

DIAGNOSTIC STUDIES
- ALT and AST may be elevated; levels peak (400 to several thousand U/L) during the icteric phase, then progressively decrease during the convalescent phase
- Serum bilirubin normal to markedly elevated; clinical jaundice evident at levels >2.5
- Alkaline phosphatase may be normal or mildly elevated
- Prothrombin time; if prolonged, may indicate serious disease
- CBC may reveal an increased number of atypical-appearing lymphocytes
- Urinalysis may be positive for protein and bilirubin
- Above tests may be normal in patients with chronic hepatitis C
- Serologic tests for viral hepatitis (see Table 9–7)
- Liver biopsy if diagnosis is uncertain; gold standard for severity and activity of chronic hepatitis

Differential Diagnosis
- Cytomegalovirus (CMV), herpes simplex
- Coxsackie virus
- Toxoplasmosis
- *Candida*, *Mycobacteria*
- *Pneumocystis*
- *Leptospira*
- Use of hepatotoxic agents
- Alcoholic hepatitis
- Ischemic hepatitis
- Acute cholecystitis
- Common bile duct stone
- Ascending cholangitis
- Cirrhosis

Table 9–7. Viral Hepatitis Diagnostic Criteria

Virus	Symptoms	Contagious Interval	Diagnosis Positive Labs
Hep A	Children either asymptomatic or very mild, nonspecific symptoms Adults usually symptomatic with 1–2 week prodrome of anorexia, nausea, malaise, fever, then jaundice	1–3 weeks before illness lasting through first week of illness	*Acute:* Anti-HAV IgM Anti-HAV IgG develops later in disease and stays for life
Hep B	In young children usually asymptomatic Adult symptoms range from asymptomatic seroconversion to acute illness with anorexia, nausea, malaise, jaundice, arthralgias, arthritis, macular skin rash, to fatal hepatitis	All persons with HbsAG are infectious	*Acute:* HBsAG HBcAG IgM anti-HBc If HBeAG positive, indication of more serious disease Recovery: HBsAG Anti-HBs Anti-HBc Chronic: HBsAG Anti-HBc
Hep C	Asymptomatic in children Adults often mild disease, difficult to distinguish from hep A and hep B Jaundice in only 25%	All persons with HCV antibody or HCV-RNA are considered contagious	*Acute:* ELISA II RIBA Chronic: Serum anti-HCV antibody
Hep D	Occurs either as a co-infection with HBV or as a superinfection in chronic HBV Same signs and symptoms as for hep B	Similar to hepatitis B	*Acute:* Anti-HDV
Hep E and G	More common in adults than children Acute illness: Jaundice, malaise, anorexia, abdominal pain, arthralgias, fever	Exact interval unknown but for at least 2 weeks after acute illness	Based on exclusion of other hepatitis viruses

Management
NONPHARMACOLOGIC TREATMENT
- Activity as tolerated; high-calorie, small, palatable meals, hydration to 4,000 cc daily
- Avoid hepatotoxic agents (i.e., acetaminophen and alcohol)
- Colloid baths and lotions to decrease pruritus if present

PHARMACOLOGIC TREATMENT
- For acute, uncomplicated hepatitis A & B, no pharmacologic treatment is indicated
- Acute Hepatitis C, medications are effective
- Antiemetics for nausea and vomiting if needed
- Use oxazepam if a benzodiazepine is indicated; avoid morphine sulfate
- Both chronic hepatitis B and C are treated with recombinant human interferon alfa and/or nucleoside analogs (lamivudine and ribavirin) if there is evidence of liver impairment
- Post-exposure hepatitis B
    - Unvaccinated persons: Immune globulin (HBIG) 0.06 mL/kg IM given as soon as possible (within 7 days of exposure), followed by initiation of the HBV vaccination series (above), prevents illness in approximately 75%
    - Recommended after direct transmucosal or parental exposure with HBsAg-infected blood or body fluids; HBIG (0.5 mL IM) is given to all newborns of HBsAg-positive mothers within 12 hours of birth
- Post-exposure hepatitis A
    - All household and sexual contacts, give 0.02 mL/kg of immune globulin as soon as possible (within 2 weeks) and begin HAV vaccine

LENGTH OF TREATMENT
- In chronic hepatitis B, treatment is continued until loss of HBeAg, loss of HBV-DNA, loss of HBsAg, and normal ALT level
- In chronic hepatitis C, treatment is continued until viral replication is inhibited, normal ALT levels, loss of HCV-RNA, reduction of hepatic inflammation, and improvement in liver histology

Special Considerations
- HBV: Transmitted vertically (mother to infant) in <10%
- HEV: High mortality rate in pregnancy (10%–20%)
- Lactation: HBV transmission uncertain; HCV transmission unlikely

When to Consult, Refer, Hospitalize
- Consult with physician or specialist for all cases of hepatitis B, C, D because of high incidence of chronic hepatitis development
- Refer to a gastroenterologist and/or an infectious disease specialist for uncertain diagnosis, symptoms of fulminant hepatitis, and chronic hepatitis

Follow-Up

- Hepatitis A patients should follow up in 2 weeks to reevaluate condition
- Hepatitis B, C, D require frequent follow-up during acute stage, then 4–8 week intervals if chronic illness develops

  EXPECTED COURSE
  - Acute hepatitis usually resolves over 4–8 weeks

  COMPLICATIONS
  - Hepatic necrosis, chronic active or chronic hepatitis, cirrhosis, hepatic failure, hepatocellular carcinoma (HBV and HCV)
  - Fatal fulminant hepatitis (HAV)
  - Chronic hepatitis B and C increase risk for development of cirrhosis

Physiologic Jaundice in the Healthy-Term Newborn

Description

- Increased levels of unconjugated serum bilirubin (>2.0 mg/dL) that occurs 3–5 days after birth and causes jaundice
- Pathologic jaundice occurs when there is erythrocyte destruction due to ABO or Rh incompatibility, G6PD deficiency, or other pathologic conditions

Etiology

- Overproduction of bilirubin and delayed conjugation of bilirubin caused by:
  - Increased rate of hemolysis
  - Increased production of bilirubin secondary to increased red blood cell volume, increased and inefficient red cell production, and inefficient hepatic breakdown of bilirubin

Incidence and Demographics

- About 60% of infants will have clinical physiologic jaundice with peak bilirubin level 5–6 mg/dL
- Approximately 3% of newborns will have more severe jaundice with serum bilirubin levels in the range of 13–15 mg/dL; 2% of breastfed infants will have a 2–8 week course of detectable physiological jaundice with an unconjugated bilirubin level in the range of 10–15 mg/dL

Risk Factors

- Breastfeeding, poor feeding
- Frequently recurs in siblings

Prevention and Screening

- Educate parents on normal feeding, adequate urine output
- Parents must be aware that normal physiologic bilirubin levels will not peak until 72–96 hours of age for full-term infant
- Teach parents how to assess for the presence of jaundice

Assessment
HISTORY
- Question parents about when first noticed, where on body, pattern of spread
- Evidence of yellow tinge to skin and sclera noticed on third to fifth day, declining in 1 week, longer if premature
- Other symptoms: Lethargy, poor feeding, dark stools and urine, decreased urine
- Obtain complete feeding and voiding history to ensure adequate hydration
- Review history of Rh and ABO status of the mother, pregnancy and delivery history, family history of jaundice, any history of infant deaths for suspicion of pathologic jaundice

PHYSICAL EXAM
- Vital signs, weight
- Observe skin color, noting how far down the trunk jaundice has progressed (begins in face and moves downward as bilirubin levels rise)
- Blanch the skin to observe jaundice
- Abdominal exam: Should have normal liver

DIAGNOSTIC STUDIES
- Total bilirubin level, including conjugated, necessary for severe and rapid-onset jaundice
- Direct Coombs' test, G6PD enzyme assay done if physiologic jaundice suspected
- Hematocrit
- Blood type, Rh

Differential Diagnosis
- Sepsis
- Galactosemia
- Hemolytic disease

Management
NONPHARMACOLOGIC TREATMENT
- Phototherapy may be necessary: Light enhances bile excretion; home phototherapy can occur in uncomplicated cases
- Guidelines for initiation vary with age of infant, presence of risk factors (i.e., breastfed infants are expected to reach higher levels), hydration status, gestational age
- Generally, consider in full-term infants with total serum bilirubin levels 12–15 at 24–48 hours old, 15–18 at 48–72 hours old, or 17–20 at >72 hours old
- Breastfeeding can continue and supplementation with water is not necessary, but more frequent feeding should occur

PHARMACOLOGIC TREATMENT
- None

LENGTH OF TREATMENT
- Monitor total bilirubin levels daily, continue treatment until levels stabilize or begin to fall

Special Considerations
- When phototherapy is instituted, the infant's eyes must be protected from the light, temperature should be monitored, and extra fluid should be given to replace that lost from evaporation

When to Consult, Refer, Hospitalize
- Consult with physician or refer to neonatal specialist if pathologic jaundice suspected or have feeding difficulty, behavior changes, apnea, fever, or temperature instability
- Suspect pathologic jaundice if occurs in first 24 hours of life: Total bilirubin rises more than 5 mg/dL per day; total bilirubin exceeds 15 in full-term infants (10 in premature infants); jaundice lasts longer than 10 days in full-term infants (21 days in premature infants); direct bilirubin exceeds 1.5 mg/dL

Follow-Up
EXPECTED COURSE
- Physiologic jaundice resolves approximately 1 week after birth

COMPLICATIONS
- Kernicterus: Staining of brain cells by the bilirubin, which can result in death, CNS damage, long-term problems with hearing, cerebral palsy, dental problems
- Once common, this is now extremely rare and unlikely to occur with total bilirubin levels <30 mg/dL

OTHER RELATED CONDITIONS

Failure To Thrive

Description
- Failure to thrive (FTT) in children is a symptom that occurs when children do not follow normal growth patterns for their age. It can be a sign of an underlying illness, secondary to a functional problem, or of mixed origin.

Etiology
- Organic FTT is a failure to receive the nutrients needed to grow
  - Genetic, congenital, or chromosomal disorders (fetal alcohol syndrome, congenital rubella), neuropathology
  - Malabsorptive disorders; inadequate caloric intake
  - Endocrine disorders, excessive catabolism, metabolic needs greater than intake; chronic illness
- Nonorganic causes of FTT exist that also impact growth:
  - Multiple psychosocial factors, including poor parent-child interaction

Incidence and Demographics
- 25% are from organic causes; 50% are nonorganic; 25% have mixed etiologies
- 5%–10% prevalence in urban areas

Risk Factors
- High-risk parents: Young, IV drug users, noncompliant history
- FTT secondary to other chronic illness; parental psychosocial influences; developmental delays

Prevention and Screening
- Measure and plot growth parameters at all visits; follow closely child who drops one standard deviation
- Prenatal and postnatal anticipatory guidance

Assessment
HISTORY
- Prenatal as well as perinatal history; review of growth since birth; developmental history
- Careful family and social history
- Careful diet history including formula changes, calorie count, assessment for inappropriate foods
- Emotional tone of the family during the interview process
- Review of systems for any underlying illness

PHYSICAL EXAM
- General appearance of the child
- Growth parameters: Weight that crosses two standard deviations or falls below fifth percentile for age and sex (after correcting for parents' stature, prematurity, and growth retardation at birth) meets criteria for FTT
- Developmental milestones may be delayed
- Bruises, scars, or unexplained injuries that may be sign of neglect or abuse
- Systematic exam, especially heart, lungs, abdomen, neurologic, facial structure for underlying disorder

DIAGNOSTIC STUDIES
- First get CBC, fasting chemistry panel, urinalysis to look for underlying disorder
- Thyroid function tests, stool culture and for ova and parasites, sweat chloride test for evaluation of cystic fibrosis
- Consider TB test, HIV serology, skeletal survey for bone age, wrist film if abuse suspected

Differential Diagnosis
- Chromosomal/genetic disorders
- Hypothyroidism
- Cystic fibrosis
- Chronic diarrhea
- Lactose intolerance
- GERD
- HIV
- UTI
- Dental caries

Management

NONPHARMACOLOGIC TREATMENT

- Treat underlying cause
- Involve the parents in the work-up, building a trusting relationship for future discussions
- May require more frequent visits for weight monitoring
- Multidisciplinary approach to therapy; parent education and coaching at mealtime
- Provide home resources to evaluate other problems as well as to provide support, teaching
- High-calorie, high-protein diet calculated to provide 1½ to 2x the daily caloric need

PHARMACOLOGIC TREATMENT

- Vitamin supplement

LENGTH OF TREATMENT

- Close monitoring of weight is necessary for months

Special Considerations

- Parents at risk should be identified and intervention designed for prevention with in-home support

When to Consult, Refer, Hospitalize

- Consult with physician and seek the consultation of a dietitian, social worker, and other subspecialists as needed
- Children who do not respond within 2–3 months in the primary care setting should be referred to pediatric growth specialist or program
- Hospitalize those children who present severely malnourished, septic, or if abuse is suspected

Follow-Up

- Weekly, until significant weight gain

EXPECTED COURSE

- Infants on a high-calorie diet should gain significant weight in the first week of therapy

COMPLICATIONS

- Impaired cognitive development, developmental delays
- Short stature, chronic medical problems

CASE STUDIES

Case 1. A 6-week-old infant presents to the clinic for a well-baby exam. The mother tells you about how much the baby is spitting up with every feeding. She has decreased the amount per feeding and increased the frequency but still the child spits up a large portion of the feeding. He is on Isomil and Mom is feeding 1–2 oz q 1–2 h around the clock. There is no weight loss; he has gained 6 oz since his 2-week visit. Denies projectile vomiting.

PMH: He is the product of an uncomplicated pregnancy and full-term birth. Currently on no medications.

    1. What other history would you ask?

Exam: Vital signs, growth parameters stable. HEENT: normal, Lungs: clear, Heart: RRR, no murmur. Abdomen: normal bowel sounds, soft, no masses or organomegaly

    2. What laboratory tests would you order?
    3. What other studies would you order?
    4. What is the most probable diagnosis and what treatment would you provide?

Case 2. An 18-year-old female presents with abdominal pain. She has had some vague lower abdominal cramping off and on for the last 2 months, but today the pain intensified and she was unable to attend school. She has had episodes of loose stools and that has seemed to ease the pain until today; otherwise her bowel habits have been normal.

    1. What other history questions would you ask this patient?

Exam: Alert and oriented female lying in a fetal position. Vital signs stable; abdomen: increased bowel sounds, softly distended, no masses or organomegaly, diffuse tenderness in R & LLQ, no rebound or guarding. Rectal: no masses or tenderness; hemoccult: negative; pelvic: normal.

    2. What laboratory tests would you order?
    3. What other studies would you consider?
    4. What is the likely diagnosis if laboratory tests are normal and what treatment would you provide?

Case 3. A family of three presents to you complaining of vomiting and diarrhea times 2 days. It started with the 3-year-old son and then the mother and now the father. They are most concerned about their son because he has not eaten or drank anything since yesterday and has had a fever of 101°F. He is otherwise healthy and has had no past medical illness other than an occasional cold.

    1. What other questions would you ask this family?

Exam: 3-year-old black male appears lethargic. Temp: 101.4°F, Pulse: 120, Resp: 22
HEENT: normal, Heart: RRR, no murmur, Lungs: clear.
Abdomen: Increased bowel sounds; soft; no masses, tenderness, or organomegaly.

    2. What laboratory tests would you order?
    3. Are any other diagnostic studies warranted at this time?
    4. What likely diagnosis and treatment would you provide?

REFERENCES

American Academy of Pediatrics. (2006). *The 2006 red book: Report of the Committee on Infectious Disease*. Elk Grove, IL: Author.

American Gastroenterology Association. (2005). Guidelines: Elevation of liver chemistry tests. *Gastroenterology, 122*, 1364.

American Gastroenterological Association. (1997). Medical position statement: Irritable bowel syndrome. *Gastroenterology, 112*, 2118–2119.

Behrman, R. E., Kliegman, R. M., & Jenson, H. B. (2004). *Nelson textbook of pediatrics* (17th ed.). Philadelphia: W. B. Saunders Co.

Bishop, W. P., DiLorenzo, C., Leoning-Baucke, V., Pashankar, D. S., & Tucker, N. T. (2004). New paradigm in the diagnosis and management of constipation. *Pediatric News [Supplement]*, 1–12.

Burns, C. E., Barber, N., Brady, M. A., & Dunn, A. M. (Eds.). (2004). *Pediatric primary care: A handbook for nurse practitioners* (3rd ed.). Philadelphia: W. B. Saunders Co.

Centers for Disease Control and Prevention. (2008). *Enterobiasis (Enteroblus vermicularis)*. Retrieved August 27, 2007, from www.dpd.cdc.gov/DPDx/HTML/Enterobiasis.htm

D'Agostino, J. (2006). Considerations in assessing the clinical course and severity of rotavirus gastroenteritis. *Clinical Pediatrics, 45*(3), 203.

De Nardi, P., Ortolano, E., Radaelli, G., & Staudacher, C. (2006). Comparison of glycerine trinitrate and botulinum toxin-a for the treatment of chronic anal fissure: Long-term results. *Diseases of the Colon and Rectum, 49*, 427.

Drossman, D. A,. Camilleri, M., Mayer, E. A., & Whitehead, W. E. (2002). AGA technical review on irritable bowel syndrome. *Gastroenterology, 123*, 2108.

Edmunds, M. W., & Mayhew, M. S. (2004). *Pharmacology for the primary care provider* (2nd ed.). St. Louis, MO: Mosby.

Gilbert, D. N., Moellering, R. C., Jr., Eliopoulos, G. M., Sande, M. A., & Chambers, H. F. (Eds.). (2008). *The Sanford guide to antimicrobial therapy* (33rd ed.). Hyde Park, VT: Antimicrobial Therapy, Inc.

Goroll, A. H., May, L. A., & Mulley, A. G. (Eds.). (2006). *Primary care medicine: Office evaluation and management of the adult patient*. Philadelphia: Lippincott Williams & Wilkins.

Hommes, D., Baert, F., van Assche, G., Caenepeel, F., & Vergauwe, P. (2007). Management of recent onset Crohn's disease: A controlled, randomized trial comparing step-up and top-down therapy. *Gastroenterology, 129*, 371.

Jemal, A., Siegel, R., Ward, E., Murray, T., Xu, J., Smigal, C., & Thun, M. J. (2006) Cancer statistics, 2006. *CA: A Cancer Journal for Clinicians, 56*, 106.

Katz, D. A. (2001). Evaluation and management of inguinal and umbilical hernias. *Pediatric Annals, 30*(12), 729–735.

Kornbluth, A., & Sachar, D. B. (2004) Ulcerative colitis practice guidelines in adults (update): American College of Gastroenterology, Practice Parameters Committee. *American Journal of Gastroenterology, 99*, 1371.

Malfertheiner, P., Megraud, F., O'Morain, C., Bazzoli, F., El-Omar, E., Graham, D., et al. (2007). Current concepts in the management of Helicobacter pylori infection: The Maastricht III Consensus Report. *Gut, 56*, 772.

Mamula, P., Mascarenhas, M. R., & Baldassano, R. N. (2002). Biological and novel therapies for inflammatory bowel disease in children. *Pediatric Clinics of North America, 49*(1), 1–24.

Morrison, W. (2007). Infantile hypertrophic pyloric stenosis in infants treated with azythromycin. *Pediatric Infectious Disease Journal, 26*, 186.

North American Society of Pediatric Gastroenterology, Hepatology and Nutrition. (2003). *Pediatric gastroesophageal reflux clinical practice guideline summary.* Retrieved February 4, 2008, from http://www.cdhnf.org/openbinfile.php?app=pdf&subfold=pdf&name=GERD_8_pg_brochure_031604.pdf

Patel, A. S., Pohl, J. F., & Easley, D. J. (2003). Proton pump inhibitors and pediatrics. *Pediatrics in Review, 24*(1), 12-15.

Pietzak, M. M., & Thomas, D. W. (2003). Childhood malabsorption. *Pediatrics in Review, 24*(5), 195–206.

Rafferty, J., Shellito, P., Hyman, N. H., & Buie, W. D. (2006). Practice parameters for sigmoid diverticulitis. *Diseases of the Colon and Rectum, 49,* 939.

Rowe, S. M., Miller, S., & Sorscher, E. J. (2005). Cystic fibrosis. *New England Journal of Medicine, 352,* 1992.

Ruhl, C. E., & Everhart, J. E. (2005). Coffee and caffeine consumption reduce the risk of elevated serum alanine aminotransferase activity in the United States. *Gastroenterology, 128,* 24.

Sampayo, E. M., & Adams, H. M. (2003). Rotavirus infections. *Pediatrics in Review, 24*(9), 322–323.

Stansbury, A. (2004). GER and GERD in children. *American Journal for Nurse Practitioners, 8*(3), 37–44.

Tierney, L. M., McPhee, S. J., & Papadakis, A. (2008). *Current medical diagnosis and treatment* (44th ed.). Norwalk, CT: Appleton & Lange.

Uphold, C. R., & Graham, M. V. (2003). *Clinical guidelines in family practice* (4th ed.). Gainesville, FL: Barmarrae Books, Inc.

Van den Berg, M. M., Benninga, M. A., & Di Lorenzo, C. (2005). Epidemiology of childhood constipation: A systematic review. *American Journal of Gastroenterology, 101,* 2401.

Zaslavsky, C., De Barros, S. G. S., Gruber, A. C., Maciel, A. C., & Da Silveira, T. R. (2004). Chronic functional constipation in adolescents: Clinical findings and motility studies. *Journal of Adolescent Health, 34*(6), 517–522.

Zeiter, D. K., & Hyams, J. S. (2002). Recurrent abdominal pain in children. *Pediatric Clinics of North America, 49*(1), 53–71.

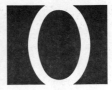

Renal and Urological Disorders

Barbara Rideout, MSN, APRN-BC

GENERAL APPROACH

- Kidney pain is commonly located in the area of the costovertebral angle (CVA). Radiation to the umbilicus or the testicle or labia is possible.
- Pain associated with infection is typically constant.
- The normal urinary tract is sterile, and the immunocompetent patient is resistant to bacterial colonization. Urinary tract infection (UTI) is, however, the most common bacterial infection in all age groups.
- Urinary tract infection is also the most common nosocomial infection.
- UTI should be part of differential diagnoses in any febrile infant or child.
- UTI is a marker in young children for abnormalities of the urinary tract. Imaging tests should be conducted in all boys of any age with first UTI, in girls younger than 5 years with first UTI, older girls with recurrent UTI, and any child with pyelonephritis to identify abnormalities that may lead to renal damage (e.g., vesicoureteral reflux [VUR]).
- Limit antibiotics to category B if patient is pregnant or lactating; most antibiotics enter breast milk.
- Refer unusual presentations of disease as well as those that do not respond to standard treatment.

Red Flags

- Wilms' tumor: Embryonal malignant tumor of the kidney in children <5 years can be asymptomatic and present with abdominal mass felt in flank over to midline. Consult with a physician for prompt work-up and appropriate referral. Do not be aggressive with abdominal exam in these patients.
- Patients with signs of UTI who are hemodynamically unstable, severely dehydrated, or unable to take oral medications require hospitalization
- Gross hematuria without evidence of acute UTI should be considered an indication of malignancy until proven otherwise

Asymptomatic Bacteriuria

Description

- Significant bacterial counts in urine of a patient who has no other symptoms; more common with female gender, aging, perimenopausal status, pregnancy, structural abnormalities in tract, prostatic hypertrophy, asymptomatic calculi, indwelling urinary catheter

Etiology

- Most commonly caused by Gram-negative bacteria such as *E. coli*

Incidence and Demographics

- Incidence increases with age: 1% in school-age females to 20% in women over 80
- Increased incidence in women with diabetes, 8%–14%
- Rare in men under age 75

Risk Factors

- Indwelling catheters
- Pregnancy
- Diabetes mellitus
- Spinal cord injury

Prevention and Screening

- Screen, culture, and treat asymptomatic bacteriuria in pregnant women, before TURP and other urologic procedures with mucosal bleeding, and to improve urinary incontinence in the elderly
- Increase fluids to flush urinary tract
- Empty bladder fully and frequently to avoid stasis

Assessment

- Urinalysis reveals bacteria and white blood counts (WBC); urine culture may be positive for bacteria in absence of a contaminated specimen or symptomatic UTI

Differential Diagnosis

- Cystitis
- Urethritis
- Acute pyelonephritis

Management
- Antibiotic therapy is controversial except in immunosuppressed patients (as in AIDS), malignancy, or pregnancy to prevent acute pyelonephritis
- 2005 Infectious Disease Society of America (ISDA) guidelines call for treating symptomatic women if two consecutive clean-catch voided urines have the same bacterial strain at 105 cfu/mL. In asymptomatic patients, treatment should be considered if a single cathed specimen contains one bacterial strain >102 cfu/mL.

Special Considerations
- U.S. Preventive Services Task Force recommends screening for asymptomatic bacteriuria with urine culture for pregnant women at 12–15 weeks of gestation

When to Consult, Refer, Hospitalize
- Consult urology if frequent recurrence or non-responsiveness to treatment
- Hospitalize for urinary sepsis may be necessary in elderly

Follow-Up
- If treated with antibiotics, follow up 1–2 weeks after completion of course with repeat urinalysis or culture

Hematuria

Description
- The presence of red blood cells (RBCs) in the urine
- May be microscopic (>3 RBCs/high-power field) or gross (visible to naked eye)

Etiology
- Infection: Proximal (renal) or distal (urethral) in location
- Renal calculi, tumors, trauma, polycystic renal disease, neoplasms in persons over 50, hydronephrosis, renal vascular diseases
- Most commonly seen in inflammation or infection of prostate or bladder, stones, and in older patients with malignancy or benign prostatic hypertrophy (BPH)
- Medications (anticoagulants-heparin, warfarin, aspirin)
- Benign prostatic hypertrophy, prostatitis, epididymitis
- Coagulopathies, sickle cell disease
- Strenuous exercise
- Vascular glomerular abnormalities, familial nephritis (Alport syndrome)
- Granulomatous diseases (tuberculosis)
- Connective tissue diseases (lupus)
- Trauma

Incidence and Demographics
- Ranges from 1%–16% in the general population
- Higher risk in elderly men who are at high risk for obstructive and other urologic diseases

Risk Factors
- UTIs

- Renal calculi
- Environmental exposure to elements that can cause bladder cancer

Prevention and Screening
- Urinalysis in high-risk patients at annual physical examination

Assessment
- Complete history and physical exam to determine underlying disorder
- Urinalysis, microscopic exam of urinary sediment, urine culture
  - If accompanied by red cell casts and/or marked proteinuria, glomerular origin probable
  - 3-tube test may help identify source of bleeding; tube 1 from initial stream, tube 2 from mid-stream and tube 3 from end-stream; blood in tube 1 indicates origin from urethral lesion, in tube 2 from bladder, and tube 3 from bladder trigone
- Renal function studies (BUN and creatinine)
- CBC/differential, erythrocyte sedimentation rate (ESR)
- Additional testing based on presentation: Intravenous pyelogram (IVP), renal ultrasound, or cystourethrogram
- STD cultures, gram stain

Differential Diagnosis
- Hemorrhagic cystitis
- Bladder cancer
- Ingestion of dyes and pigments
- Glomerulopathy
- Pyelonephritis
- Renal calculi
- Pelvic inflammatory disease

Management
- Determine cause using appropriate diagnostic tests, usually referred for treatment depending on cause.

Special Considerations
- Persons who ingest large amounts of beets and foods containing red dye may have pseudohematuria

When to Consult, Refer, Hospitalize
- Refer for persistent, unexplained hematuria, if it does not resolve with treatment for infection, need for invasive testing, or renal biopsy

Follow-Up
- Regular urinalysis to assess for signs of recurrence recommended. An isolated incidence is often an early sign of a more lethal problem.

UROLOGIC DISORDERS

Urinary Tract Infection (UTI, Cystitis)

Description
- Lower UTI is infection of one or more of the urinary tract structures but most commonly is used to refer to cystitis, inflammation or infection of the bladder. If acute, usually one organism is identified; if chronic, two or more organisms may be found.

Etiology
- Most commonly caused by *E. coli* (80%–90%), other Gram-negative bacteria from gastrointestinal tract (*E. coli, Proteus mirabilis, Klebsiella pneumoniae, Enterobacter sp.*).
- A Gram-positive organism (*Staphylococcus saprophyticus*) is common in sexually active young women but an uncommon cause of infection in men. If found in men it is truly a urinary pathogen.
- Symptomatic women with pyuria but without significant bacteriuria ("sterile pyuria") may have infection with *Chlamydia trachomatis.*
- Viruses may be associated with hemorrhagic cystitis.
- Most UTIs (>95%) are caused by ascending infections from urethra.

Incidence and Demographics
- Most common of all bacterial infections in women
- In first 2 months of life, incidence is higher in males, especially (95%) those uncircumcised
- May be associated with bacteremia in the first 3 months of life
- After 1–2 years of age, females are 10–20 times more likely to experience a UTI than males secondary to shorter urethra, closer proximity to perirectal area
- Reccurrence will occur in 50%–75% of females
- Vesicoureteral reflux is found in approximately 20% of females after first UTI, 40%–45% of those with recurrent UTIs

Risk Factors
- Female; sexual activity; history of prior UTI; diabetes mellitus or other immunocompromised state; pregnancy; use of spermicides, diaphragm, or oral contraceptives
- Structural urinary tract abnormalities (strictures, stones, tumors, neuropathic bladder)
- Procedures such as catheterization or recent surgery
- Aging issues: Relaxation of pelvic supporting structures, BPH or prostatitis, incontinence of urine/stool, cognitively impaired
- Dysfunctional voiding pattern or infrequent voiding
- Chronic constipation in children

Prevention and Screening
- In women who experience three or more UTIs, voiding immediately after intercourse and avoiding use of a diaphragm may be helpful
- Drinking cranberry juice or taking cranberry pills to reduce pyuria and bacteriuria
- Education of parents and children regarding hygiene, tips on toilet training; education of adolescents regarding sexual intercourse
- Low-dose oral antimicrobial prophylaxis can be considered for recurrent infections

- Post-coital treatment with a single-dose antibiotic is an option
- In post-menopausal women, systemic or topical estrogen therapy markedly reduces the incidence of recurrent UTI

Assessment

HISTORY
- Dysuria, urgency, frequency, nocturia, hematuria, suprapubic discomfort
- Low-grade fever and enuresis in children
- Lower abdominal or back pain, fever, chills, and lassitude (may indicate pyelonephritis)
- Presence of vaginal or urethral discharge or odor, pruritus, dyspareunia, external dysuria without frequency may indicate vaginitis or urethritis
- Perianal itching (may indicate pinworms)
- Mental status change in the elderly may be the only symptom of UTI

PHYSICAL EXAM
- Fever (in children), suprapubic tenderness to palpation
- CVA tenderness if pyelonephritis
- Assess signs of hydration status in children
- Inspection of genitalia in children for trauma, anomalies, meatal stenosis, phimosis
- Pelvic examination recommended in adolescents and adults to rule out vaginitis
- In elderly, mental status changes or new onset of falls may be the only signs of infection

DIAGNOSTIC STUDIES
- First infection: Clean catch urinalysis, treat if positive; in children, always obtain culture from mid-stream
- May obtain urine by catheterization or SPA (suprapubic bladder aspiration) in infants and children
- Hematuria is common in women with UTI, not in women with vaginal infections
- Repeat or refractory infections: Consider urine culture and sensitivity, renal/bladder ultrasound, cystourethroscopy, or IVP; nonresponse to appropriate antimicrobial therapy is the most useful indicator for radiologic/urologic examinations
- Radiographic follow-up with a renal and bladder ultrasound and a voiding cystourethrogram (VCUG) should be obtained for all children under 5 years with a documented UTI, all males with a UTI, and all females with a febrile UTI to evaluate for vesicoureteral reflux and structural abnormalities; the VCUG should be done after 3–4 weeks since mucosal changes (edema) during an infection may result in a transient reflux
- Dimercaptosuccinic acid (DMSA) scan may be recommended for patients with pyelonephritis to detect renal scarring
- Voiding cystourethrogram is a dynamic test for stricture/reflux; a normal renal ultrasound does not exclude VUR
- For systemic symptoms, CBC and possibly BUN and creatinine

Differential Diagnosis
- Urethritis
- Diabetes
- Pyelonephritis
- Renal calculi
- Vaginitis
- Encopresis
- Female urethral syndrome
- Chemical vaginitis
- Prostatitis
- Meatal stenosis
- Dysfunctional voiding
- STDs
- Balanitis
- Sexual abuse
- Foreign body
- Pinworms
- Diaper dermatitis

Management

NONPHARMACOLOGIC TREATMENT
- Hygiene measures (front-to-back wiping, care of uncircumcised penis)
- More frequent and complete voiding, voiding after coitus
- Hydration, cranberry juice (will help prevent strains of *E. coli* from adhering to bladder)

PHARMACOLOGIC TREATMENT
- Adolescents and adults:
  - See Table 10–1 for antibiotic regimens
  - Short-course treatment with trimethoprim-sulfamethoxazole or a fluoroquinolone are the treatments of choice and are superior to the beta lactams (Augmentin)
  - For pain relief, consider use of urinary analgesic phenazopyridine (Pyridium), 100–200 mg tid or Uristat, 190 mg tid po; for 2 days maximum therapy; inform patient drug will turn urine orange and possibly affect contact lenses; not recommended for children
- Infants and children:
  - See Table 10–2 for antibiotic regimens
  - It is important to know antimicrobial susceptibility profile of uropathogens causing uncomplicated UTIs in community to guide therapeutic decisions; there is an increasing resistance among uropathogens to Bactrim
  - Fluoroquinolones not recommended in children <18 years because of possible adverse effects on developing cartilage
  - Prophylaxis of UTIs in infants and young children during vesicoureteral reflux work up and, if reflux is confirmed, with low-dose sulfa, nitrofurantoin, or other antibiotic in consultation with a physician

Table 10–1. Standard UTI Treatment in Adults

Drug	Dosage
Trimethoprim-sulfamethoxazole (Bactrim)	160/800 mg po single dose or DS bid
Cephalexin (Keflex)	250–500 mg po q6h
Ciprofloxacin (Cipro)	250–500 mg po q 12 h
Nitrofurantoin (Macrodantin)	100 mg po q 12 h or 50 mg po qid
Norfloxacin (Noroxin)	400 mg po q 12 h
Ofloxacin (Floxin)	200 mg q 12 h

Table 10–2. Standard UTI Treatment in Infants and Children

Drug	Dosage	Recommendations & Comments
Trimethoprim-sulfamethoxazole (Bactrim/Septra)	8–12 mg/kg/day TMP and 40–60 mg/kg/day SMZ q 12 h	Not recommended for infants <2 months
Nitrofurantoin (Furadantin Suspension)	5–7 mg/kg/d q6h	Must give with food; not recommended for infants <2 months
Cephalexin (Keflex)	500 mg bidh	Increasing resistance; use in children over age 15 years
Cefixime (Suprax)	8 mg/kg/day one dose	Expensive
Ceftriaxone sodium (Rocephin)	50–75 mg/kg/day IM q 12 h (2 divided doses)	May start febrile, ill-looking child on this, pending culture
Amoxicillin (Amoxil)	40 mg/kg/day q8h	Increasing resistance
Amoxicillin and clavulanate potassium (Augmentin)	30–50 mg/kg/day q 12 h	Abdominal discomfort; generic, diarrhea common

LENGTH OF TREATMENT
- In healthy young women, a 3-day course of therapy is superior to single-dose since early recurrence is more common after single-dose therapy; Nitrofurantoin requires a 5-day course; amoxicillin and Augmentin require 7–10 days.
- Short-course therapy is not recommended if symptoms have been present for >7 days, if there is a high probability of deep-tissue infection, for any man with UTI, in presence of underlying structural or functional defect of the urinary tract, immunosuppressed individuals, or patients with indwelling catheters
- In cases of recurrent infection, assume patient has covert renal infection and retreat for a minimum of 14 days
- Males <50 years with the following risk factors usually receive 10–14 day course; homosexual, men having intercourse with women colonized with uropathogens, AIDS with CD4+ lymphocyte count <200/mm3
- Males >50 years may require 4–6 weeks and as many as 12 weeks of treatment to sterilize the urinary tract if the prostate is source of infection
- Infants and children: Treat for 10 days or until imaging studies are completed and assessed

Special Considerations
- Geriatric patients: May or may not demonstrate symptoms other than mental status change
- Pregnancy/lactation: Consult with OB for management in pregnancy. Always obtain urine culture and sensitivity. Treat with amoxicillin 500 mg po qid for 7–14 days, amoxicillin 500 mg po tid for 7–10 days, or cephalexin (Keflex) for 10–14 days. May need prophylactic antibiotics for duration of pregnancy (history of acute pyelonephritis during pregnancy, bacteriuria during pregnancy with recurrence after treatment, and history of recurrent UTI before pregnancy requiring prophylaxis in past)

When to Consult, Refer, Hospitalize
- Consult or refer to adult/pediatric urologist for recurrent infections if suspect anatomic abnormality
- Hemodynamically unstable patients, or those in whom urosepsis is a potential concern, may require hospitalization or intravenous antibiotics
- Hospitalize if signs of pyelonephritis in children or pregnant woman for IV antibiotics

Follow-Up
- Repeat urine culture 3–4 days after completion of therapy in children
- Radiographic follow-up with a renal and bladder ultrasound and a VCUG should be obtained for all children under 5 years with a documented UTI, all boys of any age with a UTI, and all girls with a febrile UTI to evaluate for vesicoureteral reflux
  - EXPECTED COURSE
    - If using correct antibiotic (per culture and sensitivity), signs and symptoms should dissipate within 48–72 hours
    - Many providers routinely check urinalysis after therapy for test of cure; helps differentiate inadequately treated infection from recurrence

  - COMPLICATIONS
    - Pyelonephritis, recurrent or relapse of infection, sepsis (esp. in elderly), renal abscess
    - In children, VUR graded according to the International Reflux Study, grade I–V; grade IV–V usually requires surgical correction and should be referred to a pediatric urologist; grade I–III have an 80%–85% chance of spontaneous resolution; VUR can result in renal scarring and loss of renal function

Acute Pyelonephritis

Description
- Acute bacterial infection of soft tissue of the renal parenchyma and pelvis, or other portion of upper urinary tract, typically producing signs and symptoms of systemic toxicity

Etiology
- 75% due to *E. coli* organism
- 10%–15% are due to other Gram-negatives (*P. mirabilis, K. pneumoniae, Enterobacter*)
- 10%–15% due to *S. aureus* or *saprophyticus*
- Most common route of infection is ascension from bladder

Incidence and Demographics
- 15.7/100,000 cases annually in U.S.
- Frequently in women 18–40

Risk Factors
- Urinary tract abnormalities or instrumentation, stones, catheters, diabetes or other immunocompromised states, recent pyelonephritis, BPH, pregnancy, fecal incontinence
- Recent lower UTI

Prevention and Screening
- Hygiene, hydration, voiding after coitus
- Prophylactic antibiotics if infected recurrently or frequently
- Screening pregnant women for asymptomatic bacteriuria

Assessment
HISTORY
- Fever often >102°F, shaking chills, flank pain, myalgias, abdominal pain
- Hematuria, dysuria, frequency, urgency
- Nausea and vomiting

PHYSICAL EXAM
- CVA tenderness, fever

DIAGNOSTIC STUDIES
- Urinalysis: Bacteria and WBCs visible on microscopy, may also see casts; leukocyte esterase and nitrites on dipstick, possible proteinuria, pyuria
- CBC: May have elevated WBCs
- Urine culture and sensitivity should be performed on all patients
- A Gram stain should be performed prior to instituting therapy to determine if Gram-negative as well as Gram-positive organisms are present
- Voiding cystourethrogram, IVP, renal scan, cystoscopy may be indicated if structural abnormality suspected; if renal abscess suspected, order abdominal/pelvic CT

Differential Diagnosis
- Stones
- Prostatitis
- TB of the kidney
- Acute low back pain
- Tumors

Management
NONPHARMACOLOGIC TREATMENT
- Fluids

PHARMACOLOGIC TREATMENT
- See Table 10–3 for oral doses of antibiotic therapy
- Parenteral antibiotics may be indicated for Gram-positive cocci, complicated

histories, previous episodes of pyelonephritis, or recent urinary tract manipulations

- If no nausea or vomiting, may use Ceftriaxone 1 gm IM or Gentamycin 3–5 mg/kg body weight IM in office to avoid hospitalization; MUST see patient back in office in 24 hours

LENGTH OF TREATMENT

- Treat 14 days
- In the otherwise healthy patient with mild disease, outpatient treatment with oral antimicrobials (trimethoprim-sulfamethoxazole or a fluoroquinolone for 14 days) is possible if the patient has no nausea or vomiting, no signs of volume depletion, no evidence of septicemia, and is reliable in following medical advice
- Otherwise, parenteral therapy should be initiated, then switch to oral therapy for 14 days once the patient has been afebrile for 24 hours (usually within 72 hours of starting treatment)
- Infants, children, pregnant women usually hospitalized for initial therapy with IV antibiotics
- If develops chronic pyelonephritis, therapy required for 3–6 months

Table 10-3. Oral Treatment for Acute Pyelonephritis (Mild)

Drug	Dosage
Trimethoprim-sulfamethoxazole (Bactrim)	160–800 mg bid
Ciprofloxacin (Cipro)	500 mg bid or 1 g extended release (XR) daily
Ofloxacin (Floxin)	200–300 mg q 12 h

Special Considerations

- Elderly patients should be hospitalized and started on an aminoglycoside with dosage adjusted for weight and renal function
- Pregnancy: Sulfa drugs and fluoroquinolones contraindicated; use beta lactams, aminoglycosides, or both

When to Consult, Refer, Hospitalize

- Inpatient management required if patient appears toxic or is elderly, hemodynamically unstable, immunocompromised, pregnant, or unable to tolerate oral antibiotic therapy
- If fever persists >3 days, suspect abscess or obstruction, refer to urologist

Follow-Up

- Recheck patient in office in 24 hours
- Repeat culture 2 weeks after completion of therapy and again at 12 weeks
- In children, after completion of treatment course, a prolonged 1–3 month course of oral therapy is then instituted with follow-up urine cultures at frequent intervals for the next year
  EXPECTED COURSE
  - Good prognosis: Should resolve within 72 hours of institution of appropriate therapy

COMPLICATIONS
- Sepsis, preterm labor in pregnancy, chronic renal insufficiency, chronic pyelonephritis, renal abscess, death
- Without demonstrable obstruction or recurrent acute infection, asymptomatic renal bacteriuria has not been clearly established as harmful and repeated courses of antimicrobials or suppression therapy are not indicated
- If obstruction cannot be eliminated and recurrent UTI is common, long-term therapy is useful

Urinary Incontinence (UI)

Description
- A general term used to describe the involuntary loss of urine; further classified based upon causation
- 5% will have infections or other diseases causing urinary incontinence
- 10%–25% will also have fecal incontinence

Etiology
- Urge incontinence: Involuntary loss of large amount urine preceded by strong, unexpected urge to void
  - Unrelated to activity or position and indicative of detrusor instability
  - May be due to aging, Parkinson's, stroke
- Stress incontinence: Involuntary loss of small amounts of urine
  - Associated with activities that increase intra-abdominal pressure including coughing, sneezing, lifting, and certain exercises
  - Urine does not leak when patient is lying down
  - May be due to aging, pelvic floor muscle weakness (e.g., cystocele, rectocele), perineal trauma, prostatitis/pelvic surgery, and estrogen deficiency in women
- Overflow incontinence: From chronic urine retention
  - Results from the chronically distended bladder receiving an additional increment of urine to exceed intravesical pressure and release small amount of urine
  - May be due to prostatic enlargement, anticholinergics, tricyclic antidepressants, diabetic neuropathy, outflow obstruction, multiple sclerosis
- Functional incontinence
  - Physical or cognitive disability, sedating medications that make it difficult to use the bathroom
- Total incontinence
  - Loss of urine at all times in all positions
  - Due to sphincteric inefficiency from surgery, nerve damage, tumor infiltration, or fistula formation
- Transient incontinence
  - May be due to delirium, infection, atrophic vaginitis, urethritis, or drugs (sedatives, hypnotics, diuretics, opioids, calcium channel blockers, anticholinergics, antidepressants, antihistamines, decongestants, and others
  - Other less common etiologies include diabetes mellitus or insipidus, restricted mobility, stool impaction, depression
- Mixed: Two causes present
  - Stress and urge incontinence
  - Urge and functional

Incidence and Demographics
- Problem for 5%–15% of elderly patients in community setting and up to 50% of nursing home residents
- Overall affects 12 million adults; females affected more than males; 22%–45% of persons with incontinence ever seek care

Risk Factors
- Elderly, estrogen deficiency, prostatic hypertrophy, multiparity, dementia, diabetes, Parkinson's, myelodysplasia, multiple sclerosis (MS), spinal cord injury or lesion, stroke, immobility, pregnancy, use of diuretics

Prevention and Screening
- Kegel exercises, regular pelvic examination to detect pathology early
- Avoid constipation
- Regular rectal exam for detection of BPH and initiation of therapy before symptom presents

Assessment
- Confirm urinary incontinence and identify factors that might contribute or exacerbate symptom
  - HISTORY
    - Urgency, leaking, dribbling, burning, hesitancy, nocturia, irritation
    - Double vision, muscle weakness, paralysis, or poor coordination suggest neurologic disorders
    - Assess exposure to medications (particularly potassium-sparing diuretics) and other provoking factors (caffeine, alcohol, physical activity, cough, laughing, sounds of water, hands in water)
    - 3 IQ tool aids provider in differentiating stress and urge incontinence; ask patient, "In past 3 months have you leaked urine?", "How often?", and "Which of the above provoking factors caused leakage more often?"

  - PHYSICAL EXAM
    - To detect anatomic and neurological abnormalities
    - Examine abdomen (with full bladder if possible) for masses, suprapubic tenderness or fullness
    - Pelvic exam to assess perineal skin, cystocele/rectocele, uterine prolapse, pelvic mass, perivaginal muscle tone, atrophic vaginitis
    - Estimate post-voiding residual by abdominal palpation and percussion and/or bimanual exam
    - Rectal exam for perineal sensation, resting and active sphincter tone, rectal mass, and fecal impaction; assess consistency, size, and contour of prostate
    - Neurological exam with deep tendon reflex, sensation, gait
    - Mental status exam in elderly
    - Musculoskeletal exam for secondary causes such as weakness, ambulation problems

DIAGNOSTIC STUDIES
- Provocative stress testing if stress incontinence is suspected
- Urinalysis, and culture to rule out UTI
- 24-hour voiding record: Include type of fluid ingested and when, time and volume voided
- Observe voiding to detect problems with hesitancy, dribbling, or interrupted stream
- Renal function studies may reveal decreased function
- Urine cytology
- Cystograms may demonstrate fistula sites
- Stress cystograms may show descent of bladder neck on straining
- Measure post-void residual urine (<50 mL is normal)
- Pelvic ultrasound may reveal source of obstruction
- Cystometry with flow rates may be needed

Differential Diagnosis
- Vaginal reflux
- UTI
- Vaginitis
- Urethritis
- Effect of medication or psychiatric illness

Management
NONPHARMACOLOGIC TREATMENT
- Use a voiding diary for 3 days to provide information about voiding habits as a diagnostic technique
- General:
  - Good personal hygiene
  - Dietary modifications (avoid caffeine and alcohol)
  - Limit use of diuretics
  - Eliminate constipation
- Behavioral techniques:
  - Bladder training for urge UI, may also work for stress UI
  - Pelvic muscle exercises (Kegel) for stress UI
    » Biofeedback for stress UI
    » Vaginal cone for stress UI
  - Habit training or timed voiding for functional UI
- Surgical:
  - Overflow incontinence from anatomic obstruction (e.g., BPH)
  - Stress incontinence from anatomically reversible condition (prolapse, cystocele)
- Other measures:
  - Intermittent catheterization; useful in overflow incontinence
  - External collection catheters
  - Incontinence pads or garments
  - Pessaries for prolapsed uterus

PHARMACOLOGIC TREATMENT
  • Treat UTI if present; otherwise, see Tables 10–4 and 10–5

LENGTH OF TREATMENT
  • Indefinitely or until surgical correction

Table 10-4. Pharmacologic Treatment for Urge Incontinence

Class	Drug	Dosage
Anticholinergic & Antispasmodic	Oxybutynin (Ditropan) or Tolterodine (Detrol)	2.5–5.0 mg tid or qid or 2 mg bid
	Darifenacin (Enablex)	7.5–15 mg daily
	Tropsium chloride (Santura)	20 mg daily to bid
	Solifenacin succinate (VESicare)	5–10 mg daily
	Oxytrol patch 0.3 mg patch twice a week	
Anticholinergic Agent	Dicylomine	10–20 mg tid
Tricyclic Agents	Imipramine (Tofranil)	Initial: 10–25 mg qd, big, or tid
SSRIs	Duloxetine (Cymbalta)	40 mg bid

Table 10-5. Pharmacologic Treatment for Stress Incontinence

Class	Drug	Dosage
Hormone Therapy	Conjugated estrogen (Premarin)	0.5–2 mg/day po vaginally daily, then 3 x per week, then 2 x per week
	Progestin (Medroxyprogesterone) (if uterus present)	2.5–10 mg/day either continuously or intermittently
Tricyclic Antidepressant	Imipramine (Tofranil)	10–25 mg qd to qid, may not tolerate due to sedation

Special Considerations
• More central nervous system (CNS) effects with oxybutynin (headaches, cognitive impairment) plus dry mouth, constipation. Caution patient to avoid alcohol when taking this medication.
• Tolterodine does not cross blood-brain barrier; less constipation, dry mouth
• Pregnancy: Stress incontinence is common in pregnancy. It should be treated with good hygiene, frequent voiding, and Kegel exercises
• Lactation: Avoid pharmacologic agents that could be transmitted via breast milk
• Overactive bladder (OAB) without incontinence (OAB-dry) may be part of the urge incontinence continuum. Limited data on behavioral or pharmacologic treatment.
• OAB-dry may respond to lifestyle changes, bladder retraining, and antimuscarinics

When to Consult, Refer, Hospitalize
- Consult specialist for patients with stress and urge incontinence who fail to respond to behavioral therapy and initial drug treatment
- Refer if any neurologic abnormalities coexist
- Refer for overflow incontinence evaluation and treatment
- Refer to urologist for cystoscopy for persistent RBCs on urinalysis

Follow-Up
- Weekly visits until most symptoms controlled, then as needed
  EXPECTED COURSE
  - Long-term prognosis depends on patient compliance and follow-up

  COMPLICATIONS
  - UTI, renal failure, skin breakdown, hydronephrosis, depression, social isolation

Enuresis

Description
- Persistent involuntary loss of urine in girls older than 5 and boys older than 6 years
- Most commonly occurs during sleep
- Termed "primary enuresis" in a child who has never achieved nighttime continence
- Secondary enuresis is return of involuntary urination after nighttime continence has been achieved

Etiology
- Usually multifactorial
- Appears to run in families. Has been linked to specific genetic markers (e.g., chromosome 8, 12, 13, 22, and ENUR 1 gene on chromosome 13). 77% risk if both parents had enuresis, 44% for one parent, and 15% if neither.
- 20% of children with nighttime incontinence also have daytime problems
- Primary enuresis may be due to food allergies, disorders of the urinary or nervous systems, psychological factors, reduced bladder capacity, lack of normal increase in nocturnal antidiuretic hormone (ADH) secretion
- Primary nocturnal enuresis (PNE) is primarily an arousal disorder with failure of the CNS to recognize bladder fullness or contraction and/or failure to inhibit bladder contraction or sphincter relaxation, detrussor instability
- Secondary enuresis may be due to bacteriuria, UTI, inability to concentrate urine secondary to insufficient ADH or a renal tubular defect, a pelvic mass or spinal cord malformation, meatal stenosis, ectopic ureter, glycosuria as in diabetes mellitus or diabetes insipidus, possible sleep disorder

Incidence and Demographics
- Occurs in approximately 15% of children; by age 18, incidence has decreased to 1%
- Multifactorial, though most children outgrowing monosymptomatic nocturnal enuresis (MNE) indicate maturational delay
- Genetic predisposition: If both parents have a history then child has approximately 75% chance of developing enuresis; one parent, 45% chance; neither parent, 15% chance

Risk Factors
- Males > females; first born
- Family history in at least one parent
- Institutionalized

Prevention and Screening
- Ask patient and parent at each well-child visit

Assessment

HISTORY
- Bed-wetting at least one night per month, with no daytime wetting (PNE)
- May increase during times of emotional stress
- Family's/child's response to PNE
- Family history
- Social history may contribute to secondary NE

PHYSICAL EXAM
- Genitourinary exam (abnormal structure or function), perianal excoriation or vulvovaginitis (may be caused by pinworms)
- Abdominal exam (palpable bladder, stool)
- Neurological exam (reflexes, perineal sensation, gait; examine lower back/spine for sacral dimpling, cutaneous abnormalities)
- Poor growth patterns
- Hypertension may indicate renal disease

DIAGNOSTIC STUDIES
- Urinalysis, culture, include specific gravity
- If abnormal PE or complicated UTI: 24-hour urine, intravenous pyelogram (IVP)/sonogram of kidneys, CT, or MRI
- Voiding cystourethrogram with significant daytime complaints

Differential Diagnosis
- Urinary tract structural abnormalities
- UTI
- Neurologic dysfunction
- Spinal cord malformations (hair tuft, abnormal gluteal folds)
- Tumors
- Diabetes mellitus or insipidus
- Pinworms
- Psychogenic polydipsia
- Encopresis
- Unrecognized medical disorders: sickle cell anemia
- Seizures, hyperthyroidism,
- Chronic renal failure (CRF)

Management

- If normal exam, positive UTI, treat UTI
- If history consistent with secondary enuresis, and post-treatment urinalysis is normal, return only if enuresis continues
- If abnormal exam, complicated UTI, consult/refer
- If normal exam, negative urinalysis, treatment below

NONPHARMACOLOGIC TREATMENT

- Behavioral or motivational therapy: Behavior modification with reward system (25% success rate)
- Conditioning therapy: Bladder stretching and strengthening exercises (encourage less frequent urination by holding as long as possible at least once a day, have patient start and stop flow of urine when urinating) have a 30% success rate
- Voiding and stooling diaries, fluid intake diary
- Enuresis alarms: Requires a committed and motivated family and takes 12–16 weeks to be effective; alarms have a 70% success rate and the lowest rate of relapse (30%)
- Counseling and behavior modification
- Anticipatory guidance in relation to toilet training
- Encourage daytime fluids and encourage less frequent urination to help increase bladder size
- Avoid fluids 2 hours prior to bedtime
- Protect bed; use diapers, pull-up pants to reduce laundry load when necessary
- Bladder stretching exercises may be helpful

PHARMACOLOGIC TREATMENT

- Tricyclic antidepressants: imipramine (Tofranil) or desipramine (Norpramin) 1–2 mg/kg hs to maximum of 50 mg. Not recommended and seldom used today because of CNS toxicity and narrow therapeutic range where toxic effects are easily reached with minor dose adjustments.
- Desmopressin (DDAVP): Decreases urine production; now comes in pill form, which is preferred over intranasal route (inconsistent dosage, frequent nasal irritation, nosebleeds). Not for children <6 years old. Starting dose: 0.2 mg at hs. For children >6 years who have difficulty swallowing pills, 20 mcg intranasally hs depending on product availability. May take several days to begin working. Safety has been shown for use up to 6 months. However, check blood pressure, serum electrolytes if used beyond 3 months. Stress importance of continuing to restrict nighttime fluids to decrease risk of fluid overload that rarely can cause water intoxication and hyponatremia. Side effect is primarily headache.

LENGTH OF TREATMENT

- Taper medications when problem seems to be resolving
- DDVAP may be used for a 3-month trial to break the cycle of intermittent wetting and allow child to develop the habit, feelings associated with dry nights
- DDVAP may be used short-term for camping trips, vacations, sleepovers; start a few days in advance

When to Consult, Refer, Hospitalize
- Emotional disturbance may require referral
- Genitourinary dysfunction or neurological symptoms warrant referral to specialist if clinical or radiographic findings suggest renal or urologic abnormality or bladder instability
- Neurosurgery should be consulted if evidence of occult spinal dysraphism

Follow-Up
EXPECTED COURSE
- Usually self-limiting problem

COMPLICATIONS
- Emotional distress, social isolation, depression

Urolithiasis/Nephrolithiasis

Description
- Stones occurring within the urinary tract; nephrolithiasis is stones within kidney
- Stones are initially formed in the proximal urinary tract and then pass distally
- Usually arrested in the ureter and cause pain, infection, and obstruction
- Most composed of calcium (80%), uric acid (5%), cystine (2%), or struvite

Etiology
- Supersaturation of urine with stone-forming salts
- In many instances, may be a manifestation of systemic disease (e.g., bone diseases, immobilization, hyperthyroidism, primary hyperparathyroidism, hypervitaminosis D, renal tubular acidosis, mild-alkali syndrome, gout, others), but idiopathic hypercalciuria responsible for about 50% in adults
- Up to 98% of stones <0.5 cm in diameter will pass spontaneously, especially in the distal ureter
- Calcium stones are the most common. When they cause obstruction it tends to be acute and intermittent, producing no long-term effects on renal function
- Cystine and struvite stones are more likely to be associated with renal damage
- Struvite stones form in alkaline urine; may be seen with chronic proteus species infections

Incidence and Demographics
- 1%–3% of population present with urolithiasis at some point during lifetime
- Most occur at age 30–50 years
- Male-to-female ratio 3:1 (calcium stones; struvite stones are more common in females)

Risk Factors
- Cystinuria, genetic defects, renal tubular acidosis, low water intake, high-protein diet, excessive oxalate intake, sedentary lifestyle
- Middle age, Whites, family history, obesity, diabetes mellitus, chronic diarrhea, malabsorption, history of bowel or bariatric surgery, pathologic skeletal fractures, gout, Paget's
- Certain medications: Vitamins A, C, D, loop diuretics, ammonium chloride, acetazolamide, alkali, antacids

Prevention and Screening
- Adequate fluid intake
- If prone to calcium stones, restrict protein, sodium, dairy products and other oxalate rich foods
- If prone to uric acid stones, alkalinization of urine may prevent formation

Assessment
HISTORY
- May be asymptomatic even with severe obstruction or present with acute back and flank pain that comes and goes
- Obstruction of the ureter: Acute, colicky flank pain which may be episodic in nature; anterior radiation of pain; nausea and vomiting; diaphoresis; patient constantly moving to relieve pain
- Progression of stone: Pain referred to ipsilateral testis or labia; urinary urgency or hesitancy
- Ingestion of large amounts of fluids or diuretic use may precipitate an attack
- May be associated with dysuria, frequency, hematuria, diaphoresis, restlessness, chills and fever, nausea, and/or vomiting

PHYSICAL EXAM
- Acute obvious discomfort, pacing, grimacing, unable to get comfortable
- Fever, tachycardia, tachypnea, diaphoresis, restlessness, CVA tenderness
- Be alert to signs of systemic disease (e.g., lymphadenopathy, organomegaly, adenopathy)

DIAGNOSTIC STUDIES
- Urinalysis, culture, CBC, BUN, creatinine
- Urinalysis that shows hematuria with or without proteinuria suggests calculus or tumor
- Plain film of the abdomen (KUB) will show calculi (85%–90% of which are radiopaque) in the renal pelvis, along the course of the ureter or in the bladder; Limitations: Overlying bowel gas and rib cartilage calcification may make interpretation difficult
- Ultrasound is the preferred screening modality when obstruction is suspected (high sensitivity for hydronephrosis) and in pregnancy to assess renal colic; however, it can only suggest (not reveal) the presence of obstruction
- Spiral CT is now preferred imaging because it visualizes both radiopaque and radiolucent stones
- If recurrent, refer/consult for additional work-up

Differential Diagnosis
- Acute pyelonephritis
- Lower urinary tract infection

Management
- For small stones (<0.5 cm), observe and treat pain
- Strain urine by pouring through gauze (or coffee filter) to collect stones or sediment as they pass; stone analysis is required

- For larger stones, may refer for extracorporeal shock wave lithotripsy, ureteroscopy, percutaneous nephrolithotomy, or open surgery for removal of stone
- Difficulties in tolerating pain or other factors may mandate treatment with shock wave lithotripsy or ureteroscopy in a patient who otherwise might be expected to pass the stone

  NONPHARMACOLOGIC TREATMENT
  - Increase fluid intake to maintain urinary output at 2–3 L/day, increase fiber in diet
  - Decrease animal fat in diet

  PHARMACOLOGIC TREATMENT
  - Pain management with NSAIDS and opioids as required
    – Acetaminophen/codeine (Tylenol #3) 1–2 tabs q4h prn
    – Hydrocodone/acetaminophen (Vicodin) 1–2 tabs q4h prn
    – Oxycodone/acetaminophen (Percocet) 1–2 tabs q4h prn
    – Ketorolac (Toradol) 30–60 mg IM initially, then 30 mg tabs q6h prn
    – Morphine 5–10 mg IM q4h prn
    – Other drugs: Meperidine, dilaudid
  - Antiemetics as needed

Special Considerations
- For prevention of recurrence of all types of stones, stress importance of adequate hydration: 2–3 L per day, dividing intake evenly to produce dilute urine at all times
  – Avoid apple and grapefruit juices
  – Avoid long periods of immobilization
- To prevent recurrence of calcium stones, limit protein, oxalate, and sodium intake; HCTZ 50 mg qd (rule out hyperparathyroidism before prescribing)
- To prevent recurrence of oxalate stones, restrict dietary oxalate (tea, rhubarb, leafy green vegetables, peanuts)
- To prevent recurrence of uric acid stones, restrict protein, consider allopurinol if serum uric acid is elevated, sodium bicarbonate

When to Consult, Refer, Hospitalize
- Refer to urologist if obstruction suspected or if symptoms persist over 3–4 days
- Hospitalize if infection present, stone is >6 mm in diameter, excessive nausea and vomiting, intractable pain, gross hematuria

Follow-Up
- Plain films of abdomen at 1–2 week intervals to monitor progress of stone in ureter
- Continue to strain urine until stone is passed. Monitor potassium and blood pressure in patients taking hydrochlorothiazide

  EXPECTED COURSE
  - 98% will pass spontaneously
  - Usually resolves within 4 weeks
  - Recurrences within 5 years are common in up to 50% of patients

  COMPLICATIONS
  - Complete urinary obstruction, hydronephrosis, renal failure, infection

RENAL DISORDERS

Acute Glomerulonephritis

Description
- Glomerular injury and inflammation as a result of an immune response, usually to a streptococcal infection. Follows an immunologic injury (i.e., deposition of antigen-antibody complexes from the bloodstream in the glomeruli). Presents with hematuria, edema, hypertension, proteinuria.

Etiology
- Characterized by diffuse inflammatory changes in the glomeruli and clinically by the abrupt onset of hematuria with RBC casts and mild proteinuria 1–2 weeks after a streptococcal infection
- Range of latent period (from onset of infection to onset of nephritis) is 7–21 days

Incidence and Demographics
- 20/100,000 cases in U.S. annually
- On the decline in developed countries but continues to occur in undeveloped nations at same rate

Risk Factors
- More common in children (peak ages 2–6 years)
- Multiple causes: Most common in children is recent Group A beta hemolytic streptococcal infection, such as pharyngitis or impetigo; only a few strains cause this kidney problem (type 12 and type 49)

Prevention and Screening
- Early and aggressive treatment of streptococcal infections

Assessment
HISTORY
- Edema, particularly of face, hands and feet; malaise; fever; abdominal or flank pain
- Skin or pharyngeal streptococcal infection within past 2–3 weeks; often cannot identify exact cause
- Abrupt onset of hematuria, oliguria or anuria

PHYSICAL EXAM
- Edema (90%), hypertension (75%), fever, abdominal tenderness

DIAGNOSTIC STUDIES
- Urinalysis will demonstrate proteinuria, hematuria
- Throat and skin cultures may be positive for streptococcal organism
- Total serum complement is decreased
- Antistreptolysins O (ASO) titer is increased in 60%–80% of cases

Differential Diagnosis
- Systemic lupus
- Anaphylactoid purpura
- Subacute bacterial endocarditis
- Congestive heart failure

Management
NONPHARMACOLOGIC TREATMENT
- Treat as inpatient until edema and hypertension are under control
- Restrict fluid: Restrict to replacement of insensible losses plus two-thirds of the urine output until diuresis; use no-salt-added diet
- Restrict protein in presence of azotemia and metabolic acidosis
- Avoid high-potassium foods
- May need dialysis

PHARMACOLOGIC TREATMENT
- Streptococcal infection: Penicillin IM or po for 10 days
- Acidosis: Sodium bicarbonate 1.2–2.4 grams per day if symptomatic or if serum bicarbonate <15
- Hypertension:
    - Diuretics: Furosemide (Lasix) 0.5–1 mg/kg IV or 2 mg/kg po bid or tid
    - Vasodilators: Apresoline (Hydralazine) 0.25–1.0 mg/kg qid or nifedipine (Procardia) 0.25 mg/kg/po prn or qid

LENGTH OF TREATMENT
- Usually a spontaneous diuresis occurs within 7–10 days after onset of illness; then supportive care is no longer required

Special Considerations
- Caution in elderly as frank heart failure occurs in 40%

When to Consult, Refer, Hospitalize
- Consult with physician for inpatient management in acute stage, or if significant edema/hypertension

Follow-Up
- Several times per week until resolves
    EXPECTED COURSE
    - Most cases are self-limited and resolve in 2–3 weeks; second episodes are rare
    - 95% of patients recover fully
    - More morbidity in those with pre-existing renal disease
    - Proteinuria may persist for as long as 2 years

    COMPLICATIONS
    - The most common long-term sequelae is mild hypertension
    - Hypertensive encephalopathy or retinopathy
    - Rapidly progressive glomerulonephritis, acute renal failure, nephrotic syndrome, chronic heart failure (CHF)

Renal Insufficiency and Failure

Description
- Compromise of renal function as evidenced by a decrease in glomerular filtration rate (GFR)
- Characterized by elevated BUN and creatinine and greatly diminished capacity for dealing with water solute fluctuations, but otherwise can maintain homeostasis
- Chronic renal insufficiency: Serum creatinine 1.5–3.0 mg/dL
- Chronic renal failure: Serum creatinine >3.0 mg/dL
- First finding is often simply an abnormal urinalysis (proteinuria, hematuria, pyuria, casts)
- Patient may be asymptomatic, but may have extra-renal symptoms of edema, hypertension, or signs of uremia

Etiology
- Diabetes, hypertension, glomerulonephritis, polycystic renal disease, obstructive uropathy, amyloidosis
- Congenital anomalies, infection, collagen vascular disease, nephrotoxins, ischemia, acute renal failure
- Deterioration may continue after initial insult resolves

Incidence and Demographics
- 2.8 per 100,000 people in U.S. with renal insufficiency or failure
- Males > females, increased incidence in non-Caucasians

Risk Factors
- Poorly controlled chronic conditions mentioned above, especially hypertension, diabetes
- Chronic NSAID use, especially in patients with hypertension
- Aging

Prevention and Screening
- Early treatment of above-mentioned conditions
- ACE inhibitors have been demonstrated to decrease progression to renal failure in both diabetic and nondiabetic patients. Hypertension need not be present to consider captopril (Catapres) 25 mg bid or tid early in the course of renal insufficiency, particularly for diabetic patients
- Protein restriction may reduce progression of chronic renal disease
- Blood pressure control in crucial

Assessment
- Patients may remain asymptomatic until GFR is less than 10% of normal
  HISTORY
    - Early manifestations may include nocturia because of inability to concentrate urine
    - Later patients may complain of anorexia, fatigue, weakness, edema, pruritus, nausea, vomiting, constipation or diarrhea, shortness of breath, hiccups, lethargy, insomnia, stocking-glove paresthesias

PHYSICAL EXAM
- Hypertension, increased skin pigmentation, edema, decreased deep tendon reflexes, pallor, uremic frost of skin, muscle twitching, stocking-glove sensory deficit

DIAGNOSTIC STUDIES
- Urine for micro albumin: First indication
- Urinalysis: Hematuria, proteinuria, casts
- Elevated 24-hour urine creatinine
- Elevated serum BUN, creatinine, potassium, phosphate, uric acid, and sodium
- Decreased serum calcium and hemoglobin/hematocrit
- Prolonged bleeding time due to platelet dysfunction
- Acidosis is usually present

Management
- Conservative management is designed to prolong the symptom-free period

NONPHARMACOLOGIC TREATMENT
- Dietary restrictions: Required to maintain appropriate fluid and electrolyte balance
- Maintain calorie intake at 40–50 cal/kg daily
- Protein is restricted to 20–25 g per day of balanced amino acids; may reduce acidosis and symptoms from elevated BUN (hiccups, nausea, pruritus) and may slow disease progression
- Monitor for both hypo- and hyperkalemia and avoid potassium-sparing diuretics; treat hyperkalemia >6 mEq/L and watch for ECG changes, especially above 6.5 mEq/L
- Potassium restriction to 2 g/day may be required
- Monitor both serum phosphate and calcium levels; limit phosphate intake
- Mild to moderate renal insufficiency, no need to restrict fluids or sodium
- If poorly controlled hypertension or CHF present, restrict fluids and sodium (2 g daily)
- In presence of oliguria, restrict fluids and sodium; intake should equal urine output and insensible losses

PHARMACOLOGIC TREATMENT
- For nausea, 5–10 mg prochlorperazine po qid
- For CHF, diuretics such as furosemide to remove excess free water if kidneys lose ability to regulate sodium
- For CHF also consider use of an ACE inhibitor (12.5–25 mg captopril bid or tid) but monitor renal function closely
- CHF usually not problematic until late in course
- Acidosis may require treatment with sodium bicarbonate if symptomatic (fatigue, tachypnea, lethargy) or <15 mEq/L with 600 mg of sodium bicarbonate bid initially; titrate to maintain levels of 16–20 mEq/L; be sure to follow serum potassium and calcium levels as both may decrease
- Patients may develop aldosterone resistance and may require more aggressive therapy such as fludrocortisone and potassium-binding resins
- Correct hyperphosphatemia with calcium citrate (667 mg tid before meals) to prevent development of renal osteodystrophy; if symptomatic or severe

hypocalcemia despite normal phosphate levels, add calcium carbonate 600 mg bid and vitamin D supplementation, calcitriol 25 mcg daily
- Anemia may require erythropoietin treatment, 1,000–6,000 units three times a week sq; monitor Hgb, hct, reticulocyte count and serum ferritin; make sure patient is not iron deficient before starting therapy; replace Fe+ as needed with 325 mg ferrous sulfate daily; severe anemia (e.g., with angina, high output failure) may require transfusion
- Bleeding can be treated with FFP or cryoprecipitate
- Bleeding in uremia has been treated with conjugated estrogens

LENGTH OF TREATMENT
- May require indefinite treatment

Special Considerations
- Geriatric patients: highest incidence, highest morbidity and mortality, exacerbated by many age-related conditions

When to Consult, Refer, Hospitalize
- Consult with physician for patient with chronic renal insufficiency who has abnormal laboratory tests beyond baseline (creatinine, serum albumin, creatinine clearance, electrolytes, calcium, phosphate, CBC, platelets) and when patient's symptoms and physical exam indicate
- For increases in proteinuria, follow with 24-hour urine for protein; refer/consult if abnormal
- Refer to nephrologist for dialysis and/or transplantation when the above therapies are no longer effective

Follow-Up
- Monthly
  EXPECTED COURSE
  - Progressive disease

  COMPLICATIONS
  - Anemia, congestive heart failure, pericardial tamponade, electrolyte imbalance, acidosis

CASE STUDIES

Case 1. A 49-year-old woman with a history of hypothyroidism complains of mid-back pain for 2 days. This is pain that she has never experienced in the past. She also complains of urinary frequency, dysuria, and intermittent nausea.

PMH: Gravida 2 Para 2. Multiple UTIs during early reproductive years. Medications include Synthroid 100 mcg, Prempro. She has a 15 pack-year smoking history.

   1. What additional history will you need?

Exam: Vital signs stable, afebrile, appears in moderate distress, positive left-sided CVA tenderness.

   2. What are the differential diagnoses?
   3. What diagnostic studies will you consider?

Results: Urinalysis shows 2+ hematuria with 1+ proteinuria, negative leukocytes, negative nitrates. A KUB was then ordered and demonstrated a small stone in distal ureter, 4 mm.

   4. What treatment will you consider?

Case 2. A 25-year-old female, recently married, comes in complaining of painful urination for 2 days. She has no fever. She uses a diaphragm for birth control.

HPI: No medications. Reports burning, frequency, hematuria, urgency. PMH significant for one urinary tract infection at age 19. Otherwise in good health.

   1. What are the differential diagnoses?

Exam: Vital signs are stable, afebrile, mild suprapubic tenderness. Normal pelvic exam.

   2. What diagnostic studies will you order?
   3. What risk factors can you identify?
   4. What treatment measures will you prescribe?
   5. What follow-up is necessary?
   6. What will you do if this patient follows up 2 weeks later with another UTI?

Case 3. A 10-year-old boy comes in with his parents to discuss bedwetting. He has daytime continence but has always had nocturnal enuresis once or twice a week. He has been diagnosed with attention-deficit disorder, but is not receiving any drug treatment; however, he has recently been placed in a special education class in school. Episodes of enuresis are now occurring almost nightly.

HPI: Normal gestation, normal labor and delivery. No serious childhood illnesses. No history of UTI. No medications, no allergies.

   1. What additional history would you like?

Exam: Physical exam and neurological exam are normal (i.e. no anatomic abnormalities, normal gait and reflexes).

   2. What are the differential diagnoses?
   3. What diagnostic studies will you order?
   4. What treatment would you consider?

REFERENCES

Agency for Healthcare Research and Quality. (2007). *Guide to clinical preventive services* (AHRQ Publication No. 07-05100). Rockville, MD: Author. Retrieved March 1, 2008, from http://www.ahcpr.gov/clinic/uspstfix.htm

American Academy of Pediatrics. (2006). *The 2006 red book: Report of the Committee on Infectious Disease.* Elk Grove, IL: Author

American College of Obstetricians and Gynecologists. (2005). *Urinary incontinence in women* (ACOG practice bulletin No. 63). Washington, DC: Author.

American Urological Association, (2007). *Prostate cancer clinical guideline update panel: Guideline for the management of clinically localized prostate cancer: 2007 update.* Linthicum, MD: American Urological Association Education and Research, Inc.

Arcangelo, V. P., & Peterson, A. (2005). *Pharmacotherapeutics for advanced practice: A practical approach.* Philadelphia: Lippincott Williams & Wilkins.

Benner, B. M. (Ed.). (2008). *Brenner and Rector's the kidney.* Philadelphia: Elsevier Health Sciences.

Burke, M., & Laramie, J, (2003). *Primary care of the older adult: A multidisciplinary approach.* Philadelphia: Elsevier Health Sciences.

Burns, E. E., Dunn, M., & Brady, A. (2004). *Pediatric primary care: A handbook for nurse practitioners* (3rd ed.). Philadelphia: Elsevier Health Sciences.

Gilbert, D. N., Moellering, R. C., Jr., Eliopoulos, G. M., Sande, M. A., & Chambers, H. F. (Eds.). (2008). *The Sanford guide to antimicrobial therapy* (33rd ed.). Hyde Park, VT: Antimicrobial Therapy, Inc.

Goroll, A. H., May, L. A., & Mulley, A. G. (Eds.). (2006). *Primary care medicine: Office evaluation and management of the adult patient.* Philadelphia: Lippincott Williams & Wilkins.

Griffith, H. W., & Dambro, M. R. (2008). *The 5 minute consult.* Malvern, PA: Lea & Febinger.

Grodstein, F., Fretts, R., Lifford, K., Resnick, N., & Curhan, G. (2003). Association of age, race, and obstetric history with urinary symptoms among women in the Nurses' Health Study. *American Journal of Obstetrics and Gynecology, 189,* 428–434.

Hanson, S. M., & Gedalay-Duff ,V. (2005). *Family health care nursing: Theory, practice and research.* Philadelphia: F. A. Davis.

Harris, S. S., Link, C. L., Tennstedt, S. L., Kusek, J. W., & McKinlay, J. B. (2007). Care seeking and treatment for urinary incontinence in a diverse population. *Journal of Urology, 177,* 680.

Hooton, T. M., Besser, R., Foxman, B., Fritsche, T. R., & Nicolle, L. E. (2004). Acute uncomplicated cystitis in an era of increasing antibiotic resistance: A proposed approach to empirical therapy. *Clinical Infectious Diseases, 39,* 75.

Karlowsky, J. A., Thornsberry, C., Jones, M. E., & Sahm, D.F. (2003). Susceptibility of antimicrobial-resistant urinary Escherichia coli isolates to fluoroquinolones and nitrofurantoin. *Clinical Infectious Diseases, 36,* 183.

Liu, C. C., Wang, C. J., Huang, S. P., Chou, Y. H., Wu, W. J., & Huang, C. H. (2004). Relationships between American Urological Association symptom index, prostate volume, and disease-specific quality of life question in patients with benign prostatic hyperplasia. *Kaohsiung Journal of Medical Science, 20*(6), 273–278.

MacFarlane, M. T. (2006). *Urology.* Philadelphia: Lippincott Williams & Wilkins.

Mardon, R. E., Halim, S., Pawlson, L. G., & Haffer, S. C. (2006). Management of urinary incontinence in Medicare managed care beneficiaries: Results from the 2004 Medicare Health Outcomes Survey. *Archives of Internal Medicine, 166,* 1128.

Miller, L. G., & Tang, A. W. (2004). Treatment of uncomplicated urinary tract infections in an era of increasing antimicrobial resistance. *Mayo Clinic Proceedings, 79*(8), 1048–1053.

Nicolle, L. E., Bradley, S., Colgan, R., Rice, J. C., Schaeffer, A., Hooton, T. M., et al. (2005). Infectious Diseases Society of America guidelines for the diagnosis and treatment of asymptomatic bacteriuria in adults. *Clinical Infectious Diseases, 40,* 643.

Staskin, D., Hilton, P., Emmanuel, A., Goode, P., Mills, I., Shull, B., et al. (2005). Initial assessment of incontinence. In P. Abrams, L. Cardozo, S. Khoury, A. Wein (Eds.), *Incontinence* (3rd ed.; p. 485). Plymouth, MA: Health Publications.

Stoller, M. L., & Carroll, P. R. (2008). Urology. In L. M. Tierney, Jr., S. J. McPhee, & M. A. Papadakis (Eds.), *Current medical diagnosis and treatment* (47th ed.). New York: Lange Medical Books/McGraw-Hill.

Tan, T. L. (2003). Urinary incontinence in older persons: A simple approach to a complex problem. *Annals of the Academy of Medicine Singapore, 32*(6), 731–739.

U.S. Preventive Services Task Force. (2007). *Guide to clinical preventive services: Periodic updates.* Alexandria, VA: International Medical Publishing, Inc.

Wallach, J. (2007). *Interpretation of diagnostic tests* (8th ed.). Philadelphia: Lippincott, Williams & Wilkins.

Female Reproductive System Disorders and Concerns

Barbara Siebert, MSN, CRNP, FNP-BC

GENERAL APPROACH

- Because of the high number of women who seek health care, the primary care clinician must be prepared to handle a broad variety of women's health concerns.
- The clinician may view women's health concerns around common groupings: menstrual cycle, normal changes (menopause), variations (PMS), abnormalities of that cycle (abnormal bleeding) and fertility issues.

Red Flags

Ovarian Cancer

- High-risk women: Familial cancer syndromes; history of breast, colon, or uterine cancer; two first-degree relatives with ovarian cancer; smokers
- Presentation with ovarian cancer is vague: Mild, nonspecific gastrointestinal symptoms; dyspareunia; abdominal pain; bloating; urinary symptoms; dyspepsia; abdominal fullness; increasing abdominal girth; cramping; irregular vaginal bleeding; fatigue; or pelvic pressure; 60%–75% present with advanced disease
- In a recent study, predominance of the following symptoms differentiate cases of ovarian cancer versus controls: unusual bloating (71%) unusual abdominal or lower back pain (52%); fullness, abdominal pressure, and lack of energy (43%)
- Weight loss and anorexia are poor prognostic signs
- Physical exam findings occur late in disease: Palpable adnexal mass; ascites (poor prognostic sign)
- If suspicious, get transvaginal sonography. May consider getting CA-125 as you refer to GYN oncology specialist.

- Refer women in high-risk groups to OB/GYN/oncologist—premenarchal or postmenopausal females with a palpable ovary, persistent ovarian cyst >5 cm (beyond 6 weeks) among reproductive-age women

Endometrial Cancer

- Risks include any condition leading to unopposed estrogen, including prolonged anovulation, oligomenorrhea nulliparity, obesity, diabetes, early menarche/late menopause, endometrial hyperplasia, hormone replacement therapy with estrogen alone, smokers, polycystic ovary syndrome (PCOS), tamoxifen therapy; if diagnosed in early stages, 5-year survival is 85%–95%
- 80%–90% present with painless abnormal bleeding pattern as cardinal sign but may also present with a watery vaginal discharge
- Pelvic pain, pressure, or mass present late in disease (entire uterus may be boggy, enlarged)
- Refer if Pap smear reports atypical glandular cells of undetermined significance (AGCUS); transvaginal ultrasound reports endometrial stripe >10 mm among postmenopausal women
- Any postmenopausal vaginal bleeding merits a referral to gynecology for further work-up; women over 35 or with risk factors should have a pelvic ultrasound and/or an endometrial biopsy. Younger women with vaginal bleeding unresponsive to therapies merit pelvic ultrasound and/or endometrial biopsy.

Vulvar Cancer

- Pruritus most common symptom, followed by burning or dysuria, bleeding, pain, or discharge
- Common areas for lesions include labia majora, clitoris, and periurethral areas but may occur anywhere on vulva
- Suspicious findings include changes in pigmentation or tissue that is thickened, reddened, ulcerated, nodular, fissured, or with abnormal raised areas
- Refer any lesions that fail to spontaneously resolve in several weeks or with therapy; promptly refer new lesions among women >60 years of age

Vaginal Cancer

- Frequently secondary to cervical or endometrial cancer, diethylstilbestrol (DES) exposure
- Signs and symptoms include bleeding from the vaginal wall, chronic pruritus, vaginal or pelvic pain
- Usually found in proximal one-third of posterior vagina; most lesions raised, granular, friable; lesions may be palpable but not visible
- Refer all lesions for biopsy if history of DES exposure

Ectopic Pregnancy

- Represents 1%–2% of pregnancies but accounts for 13% maternal deaths
  - Majority of ectopics implant in the tubes (97%)
  - Most common time for rupture is during the first 8–12 weeks
- Risk factors include history of sexually transmitted diseases (STDs; especially multiple episodes), pelvic inflammatory disease (PID), adhesions, history of intra-uterine device (IUD) use, tubal ligation failure, pelvic or abdominal surgery, prior history of ectopic gestation, inconsistent or nonuse of birth control methods, infertility therapy
- Classic symptoms are amenorrhea, abdominal pain, abnormal bleeding

- Commonly see late menses which is lighter than normal OR amenorrhea of 4–6 weeks duration followed by erratic vaginal bleeding (75%)
- Abdominal tenderness (95%); adnexal tenderness (87%–99%), adnexal mass (33%–53%); cervical motion tenderness in almost all cases
  - Peritoneal signs: Involuntary guarding, rigidity (75%)
- Late and more ominous signs indicating potential rupture are syncope or orthostatic blood pressure changes (shock, 2%–17%), shoulder pain similar to cholecystitis (10%), increase in vaginal bleeding (dark red or bright red), and a significant worsening of abdominal pain
  - If urine or serum beta-HCG is positive: Get series of quantitative serum HCG (low and not doubling every 24–48 hours indicates ectopic); if urine is negative, get serum (neg. serum rules out ectopic)
  - Transvaginal ultrasound may be done to rule out intrauterine pregnancy over 6 weeks from last menstrual period (LMP)
  - If condition is stable, refer to gynecologist for possible medical treatment with methotrexate, laparoscopy, or laparotomy
- Transfer to emergency facility for signs of rupture
- RhoGAM 300 mcg also needs to be given to an Rh-negative woman

Toxic Shock Syndrome
- Caused by strain of *Staphylococcus aureus*; risk factors include menstruation (especially with tampon use), skin and respiratory infections, post surgery, postpartum
- Signs and symptoms: 2–3 day prodrome including but not limited to malaise, myalgias, fever (>102°F), erythematous rash (particularly palms and soles), vomiting, watery diarrhea, or abdominal pain followed by signs of shock and organ failure
- Consult with physician promptly for hospitalization or immediate transfer to emergency facility

Contraception

Description
- The voluntary control of childbearing
- In the U.S., over 3.5 million women unintentionally become pregnant each year. These pregnancies occur because of both birth control failures and nonuse of method.
- Most popular methods in the U.S. are oral contraceptives, female sterilization, condoms, and male sterilization. Many forms of contraception do not decrease risk of sexually transmitted infections.
- Abstinence is the only method with 100% safety and efficacy for preventing pregnancy and STDs.
- Surgical sterilization via tubal ligation has efficacy >99%; should be considered irreversible.
- Choice of contraceptive method is based on lifestyle, developmental level, efficacy, and safety characteristics of sexual relationships. Adolescents are typically sexually active 6 months prior to seeking counseling and information regarding contraception; contraception failure rates are highest among adolescents.
- By high school graduation, approximately 65% of all adolescents are sexually active and 20% of adolescents surveyed have had multiple (>4) sexual partners.
- Provider must know state regulations regarding adolescent confidentially when seeking contraception.

Spermicides

- Spermicides (gels, creams, suppositories; vaginal film, foam) usually contain nonoxynol-9, are sold over the counter with specific instructions for each type
- **Warning:** The Centers for Disease Control (CDC) has indicated that vaginal spermicides that contain nonoxynol-9 (N-9) are not effective in the prevention of STDs and HIV. Furthermore, frequent use of spermicides containing N-9 has been associated with disruption of the genital epithelium, which might be associated with an increased risk for HIV transmission. Therefore, N-9 is not recommended for STD/HIV prevention.
- Can be effective if used consistently but first-year failure rate of typical users is 21%
- More effective when combined with barrier method
- May irritate vagina or urinary tract; alters normal vaginal flora or may alter normal vaginal barriers (mucus, flora, pH) that protect from infection; no major contraindications, no systemic side effects

Nonprescription Barrier Methods

- Over-the-counter barriers: Female or male condoms, prevent sperm from physically entering woman
- Up to 97% effective if perfect use (99% if combined with spermicide)
- Screen for latex allergy (nonlatex products may offer less STD/HIV protection)
- Latex condoms are good choice for protection from STDs and HIV when used appropriately. They require partner cooperation support (see Chapter 12 for steps on male condom use).
- Contraceptive sponge:
  - Nonprescription barrier method of reversible birth control; inserted deep into the vagina before intercourse; made of solid polyurethane foam containing nonoxynol-9 spermicide; soft, round, and about 2 inches in diameter; has a nylon loop attached to the bottom for removal
  - Covers the cervix and blocks sperm from entering the uterus; continuously releases spermicide that immobilizes sperm; cannot reduce the risk of sexually transmitted infections
  - *Advantages:*
    - No prescription or fitting is need
    - Can be used during breast-feeding
    - Portable
    - Does not affect a woman's natural hormones
    - Does not interrupt sex play
  - Method of use: Before inserting the sponge, wet it with at least two tablespoons of clean water. Gently squeeze the sponge. The spermicide will become active when the sponge is thoroughly wet. Fold the sides of the sponge upward and away from the loop on the bottom to make it look long and narrow. Then slide the sponge as far back into vagina as fingers will reach. The sponge will unfold and cover the cervix once released. To make sure the cervix is covered, slide a finger around the edge of the sponge and check its position. The nylon loop on the bottom of the sponge should also be felt.

- Can be inserted up to 24 hours before intercourse; must be left in place for at least 6 hours after the last act of intercourse; during that time, intercourse may be repeated without additional preparation during the first 24 hours. It should not be worn for more than 30 consecutive hours. Use sponge only once, then discard.
- To remove the sponge, insert a finger inside the vagina and through the loop. Pull the sponge out slowly and gently.
- *Contraindications for use*: Allergy to polyurethane, spermicide, or sulfa drugs; current menstruation; current reproductive tract infection; difficulty with insertion; discomfort with touching one's genitals; history of toxic shock syndrome; recent abortion, childbirth, or miscarriage; vaginal obstructions; women should not use the sponge during any kind of vaginal bleeding, including menstruation.
- *Disadvantages*: Few side effects reported. Sponge may be difficult to remove. If the sponge cannot be removed, or if it breaks into pieces that can not be completely removed, instruct patient to be seen by her healthcare provider immediately. Some women may notice vaginal irritation. Sponge users may be at slightly increased risk of toxic shock syndrome, which is also associated with the prolonged use of highly absorbent tampons.

Emergency Contraception
- Emergency contraception used within short interval after coital event to reduce chance of pregnancy
- Depends on the current point along the menstrual cycle
- Typically prevents luteinizing hormone (LH) surge and thus ovulation; alters endometrium to prevent implantation
- Preven: 4-pill system, 50 mcg ethinyl estradiol/0.5 mg levonorgestrel, take 2 pills within 72 hours of intercourse and 2 pills 12 hours later; approximately 75% effective, may cause nausea and vomiting
- Plan B: 2-pill system, 0.75 mg levonorgestrel, take 1 pill with 72 hours of intercourse and 1 pill 12 hours later, much less nausea and vomiting reported than seen with Preven
- Contraindicated in pregnancy; first screen for pre-existing pregnancy with serum or urine HCG
- Education regarding correct emergency contraceptive regimen
- Emergency contraception needs to be initiated within 72 hours of need, preferably within 24 hours to increase effectiveness
- Nausea (30%–50%) and vomiting (15%–20%) are the most common complaints associated with emergency contraception with combination pills; take pills with food, not on an empty stomach
- Advise the patient to return for pregnancy test if no menses in next 3–4 weeks
- Emergency follow-up is recommended if patient experiences severe abdominal pain or other severe side effects possibly related to the treatment, ectopic gestation, or miscarriage
- The ParaGard IUD may also be inserted within 5 days after unprotected vaginal intercourse to reduce the risk of pregnancy by 99.9%
- Plan future contraceptive methods

Natural Family Planning

- Efficacy is variable but can be high if couple is very dedicated.
- Several visits or specialized classes are recommended to provide instructions for use of one or more of the natural family planning methods, for practicing the record-keeping, and learning to observe the signs correctly; instructor should be specially trained.
- Calendar rhythm method: Uses calendar charting to calculate a woman's fertile period, averaging longest and shortest cycles, and identifying times of likely ovulation
- Basal body temperature (BBT) method: Daily a.m. basal body temperatures are monitored for a sustained rise (0.4°F –0.8°F degrees) at ovulation that continues until next menses
- Ovulation or "billings" method: Daily cervical mucus changes are observed for characteristics at ovulation (sticky and pasty precedes ovulation, silky and stretchy occurs at ovulation)
  - A variety of factors may interfere with the cervical mucus characteristics: douching, spermicides, vaginal infections, lubricants, semen, vaginal medications, normal lubrication of sexual arousal
- Symptothermal method: Combines mucus and cervical changes and recognition of ovulation symptoms with BBT; charted daily and used to assess fertile times
- Needs cooperation between partners and agreement about any backup methods. Typically, the ovum is viable for 24 hours and sperm up to 72 hours; however, ova can survive up to 72 hours and sperm can survive 72 or more hours, so must factor this into fertile interval planning; needs regular cycles to be most successful. Studies have shown that conception can occur up to 6 days prior to ovulation and 1 day after.

Prescription Barrier Methods

- Diaphragms, caps, and shields are soft latex or silicone barrier devices that cover the entire cervix, blocking the opening to the uterus to prevent sperm from physically entering the cervix. Used with spermicidal jelly or cream to enhance contraceptive effect.
- Diaphragm is a shallow, dome-shaped cup with a flexible spring rim. There are several types of diaphragms as determined by the spring rim: coil, flat, or arcing. Coil-spring and flat-spring diaphragms become a flat oval when compressed for insertion. Arcing diaphragms form an arc or half moon when compressed and are the easiest to insert. Efficacy may reach 96% if used properly.
- Use with 1 teaspoon of spermicidal jelly; insert to back of vagina and tuck behind the pubic bone, ensuring the cervix is covered; must stay in place 6 hours after last act of intercourse; if intercourse is repeated or occurs more than 6 hours after insertion, leave the diaphragm in place and apply more spermicide; do not leave the diaphragm in place for more than 24 hours.
- Cervical cap (FemCap) is a silicone rubber cup-shaped device that fits securely in the vagina to cover the cervix; efficacy may reach 94% if used properly. Cannot use cervical cap if short or irregular cervix, post cervical conization, or abnormal Pap smear.
- Use with spermicidal jelly; insert cap into the vagina and onto the cervix, ensuring the cervix is completely covered; with each act of intercourse, check that cap is still covering the cervix; apply more spermicide if needed; cap must stay in place 6 hours after the last intercourse; do not leave cap in place for more than 48 hours.
- Lea's Shield is a silicone rubber cup that covers the cervix with an air valve and a loop to aid in removal.

- Use with spermicidal jelly, coating the inside of the bowl around the hole, the front of the rim, and outer part of the valve with spermicide; insert the shield into the vagina with the valve facing down and the thickest end inserted first; push the shield up as far in the vagina as is possible; be sure that the loop is not sticking out of vagina; the air between the cervix and shield will be vented out through the valve to create a proper fit; the valve may be pressed a few times after insertion to be sure that the air is removed; with each act of intercourse check that the shield is still covering the cervix; apply more spermicide if needed; the shield must stay in place 8 hours after the last intercourse; do not leave in place for more than 48 hours.
- Fitting or sizing done by a clinician to determine the correct size for diaphragm and cap.
- No major contraindications, no systemic side effects; may increase urinary tract infections (UTIs) in some women.
- Protection may be increased by ensuring cervix is covered before each act of intercourse; spermicide used as recommended; using a latex condom.
- Diaphragms, caps, and shields offer no protection against sexually transmitted infection. Use a latex condom to reduce the risk of infection.
- Diaphragms are available in many sizes and designs. A new size may be needed after any of the following: full-term pregnancy; abdominal or pelvic surgery; miscarriage, or abortion after 14 weeks of pregnancy; a 20% change in weight.
- FemCap is available in three sizes: small, for women who have never been pregnant; medium, for women who have had an abortion or a cesarean delivery; large, for women who have given birth vaginally.
- The shield only comes in one size.
- Warning signs: Toxic shock syndrome (TSS): Rare cases of toxic shock syndrome have been reported with diaphragm, sponge, and other cervical barrier method use. The symptoms of TSS include a sunburn-type rash; diarrhea; dizziness, faintness, weakness; sore throat; aching muscles and joints; sudden high fever; vomiting.
- Contraindications to use: Allergy to latex, silicone, or spermicide; childbirth in the last 6 weeks (10 weeks for FemCap); difficulty with insertion; discomfort with touching one's genitals; history of toxic shock syndrome; recent cervical surgery; recent abortion after the first trimester (after any recent abortion for FemCap); uterine prolapse; vaginal obstructions.
- A woman may have inability to use a diaphragm if she has frequent urinary tract infections; poor vaginal muscle tone.
- Inability to use FemCap if she has breaks in the vaginal or cervical tissue; cancer of the uterus, vagina, or vulva; a reproductive tract infection; poor vaginal muscle tone.
- Inability to use a shield if she has breaks in the vaginal or cervical tissue; frequent urinary tract infections; a reproductive tract infection.
- Diaphragm, cap, or shield should never be used during any kind of vaginal bleeding, including menstruation.
- Advantages: Can be used during breastfeeding; portable; generally cannot be felt by either partner; immediately effective and reversible; no effect on a woman's natural hormones; no interruption of sex play; can be inserted hours ahead of time.
- Disadvantages: Cannot be used during menstruation; may be difficult for some women to insert; may be pushed out of place by some sexual positions; must be in place every time a woman has vaginal intercourse; diaphragms and caps may require refitting.
- Use of the spermicide nonoxynol-9 many times a day by people at risk for HIV may irritate tissue and increase the risk of HIV and other sexually transmitted infections.

- Care of diaphragms, caps, and shields: Diaphragm and cap may last 2 years and the shield may last 6 months; wash with warm soapy water and air dry; do not use powders; never use oil-based lubricants such as petroleum jelly (Vaseline), creams, or lotions as they will damage latex; examine devices for small holes or fill the cup of the diaphragm or cap with water and look for leaks; diaphragms, caps, and shields can still be used if the rubber becomes discolored. However, if the rubber puckers, especially near the rim, it has become too thin.

Intra-Uterine Device (IUD)

- IUDs are small, T-shaped contraceptive devices made of flexible plastic; can be imbedded with progestin or wrapped with copper; sit in uterine cavity and prevent implantation of fertilized ovum; >99% effective, no user error or inconsistency.
- Two types are now available in the U.S.: ParaGard (Copper T 380A) contains copper and can be left in place for 10 years; Mirena continuously releases a small amount of the hormone progestin and is effective for 5 years.
- Hormonal IUD thickens cervical mucus, disrupts the pattern of ovulation, and impairs uterine and tubal motility.
- Levonorgesterol Intra-Uterine System: Mirena approved December 2000, T-shaped polyethylene device; reservoir contains Levonorgesterol 52 mg; delivers 20 mcg/day of the progestin; approved for 5 years of use; decreases bleeding and cramping; 20% become amenorrheic; must be inserted by a trained clinician; irregular bleeding/ spotting first 3 months; abdominal pain, back pain, breast pain, mood changes, acne, headaches, and nausea may occur; must be comfortable checking string monthly.
- Copper-based IUD: ParaGard (Copper T 380A) contains copper and can be left in place for 10 years; causes increased copper in ions, enzymes, and prostaglandins that alters tubal and uterine transport, interfering with fertilization and destroying sperm.
- Choose candidates based on careful assessment of risk factors (PID risk related to multiple partners; history of heavy menses; dysmenorrhea); need special training for insertion.
- May be inserted any time in woman's cycle if negative HCG midcycle and no unprotected coitus since LMP; post abortion 2–3 weeks after uncomplicated procedure; immediately to 3 months postpartum.
- Common complaints for nonhormonal IUD include dysmenorrhea and increased blood flow.
- Should consider IUD removal in addition to antibiotic therapy when treating endometritis, STD, PID
- ParaGard is effective immediately after insertion.
- Mirena is effective immediately if inserted within 7 days of LMP. If Mirena is inserted at any other time of the menstrual cycle, patient will need to use another method of birth control if vaginal intercourse occurs during the first week after insertion. Protection will begin after 7 days.
- Highest risk of perforation is at time of insertion; early IUD warning signs:
  - **P**: Period late, abnormal spotting, bleeding
  - **A**: Abdominal pain, or pain with intercourse
  - **I**: Infection exposure (STDs), abnormal discharge, itching, pain
  - **N**: Not feeling well, fever, chills, fatigue
  - **S**: String missing, shorter, or longer (check monthly)

Hormonal Contraception

- The first question to be decided is whether the presence of estrogen is medically acceptable and not contraindicated.

Oral, Transdermal, Vaginal, Injectable Progestin, and Progestin Implants

- Hormonal methods interfere with negative feedback loop with steady hormonal doses, which inhibit ovulation, decrease endometrial lining (less flow, less area to implant in), and alter cervical mucus.
- Estrogen effects: Follicle-stimulating hormone (FSH) and LH are suppressed, ovary is not stimulated, secretions and cellular structure of endometrium are altered.
- Progestin effects: Inhibits FSH and LH, which suppresses ovulation, thickens cervical mucus so sperm transport is inhibited; decidualized endometrial bed inhibits implantation.
- Contraindications: Thrombophlebitis; thromboembolic disease; cerebrovascular accident (CVA); coagulopathies; uncontrolled hypertension (may use progestin-only pills); vascular disease (coronary artery disease [CAD], peripheral vascular disease [PVD]); breast cancer; estrogen-dependent neoplasia; hepatic adenoma/cancer; pregnancy; impaired renal function/hepatitis; diabetes with nephropathy, neuropathy, retinopathy, or other vascular disease; lactation <6 weeks postpartum; major surgery with immobilization; hypertension (160+/100+); smoking (age >35 smoking >20 cigarettes/day); migraines with focal neurological symptoms that worsen with any hormonal contraceptive use. Usually not given to smokers.
- Relative contraindications, exercise caution: Undiagnosed vaginal bleeding, active gallbladder disease, family history of hyperlipidemia/myocardial infarction (MI) <age 50, smoking (age >35 and smoking >15 cigarettes/day).
- No significant adverse fetal effects have been documented regarding exposure prior to and early in pregnancy.
- Highly effective (>98%) when used correctly; reversible, widely studied for years, menstrual benefits (especially with endometriosis).
- No STD protection.
- The most common side effects: Acne (with high androgenic activity pills), light/no menses (rule out pregnancy), breakthrough bleeding or spotting between periods, breast pain (mastalgia), depression, headaches, libido changes, nausea, weight changes.
- Serious side effects include stroke, pulmonary embolus, thrombophlebitis, hepatitis; stroke risk increased in smokers.
- Some drugs reduce oral contraceptive levels (Carbamazepine, Dilantin, Rifampin).
- These antibiotics *do not* decrease steroid levels in women using oral contraceptives: ampicillin, clarithromycin, metronidazole, quinolone antibiotics (ciprofloxacin, ofloxacin), doxycycline, tetracycline, fluconazole.
    - ORAL CONTRACEPTIVES (OCS)
        - Multiple dosage arrangements available combining estrogens and progestins in fixed amounts during 21 days of the cycle, or varying amounts of progestin and sometimes estrogen. Side effects (breakthrough bleeding) and beneficial effects (acne reduction) based on the estrogenic, progestational, androgenic, endometrial, and lipid biological activity of each type.
        - Seasonale is a contraceptive taken for 91 days—81 days of hormonal pills followed by 7 days of placebo. Each pill contains levonorgesterol 0.15 mg and ethinyl estradiol 0.03 mg. Women taking Seasonale have only 4 menstrual periods per year.

- Low-dose estrogen OCs (20–25 mcg) decrease estrogen side effects; possible increased breakthrough bleeding; decreased suppression of cyst formation/reduction; decreased margin of error for noncompliance.
- Progestin-only OCs: Failure rate is five times that of combined OCs; taken continuously with no placebos; breakthrough bleeding more common especially if pills are missed or taken late; need backup method for missed or late pills.
- Warning signs of problems with OCs:
  - Abdominal pain (severe)
  - Chest pain (severe, cough, short of breath, sharp pain when inhaling)
  - Headache (severe), dizziness, weakness, numbness, especially if one-sided
  - Eye (visual blurring, visual loss), speech problem
  - Severe leg pain (calf or thigh)
- Use pill with the least bleeding side effects, better lipid profiles, less estrogenic effects.
- Start first pill within 7 days of LMP. A pregnancy test is not necessary for the first cycle since the pill is easily withdrawn and has an excellent safety record in early pregnancy over the past 40 years.
- Use alternative contraception in addition to OCs during first 2 weeks, unless started on first day of menses; also use alternative contraception if missed pills, late pills, use of certain drugs used with pills.
- With combined forms OCs: If one pill is missed, take it immediately or 2 pills together the next day; if 2 days of pills are missed, take 2 pills immediately and 2 pills the following day, avoid intercourse on days when pills are missed or use condoms for 7 days. If more than 2 days of pills are missed in a row, discard the pack, use another form of birth control such as condoms, and start a new pack within 7 days of the onset of the next menses.
- With progestin-only forms: If minipill is even 2–3 hours late, use backup method. Report severe headache, or severe lower abdominal pain that may indicate pregnancy or ruptured cyst.
- In the first 2–3 weeks postpartum, avoid combination OCs due to clotting risk; progestin-only pill may be used; OCs pose no apparent harm to the neonate but lactation may be impaired.
- Thorough history and physical exam with attention to the breasts, blood pressure, abdomen, pelvic organs, cervical cytology should be done on initiation of the pill and at least yearly.

TRANSDERMAL PATCH

- Ortho Evra Transdermal Contraceptive Patch contains norelgestromin 150 mcg and ethinyl estradiol 20 mcg, both released per 24 hours. The patch is applied to abdomen, buttock, upper outer arm, or upper torso (except breasts) weekly 3x, followed by a patch-free week causing withdrawal bleeding/menses to occur. A backup method should be used the first week after starting the patch.
- Same indications, risk factors, mechanisms, and side effects as OCs.
- May be less effective in women who weigh more than 198 pounds.
- About 2%–4.7% of patches have to be replaced due to detachment.
- No powder, lotion, or other products should be applied around the site of the patch.
- May bathe, exercise, and swim.

- 3% discontinuation rate due to application-site reaction.
- Increased breakthrough bleeding first 1–2 cycles.

VAGINAL RING CONTRACEPTIVE
- NuvaRing: Etonogestrel 120 mcg and ethinyl estradiol 15 mcg, both amounts released each day; 21 days on/7 days off; flexible donut-shaped ring (2 inches); ethylene vinylacetate copolymer (not latex).
- Insert one ring vaginally on day 1–5 of menstrual cycle. Leave in place for 3 weeks, then remove and discard for 1 week allowing menses to occur; insert new ring following menses and repeat 3 weeks in and 1 week out pattern; backup method recommended during initial week.
- If ring falls out for <3 hours it may be reinserted.
- Same indications, risk factors, mechanisms, and side effects as OCs; may cause some irregular bleeding, leukorrhea, vaginitis, foreign body sensation, coital problems, and expulsion.
- Cautious use in women with vaginal abnormalities (rectoceles, stenosis, cervical prolapse).

DEPO MEDROXYPROGESTERONE ACETATE (DMPA)
- Depo-Provera: Progesterone only, 150 mg IM injection every 12–13 weeks, may use deltoid or gluteal muscles, do not rub site after injection; given within first 5 days of menses; cannot be immediately reversed, may take 6–18 months for return of fertility; recommend a urine HCG prior to administering first two DMPA injections to rule out pregnancy.
- Amenorrhea, spotting, irregular bleeding are most common first 3 months.
- Start Depo Provera at 30 days postpartum.
- NOTE: Lunelle is no longer available in the U.S.
- Frequently causes weight gain, headaches, mood changes, menstrual irregularities (amenorrhea in 60%–70%), hair loss/thinning, lowering of high-density lipoprotein (HDL), decreased bone density.
- Contraindications: Absolute: Pregnancy and unexplained vaginal bleeding.
- Contraindications: Relative: Weight gain issues, headaches, and liver or gallbladder disease.

IMPLANON
- Single rod, progestin-only subdermal implant; effective for up to 3 years; packaged as a sterile, disposable, preloaded applicator; rod is 4 cm x 2 cm; solid core imbedded with etonogestrel; initial release is 60–70 mcg/day, after a few weeks 40–50 mcg/day, end of the third year 25–30 mcg/day; not radio-opaque, may cause irregular bleeding.
- Inserted subdermally in the grove between the bicep and tricep muscles; clinician may insert/remove device after completing a training program.
- Inhibits ovulation, increases viscosity of cervical mucus; drug below detectable levels within 1 week of removal, >90% women ovulated well within 3 months post removal.
- Contraindications: pregnancy, current or past history of thrombotic disease, undiagnosed vaginal bleeding, history of breast cancer, hypersensitivity to any of the components, not recommended with hepatic enzyme inducer drugs.

ESSURE PERMANENT BIRTH CONTROL SYSTEM
- Essure micro-insert is placed in proximal portion of each fallopian tube lumen; micro-insert expands upon release and anchors itself in the tube; subsequent benign local tissue in-growth over a 3-month period; scarring blocks fallopian tube, device permanently anchored in occluded fallopian tube, resulting in permanent contraception; provider must be an experienced hysteroscopist.
- Candidates: Women who prefer this approach to laparoscopy; especially for women with obesity (BMI of >45), abdominal mesh that prevents laparoscopy, permanent colostomy, multiple abdominal/pelvic surgeries (adhesions), use of anticoagulation medications, medical problems that contraindicate general anesthesia.
- Menstrual function: Some transient or recurrent menstrual changes that may or may not be related to Essure, women reported both heavier and lighter than normal menstrual flow, few persistent changes in menstrual function.
- Post-placement follow-up: *Low-pressure* hysterosalpingogram (HSG) is recommended 3 months after Essure; if tubal occlusion is not demonstrated, repeat HSG 3 months later.
- Benefits: No incisions or general anesthesia required; micro-insert contains no hormones; use in patients not eligible for incisional surgery (morbid obesity, prior abdominal/pelvic surgery).

CONDITIONS OF THE MENSTRUAL CYCLE

Normal Menstrual Cycle
- Complex rhythmical, hormonal interchange among the hypothalamus, pituitary gland (the hypothalamic-pituitary axis), ovaries, and uterine endometrium
- Cycle requires intact hormonal feedback, functional organs, and open cervical and vaginal orifices
- Cycle divided into two phases: Follicular phase (starts with day 1 of menses and ends with luteinizing hormone [LH] surge) and luteal phase (begins with pre-ovulatory LH surge and ends with menses)
- Low estrogen level causes the hypothalamus to produce pulsatile waves of gonadotropin-releasing hormone (GnRH)
- GnRH causes anterior pituitary to produce follicle-stimulating hormone (FSH) and LH
- Ovary responds to FSH production and higher level of estrogen (estradiol) with follicle stimulation to prepare the ovum. Estrogen also produces proliferation of the endometrial lining.
- Rising estrogen provides feedback to the pituitary; LH surges; stimulates release of the egg follicular material (ovulation)
- Estradiol continues to rise and progesterone starts increasing
- Progesterone thickens and stabilizes the endometrial lining (if the zygote needs to implant, the endometrium is ready). From LH surge to endometrial shed (menses) is approximately 14 days for most women.
- A negative feedback cycle occurs as rising estrogen and progesterone levels "switch off" the stimulating hormones from the pituitary/hypothalamus
- Corpus luteum begins to shut down, estrogen and progesterone production falls, and the endometrial tissue loses hormonal support

- Ischemia and vasoconstriction ensues 4–24 hours before menstruation and causes degeneration of the endometrium, which eventually sloughs away
- Average age of menarche 12 years; range 10–16 years
- Average duration of menses is 2–7 days and average interval between menstrual periods is 28 days +/- 7 days. The normal amount of blood loss per menstrual period is approximately 30 mL.
- If a conceptus implants in the endometrial lining, the BhCG produced will help the ovary maintain the corpus luteum, which helps maintain the progesterone levels, which maintains the protective endometrial lining and supports the developing gestation. The "negative feedback loop" is thus short-circuited.

Premenstrual Syndromes (PMS)

Description
- Clusters of mood and behavioral symptoms (somatic and/or affective) occurring or worsening cyclically during the luteal phase (between ovulation and onset of menstruation), followed by resolution after menses
- Must have some negative impact on one or more aspects of the patient's life (work, social, lifestyle, interpersonal relationships)
- Premenstrual symptom clusters occur within a continuum
  - Premenstrual syndrome (PMS), a mild to moderate form
  - Premenstrual dysphoric disorder (PMDD) is a subset of PMS; more severe with major impairment
- Diagnosis of exclusion (see differential list)

Etiology
- Precise pathogenesis unknown; presumed to relate to hormonal fluctuations preceding menses
- Psychophysiologic disorder tied to menses by unknown biological link
- May be increased sensitivity of one or more neurotransmitters to the cyclic fluctuation of ovarian hormones, particularly for PMDD theorized to be due to neurotransmitter dysregulation
- Deficit of serotonin may play a role

Incidence and Demographics
- 90% of all women report at least one premenstrual symptom
- 10% of these women report adverse lifestyle impact of symptoms and have severe PMS or PMDD
- These syndromes most frequently affect 25–45-year-old parous women
- Symptom onset often in adolescence; affects approximately one-third of premenopausal women

Risk Factors
- Strongly associated with a past history of mood disorders (including depression and anxiety)
- Familial trend in female relatives

Prevention and Screening

- Balanced diet; regular exercise; decreased alcohol intake; elimination of caffeine, sodium to reduce symptoms; smoking cessation; and adequate sleep

Assessment

HISTORY

- PMS and PMDD are diagnoses of exclusion
- Begin 7–10 days before menses, after ovulation
    - Fatigue/lack of energy, sleep changes
    - Depression, affective lability, panic attacks, anxiety, lethargy, persistent marked anger or irritability, changes in libido, difficulty concentrating, feelings of being overwhelmed or out of control
    - Breast tenderness
    - Abdominal bloating, thirst, and appetite changes
    - Other: Headaches, edema, joint or muscle pain, weight gain
- Anxiety may peak 1–2 days before menses
    - Severe emotional symptoms predominate for PMDD; symptoms also tend to become more severe and of greater duration with time; in mild or moderate PMS, symptoms do not cause functional impairment; neither the affective nor somatic symptoms predominate

PHYSICAL EXAM

- Affect, speech, mood, mental status, depression scale to evaluate for other mood disorder
- General appearance, skin, thyroid exam to look for signs of adrenal or thyroid disorder
- Cardiac exam for changes with thyroid disorder, substance abuse
- Musculoskeletal exam for trigger points of fibromyalgia
- Complete pelvic examination screening for focal pain, masses
- Complete neuro exam to evaluate headache, mood changes

DIAGNOSTIC STUDIES

- Thyroid-stimulating hormone (TSH) cortisol level as indicated to rule out thyroid adrenal disorders; prolactin if headache severe
- Consider CBC, glucose and serum chemistries, liver function tests, renal function to evaluate lethargy
- If perimenopausal or premature menopause is suspected: FSH, estradiol, progesterone, testosterone, and Dehydroepiandrosterone sulfate (DHEA-S) hormone testing may be indicated
- Can do Self-Rating Scale for PMS (Steiner, Haskett, & Carroll, 1980) or calendar of symptoms; must have 2 months of charting of symptoms
- To differentiate PMDD from PMS, see Table 11–1

Table 11-1. DSM-IV Criteria for Premenstrual Dysphoria Disease (PMDD)

Patients must have 5 or more of the following symptoms, and 1 of them must be from Column 1. None of the symptoms can be an exacerbation of another disorder.

Column 1

- Feeling sad, hopeless, or self-deprecating
- Feeling tense, anxious, or "on edge"
- Marked lability of mood interspersed with frequent fearfulness
- Persistent irritability, anger, and increased interpersonal conflicts

Column 2

- Decreased interest in usual activities, which may be associated with withdrawal from social relationships
- Difficulty concentrating
- Feeling fatigue, lethargic, or lacking in energy
- Marked changes in appetite, which may associated with binge eating or craving certain foods
- Hypersomnia or insomnia
- A subjective feeling of being overwhelmed or out of control
- Physical symptoms such as breast tenderness or swelling; headaches, joint, or muscle pain; sensations of bloating or weight gain with tightness of fit of clothing, shoes, or rings
- Symptoms interfere with work or usual activities or relationships

Differential Diagnosis

- Thyroid disorders
- Substance abuse
- Adrenal disorders (Cushing's)
- Depression (often with suicide ideation)
- Dysthymia
- Anxiety disorders
- Fibromyalgia
- Chronic fatigue syndrome
- Irritable bowel syndrome
- Personality disorders
- Sleep disorders
- Chronic pelvic pain syndromes
- Perimenopause
- Menopause

Management

- Focus therapeutic management on self-care approaches and lifestyle modification. No treatment of PMS has been validated by evidence-based studies. However, the following lifestyle changes are reported effective for some patients with PMS.
  - NONPHARMACOLOGIC TREATMENT
    - During evaluation, consider discontinuing all self-remedies such as vitamins and supplements
    - Menstrual charting for symptom assessment during management

- Aerobic exercise 3–4x weekly, especially during luteal phase
- Stress reduction
- Reduction of alcohol, caffeine, sugar, sodium during most symptomatic times
- Balanced diet
- Adequate sleep
- Smoking cessation

PHARMACOLOGIC TREATMENT
- Calcium Carbonate 1,200 mg daily
- Dietary supplements: Vitamin B6 100 mg/day, vitamin E 400 IU/day, and magnesium 200–400 mg/day
- SSRIs, tricyclic antidepressants, benzodiazepines helpful in clinical trials; SSRIs are the drug of choice for PMDD
- NSAIDs effective for pain and cramping components
- Evening primrose oil, oral contraceptives (OC), progesterone, MAO inhibitors, bromocriptine, vitamins, lithium, spironolactone not demonstrated in clinical trials to reduce PMS symptoms
- Use of monophasic OCs continuously (tricycling is taking 3 or 4 months of 21-day packets without placebo interval) or with first day start (begin new packet with first day of menses) may improve PMS but recurrence is common with discontinuation of OC; new continuous-use Seasonale may also be helpful in reducing symptoms
- Psychological support is helpful for severe manifestations affecting functioning

LENGTH OF TREATMENT
- Therapy is based on patient response; expect long intervals of treatment

Special Considerations
- Accurate identification of premenstrual syndromes requires ruling out other disorders and careful evaluation of menstrual charts and symptom diaries for at least 3 months
- Placebo effect very potent: Confidence in clinician, improved understanding of condition, eliminates some fears, provides some hope, improves self-control
- Complimentary therapies may offer variable efficacy although clinical trials are lacking to support these modalities

When to Consult, Refer, Hospitalize
- Psychological counseling may be indicated

Follow-Up
- After charting symptoms for 2–3 cycles; follow-up every 3–4 months to assess or evaluate effectiveness of therapy
    EXPECTED COURSE
    - In the absence of treatment, signs and symptoms expected to persist as long as the woman has ovulatory menstrual cycles; spontaneous remission occurs with menopause and otherwise anovulatory cycles

    COMPLICATIONS
    - None

Amenorrhea

Description
- Absence of menses
  - *Physiologic amenorrhea* occurs with pregnancy, lactation, and menopause
  - *Primary amenorrhea* is lack of menarche by 14 years of age with the absence of secondary sex characteristics, or lack of menarche by age 16 regardless of presence of secondary sex characteristics
  - *Secondary amenorrhea* is a minimum of 3 missing cycles or 6 months of cessation of menses after menarche established

Etiology
For primary amenorrhea
- Constitutional delay of puberty
  - Müllerian agenesis (2nd most common cause of primary amenorrhea) includes:
    - 46,XX-Rokitansky-Kuster-Hauser syndrome: Absent vagina and uterus but ovaries and sexual hair normal
    - 46,XY-androgen sensitivity syndrome (testicular feminization): X-linked recessive defect; uterus and adnexa absent with testes and blind pouched vagina; breasts well-developed but scant sexual hair; elevated testosterone
- Müllerian fusion anomalies: Müllerian duct fails to fuse with urogenital sinus resulting in transverse septum of vagina usually located in middle or upper vagina; normal uterine development
- 45,XO-Turner syndrome: Ovarian dysgenesis, most common chromosomal abnormality causing gonadal failure and primary amenorrhea
- Gonadal dysgenesis: Lack of mature breast/pubic hair development, but some initial stages of development may be present
- Approximately 30% of patients with primary amenorrhea have associated genetic abnormality
- Congenital defects in steroid synthesis
- Late-onset congenital adrenal hyperplasia
  - Depending on onset, some disorders classified under secondary amenorrhea may present as primary amenorrhea

For secondary amenorrhea
- Pregnancy is the most common cause of secondary amenorrhea. After pregnancy the next five most common causes are polycystic ovary syndrome (PCOS), hypothalamic amenorrhea, thyroid dysfunction, hyperprolactinemia, and ovarian failure.
- Hormonal contraception such as depo medroxyprogesterone (Depo-Provera), combined with oral contraceptives
- Hypothalamic dysfunction, including excessive exercise, severe drop in body fat (<22%) as in anorexia nervosa, severe malnutrition, severe systemic illness, and stress
- Pituitary dysfunction (adenoma, idiopathic hyperprolactinemia)
- Other endocrine causes: Severe hypo- or hyperthyroidism, adrenal disorders, diabetes
- Ovarian dysfunction: Premature ovarian failure; polycystic ovary disease (characterized by amenorrhea, obesity, infertility, and hirsutism)
- Other medications: Phenothiazines, antidepressants, antihypertensives, complication of chemotherapy or radiation therapy, systemic steroids, GnRH agonists

- Surgical: Oophorectomy, hysterectomy
- Outflow tract obstruction: Severe cervical stenosis, severe endometrial scarring and obliteration of endometrium, vaginal scarring, labial fusion

Incidence and Demographics
- Incidence for primary amenorrhea is 0.3%
- Incidence for secondary amenorrhea is 3.3%

Risk Factors
- Varies according to the underlying etiology
- Endocrine disorders, stressful life events, and a variety of medications may produce amenorrhea: phenothiazines, antidepressants, antihypertensives, chemotherapy, systemic steroids, GnRH agonists

Assessment
HISTORY
- Assess first for pregnancy, then galactorrhea (in addition to amenorrhea)
    - Gynecologic history: Infertility, PID, STDs, surgical procedures such as dilation and curettage (D&C), cryotherapy, ovarian wedge resection (for polycystic ovary disease), myomectomy, hysterectomy
    - Pubertal development history
    - Menstrual history with attention to past episodes of erratic bleeding or absence of bleeding
    - Update obstetrical history; update contraceptive history
    - Endocrine: Thyroid, diabetes signs and symptoms
    - Headaches, visual changes
    - Acne, hirsutism (include adolescent as well as family history)
    - Emotional stress: Recent major life events such as divorce, death
    - Depression or other psychological symptoms
    - Nutritional patterns, weight changes, history of eating disorder
    - Family history of genetic anomalies
    - Athletes who exercise excessively

PHYSICAL EXAM
- Weight changes since last visit, body habitus/height
- Observe for common anomalies associated with gonadal dysgenesis such as neck folds and low-set ears
- Secondary sexual characteristics and Tanner staging—pubic and axillary hair patterns, breast development, genital appearance
- Eyes: Impaired visual fields, ptosis, nystagmus, papilledema
- Skin: Hirsutism, acne, hyperpigmentation, vitiligo, fat distribution
- Thyroid: Tenderness, nodules, enlargement
- Breasts: Galactorrhea, engorgement
- Pelvic: Assess for presence/absence of normal structures; clitoromegaly, vulvar or vaginal atrophy, imperforate hymen, uterine enlargement (pregnancy), cervical stenosis, tenderness, adnexal masses, ovary greater than 5 cm, masses

DIAGNOSTIC STUDIES
- First rule out pregnancy with a urine or serum test
- Work-up for primary amenorrhea
- If secondary sex characteristics absent or poorly developed, obtain karyotype to rule out genetic etiology
- If breast tissue absent or poorly developed and uterus present, obtain serum FSH
    - If elevated, suggests ovarian failure; obtain karyotype to rule out ovarian dysgenesis
    - If low, suggests pituitary or hypothalamic dysfunction
- If breast development present but absent uterus, obtain serum testosterone
- If results are appropriate for males, obtain karyotype to rule out testicular feminization
- If breast tissue and uterus present, obtain serum prolactin
    - If elevated, include pituitary tumor in differential diagnosis
    - If normal, begin progesterone challenge test (see below)
- If work-up negative, proceed to work-up for secondary amenorrhea
- Work-up for secondary amenorrhea (obtain serum prolactin at start of challenge): CBC, erythrocyte sedimentation rate (ESR), TSH levels, bone age, FSH and LH levels, liver function tests, BUN, creatinine levels, urinalysis (UA), urine HCG, karyotyping, DHEA-S levels, rostenedione levels, testosterone levels, adrenal suppression test for 17-hydroxyprogesterone
- Progesterone challenge: Prescribe oral Provera (medroxyprogesterone acetate [MPA]) 10 mg daily for 5 days
- Positive: Withdrawal bleeding (or spotting) within 7 days of last MPA pill; suggests adequate endogenous estrogen present to prime endometrium; suggests anovulation meaning presence of intact outflow tract; intact functioning of endometrium, ovary, pituitary, central nervous system (CNS); if prolactin is normal and there is no galactorrhea, no further work-up is needed
- Negative: No withdrawal bleeding or spotting; suggests either inadequate estrogen levels to prime uterus or absent endometrial cavity (in case of primary amenorrhea); if negative progesterone challenge, wait 2 weeks then:
    - Prescribe conjugated estrogen 1.25 mg daily for 21 days OR 2 mg estradiol po qd for 21 days, with Provera (MPA) 10 mg po for the last 5 days of the estrogen, or combination oral contraceptives (monophasic) 1 tab po for 21 days
        » Positive: Withdrawal bleeding/spotting within 14 days; there is no outflow tract problem (uterus, cervix, or vagina) but estrogen deficiency
        » Negative: No withdrawal bleeding; suggests end-organ failure possibly due to congenital malformation or distortion (e.g., intrauterine adhesions) of the uterus, vagina; need to repeat estrogen/MPA trial to confirm
            ◦ If negative, obtain serum TSH/thyroid panel, FSH, LH, and LH/FSH ratio
            ◦ If TSH elevated, suggests hypothyroidism
            ◦ If TSH low or undetectable, suggests hyperthyroidism
            ◦ If LH elevated or LH/FSH ratio >3 (especially with signs of androgen excess), include polycystic ovary syndrome in differential
            ◦ If LH normal or low, include hypothalamic/pituitary regulation defect in differential

- If low LH, low FSH, suggests hypothalamic etiology, e.g., stress, excessive exercise, anorexia, or pituitary malfunction
- If high LH, high FSH, suggests ovarian failure/menopause secondary to radiation, chemotherapy, autoimmune disease, chromosomal abnormalities
- If Cushing's suspected, check ACTH (adrenocorticotrophic hormone), DHEA-S, urinary free cortisol
- Pelvic ultrasonography if any abnormality found on physical exam (masses, absent organs, enlarged organs) or if PCOS suspected
- If galactorrhea or elevated prolactin, must get an MRI of the sella turcica to assess for adenoma or necrosis/ischemia (Sheehan syndrome); coned down x-ray of sella turcica is also appropriate

Differential Diagnosis
- Pregnancy
- Chromosomal abnormality
- Secondary causes

Management
- Treat any abnormality identified and assess in 3–6 months for spontaneous return of menses.

NONPHARMACOLOGIC TREATMENT
- Pituitary adenoma: May need surgical treatment
- Increase caloric intake if underweight, encourage adequate calcium intake, reduce exercise if excessive, help patient cope with stress, refer to eating disorder center as needed

PHARMACOLOGIC TREATMENT
- If positive MPA challenge, give MPA monthly 10 mg qd for a minimum of 10 days or progesterone (Prometrium) 100–200 mg po qd (day 14–16 until menses onset) for 3–6 cycles OR can treat with combined OCs for minimum of 3–6 cycles
- Start hormonal therapy with oral contraceptives OR hormone replacement therapy (HRT) regimen if no menstruation present for more than 6 months (or sooner if estradiol levels <20, FSH levels >20)
- Suggest NOT using progestin-only contraception until regular cycles recur
- If no withdrawal bleed occurs, further exploration is needed
- For pituitary adenoma, referral to an endocrinologist for bromocriptine (Parlodel) treatment

Special Considerations
- Endometrial biopsy is recommended if a long duration of unopposed estrogen (e.g., erratic, variable episodes of bleeding without premenstrual prodrome), amenorrhea for more than 12 months, or more than 3-month history of undiagnosed abnormal vaginal bleeding.

When to Consult, Refer, Hospitalize
- Consult with endocrinologist for pituitary adenoma, PCOS
- Refer to a gynecologist if no withdrawal bleeding occurs, for patients who do not respond to therapy, if prolonged amenorrhea recurs, for infertility management or HRT

Follow-Up
- As appropriate for cause
  COMPLICATIONS
  - Endometrial cancer is a complication of unopposed estrogen
  - Reduced bone mass with prolonged amenorrhea

Dysmenorrhea

Description
- Painful menstruation associated with the menstrual cycle may be primary (absence of pelvic pathology) or secondary (organic cause of pain may be identified)

Etiology
- Primary dysmenorrhea is menstrual pain occurring soon after menarche in absence of pathology.
  - Typically worst in first few years of menses and lessens after early 20s
  - Considered to be chiefly prostaglandin-mediated (PGE and PGF), produced within the endometrial tissue by influence of progesterone and secretory phase of cycle
  - Diagnosed by history and ruling out other causes, especially pregnancy and PID
  - Presents as crampy middle to lower abdominal pain, occurs with menses, worst the first 1–2 days; may radiate to the lower back, thighs
- Secondary dysmenorrhea is painful menstruation due to an identifiable organic cause.
  - Occurs chiefly in women years after menarche and into fourth decade
  - Associated with pain frequently but not limited to the menstrual phase, and/or the pattern of pain becomes more severe over time
  - Symptoms suggest a specific etiology such as endometriosis, tumors, adhesions, adenomyosis, leiomyomas, polyps, or infection

Incidence and Demographics
- Affects 50%–75% of menstruating women; approximately 10% suffer from severe symptoms.
- High incidence in adolescents, 60%–92%

Risk Factors
- Primary dysmenorrheal: Adolescent age
- Secondary dysmenorrheal: Varies with etiology, usually >30 years

Assessment
  HISTORY
  - History should direct the clinician to a likely etiology; emphasis on menstrual history, descriptors of pain relative to menses
  - Low midline pain, cramping in character, occurs in waves, may radiate to back or thighs, lasts one or more days with headache, diarrhea, vasomotor flushing, nausea

- Associated symptoms indicating underlying problem include fever, unilateral pain, dizziness, unusual bleeding, increased pain with coitus
- Associated symptoms with primary dysmenorrhea include fatigue, nervousness, irritability dizziness, syncope, bloating, headache, mood changes, nausea, vomiting, constipation, and/or diarrhea
- Review past medical history, surgeries, complications of pregnancy (infection), fibroids, STDs, bowel disorders

PHYSICAL EXAM
- Assess for fever or signs of shock (i.e., low blood pressure, rapid pulse)
- Abdominal masses, abdominal tenderness, guarding, or rebounding; focal abdominal pain, can identify source (e.g., LLQ suggests bowel, ureter, fallopian tube, ovary)
- Vaginal discharge, odor
- Cervical erythema, purulent mucus, friability, cervical motion tenderness
- Uterine enlargement or tenderness, masses, immobility, firmness
- Adnexal or ovarian masses, or adnexal tenderness
- Exam and diagnostic studies will be normal in primary dysmenorrhea

DIAGNOSTIC STUDIES
- Vaginal/cervical smear and wet mount to rule out STD—increased WBCs indicating STD or PID
- *Chlamydia*/gonorrhea testing
- Pregnancy test
- Pap screen may be deferred if obvious vaginal or cervical infection exists; obtain later
- Ultrasound if ectopic or intrauterine pregnancy, ovarian masses, or fibroids suspected

Diagnostic Differential
- Pregnancy
- Ectopic gestation
- Endometriosis
- STD infection
- PID
- Leiomyoma (fibroids)
- Chronic pelvic pain syndromes
- Irritable bowel syndrome (IBS) or other bowel disorder
- Fibroids
- Urinary tract disorder (calculi, UTI)
- Must always consider carcinoma

Management
NONPHARMACOLOGIC TREATMENT
- Treat causes of secondary dysmenorrhea as indicated
- For primary dysmenorrhea, evidence of interference in activities of daily living and severity of complaints determines management protocols
  - Grade 1 (mild dysmenorrhea): Little or no interference in activities of daily living, mild somatic complaints

- Grade 2 (moderate–severe dysmenorrhea): Complaints of significant interference in daily living, positive systemic somatic complaints
- Grade 3 (severe dysmenorrhea): Severely restricted activities, large degree of systemic somatic complaints
- Supportive treatment of primary dysmenorrhea: Eat regularly, use dry or moist heat to abdomen to hasten pain relief
- Transcutaneous electrical nerve stimulator (TENS) appliance may be helpful

PHARMACOLOGIC TREATMENT
- NSAIDs are the treatment of choice for primary dysmenorrhea; work most effectively when taken before the pain becomes severe
  - Take NSAIDs 2 days or more (up to 1 week) before onset of menses, at regular intervals around the clock; take with food to avoid GI upset
  - If inadequate response, increase dosage or switch to other product, allow minimum of 2–3 cycles to evaluate before switching
  - Ibuprofen (Motrin), 400–800 mg po tid–qid prn
  - Mefenamic acid (Ponstel) 500 mg po loading dose, then 250–500 mg po q6h prn
  - Naproxen (Anaprox, Naprosyn), 500 mg po loading dose, then 250 mg po q 6–8 h prn (maximum 24 hour dose = 1,250 mg)
  - Naproxen sodium extended release (Anaprox DS) 550 mg tablet po bid prn (single dose) or (Naprelan) 500 mg, 2 tablets po once daily (single dose)
  - Ketoprofen extended release (Oruvail) 200 mg caplet po daily (single dose)
  - Newest class of NSAIDs, cyclooxygenase-2 (COX-2) specific inhibitor, several drugs approved for treatment of primary dysmenorrhea; rofecoxib, valdecoxib, and celecoxib have been proven to work as well as first-generation NSAIDs
  - See Table 11–2
- Controlling menses with oral contraception can also be beneficial; options include:
  - Tricycling (take active contraceptive pills for 3 cycles without allowing withdrawal bleeding) is especially beneficial
  - Use the first-day start system
  - After 2–6 cycles some patients can discontinue OCs and will respond to NSAIDS
- Vitamin B1 100 mg (one trial)
- Magnesium (limited evidence, optimal regimen unknown)

Table 11–2. Prostaglandin Inhibitors

Drug	Initial Dose	Subsequent Dosing
Acetic Acid/Salicylic Acids		
Indomethacin	50 mg	25 mg bid
Diflunisal	500 mg	500 mg q 12 h
Diclofenac Potassium	50 mg	50 mg bid
Propionic Acids		
Ibuprofen	400–800 mg	400-800 mg q 4–6 h
Naproxen	500 mg	250 mg q 6–8 h
Naproxen sodium	550 mg	275 mg q 6–8 h
Fenamates		
Mefenamic Acid	500 mg	250 mg q6h

Adapted from "Dysmenorrhea pelvic pain in adolescents" by B. Schroeder, & J. Sanfilippo, 1999, *Pediatric Clinics of North America, 46, 559.*

Special Considerations
- Aspirin, a mild prostaglandin inhibitor, tends to increase menstrual flow while ibuprofen, a potent prostaglandin inhibitor, lessens flow and controls cramping more effectively.

When to Consult, Refer, Hospitalize
- Refer to gynecologist if poor response to NSAID therapy or need evaluation and management of secondary dysmenorrhea

Follow-Up
- Every 2–3 months as necessary to evaluate efficacy of therapy or as appropriate for underlying cause
  EXPECTED COURSE
  - Primary dysmenorrheal: Tends to improve with age and pregnancy
  - Symptoms resolve with NSAIDS or OCs within 3 cycles
  - For Grade 1, use medication for 24–72 hours; Grade 2, treat with NSAIDS for 3–4 cycles or continuous NSAIDS for 3–4 months; Grade 3, try NSAIDs, then use OC for 2–6 months then stop; retry NSAIDs
  - Secondary dysmenorrheal: Depends on cause

  COMPLICATIONS
  - Primary dysmenorrheal: None
  - Secondary dysmenorrheal: Depends on cause

Abnormal Vaginal Bleeding (AVB)

Description
- Abnormal vaginal bleeding (AVB) is defined as any vaginal bleeding that is not attributed to normal menstrual flow. It is classified as premenopausal or postmenopausal; bleeding at inappropriate times, amount, or duration.
- DUB (dysfunctional uterine bleeding) is a diagnosis of exclusion defined as painless, irregular bleeding due to anovulation.

- AVB can be classified as follows:
  - Blood loss during normal menses averages 60 cc over a maximum of 7 days
    - Menorrhagia: Menstrual periods occurring at regular intervals but of excessive duration and flow; total blood loss of >80 cc and duration >7 days
    - Metrorrhagia: Menstrual periods occurring at irregular intervals of varying flow and duration
    - Oligomenorrhea: Menstrual periods occurring irregularly at intervals of greater than 40 days, but less than 6 months
    - Hypomenorrhea: Regular menstrual periods but with reduced amount or duration, <60 cc
    - Menometrorrhagia: Irregular menstrual periods of increased amount or duration
    - Polymenorrhea: Regular menstrual periods but at intervals of less than 21 days
- A single spot of blood with ovulation is common and benign

Etiology

- Women <20 years old: Anovulation due to immature pituitary-hypothalamic-ovarian axis
  - More than 90% of AVB is anovulatory in this age range
  - Estimates suggest 55% of teens have anovulatory cycles the first year after menarche
  - Less frequent cycles and erratic ovulation may lead to AVB (mostly anovulatory), intervals of amenorrhea, and reduced fertility
- Women age 20–40 years old:
  - Usually ovulatory (less than 20% of cases are due to anovulatory problems)
  - Pregnancy, PID, OCs, DMPA, other drugs, IUDs, severe stress, thyroid disease, endometriosis, polyps, fibroids, and neoplasm
- Women >40 years old:
  - Anovulation due to perimenopause, aging, polyps, fibroids, uterine atrophy or thickening (hyperplasia), uterine cancer
  - 40% of all DUB cases occur in women over age 40, who are more likely to have disruptions in ovarian function
  - Perimenopausal women have menstrual changes including altered intermenstrual intervals (shorter, longer, or variable) and altered menstrual flow (heavier, lighter, longer, or shorter patterns)

Incidence and Demographics

- 25% of all AVB is from pregnancy-related complications

Risk Factors

- Adolescents and perimenopausal women

Assessment

HISTORY
- Complete menstrual history and patterns; STD, nipple or vaginal discharge, contraceptive patterns, abdominal pain, dyspareunia, heat/cold intolerance, bleeding or bruising, weight changes, headaches, visual problems, male pattern hair growth, drugs and medication use including oral and long-acting contraceptive use
- Abnormal bleeding is the primary symptom

PHYSICAL EXAM
- Thyroid nodules, enlargement, tenderness
- Visual field defects
- Galactorrhea: Often present with hyperprolactinemia
- Abdominal pain, guarding, rebound
- Pelvic: Polyps, lesions, cervical motion tenderness, cervicitis, cervical discharge or blood, enlarged uterus, adnexal pain or masses, infection, pregnancy
- Moon facies, truncal obesity, abdominal striae, elevated blood pressure (BP)—include Cushing's disease in differential
- Check for hirsutism

DIAGNOSTIC STUDIES
- HCG, CBC, TSH, Pap test, prolactin, *Chlamydia*, gonorrhea testing
- If indicated by history or physical exam:
  - Glucose, renal function, hepatic function, bleeding studies (platelet count, PT, PTT, bleeding time), von Willebrand factor
  - Endometrial biopsy or hysteroscopy: Need determined by history but generally more than 3–6 months of unexplained AVB despite therapies
  - Pelvic or transvaginal ultrasound: Rule out pregnancy or its related complications, assess endometrial stripe to rule out endometrial hyperplasia, other masses (e.g., fibroids)
  - Dexamethasone test, ACTH, serum and urine cortisol
  - FSH, LH, LH/FSH ratio
  - MRI of sella turcica

Differential Diagnosis
- Pregnancy
- Spontaneous abortion
- Ectopic pregnancy
- Polyps
- Hyper/hypothyroidism
- PCOS
- Gynecologic cancer (usually endometrial)
- Salpingitis (especially chronic)
- Endometriosis
- Fibroids
- IUD
- Thrombocytopenia
- Coagulopathy
- Blood dyscrasia
- Hyperprolactinemia (r/o pituitary adenoma, medications)

Management
- Main goal of management is to determine who requires intervention and who can just be monitored.
- In adolescents, advise that the problem is often self-limiting and should resolve within a year or two of menarche.
- Treat any causes identified as indicated.
- DUB is the working diagnosis if other causes are ruled out.

PHARMACOLOGIC TREATMENT
- Oral contraceptives or hormone replacement therapy for several cycles
- Monophasic combination OC with 30–35 mcg estrogen may be given 1 tab po bid–qid for 7–10 days until bleeding is controlled
- If bleeding stops within the treatment period, advise one OC qd, uninterrupted without a withdrawal bleed, for another 21 days
- Delayed withdrawal bleeding after 6–12 weeks allows gradual thinning of the endometrium, results in a lighter bleed than if withdrawal bleeding occurs within the 10 days
- Another treatment is 1.25 mg conjugated estrogens po or 2 mg estradiol po q4h for 24 hours, then a daily dose for 7–10 days
- Follow with progestin coverage allowing withdrawal bleed; treatment after this is OC cycles x 3

Medroxyprogesterone acetate (MPA or Provera)
- May be given 10 mg po for 10–14 days every month
- The first withdrawal bleed will be heavy but the woman should cycle after that
- MPA may be used monthly

Depo medroxyprogesterone acetate (DMPA, Depo-Provera)
- Give Depo-Provera 150 mg IM every 12 weeks

Other: Progestin-impregnated IUD
- Iron replacement therapy if needed for anemia
- NSAIDS (prostaglandin synthetase inhibitors): 20%–30% reduction in bleeding may occur; start NSAIDs the first day of menses and continue through the heavy flow days
  - Mefenamic acid (Ponstel) 500 mg po tid for 3 days
  - Naproxen (Naprosyn) 500 mg po bid
  - Ibuprofen (Motrin) 400 mg q6h

Special Considerations
- With postmenopausal women, any bleeding/spotting is presumed to be of malignant origin until proven otherwise.

When to Consult, Refer, Hospitalize
- Refer to gynecologist for acute menorrhagia if the bleeding is severe enough to cause volume depletion, shortness of breath, fatigue, palpitations, and other related symptoms. This level of anemia necessitates hospitalization for intravenous fluids and possible transfusion and/or intravenous estrogen therapy. Patients who do not respond to medical therapy may require surgical intervention to control the menorrhagia.

Follow-Up
- Varies according to etiology
  EXPECTED COURSE
  - Varies with etiology

  COMPLICATIONS
  - Varies with etiology

Endometriosis

Description
- Defined as endometrial glands and stroma outside of uterine endometrial cavity, sometimes well outside of pelvic cavity
- Common cause of secondary dysmenorrhea, abnormal bleeding patterns, altered fertility, dyspareunia

Etiology
- Pathogenesis poorly understood; theories include retrograde menstruation, abnormal cellular process from embryogenesis, lymphatic or vascular transplantation, autoimmune disorders

Risk Factors
- Increased risk with affected first-degree female relatives
- History of uninterrupted, prolonged menstrual cycles

Incidence and Demographics
- 3%–10% prevalence in fertile women and 25%–35% in infertile women
- Commonly diagnosed in mid-20s

Assessment
HISTORY
- Gradual onset of constant, achy pain starting on or near menses, with increasing severity for a few days and relenting only when menses starts to abate
- History of pain-free cycles then gradual pain, with recurrences for months or years with increasing intensity over time, will help rule out most acute abdominal conditions
- History of large doses of NSAID analgesics with or without narcotics can be a tip towards assessing pain severity
- Severity of symptoms may not correlate with extent of disease
- Symptoms include pain, infertility, dysmenorrhea, nonmenstrual pelvic pain, dyspareunia, low back pain, bladder pain, frequency and dysuria, irregular vaginal bleeding, partial bowel obstruction, IBS, perimenstrual chest and shoulder pain, abdominal wall pain, and nonpelvic pain

PHYSICAL EXAM
- Physical examination at time of menses may identify typical patches of enlarged tissue palpable at points of pain (some only identifiable at time of laparoscopic examination)
- There may be fixed uterine position, adnexal enlargement, cervical motion tenderness, tenderness in vaginal cul-de-sac

DIAGNOSTIC STUDIES
- Diagnosis is suggested by history and physical and tests to exclude other sources
- Lab test to rule out other causes of pain: STD screens, urinalysis, Hemoccult testing, Pap testing
- Ultrasound may show complex fluid-filled masses

- Abdominal CT or MRI may show masses but not small implants
- Confirmation can only be made by laparoscopy or surgical exploration with biopsy

Differential Diagnosis

- Leiomyomas
- STDs or PID
- Irritable bowel other GI disorders
- Adenomyosis
- Ectopic pregnancy
- Urinary tract disorders
- Chronic pelvic pain
- Nerve pain syndromes
- Musculoskeletal pain disorders
- Ruptured ovarian cyst
- Neoplasms
- Pelvic adhesions

Management

NONPHARMACOLOGIC TREATMENT

- Surgical management may involve excision of implants, lysis of adhesions, reduction of ovarian tissue, or hysterectomy with bilateral salpingo-oophorectomy (TAH-BSO)

PHARMACOLOGIC TREATMENT

- Treatment goals are pain relief, control of endometrial patch growth, preservation of fertility
- NSAIDS; additional analgesics may be necessary when menses occur
- Hormonal contraception may be used (omitting the withdrawal bleed interval) for 6–12 months (continuous use of OCs daily without placebo pills or break, Depo-Provera injections on accelerated schedule); continuous OCs may be associated with breakthrough bleeding (BTB) if taken more than 3 months continuously; patient must be informed about this possibility
- Provera tablets po 30 mg daily (side effects: change in lipid profile, depression, BTB common)

LENGTH OF TREATMENT

- Until pain relief, pregnancy, or menopause (biologic or surgical)

Special Considerations

- Calcium supplementation is advised during therapy
- Needs HRT (both estrogen progesterone, to reduce endometrial cancer risk from residual implants) and calcium supplementation after TAH-BSO

When to Consult, Refer, Hospitalize

- Refer to gynecologist if poor response to medical therapy or fertility assistance is desired
- Refer for other hormonal suppression with GnRH analogs such as leuprolide (Lupron), or androgens such as danazol (Danocrine); significant side effect profile and expense

Follow-Up

- Gynecologist should be managing any follow-up required if receiving GnRH agonists or danazol, to assess side effects and evaluate efficacy

  EXPECTED COURSE

  - After surgery or suppressive drug therapies (e.g., GnRH agonists or danazol), women may have 18–24 months of pain relief

  COMPLICATIONS

  - Infertility

Perimenopause/Menopause

Description

- Defined as age-related biologic reduction in ovarian function with end of fertility and menstrual cycle
- Biological menopause is defined as the natural failure of the ovaries after age 40–45, resulting in absence of fertility and >12 months without menses

Etiology

- The actual cause of natural menopause is unknown
- Ovary is less responsive to FSH (so pituitary increases production). Contrary to past understanding, estrogen levels remain normal or slightly elevated until cessation of menses but there is inconsistent ovulation each cycle.
- Fluctuation in estrogen level (controversial) creates menstrual cycle changes, hot flashes and sweats (vasomotor instability), sleep disturbances, fatigue, irritability, PMS, mood changes, vaginal dryness, and urinary complaints
- Perimenopause is suggested when FSH levels are greater than 20 IU/L despite continued menstrual bleeding
- Adverse postmenopausal body changes include:
  - Increased bone resorption and decreased bone formation, leading to decreased bone density (osteoporosis)
  - Rise in total cholesterol, low-density lipoprotein (LDL) and very low-density lipoprotein (VLDL); high-density lipoprotein (HDL) declines and triglycerides show no change
  - Diminished bladder control (may occur months to years later)
  - Reduced fertility (depending on the woman's reproductive needs)
- Positive postmenopausal changes include:
  - Reduction in myomas, endometriosis, adenomyosis
  - Gradual decrease in PMS-type symptoms is common: less mastodynia, bloating, edema, headache, and cyclical mood swings
  - Reduced fertility (again, depending on the woman's reproductive needs)

Incidence and Demographics

- Average age at perimenopause is 47 years with a duration of approximately 3.5 years
- Approximately 95% reach menopause at 45–55 years
- Average age of biological menopause is 51
- About 10% of women have abrupt cessation of menses and 90% of women have menstrual changes prior to menstrual cessation
- About 0.9% of women experience menopause before age 40 (premature menopause)

- Artificial menopause can occur at any time if the ovaries are removed or irradiated before biologic failure occurs

Risk Factors (for premature menopause)
- Turner syndrome (mosaic variant)
- Autoimmune endocrinopathy
- Severe systemic illness
- Chemotherapy and radiation
- Possible familial component

Prevention and Screening
- All women should be asked about menstrual history and onset of menopausal symptoms after age 40
- Assess risk for coronary heart disease (CHD), osteoporosis, breast and endometrial cancer

Assessment

HISTORY
- Obtain complete medical, GYN, and menstrual history, contraceptive use, and medication use, and family history of menopause
- Associated symptoms: Mood, sleep, hot flashes, vaginal dryness, and vaginal bleeding not related to menses

PHYSICAL EXAM
- Complete physical exam including breast and pelvic exam; uterus and ovaries become smaller
- Leiomyomata or adenomyosis reduced
- Rectovaginal exam, stool for occult blood in women >50 years

DIAGNOSTIC STUDIES
- Some experts suggest diagnosis should be based on clinical not laboratory criteria (cessation of menses, age, vasomotor symptomatology); but pregnancy test (must be done if there is any possibility), TSH, and FSH if suspect thyroid problems
- Fluctuation of FSH, LH, and estradiol levels is common until menopause
- Within 1 year after cessation of menses there is a 3–4-fold increase in FSH and a 3-fold increase in LH (confirm ovarian failure) with estradiol levels below 20 pg/mL
- Predominance of immature epithelial cells on vaginal wet mount (simple, inexpensive)
- Pap testing, mammogram, DEXA Scan, STD testing if indicated, FOB/ sigmoidoscopy; follow Periodic Health Screening and Evaluation for Adults as recommended by the US Preventive Services Task Force (USPSTF, 2006).

Differential Diagnosis
- Pregnancy
- Depression
- Thyroid and other endocrine disorders
- PMS
- Hot flashes

- Pheochromocytoma
- Cancer
- Leukemia
- Thyroid tumors
- Pancreatic tumors

Management

NONPHARMACOLOGIC TREATMENT

- Exercise and weight management
- Smoking cessation: Reduces heart disease, osteoporosis, may relieve hot flashes, may avoid early menopause
- Healthy nutritional and dietary practices including: well balanced diet consisting of fresh fruits and vegetables, whole grains, lean proteins, and low saturated fats; daily multivitamin, daily recommended dosage of calcium (1200–1500 mg/day), vitamin D (400–800 IU per day for individuals at risk of deficiency); see Chapter 14 for osteoporosis prevention
  - Limit alcohol to 1 drink/day or less, limit caffeine
  - Kegel exercises for coitus and urinary incontinence
  - Vaginal lubricants for coitus
  - In a meticulously conducted yearlong clinical trial funded by the National Institutes of Health (NIH) and published in late 2006, black cohosh, soy products, red clover and vitamin E were found to be no better than placebo for relieving hot flashes; the women given these products reported the same number of daily hot flashes as did women given a placebo

PHARMACOLOGIC TREATMENT

- Women's Health Initiative study has changed what the medical profession thought about HRT
  - Data suggest long-term estrogen, estrogen plus progestin (HRT) increase the risk of breast cancer
  - HRT has no beneficial effect on coronary heart disease (CHD)
  - HRT may increase the risk of CHD among generally healthy postmenopausal women, especially during the first year after the initiation of hormone use
  - HRT increases the risk of thromboembolic events and stroke
  - Other research suggests long-term HRT may increase chance of dementia and breast cancer
- Some women still will require hormone replacement therapy; regimen should be individualized
  - Relieves vasomotor flushing and may prevent osteoporosis; available in oral forms or transdermal patch; progestin only for those who cannot take estrogen; progestin *must* be included for women with intact uterus to protect against endometrial hyperplasia or cancer
  - Absolute contraindications: Pregnancy, thromboembolus, unexplained genital bleeding, endometrial cancer, undiagnosed breast mass, active liver disease
  - Relative contraindications include seizure disorder, hypertension, familial hyperlipidemia, migraines, gallbladder disease, past history of thrombosis

Vaginal creams for atrophic vaginitis (stop after 3–6 months; reassess)
- Estradiol 0.01% cream (Estrace) 1 g twice weekly for 3 weeks/off for 1 week
- Estropipate 1.5 mg/g cream (Ogen) 2–4 g daily for 3 weeks/off for 1 week
- Conjugated estrogens 0.625 mg/g cream (Premarin) 0.5–2 g daily for 3 weeks/off for 1 week

Vaginal ring
- Estring vaginal ring releases 7.5 mcg/24 hours, inserted deeply into upper one-third of vaginal vault by patient; remove and replace after 90 days; reassess at 3–6 month intervals

Preparations for hot flashes
- The Food and Drug Administration has approved the following drugs specifically to treat hot flashes; however, they are approved for treating other conditions as well

- **Antidepressants.** Low doses of certain antidepressants may decrease hot flashes. Antidepressants from classes of medications known as selective serotonin reuptake inhibitors (SSRIs) and serotonin and norepinephrine reuptake inhibitors (SNRIs)—including venlafaxine (Effexor), paroxetine (Paxil), fluoxetine (Prozac), citalopram (Celexa) and others—have been found to relieve hot flashes in some clinical trials. Many clinicians now consider these antidepressants the treatment of choice for moderate to severe hot flashes for patients who refuse or are not candidates for HRT. However, these medications are not as effective as hormone therapy for severe hot flashes and may cause unwanted side effects, such as nausea, dizziness, weight gain, or sexual dysfunction.
- **Gabapentin.** Gabapentin (Neurontin) is approved for treating seizures or pain associated with shingles. Some studies have found that gabapentin is moderately effective in reducing hot flashes. Side effects can include drowsiness, dizziness, nausea, imbalance when walking, and swelling.
- **Clonidine**. Clonidine, a pill or patch typically used to treat high blood pressure, may provide some relief from hot flashes. Side effects such as dizziness, drowsiness, dry mouth, and constipation are common, sometimes limiting the medication's usefulness for treating hot flashes.
  - MPA 10–20 mg qd or depo MPA (Depo-Provera) 150 mg IM q 3 months
  - Megestrol acetate (Megace) 20 mg bid
  - Progesterone (Prometrium) 100 mg qd (or 200 mg 12 days a month)
  - Transdermal clonidine 0.1 mg/d apply weekly (side effects: hypotension, dizziness, nausea, mood swings)
  - Clonidine 0.1 mg daily orally or transdermally is another option to treat vasomotor flushing

LENGTH OF TREATMENT
- Until symptoms resolve or, with HRT use, for no more than 10 years (controversial)

Special Considerations
- Do not start HRT in a woman who is being treated for ovarian or breast cancer or who has a history of either; consult with an oncologist/surgeon
- Do not use HRT as a birth control method

When to Consult, Refer, Hospitalize
- Consult or refer for all relative contraindications and questionable uses for HRT
- Consult/refer for endometrial biopsy for episodes of vaginal spotting/bleeding even though this side effect of HRT is common

Follow-Up
- 3 months after initiating HRT or as often as necessary to evaluate efficacy and side effects
- Review danger signs of HRT: Vaginal bleeding not associated with HRT use, calf pain, chest pain, shortness of breath, hemoptysis, severe headache, vision problems, breast changes, abdominal pain, and jaundice
- After HRT regimen established, annual exams
    - COMPLICATIONS
        - Postmenopausal problems include cardiovascular problems, osteoporosis, vasomotor symptoms, urogenital atrophy and incontinence, atrophic vaginitis, diminished libido

BREAST CONDITIONS

Breast Cancer, Breast Masses

Description
- Malignancy of the breast

Etiology
- Precise etiology unknown
- Noninvasive: Intraductal tumors including ductal carcinoma in situ (DCIS) or lobular carcinoma in situ (LCIS)
- Invasive: Tumor no longer contained within basement membrane
- Invasive ductal carcinoma originates from epithelial cells lining mammary ducts; subtypes include medullary, papillary, tubular, colloid
- Invasive lobular carcinoma arises from mammary lobules

Incidence and Demographics
- 1 in 8 women (lifetime risk)
- Rare in women under 25; 48% of new breast cancer cases and 56% of breast cancer deaths occur in women >65 years
- Peak age at diagnosis is age 45–65, with >75% occurring over age 50
- About 70% are invasive; invasive ductal more common than lobular (96%–97% vs. 3%–4%)
- Most common site is upper outer quadrant (49%)

Risk Factors
- Risks include female gender; living in North America, northern Europe, and older age; early menarche (before age 11) or late menarche (after age 14); late menopause (after age 55 or more than 35 years of duration of menses); nulliparity; first pregnancy after age 35 (1.5x risk); prior breast cancer (5–10x risk); obesity (may be linked to hyperinsulinemia or fat cell production of androgens converted to estrogens); android fat distribution; excess alcohol use; tobacco use; never breastfeeding; long-term estrogen use
- 20% family history (autosomal dominant with maternal linkage) relative risk (RR) 2.2 with first-degree relatives, with bilateral disease in premenopausal relatives (10.5 RR), bilateral disease in postmenopausal relatives (5.5 RR)
- 90% of women with breast cancer have NO family history
- BRCA (breast cancer recessive autosomal) carriers have risks for breast and ovarian cancers, usually early onset.

Prevention and Screening
- Protection may be conferred by exercise, dietary soy, and weight control, especially in postmenopausal years
  - Tamoxifen as prophylaxis in high-risk women (watch for endometrial abnormalities)
  - In a huge multi-center study, raloxifene (Evista), a common osteoporosis drug, was shown to be as effective as tamoxifen (Nolvadex) in preventing invasive breast cancer, but had fewer side effects as reported by the data accrued from the Study of Tamoxifen and Raloxifene, a project of the National Surgical Adjuvant Breast and Bowel Project and National Cancer Institute (NCI)
  - Further studies comparing raloxifene and an aromatase inhibitor already have been submitted to the NCI for approval; aromatase inhibitors have been shown to be more effective than tamoxifen in preventing second breast cancers
  - Breastfeeding may reduce the risk by about 4% per year; is cumulative per child
  - Women with BRCA1 mutations who breastfed for more than 1 year are less likely to have breast cancer than those who never breastfed
  - Avoid methylxanthines

Screening for Breast Cancer
- While some controversy surrounds the breast self-exam (BSE), it is still recommended
- Age 20–39: Monthly BSE and clinical breast examination q 1–3 years
- Baseline mammogram at age 35–40 or 10 years earlier than age of onset of a first-degree relative with history of breast cancer
- 40–49: Monthly BSE, annual clinical breast examination, mammography every 1–2 years
- Age >50: Monthly BSE, annual clinical breast examination, mammography every year (reduces cancer mortality by 30%–50% in women ages 50–69; over age 70 the data is conflicting; no evidence to benefit women over age 75)
- False negative rate of 10%–15%, false positive rate of 15%–20% for screening mammogram
- Clinical breast examination to find changes that may indicate a malignancy soon enough for timely intervention, and to teach or to reinforce BSE
- Yearly mammogram for women who have had breast cancer; MRI for women with history of breast cancer for close surveillance

Assessment

HISTORY

- Assess for risk factors
- Obtain detailed medical/GYN history, history of breast mass development, document all prior mammogram dates and results, contraceptive and HRT use, prior breast biopsies and breast surgery

PHYSICAL EXAM

- 55% of women have a palpable nontender mass; 35% of women have abnormal mammogram without palpable mass
- Persistent nipple itching or burning suggests Paget's disease; may present with minimal skin changes, no mass palpable, may have erosion or ulceration
- Exam shows solitary, nontender, firm to hard mass without well-defined margins, often fixed position
- Ominous signs are enlarged or tender lymphs, skin color changes, skin erosion, peau d'orange (edema), dimpling, nipple retraction, pain, breast enlargement
- Assess for nipple discharge

DIAGNOSTIC STUDIES

- Negative test results are not necessarily diagnostic in the presence of a palpable breast mass
- Fine needle aspiration
- Mammography
- Ultrasound (US)
- CBC, liver function tests (LFT), chest x-ray (CXR), estrogen/progesterone receptor determination (usually ordered once biopsy done), bone scan, CT or US to assess lymph node involvement and metastasis

Differential Diagnosis

- Fibrocystic changes
- Fibroadenoma
- Intraductal papilloma
- Lipoma
- Fat necrosis

Management

- Mastectomy (radical and modified radical) and lumpectomy when combined with radiation appear to have similar cure rates
- In addition to surgical excision:
  - Premenopausal women with positive lymph nodes often receive cytoxic chemotherapy followed by tamoxifen if estrogen receptor positive
  - Postmenopausal women with positive lymph nodes and a positive estrogen receptor assay are commonly treated with tamoxifen; less likely to benefit from chemotherapy
  - Controversial whether women with negative lymph nodes would benefit from chemotherapy (but modest success demonstrated in postmenopausal women with positive estrogen receptors)
  - High-dose chemotherapy with autologous bone marrow transplant has proven no more effective than standard treatment in many women, but still in clinical trials

Special Considerations
- Tamoxifen, toremifene, fulvestrant, letrozole, raloxifene and aromatase inhibitors may be given to women at high risk for prevention of breast cancer recurrence.

When to Consult, Refer, Hospitalize
- Refer all suspicious breast lumps and abnormal mammograms to surgeon for excision biopsy
- Additional referrals may be made to medical radiation oncologist

Follow-Up
- After diagnosis and therapy for breast cancer, a physical examination is indicated every 3–4 months for the first 5 years, and thereafter, every year
- Regular follow-up visits include chest x-rays and liver function tests
- Yearly mammogram and possible MRI for women who have had breast cancer
    - EXPECTED COURSE
        - Highly variable

    - COMPLICATIONS
        - Metastatic disease

NONINFECTIOUS BREAST DISORDERS

Benign Breast Masses

Description
- Benign mammary dysplasia also referred to as fibrocystic changes; majority not at risk for breast cancer
- Fibroadenomas are solid benign masses

Etiology
- Fibrocystic changes are the most common benign breast condition; caused by ductal dilation usually 2 mm or less; 20%–40% enlarge to palpable cysts (usually fluid-filled), may increase and decrease with menstrual cycle.
- Fibroadenomas are made of gular fibrous tissue, often located in upper quadrant, caused by an inflammatory reaction from ductal irritation, with onset late teens to early 20s.

Incidence and Demographics
- Fibrocystic breast: Most common ages 30–50
- Cysts and fibroadenomas: Most common benign breast changes, followed by duct ectasia
- Up to 50% of women affected
- Fibroadenomas often occur in younger women within 10 years of menarche

Risk Factors
- Fibrocystic disease: Caffeine, chocolate, tea, coffee, smoking, family history

Prevention and Screening
- Avoid methylxanthines

Assessment

HISTORY
- Achy, tender, or painless lumpy breasts
- More tender with menses
- Any nipple discharge; may be seen in galactocele or ductal ectasia, papilloma, or cancer

PHYSICAL EXAM
- Benign multiple breast masses, size fluctuating with menses (cystic, adenosis, fibrosis, ductal hyperplasia), occasionally with unilateral or bilateral nipple discharge; may feel 1 or 2 dominant cysts, usually 1–2 cm.
- Fibroadenomas: Unilateral mass, often solitary; well-defined, round, rubbery, mobile masses
- Fibrocystic disease: Multiple masses, tender with menses, fluctuating size, rare nipple discharge
- Axillary, supraclavicular, infraclavicular lymph nodes for enlarged nodes

DIAGNOSTIC STUDIES
- Breast ultrasonography can identify cystic structures vs. solid mass
- Suspicious masses should be evaluated by ultrasonography, mammogram
- Refer for fine needle aspiration, biopsy of suspicious areas, bloody fluid, persistent mass, or for excision

Differential Diagnosis
- Breast cancer
- Fibroadenoma
- Breast abscess
- Galactocele
- Fat necrosis
- Benign cyst
- Prolactinoma

Management

NONPHARMACOLOGIC TREATMENT
- Fibroadenoma: Watch, excise, or aspirate
- Fibrocystic disease: Reduce caffeine and chocolate in diet, supportive brassiere, oral contraceptive pills
- Evening primrose oil: Limited available research to date does not demonstrate that evening primrose oil has a significant effect on the treatment of breast cysts or mastalgia

PHARMACOLOGIC TREATMENT
- Vitamin E supplements 400 IU daily (for 2 weeks then discontinue), vitamin B6 25–50 mg daily, magnesium 200-400 mg/day supplements
- Oral contraceptives may or may not relieve symptoms
- OTC analgesics

Special Considerations
- Breast pain in postmenopausal women not on HRT should be worked up for cancer
- Despite limitations (for example, reduced mammographic sensitivity), women with implants should continue to be radiographically screened as appropriate for their age and risk factors

When to Consult, Refer, Hospitalize
- Refer to a surgeon for fine needle aspiration to confirm that cyst is fluid-filled, or excisional biopsy, or for suspicious findings as outlined above

Follow-Up
- For fibrocystic disease (with multiple or single small <1 cm cysts), reevaluate in 1–2 months soon after menses to determine efficacy of therapy, and whether further work-up required

  COMPLICATIONS
  - Usually none if benign process

Galactorrhea/Nipple Discharge

Description
- Galactorrhea is milky nipple discharge not associated with lactation

Etiology
- Duct ectasia is a collection of dilated terminal collecting ducts in the breast and is commonly associated with nipple discharge. It is not clear if the discharge causes ectasia or the other way around. The problem commonly presents when the woman is in her 40s.
- Nipple discharge is most commonly associated with endocrine alterations and/or medications (e.g., phenothiazines, oral contraceptives, tricyclic antidepressants, opiates) affecting hypothalamic inhibition of dopamine.
- The likelihood of malignancy increases when the discharge is unilateral, arises from a single duct, is accompanied by a palpable mass, is associated with a positive mammographic finding or there are positive cytologic galactotrophic findings, or when the patient is older than 50 years.
- Physiologic etiologies for galactorrhea include stress, breast stimulation, exercise, eating, and sleep; bilateral nipple discharge can be expressed in up to 80% of asymptomatic women.

Incidence and Demographics
- Occurs in the U.S. in frequencies as high as 3%–8%
- Benign discharge spontaneously resolves in as many as 73% of patients within 5 years
- About 10%–12% of breast cancers are associated with nipple discharge

Risk Factors
- Nipple discharge often results in fibrocystic changes and/or ductal ectasia

Prevention and Screening
- During clinical breast exam, gently attempt to express any fluid from the nipple

Assessment
HISTORY
- Changes are often bilateral, causing discharge from one or several nipple ducts
- Medications
- Nipple stimulation
- Lactation experience
- Menstrual cycles
- Vision problems, headaches

PHYSICAL EXAM
- Nipple discharge varies in color from white to brown
- To be clinically significant, nipple discharge must be true, spontaneous, persistent, nonlactational
- Surgically significant discharge is clear (i.e., watery), serous (i.e., clear yellow), serosanguineous, or sanguineous (i.e., bloody).
- Nipple discharge typically green to yellow to black in color if physiologic, coming from multiple ducts versus spontaneous, unilateral
- Nipple discharge often associated with duct ectasia, often thick and cheesy
- Blood discharge more likely to be associated with cancer

DIAGNOSTIC STUDIES
- Mammogram
- Subsequent to negative mammographic findings, galactography or ductography is the procedure of choice; galactography involves the retrograde injection of water-soluble radiopaque contrast material into a discharging duct with subsequent mammographic imaging
- Hemoccult tests can be used to assess the nipple discharge fluid to confirm or exclude the presence of occult blood
- Cytologic tests of the fluid can be performed; however, false-positive rates and significant false-negative rates have been reported (2.6% and 17.8%, respectively, in Leis' series)
- Prolactin, TSH
- MRI of sella turcica

Differential Diagnosis
- Breast cancer
- Fibroadenoma
- Breast abscess
- Fat necrosis
- Benign cyst

Management
NONPHARMACOLOGIC TREATMENT
- Avoid nipple stimulation
- Monthly breast self-exams encouraged

PHARMACOLOGIC TREATMENT
- None

When to Consult, Refer, Hospitalize
- As needed for suspicious findings such as positive occult blood or galactorrhea in a nulliparous woman

Follow-Up
- As indicated by breast specialist or primary care provider

Mastitis Abscess

Description
- Mastitis is inflammation of the breast tissue with possible infection. An abscess (a collection of pus) may develop but is more likely when treatment has been delayed or inadequate.

Etiology
- Occurs as a result of milk stasis
- If infection present, it is usually due to *Staphylococcus aureus*, which is generally penicillin-resistant
- Nonpuerperal infection can occur, although less common, and is usually due to *S. aureus, Bacteroides,* or *Peptostreptococcus*
- A break in the integrity of the nipple or areolar area is a risk factor but is neither adequate nor necessary for the development of infection

Incidence and Demographics
- Puerperal mastitis: 1%–33%
- Abscess from puerperal mastitis: 5%–11%

Risk Factors
- Lactation
- During lactation, any event that causes milk stasis, such as inadequate drainage of the breast; rapid weaning; oversupply of milk; pressure on the breast (e.g., from a poor-fitting bra); a blocked duct; or missed, scheduled, infrequent, or timed feeds
- Nipple trauma with skin breakdown
- Possibly also infant illness and /or maternal fatigue or stress, anemia, poor nutrition, or illness
- Eczema; these mothers are prone to colonization with *S. aureus*

Prevention and Screening
- Maintain adequate breast drainage to avoid engorgement. Teach the mother to properly latch, position her infant to maximize milk removal, and minimize nipple trauma.
- Encourage feeding demonstration.
- If weaning desired, recommend dropping one feeding every 2–3 days, taking 2–3 weeks to complete.
- Recommend avoiding abrupt weaning and/or binding of the breasts.

Assessment

HISTORY
- Painful, tender, warm, red, breast area (classic presentation is a red wedge-shaped area)
- Fever (may or may not be present)
- Nipple soreness with or without skin breakdown may be present
- Assess breastfeeding frequency, milk supply

PHYSICAL EXAM
- Local edema, erythema, induration
- Axillary lymphadenopathy
- Localized, extremely tender, fluctuant mass may develop
- May be bilateral or unilateral; (suspect *Streptococcus* Group B if bilateral in the early postpartum)
- Check nipples for increased redness, soreness, skin breakdown
- Examine skin for eczema

DIAGNOSTIC STUDIES
- Culture drainage if treatment failure, recurrent, or abscessed
- Should have mammogram and/or ultrasound if recurrent or nonpuerperal
- Ultrasound to evaluate for abscess PRN

Differential Diagnosis
- Breast trauma, breast engorgement, or plugged duct

Management

NONPHARMACOLOGIC TREATMENT
- Warm compresses, massage to promote drainage; cool compresses to reduce local pain and swelling
- Continue to breastfeed or express milk and increase the frequency to shorten symptom duration (bacteria in breast milk demonstrated not to be pathogenic to the infant)
- If possible, start on affected side, or start on unaffected side and switch after let-down occurs. If direct breastfeeding is not possible, regular pumping instead of breastfeeding should be done with a hospital grade double electric pump 8–12 times per day for 15–20 minutes. When necessary, pumping or expression can be done after feedings if the infant fails to adequately drain the breast.
- While breastfeeding, pointing the infant's chin toward the affected area may improve the drainage.
- Encourage the mother to rest, eat nutritiously, drink plenty of fluids
  - Suspect abscess if mastitis does not respond to antibiotics
  - Abscesses: Warm compresses. It is a relative contraindication to discontinue breastfeeding with an abscess as engorgement may lead to worsening of the infection (because the fluid/milk backs up into the interstitial tissue) and abrupt weaning may cause the mother to develop fever, malaise, and achiness. Maintain adequate breast milk drainage either by direct breastfeeding or with a double electric hospital grade pump.
  - Monthly breast self-exams encouraged

PHARMACOLOGIC TREATMENT
- In terms of antibiotic treatment for infectious mastitis during lactation, generally mothers with acute pain or toxicity, bacterial colony counts, white blood cell counts and culture results consistent with infection, and nipple fissures and/or severe or classic symptoms (fever, myalgias, chills along with a localized, red, hot, swollen, painful breast) should be treated with antibiotics. Mothers without these criterions should be instructed to feed frequently and maintain regular drainage of the breast as previously described. If symptoms haven't resolved within 12–24 hours, antibiotic treatment should be promptly commenced.
- For puerperal *S. aureus* infections: dicloxacillin (Dycill) 500 mg po qid or clindamycin (Cleocin) 300 mg po qid; may need to consider IV therapy if mother toxic or extensive cellulitis
- For non-puerperal infection, amoxicillin/clavulanate (Augmentin) 875/125 mg BID or IV therapy.
- Analgesics: acetaminophen, NSAIDS. (NSAIDS may be more effective. Ibuprofen and acetaminophen are compatible with breastfeeding.)

LENGTH OF TREATMENT
- Although there is no standard recommendation for treatment length, most authorities advise a 10-14 day length of treatment

Special Considerations
- When treatment for nonlactational mastitis is unsuccessful (abscess ruled out), consider squamous metaplasia.
- Monitor for candidiasis in mother or infant; treat them concurrently if it is present or develops.
- If mother is hospitalized, the infant should be in room with her.

When to Consult, Refer, Hospitalize
- Refer to physician for abscess, toxic mother with persistent fever despite oral antibiotics, extensive cellulites, or if patient needs hospitalization for IV medications.
- If abscessed, refer for incision and drainage or ultrasound-guided needle aspiration.
- Consult with a lactation specialist for breastfeeding management including oversupply, latching problems, lowered milk supply, persistent nipple pain, damaged nipples, nipple vasospasm (Raynaud's phenomenon), fussy infant, etc.

Follow-Up
- Follow-up examination to assess for resolution or identify other differentials
- Evaluate for an underlying mass if there are more than 2–3 episodes in the same area
  ### EXPECTED COURSE
  - Frequent breastfeeding and/or milk expression successfully resolves puerperal mastitis 96% of the time
  - Any lowering of the milk supply will respond to more frequent breastfeeding within a few days

COMPLICATIONS
- Development of sinus tracts
- Development of nipple soreness or burning breast pain, which may be a sign of mammary candidiasis, necessitating concurrent treatment of mother and child
- Infant thrush
- Functional mastectomy due to extensive incision and drainage; 10% of women affected by a breast abscess experience compromised lactation that includes a functional mastectomy
- Recurrent infectious mastitis may cause chronic inflammation
- Temporarily lowered milk supply

CONDITIONS OF THE VULVA, VAGINA, AND CERVIX

Abnormal Cervical Cytology

Description
- Abnormal cervical cytology (most likely via Pap smear) may indicate cervical cancer
- About 85% of cervical cancer is squamous cell carcinoma
- The Pap smear has moved cervical cancer from a top killer (U.S. in the 1940s) to a preventable disease

Etiology
- Preinvasive cancer of the intraepithelial layers (carcinoma in situ or cervical intraepithelial neoplasia [CIN]) is a common diagnosis in women of childbearing age

Incidence and Demographics
- Current lifetime risk for death by cervical cancer in the U.S. is 0.83%
- Average age at diagnosis of precancerous lesions is the mid-30s
- Average age at diagnosis of invasive cancer is the mid 40s
- 25% of invasive cervical cancers, 41% of cervical cancer deaths occur in women over age 65
- Under-screening is the number-one reason 15,700 women get cervical cancer in the U.S. and why 4,900 die from it annually
- Half of women diagnosed with invasive cervical cancer have never been screened, and another 10% have not had a Pap in 5 years
- Least likely to be screened: Elderly, poor, black, Hispanic, and uninsured women
- There is often a progression of cellular abnormalities in the single-layered cervical epithelium; an area of metaplasia occurs
  - A variety of factors leads to additional cellular abnormalities
  - Squamous cell dysplasia or cancer may occur
  - Self-contained dysplasia may invade the basement membrane and surrounding tissues
  - Degree of dysplasia can vary—no strong predictor as to which types will extend; some remain stable, others regress, some extend
  - All dysplasias must be observed serially or treated

Risk Factors

- Early onset coitus, especially within first year of menarche
- Three or more lifetime sexual partners (4x risk in prostitutes); virgins almost never get cervical cancer
- Male sexual partner who has had other partners (especially one with cervical cancer)
- More than three sexually transmitted infections
- Long-term oral contraceptive use increases risk of dysplasias and cancer
- Smoking: Nicotine and other substances bind to cells (cancer cofactor)
- Clinical history of human papillomavirus (HPV): Documented warts or positive DNA sampling
- Low socioeconomic status (less likely to be screened regularly)
- DES exposure
- HIV: Prevalence of dysplasia without HIV is 3%; with HIV 36%; with AIDS 64%; 1992 CDC surveillance criteria for AIDS include cervical cancer as an AIDS-defining illness (immunosuppression increases the risk of dysplasia). Any woman in her mid-20s or younger with advanced carcinoma in situ (CIS) or cervical cancer needs assessment for HIV.
- HPV prevalence accounts for >90% of abnormal cytology
- Herpes simplex virus (HSV), partner circumcision, parity, oral contraceptive use have not been shown to affect risk

Prevention and Screening

- Abstinence/safer sex to prevent STDs, which increase risk
- HPV Vaccine: GARDASIL, a vaccine indicated for females ages 9 to 26 for the prevention of cervical cancer, precancerous or dysplastic lesions, and genital warts caused by human papillomavirus (HPV) Types 6, 11, 16, and 18
- Is contraindicated in individuals who are hypersensitive to the active substances or to any of the excipients of the vaccine
- Does not substitute for routine cervical cancer screening, and women who receive GARDASIL should continue to undergo screening per standard of care
- Is not recommended for use in pregnant women
- Vaccination with GARDASIL may not result in protection in all vaccine recipients
- Is not intended to be used for treatment of active genital warts, cervical cancer, cervical intraepithelial neoplasia, vulvar intraepithelial neoplasia, or vaginal intraepithelial neoplasia
- Has not been shown to protect against diseases due to non-vaccine HPV types
- The vaccine-related adverse experiences observed among recipients of GARDASIL at a frequency of at least 1.0% and greater than placebo were pain, swelling, erythema, fever, nausea, pruritus, and dizziness. In addition, common postmarketing reports include vomiting and syncope
- GARDASIL should be administered in three separate intramuscular injections in the deltoid region of the upper arm or in the higher anterolateral area of the thigh over a 6-month period with the first dose at an elected date, the second dose 2 months after the first dose, and the third dose 6 months after the first dose
- Avoid initiation of tobacco use or stop smoking
- Pap smear to collect cells for analysis. Highest risk area on the uterine cervix for cancer is the "transformation zone" (TZ), where stratified squamous epithelial tissue intersects with columnar epithelial tissue

- TZ appears well outside the external os in very young women and migrates into the canal as the woman ages, or as there is disruption in the cervix (childbirth, invasive procedures, cancer treatment). With hormonal stimulation, the TZ may be more visible (hormonal contraception, pregnancy). In DES-exposed women, the TZ may extend into the vagina.
- All women who are or have been sexually active should have regular cervical cytological screening from the time sexual activity begins or they reach 21 years old. If three or more normal Paps, examine annually, screen every 3 years. Because of the prevalence of HPV and the false-negative rate of Pap smears, some clinicians will opt to screen women yearly despite this recommendation.
- If not screened for 10 years prior to age 66, screen every 3 years to age 75

Assessment

HISTORY
- There are no signs or symptoms of cervical intraepithelial neoplasia; this diagnosis is reached as a result of screening cervical cytology
- Assess the history of cervical cancer screening, management of any abnormalities
- Note any colposcopy, biopsy, any past ablative or surgical therapy
- Cervical cancer is asymptomatic until well-advanced
- Exposure to DES

PHYSICAL EXAM
- Most abnormal cytological changes are picked up on cytologic screening
- Vaginal discharge; vaginal cervical lesions; vaginal bleeding (metrorrhagia, postcoital spotting, cervical lesion or ulceration, abnormal uterine bleeding); and malodorous, bloody, nonpruritic vaginal discharge usually are caused by STDs and other conditions, which bring attention to cervical screening
  - If evidence of an infectious process, treat condition and defer Pap smear for 3–6 months
  - If inflammation noted on follow-up, obtain cervical cytology; note this on request slip

DIAGNOSTIC STUDIES
- Screening methods for cervical cancer (see Table 11–3)
- Colposcopy
- Recall that false negatives occur from sampling error (poor specimen collection) and from detection error
- Thin prep
  - Specimen obtained from nonmenstruating patient
  - Specimen should include squamocolumnar junction and endocervix
  - Cervical specimen is placed directly into preservative vial
  - Increases number of cells sampled by removing confounding mucus, blood, and debris
  - Reduces inadequate specimens or sampling error by 50%

Table 11–3. ACOG's 2004 Cervical Cancer Screening Recommendations

First Screen	Women Up to Age 30	Women Age 30 and Older
About 3 years after first sexual intercourse or by age 21, whichever comes first	Annual cervical cytology testing	Three screening options: Women who have had 3 negative results on annual Pap tests can be rescreened with cytology alone every 2–3 years **or** Annual cervical cytology testing** **or** Cytology with the addition of an HPV-DNA test; if both the cervical cytology and the DNA test are negative, rescreening should occur no sooner than three years

**Women of any age who are immunocompromised, are infected with HIV, or were exposed in utero to DES should be screened annually.

- Conventional Papanicolaou (Pap) screening
    - Has a sensitivity of 51% and a specificity of 98%
    - Most accurate and very specific for carcinoma or invasive cancer and high-grade lesions
    - Low-grade lesions often over-diagnosed: False-negative rate can be 10%–20% (vs. false–positive rate of <1%)
- Auto Pap
    - Computer-based algorithm classification of standard Pap specimen that reviews the number of abnormal cells per slide
    - Increased sensitivity (picks up more abnormals) and increased specificity (decreases the number of false positives)
- Bethesda Pap Smear Grading System updated in 2001 and is now very comprehensive
    - Specimen adequacy
        » Satisfactory for evaluation
        » Presence or absence of endocervical or transformation zone components or other quality indicators such as partially obscuring blood or inflammation
        » Unsatisfactory for evaluation (specify reason)
        » Specimen rejected or not processed (specify reason)
        » Specimen processed and examined, but unsatisfactory for evaluation of epithelial abnormalities (specify reason)
    - General categorization: Optional
        » Negative for intraepithelial lesion or malignancy
        » Epithelial cell abnormality
        » Other
    - Interpretation/result
        » Negative for intraepithelial lesion or malignancy
        » Organisms
            ○ *Trichomonas vaginalis*
            ○ Fungal organisms morphologically consistent with *Candida* species

      ◦ Shift in flora suggestive of bacterial vaginosis

      ◦ Bacteria morphologically consistent with *Actinomyces* species

      ◦ Cellular changes consistent with herpes simplex virus

» Other nonneoplastic findings (optional to report)

» Reactive cellular changes associated with:

      ◦ Inflammation (includes typical repair)

      ◦ Radiation

      ◦ Intrauterine contraceptive device

» Glandular cells status post-hysterectomy

» Atrophy

» Epithelial cell abnormalities

» Squamous cell

» Atypical squamous cells (ASC)

» ASC of undetermined significance (ASC-US)

» ASC, cannot exclude high-grade squamous intra-epithelial lesion (ASC-H)

» Low-grade squamous intra-epithelial lesion (LSIL) encompassing HPV, mild dysplasia, CIN 1

» High-grade squamous intra-epithelial lesion (HSIL) encompassing moderate and severe dysplasia, CIS/CIN 2, and CIN 3 with features suspicious for invasion

» Squamous cell carcinoma

» Atypical glandular cell:

      ◦ Endocervical, endometrial, or glandular cells (not otherwise specified [NOS] or specify in comments)

      ◦ Atypical glandular cell (NOS or specify in comments) favor neoplastic

» Endocervical adenocarcinoma in situ (AIS)

» Adenocarcinoma

      ◦ Endocervical

      ◦ Endometrial cells in a woman 40 years or older

      ◦ Extrauterine

      ◦ NOS

» Other malignant neoplasms (list not comprehensive)

» Automated review and ancillary testing (include if appropriate)

» Educational notes and suggestions (optional)

Management

NONPHARMACOLOGIC TREATMENT

- Benign with inflammation: Follow up in 3 months
- Cryotherapy (freezing) or cauterization: Appropriate for noninvasive small lesions without endocervical extension
- Laser excision: Appropriate for large visible lesions
- Loop Electrosurgical Excision Procedure (LEEP): Appropriate when CIN is clearly visible
- Cone biopsy (conization) for higher grade or invasive lesions
- Hysterectomy, radiation, or chemotherapy is not indicated unless invasion is suspected

Special Considerations
- Pap screening has a very poor positive predictive value for abnormal vaginal cytology. Vaginal cancers are only 1%–4% of gynecological malignancies; only 1.1% of women in 1996 study had abnormal cytology; none had biopsy-proven cancer
- Women who have had a hysterectomy (due to other than malignant causes) in which the cervix was removed do not require cytologic screening (<10% yield on vaginal cuff smears) but should continue to have vaginal inspection annually
- Annual cytology advised if hysterectomy done to treat cervical dysplasia, cervical cancer, uterine cancer
- Remember that a hysterectomy may NOT remove the cervix. It is important to visualize the vagina and assess for the presence of a cervix.
- If a woman happens to have two cervices, be sure to collect a Pap on each one and to label the Paps appropriately (e.g., right cervix or right Pap)
- Pregnancy changes mimic dysplasia and are sometimes indistinguishable from true neoplasia. 75% "abnormals" may regress within 6 months after the pregnancy ends. Confer with or refer to obstetrician or pregnancy specialist for abnormal cytology management in pregnancy. Be sure to obtain follow-up Pap smears during the postpartum period.
- In women at high risk for endometrial hyperplasia (postmenopausal, chronic anovulation), if endometrial cells are noted on the Pap (even without atypia), refer for endometrial sampling
- Clinical tip: Postmenopausal women with one or more unsatisfactory Pap smears due to atrophy should use topical estrogen cream for 4–6 weeks, then repeat the Pap after more than 1 week without treatment

When to Consult, Refer, Hospitalize
- Refer to gynecologist when signs, symptoms of cervical cancer.
  - Abnormal bleeding (either metrorrhagia or post-coital spotting)
  - Visible ulcer or mass on cervix, regardless of the Pap result
  - Late signs: Anemia, anorexia, urinary frequency, hematuria, weight loss, pelvic or epigastric pain
  - Late complications: Vaginal fistulas, urinary and fecal incontinence, back pain, leg edema, ureteral obstruction, eventually renal failure
- Two-thirds of deaths from cervical cancer are from the uremia; another 10%–20% die from hemorrhage
- Refer to gynecologist for abnormal Pap smear results

Follow-Up
- After ablative treatment, screening cytology should be repeated at accelerated intervals; commonly every 3–4 months for the first year, then every 6 months for the next year, then annually once a pattern of normal readings has been established
- Any recurrent abnormals need colposcopic follow-up, repeat endocervical curettage, and biopsy
  - EXPECTED COURSE
    - With appropriate management, future cancer risk is less than 5%. Many clinicians use automated cytology procedures if the patient has had therapy
    - Most treatment failures show up within 1–2 years post-procedure
    - If undetected or untreated, 15%–20% of untreated cervical lesions progress while the rest either stay stable or regress; up to 10 years from precancerous changes to invasive disease

COMPLICATIONS
- After invasion, death usually occurs in 3–5 years without treatment, or in unresponsive cancers
- Invasion moves from the cervix to the uterus, the pelvis, internal lymphs, ureters, bladder, and rectum

Atrophic Vaginitis

Description
- Thinning fragility of vaginal and vulvar epithelium

Etiology
- Estrogen deficiency (estradiol levels less than 20 pg/mL)
- Estrogen along with glycogen maintain a healthy pH of the vaginal environment between 3.8 and 4.2; estrogen deficiency causes an increased pH, disrupting the normal ecosystem
- Estrogen deficiency also causes thinning and dryness of vaginal epithelium with loss of natural folds (rugae) in vaginal wall, predisposing the vagina to overgrowth of colonizing organisms or invasion of pathogens; vagina becomes friable, prone to inflammation

Incidence and Demographics
- 40% of postmenopausal women not on HRT
- Premenopausal women with low estrogen levels

Risk Factors
- Antibiotic use and anti-estrogenic medications
- Stress and conditions suppressing immune function (e.g., diabetes mellitus and HIV)
- Premenarche, lactation, and menopause

Prevention and Screening
- All perimenopausal and postmenopausal women should be asked about signs and symptoms during their annual exams

Assessment
HISTORY
- Complaints include vaginal itching, thin watery discharge or discomfort with coitus, reduced libido, urinary urgency, dysuria; may be asymptomatic
- Obtain history of menopause, use of HRT, vaginal therapies, coital lubricants, UTI history, diabetes

PHYSICAL EXAM
- Exam: Lighter pink vagina, fewer rugae, smaller labia, dry to little discharge
- Vaginal pH 5.5–7 (a rise over premenopausal levels of approximately 4.0)

DIAGNOSTIC STUDIES
- Pap, wet prep, maturational index: more parabasal cells and fewer intermediate and superficial cells (changes consistent with reduced estrogen)
- Abnormal amount of WBCs (greater than 10 per high power field [HPF]) on wet prep

• Any vaginal specimen with blood should prompt a work-up for cervical or uterine bleeding sources; there should be minimal trauma during the examination to create vaginal bleeding (except the use of a cytobrush, which often causes slight spotting)
• Urinalysis negative

Differential Diagnosis
• Infectious vaginitis (trichomoniasis, yeast)
• Bacterial vaginosis
• Vulvar or vaginal cancer
• Diabetes
• Trauma or foreign body
• Contact irritation

Management
NONPHARMACOLOGIC TREATMENT
  • Vaginal lubricants for coitus or comfort

PHARMACOLOGIC TREATMENT
  • Estrogen therapy (topical cream, oral, transdermal) unless contraindicated
  • See menopause entry for oral and transdermal regimens (in lactating women use topical first because oral/transdermal routes may decrease milk supply)
  • Topical regimen is conjugated estrogen cream (Premarin) 2–4 g intravaginally qd in cycles of 3 weeks on, 1 week off; maintenance dose is once a week

LENGTH OF TREATMENT
  • Indefinitely as needed

Special Considerations
• Postmenopausal women not on HRT also should be evaluated for other complications from estrogen deficiency

When to Consult, Refer, Hospitalize
• If signs and symptoms do not resolve with treatment, refer for biopsy

Follow-Up
• Reevaluate in 1–2 months after treatment to assess for side effects and treatment response
• Reevaluate breastfeeding women after weaning
  EXPECTED COURSE
    • Resolves with ongoing or periodic treatment; typically takes 4–6 weeks for symptoms to resolve

  COMPLICATIONS
    • Superimposed infection

Bartholin Gland Cysts and Abscesses

Description
- Obstruction of a Bartholin gland (greater vestibular gland) causing simple cyst, or possible inflammation and infection; causing pain, swelling, and abscess formation

Etiology
- Obstruction of duct with retained mucus, causing simple cyst; contributing factors include trauma, infection, epithelial hyperplasia, congenital atresia
- Infection usually polymicrobial
- Most cysts remain minimally symptomatic <4 cm
- Infected cysts contain mixed vaginal flora, *N. gonorrhoeae*, *C. trachomatis*, *E. coli*; become enlarged, acutely painful
- Can result in chronic ductal stenosis and residual distension; frequently recurrent

Incidence and Demographics
- Most common vulvar mass

Risk Factors
- History of gonorrhea or *Chlamydia*, at risk for STDs

Prevention and Screening
- Prevention of STDs

Assessment
HISTORY
- Previous episodes; prior surgical treatment (incision and drainage, marsupialization, Word catheter placement), STDs
- Symptoms are pain on the sides of the introitus, dyspareunia, painful sitting or walking

PHYSICAL EXAM
- Physical exam may show swelling on sides of the introitus, fluctuant mass at 4 o'clock or 8 o'clock or both; if active infection, there may be redness, tenderness, edema; size can vary up to 4 cm

DIAGNOSTIC STUDIES
- If drainage present or if incision and drainage performed, wound cultures, testing for gonorrhea, *Chlamydia* are performed
- Consider cervical testing for gonorrhea, *Chlamydia*

Differential Diagnosis
- Inclusion cysts
- Lipoma
- Fibroma
- Hematoma
- Bartholin gland cancer (rare)

Management

NONPHARMACOLOGIC TREATMENT
- Warm soaks can alleviate pain, promote spontaneous ductal opening
- Cyst needs no treatment if not symptomatic
- Treatment of large, painful cyst is to perform incision and drainage
- Word catheter can be inserted at time of incision and drainage; it can be sutured or taped into place and is allowed to drain over four weeks

PHARMACOLOGIC TREATMENT
- Antibiotic treatment for Gram-negative and anaerobe coverage (e.g., amoxicillin/clavulanate or TMP/SMX and metronidazole) as well as STDs if culture positive

Special Considerations
- For women over 40 or postmenopausal, complex excision under general anesthesia is warranted to rule out carcinoma

When to Consult, Refer, Hospitalize
- Refer as needed for symptomatic or infected cyst that requires incision and drainage or other procedure
- For recurrent cyst, refer for excision of cyst and marsupialization to establish new ductal opening; laser incision can also be used
- Incision and drainage and placement of the Word catheters is not a beginner skill. Patients should be referred to either the collaborating physician or a gynecologist

Follow-Up
- If incision and drainage are done, follow up in 10 days; if Word catheter inserted, follow up in 4 weeks
  EXPECTED COURSE
  - Abscesses often recur after incision and drainage

  COMPLICATIONS
  - Recurrent abscess

Bacterial Vaginosis

Description
- A mild vaginal infection caused by overgrowth of two or more organisms as a result of increased pH and subsequent replacement of normal flora lactobacillus; not considered an STD

Etiology
- Cause not clearly known, but symptoms caused by an overgrowth of one or more anaerobic bacteria (e.g., *Prevotella* sp., Mobiluncus sp.) *Gardnerella vaginalis*, *Mycoplasma hominis*, replacing normal flora *Lactobacillus* sp.
- Primarily occurs in sexually active adolescents and adult women but not sexually transmitted
- Women who have never been sexually active rarely affected

Incidence and Demographics
- *Gardnerella vaginalis* predominant organism
- The most prevalent vaginitis (symptomatic) in sexually active adolescents adults

Risk Factors
- Sexual activity, increased with multiple partners
- Co-infection with STD

Prevention and Screening
- Wearing of all-cotton underwear and loose clothes
- Avoid douching or use of tampons to decrease bacteria overgrowth
- Advise use of condoms

Assessment
HISTORY
- Malodorous (fishy odor) vaginal discharge, primarily following coitus or before menstruation
- Itching and burning usually not present unless co-infection with another pathogen
- May report vaginal irritation secondary to presence of discharge

PHYSICAL EXAM
- Introitus, presence of homogenous discharge
- Speculum exam, presence of homogenous discharges coating vaginal walls and foul (fishy) odor
- Cervix bimanual exam is normal: Cervix without inflammation, discharge, or CMT

DIAGNOSTIC STUDIES
- Criteria for positive diagnosis (must have three):
  - Thin, white-gray homogeneous vaginal discharge adherent to vaginal wall
  - Vaginal pH >4.5
  - Positive potassium hydroxide (KOH) "whiff" test: Fishy odor when 10% KOH applied to discharge
  - Characteristic clue cells on microscopic exam

Differential Diagnosis
- *Trichomonas* vaginitis
- Cervicitis caused by *Chlamydia* or gonorrhea
- Vulvovaginal candidiasis

Management
- Only women with symptomatic disease need treatment
- Treatment of men not needed because it has not been shown that treatment alters course or relapse/re-infection rate. Intravaginal route may be preferred due to decrease in systemic side effects.

NONPHARMACOLOGIC TREATMENT
- Abstain from sexual intercourse during pharmacological treatment
- Avoid alcohol or any alcohol-containing products while taking metronidazole as interaction produces a disulfiram-like reaction that is very profound

PHARMACOLOGIC TREATMENT
- Metronidazole (Flagyl) 500 mg orally bid x 7 days, OR
- Metronidazole gel 0.75%, one applicator (5 g) intravaginally hs x 5 days, OR
- Clindamycin cream (Cleocin) 2%, on applicator (5 g) intravaginally hs x either 3 or 7 days
- Alternative treatment: Metronidazole 2 g po as single dose OR
- Clindamycin 300 mg po bid x 7 days

LENGTH OF TREATMENT
- 3–7 days

Special Considerations
- Intravaginal treatment preferred for lactating women
- Treatment of high-risk pregnant women (previous premature delivery) who are asymptomatic might reduce premature delivery; screening and treatment suggested early in second trimester
- Low-risk pregnant women who have symptomatic bacterial vaginosis should be treated; use lower doses to minimize exposure to fetus
- Clindamycin vaginal gel not recommended during pregnancy; use associated with increase in premature deliveries
- Patients allergic to metronidazole should not be given vaginal gel
- Recent meta-analysis of metronidazole does not indicate teratogenicity in humans
- Pregnant women: For high or low risk, metronidazole 250 mg po tid x 7 days

When to Consult, Refer, Hospitalize
- Consult for recurrent or refractory infection

Follow-Up
- None needed except for pregnant women, 1 month following treatment
  EXPECTED COURSE
    - Most respond promptly

  COMPLICATIONS
    - Abnormal vaginal discharge, mucopurulent cervicitis, urinary tract infections, postoperative infections, cervical dysplasia, nonpuerperal endometritis, PID
    - Obstetric: Chorioamnionitis, premature labor, premature rupture of membranes, postpartum endometritis

Vaginal Candidiasis

Description
- Vaginitis caused by the *Candida* species not considered to be a sexually transmitted infection
- Also known as *moniliasis* or *yeast*

Etiology
- A dimorphic fungi existing as either oval, budding yeast cells or chains of cells (hyphae)
- Normal flora in the vagina and skin
- Symptomatic infection typically occurs when the vaginal environment is disturbed, resulting in fungal overgrowth

Incidence and Demographics
- About 75% of all women will have at least one episode
- Second most common cause of vaginitis (after bacterial vaginosis); 25% of all vaginal infections
- Majority caused by *Candida albicans* (75%–85%) with C. *glabrata* C. *tropicalis* responsible for remaining
- C. *glabrata* and *tropicalis* increasing in prevalence; more often causing recurrent infections

Risk Factors
- Antibiotic, corticosteroid, or anti-estrogen medications
- Sexual intercourse, oral/vaginal sex, anal/vaginal sex, contraceptives, pregnancy
- Douching, tight-fitting undergarments, obesity
- Stress and immunosuppressive disorders (e.g., HIV and diabetes mellitus)

Prevention and Screening
- Advise all women of possibility of candidiasis with antibiotic, corticosteroid and antiestrogen use
- Advise against douching

Assessment

HISTORY
- Thick, white, nonodorous, cheesy vaginal discharge with or without pruritus
- Pruritus may be only symptom without discharge
- Soreness with coitus (dyspareunia); may also be the only symptom
- Obtain medication history, including recent use of over-the-counter antifungals, vaginal hygiene habits

PHYSICAL EXAM
- Varying amounts of thick, white discharge without odor
- Discharge adherent to vaginal walls
- Discharge may be scant but vulvar erythema and edema present with excoriations sometimes severe enough to preclude an adequate speculum exam

DIAGNOSTIC STUDIES
- Litmus paper for pH: <4.5
- Wet prep: pseudohyphae may be present on normal saline slide; KOH slide demonstrates fungal hyphae, maybe spores
- STD screen as appropriate
- Fungal cultures only necessary for recurrent episodes

Differential Diagnosis
- Bacterial vaginosis
- Trichomoniasis
- Atrophic vaginitis
- *Chlamydia* or gonorrhea

Management
- Pharmacologic treatment required only if symptomatic
- May presumptively treat (wet mount not very sensitive) if sole complaint is pruritus

NONPHARMACOLOGIC TREATMENT
- Proper perineal hygiene
- Wear looser-fitting undergarments (preferably cotton), especially in the summer
- Avoid alcohol and large amounts of concentrated sugars
- Oatmeal baths may reduce itching
- Sexual hygiene

PHARMACOLOGIC TREATMENT
- Fluconazole 150 mg po, one-time dose
- Clotrimazole 1%, 5 g intravaginally hs x 7
- Miconazole 2% cream, 5 g intravaginally hs x 7
- Terconazole 0.4% cream, 5 g intravaginally hs x 7
- Butoconazole 2% cream, 5 g intravaginally hs x 3
- Many of the above creams can be also given as a 1-, 3-, 10- or 14-day treatment; also available in suppository form
- Clotrimazole, miconazole, and butoconazole available over the counter

LENGTH OF TREATMENT
- 1–14 days, depending upon prescribed course

Special Considerations
- 7-day treatment recommended for pregnant women with history of recent candidiasis
- Pregnant women should not use fluconazole
- For acutely symptomatic women, creams and suppositories yield quicker relief than oral fluconazole

When to Consult, Refer, Hospitalize
- Refer to gynecologist for persistent or recurrent infection

Follow-Up
- Only indicated if signs and symptoms fail to resolve within 2 weeks or recur
  - EXPECTED COURSE
    - Usually resolves without problem

  - COMPLICATIONS
    - Refractory candidiasis

ABNORMAL GROWTHS OF UTERUS AND OVARIES

Leiomyomas

Description
- Leiomyomas (uterine fibroids, myomas, fibroid "tumors")
- Benign uterine smooth muscle connective tissue growth responsive to estrogens
- Discrete, firm, roundish, often multiple in various anatomic locations—intramural, submucous, subserous, intraligamentous, pedunculated, cervical
- Mostly asymptomatic and found incidentally on examination

Etiology
- Benign tumors represent localized proliferation of smooth muscle cells surrounded by a pseudocapsule of compressed muscle fibers. Etiology unknown.

Incidence and Demographics
- Occurs in 4%–11% of women; increases with age (20% of women over 35 and 40% of women over 50)

Assessment
  HISTORY
  - Occasionally causes menorrhagia (with degeneration calcification), dysmenorrhea, pelvic pain, bladder pressure, back pain (enlargement encroaches on adjacent structures, possible torsion), increasing pain in pregnancy, pregnancy losses (cavity distortion)

  PHYSICAL EXAM
  - Enlarged firm irregular uterus, mobile, mostly nontender, and negative other exam findings; clinically useful to document size of uterus comparable to gestational size ("10–12 weeks size"; "umbilicus minus 1 cm") for comparative evaluation over time

  DIAGNOSTIC STUDIES
  - Labs: HCG, CBC (iron deficiency anemia), screening Paps and other health maintenance as indicated
  - Pelvic ultrasonography can identify characteristic fibroid changes (hypoechoic,

no cysts, uniform structure), map number location, measure size, assess normalcy of adjacent structures (endometrial thickness); helpful to rule out other concerns (ovarian cysts)

Differential Diagnosis
- Pregnancy
- Endometriosis
- Endometrial carcinoma
- Ovarian cysts
- Uterine cancer
- Abnormal vaginal bleeding
- Adenomyosis
- Cervical cancer
- Ovarian cancer
- Leiomyosarcoma (0.5% of fibroids; very rare under age 40)

Management
NONPHARMACOLOGIC TREATMENT
- Heat, rest, regular complete voiding if causing pressure on bladder

PHARMACOLOGIC TREATMENT
- No treatment needed if asymptomatic
- Iron replacement therapy if needed; hormonal contraception may reduce bleeding but unclear if reduces fibroid size—may increase size in some
- NSAIDs work well for chronic pain
- Analgesics with narcotics only if unremitting pain; needs gynecological consultation
- Reduce size medically (Depo-Provera, Lupron), then surgical treatment may be indicated

Special Considerations
- Patients may become pregnant in the presence of a leiomyoma.
- Pregnancy in conjunction with leiomyoma is usually unremarkable with a normal antepartum course, labor and delivery. These patients need careful surveillance.
- The risk of spontaneous abortion or preterm labor following myomectomy is high. Use of prophylactic B-adrenergic tocolytics are sometimes indicated.
- Vaginal birth after myomectomy is controversial.

When to Consult, Refer, Hospitalize
- Fertility concerns should be referred to gynecologist for management.
- Consult with gynecology about options to reduce bleeding (lepride, surgical excision, myomectomy embolization therapy, hysterectomy), if endometrial sampling is indicated.

Follow-Up
- When symptomatic and at yearly exam
- Should monitor growth with pelvic ultrasound every 6 months until stable
  EXPECTED COURSE
  - Reduces in size, symptoms after pregnancy and menopause

COMPLICATIONS
- Urinary incontinence, pregnancy loss, anemia

Benign Ovarian Growths

Description
- Functional cysts (corpus luteum cysts, theca lutein cysts) and follicular cysts produce hormones
- Very common in adolescents, may have PMS-type prodrome, delayed menses until resolved
- Dermoid cysts (benign teratoma) are growths from germ cells; surgical excision prevents rare cancerous changes

Etiology
- Can occur when ovarian follicle enlarges and does not rupture or when the corpus luteum does not regress in the absence of pregnancy
- Theca lutein cysts may develop with high levels of HCG or with ovulation induction
- May grow as large as 10–15 cm but rarely larger than 6–8 cm

Incidence and Demographics
- 70% of ovarian masses are functional

Risk Factors
- Oral contraceptives tend to be protective (but benign growths still occasionally occur)

Prevention and Screening
- Screening only necessary if undergoing ovulation induction

Assessment
HISTORY
- Discomfort with or without menstrual cycle alterations; may be incidental to visit
  - Functional or follicular cysts often have hormonal effects
  - May be bloating, dyspareunia, abdominal pressure, menstrual irregularities
  - Always ask about LMP

PHYSICAL EXAM
- Exam is often unremarkable if growth small; may note unilateral or bilateral adnexal mass; tenderness may be elicited

DIAGNOSTIC STUDIES
- HCG: Rule out ectopic pregnancy; other tests as indicated by history and physical exam
- Pelvic ultrasound: Fluid component, hypoechogenic, single cyst or simple septated area, no free fluid in cul de sac

Differential Diagnosis
- Ovarian cancer
- Pregnancy
- Endometrioma
- Leiomyoma
- Urinary tract disorder
- Bowel disorder
- PID
- STD
- Ectopic gestation
- Polycystic ovary syndrome

Management

NONPHARMACOLOGIC TREATMENT
- Between menarche and menopause, an asymptomatic, mobile, lateral simple cystic mass less than 5–6 cm confirmed by sonography can be observed; spontaneous resolution is expected; most functional cysts or follicular cysts will regress or resorb without intervention
- Surgical evaluation should occur for masses that persist >6 weeks, enlarge, or are >10 cm for dermoid cysts

PHARMACOLOGIC TREATMENT
- Oral contraceptives may be used to assist regression of functional and follicular cysts
- Manage pain with NSAIDs or other analgesia

Special Considerations
- Some may rupture, causing acute pain

When to Consult, Refer, Hospitalize
- Refer to gynecologist if markedly tender, >6 cm, increases in size, or persists beyond 6 weeks

Follow-Up
- Reevaluate size with ultrasound in 4–6 weeks

COMPLICATIONS
- Usually none

POLYCYSTIC OVARY SYNDROME (PCOS)/POLYCYSTIC OVARIAN DISEASE (PCOD)

Stein-Leventhal Syndrome

Description
- Classical presentation of hyperandrogenism (obesity, hirsutism, acne), menstrual irregularities (oligomenorrhea since menarche, amenorrhea, erratic menorrhagia, or metrorrhagia), erratic fertility patterns or infertile, insulin resistance, and hyperinsulinemia
- Polycystic ovaries are the end point to the process, not the diagnostic focal point

Etiology
- PCOS is a result of a complex disruption of the hypothalamic-pituitary-ovarian axis and ovarian function; characterized by higher tonic levels of LH and low or low-normal FSH levels
- Familial pattern (autosomal dominant)

Incidence and Demographics
- Commonly begins in adolescence (post menarche)

Risk Factors
- Android pattern obesity

Prevention and Screening
- No prevention identified; no routine screening

Assessment
HISTORY
- History of oligomenorrhea, amenorrhea, erratic vaginal bleeding, infertility
- Cosmetically disturbing hirsutism; acne

PHYSICAL EXAM
- Central obesity common although some are normal weight
- Maybe adnexal mass

DIAGNOSTIC STUDIES
- LH (high normal), FSH (low normal), serum testosterone (elevated), DHEAS (elevated), prolactin (to rule out pituitary tumor)
- Fasting serum glucose (check serum insulin levels later if needed), lipid profile
- Overnight dexamethasone suppression test
- Pelvic ultrasound NOT diagnostic
- MRI is NOT diagnostic
- Consider endometrial biopsy when prolonged erratic bleeding to rule out endometrial cancer

Differential Diagnosis

- Adrenal: Tumor, Cushing's, adult-onset adrenal hyperplasia
- Hairan syndrome (hyperandrogenism, insulin resistance, acanthosis nigrans)
- Ovarian: Tumor, ovarian insensitivity syndrome
- Hepatic disease (alters estrogen clearance metabolism)
- Thyroid disease (may affect feedback loops)
- Prolactinoma

Management

NONPHARMACOLOGIC TREATMENT
- Exercise and weight loss: Goal of body mass index <27
- Exercise and weight loss will improve lipid profile, reduce hyperinsulinemia (insulin resistance uncommon with low BMI), improves fertility, improves menstrual cycles, reduces hirsutism
- Occasionally, ovarian wedge resection needed

PHARMACOLOGIC TREATMENT
- Monthly Provera 10 mg daily for 10–14 days at end of each month OR
- Oral contraceptives: Cycling will occur (reduce endometrial danger), may protect lipids, will not increase glucose
- Control of lipids, blood glucose
- Bromocriptine (Parlodel) if high prolactin
- Metformin (Glucophage) improves insulin sensitivity, lowers LH, lowers androgen, and improves fertility

Special Considerations

- Androgen-excess–related insulin resistance (reduced glucose response to insulin amount or "syndrome X"), which spurs hyperinsulinemia (ratio of fasting glucose to fasting insulin levels less than 3.0), increased risk of diabetes mellitus
- Also associated with hypertension, coronary artery disease, increased triglycerides, and decreased HDL levels

When to Consult, Refer, Hospitalize

- Consult with gynecologist for fertility issues and treatment with clomiphene (Clomid) to induce ovulation; anti-androgen or other hormonal therapy
- Consult with endocrinologist for obesity, insulin resistance, lipid issues

Follow-Up

- Close follow-up for screening of excessive endometrial buildup, breast cancer screening
- Follow up lipids, oral glucose tolerance testing at regular intervals

COMPLICATIONS
- Osteoporosis risk
- Endometrial hyperplasia/carcinoma
- Has been associated with failure of lactogenesis II and low milk supply

OTHER CONDITIONS

Pelvic Inflammatory Disease (PID)

Description
- Ascending infection and inflammation within the upper genital tract in women

Etiology
- PID has a polymicrobial etiology with the most common pathogens being *Neisseria gonorrhoeae, Chlamydia trachomatis* in acute PID; mixed with anaerobes, *Bacteroides* sp., staphylococci, streptococci, *Enterobacter* sp., *Haemophilus influenzae*, and others
- Part of an ascending continuum of cervicitis, endometritis, salpingitis, and finally pelvic peritonitis

Incidence and Demographics
- Most prevalent at ages 16–25, matching incidence in STD trends
- Diagnosed in 2%–5% of women in STD settings

Risk Factors
- Sexually active with multiple partners, change in partner within past year
- Infected partner, history of STD, prior PID
- IUD, genital surgical instrumentation (D&C, induced abortion)

Prevention and Screening
- May do STD screen for women with a new sexual partner, especially if <25 years of age

Assessment
HISTORY
- Sexual partner practice history, history of STDs prior PID, contraception, gynecologic procedures, and vaginal douching
- Presentation may be mild or subclinical in nature, which should increase suspicion
- Speed of symptomatology is dependent on the infectious organisms involved
- Mild to moderate: Mid-abdominal pain may be first, with dyspareunia and unusual vaginal discharge; may have some mid-cycle spotting; usually no anorexia; pain worsens with menses
- Severe: Increasing bilateral pain, fever and nausea with occasional vomiting as the infection worsens and progresses beyond the salpinges and into the abdominal cavity
- Fitz-Hugh-Curtis syndrome: Perihepatitis including fever, chills, and pleuritic right upper quadrant pain; accounts for about 5% of PID

PHYSICAL EXAM
- Classic triad of lower abdominal pain, adnexal tenderness (unilateral or bilateral), cervical motion tenderness; only one-third have fever >101°F
- Direct abdominal tenderness (with or without rebound)
- Cervix: Cervicitis (edema friability); note blood, ulcerations, nodules
- Vaginal discharge may or may not be present, may be mucopurulent

- Mild to moderate uterine tenderness
- Adnexal masses may or may not be palpable
- Pain response to cervical motion may be acute, startling ("chandelier sign")
- Enlarged, tender inguinal lymph nodes are often a sign of an STD or a pelvic infection; diffuse, systemic adenopathy with flu-like symptoms, consider possibility of primary HIV infection

DIAGNOSTIC STUDIES
- Diagnosis chiefly based on history and physical and less on labs, save for etiologic agent identification
- HCG, gonorrhea, *Chlamydia* testing
- If lesions noted, assess for herpes, syphilis
- Counsel to consider HIV screening
- Consider cervical cytology screening after the acute infection phase is passed to minimize confounding changes affecting cytological accuracy
- ESR nonspecific and not reliable; WBCs not reliable
- Vaginal wet preps should have >10 WBC/HPF; look for trichomonads, which can confound the work-up; confirm sexual transmission, or bacterial vaginosis, which can be an associated condition
- Transvaginal ultrasound can rule out pregnancy (ectopic) and identify tubal masses or ovarian abscess

Differential Diagnosis
- Appendicitis
- Ectopic gestation
- Endometriosis
- Ovarian cyst (ruptured)
- Leiomyoma
- Acute enteritis
- Severe UTI/pyelonephritis
- Colitis
- Renal calculi

Management
NONPHARMACOLOGIC TREATMENT
- Counsel on safer sex measures

PHARMACOLOGIC TREATMENT
- 2006 CDC criteria for empiric treatment can be based on finding classic triad; urgent treatment is preferred even without specific lab results rather than risk a lifetime of chronic pelvic pain, scarring, infertility
- Outpatient treatment is best with a multiple drug regimen that covers several pathogens, including gonorrhea, *Chlamydia*:
  - Levofloxacin 500 mg po qd x 14 days OR
  - Ofloxacin (Floxin) 400 mg po bid x 14 days with or without Metronidazole (Flagyl) 500 mg po bid x 14 days OR

– Ceftriaxone (Rocephin) 250 mg IM once and doxycycline 100 mg po bid x 14 days; consider adding Metronidazole 500 mg po bid x 14 days or Clindamycin 300 mg po bid x 14 days to cover anaerobes not covered well by second option
– Concurrent treatment of all sexual partners (and the partners' sexual partners) is highly advisable

LENGTH OF TREATMENT
- 14 days is standard regimen

Special Considerations
- Quinolones should not be used in persons with a history of recent foreign travel or partners' travel, infections acquired in California or Hawaii, or infections acquired in other areas with increased Quinolone Resistance Nisseria Gonorrhea prevalence.
- Minimal signs or symptoms does not correlate with minimal tubal scarring or other adverse sequelae
- Avoid alcohol or any alcohol-containing products while taking metronidazole as interaction produces a disulfiram-like reaction that is very profound

When to Consult, Refer, Hospitalize
- Inpatient treatment is best for a very young or unreliable patient, pregnant patient, fever >101°F, WBC >11,000/mm3, evidence of peritonitis, suspected pelvic abscess, decreased bowel sounds, and anorexia; for a patient with escalating symptoms despite treatment; for nonresolving symptoms after 72 hours of treatment; or for severely immunocompromised patients

Follow-Up
- Close follow-up within 3 days to assess treatment efficacy and compliance, with follow-up again after treatment complete
    - EXPECTED COURSE
        - Signs and symptoms of acute infection should resolve by completion of antibiotic treatment

    - COMPLICATIONS
        - If untreated, 15% develop tubo-ovarian abscesses (TOA) and many have chronic infection
        - After one episode, about 15% of women are infertile; rate doubles with each episode
        - 6- to 10-fold increase in risk for ectopic gestation following one episode
        - May produce chronic pelvic pain, dyspareunia, adhesion formation, chronic pyosalpinx, or hydrosalpinx

CARE OF THE MATERNITY PATIENT

Description
- Assessment and care of the pregnant woman from conception throughout pregnancy until birth
- Prenatal care after conception should begin as soon as possible
- Pregnancy outcome can be improved by early health intervention screening
- U.S. Public Health Service advises intensive intervention in early pregnancy if there are identified risk factors that can be modified (e.g., smoking, poor nutrition, psychosocial disorders, diabetes, drug or alcohol abuse)
- Use a biopsychosocial approach with a family focus
- Care during the prenatal period includes primary and secondary prevention
- Health promotion should be emphasized
- Childbirth and parenting education
- Adequate nutrition, smoking cessation, drug and alcohol avoidance, exercise
- Review of current medications, including over-the-counter drugs
- Review benefits of breastfeeding and the recommendation to breastfeed exclusively for the first 6 months and to continue breastfeeding with the addition of solids for a minimum of 1 year
- Pregnant women should avoid cat litter boxes and feces, eating uncooked meat (to avoid risk of toxoplasmosis); also avoid sushi (hepatitis A), non-pasteurized cheeses. Limit tuna, salmon and other high-fat fishes to once a week (due to mercury contamination).

Prenatal Screening
- To identify maternal fetal conditions that require monitoring or may be treatable
- Universal testing for all patients includes Pap smear, urinalysis, urine culture, CBC, blood type, Rh antibody testing, STD screening, hepatitis B surface antigen (HBsAg), rubella immunity, and blood glucose
- These tests are done as part of prenatal blood panel at initial visit, except for blood glucose, which is done at 24–28 weeks gestation in low-risk patients
- Group B beta hemolytic strep genital culture is done at 34–36 weeks gestation
- Hemoglobin should be checked again during last trimester to rule out anemia
- Patient is monitored for weight gain or loss, blood pressure, edema, uterine fundal growth, fetal growth, fetal heart tones, and fetal position
- Consider TSH, anti-thyroperoxidase (TPO) antibodies for undiagnosed hypothyroidism

First Prenatal Visit

Assessment
HISTORY
- Menstrual: Age at menarche, cycle, LMP, contraception
- Obstetrical/gynecological history: Pregnancies, deliveries, abortions, past pregnancy or delivery complication, newborn health/complication, STD history, sexual history, medical history, social history, breastfeeding intentions/history

PHYSICAL EXAM
- Height, weight, blood pressure, screen urine for protein and glucose
- Complete physical exam: Check skin, hair, teeth, thyroid, lungs, heart, breasts, spine, abdomen, extremities (note varicosities, edema), check neuro (presence of clonus, tremors)

- Pelvic: Cervix (note color, position, status of os, lesions, discharge), vagina, uterus (note size, position, tenderness, shape), ovaries (palpable, size, tenderness)
- Assess fundal height in centimeters; size equals dates
- Breasts should be evaluated for growth, nipple retraction/inversion, glandular tissue, elasticity of the areola, shape and symmetry in the first and last trimester. Poor growth, nipple retraction, insufficient glandular tissue, inelasticity of the areola, and marked asymmetry are lactation risk factors

DIAGNOSTIC STUDIES
- Frequently ordered as Prenatal Panel
  - CBC; hemoglobin electrophoresis to rule out sickle cell anemia in women of African decent
  - Blood type, Rh antibody screen
  - Serology: VDRL or RPR titers
  - Rubella titer
  - Hepatitis screen
  - Urinalysis, urine culture
  - Pap smear
  - STD screening: *Chlamydia*, gonorrhea, herpes if indication
  - Uterine/fetal sonogram as indicated

Management
NONPHARMACOLOGIC TREATMENT
- Patient education as appropriate to stage of pregnancy, nutrition, exercise, psychosocial evaluation, smoking cessation

PHARMACOLOGIC TREATMENT
- Prenatal vitamin with folic acid daily until 3–4 months postpartum during breastfeeding
- Iron supplements (200–300 mg/day) for patients with iron deficiency anemia (Hgb <11.0 g/dL)

When to Consult, Refer, Hospitalize
- Consult with physician for all high-risk patients for all abnormal findings during visits
- Consult with lactation specialist for history of lactation failure or abnormal breast exam

Follow-Up
- Usual schedule of prenatal visits: Every 4 weeks until 28th week of gestation, then every 2 weeks until 36th week, then weekly until delivery
- Patients with identified risk factors can be seen as frequently as needed for careful monitoring
- Follow-up visits include weight checks, blood pressure, urine screen for protein and glucose, fundal height measurement and Leopold maneuvers, fetal heart tones, edema

Return Prenatal Visits

First trimester: <13 weeks
- Review of family and social conditions
- Genetic testing, chorionic villous sampling, a-fetoprotein serum levels, amniocentesis

Second trimester: 14–28 weeks
- Fetal heart tones
- Fundus at umbilicus at 20 weeks
- Quickening: Fetal movement felt by mother at 18–20 weeks
- May order ultrasound if dates are in doubt, or fetal growth in question
- Refer for childbirth education classes
- Discuss infant feeding: Breastfeeding, bottle-feeding
- Discuss symptoms to report: Bleeding, cramping, fever, decreased fetal movement, dysuria

Third trimester: 28 weeks to birth
- Labs: Repeat hemoglobin, blood glucose, screen for STD if at risk, genital culture for group B beta hemolytic strep (linked to preterm delivery and neonatal sepsis)
- Evaluate blood pressure, weight gain/loss, edema, fundal height, fetal heart tones
- Teach signs of labor
- Repeat breast exam

Postpartum Visit
- Usually at 6 weeks postpartum; sooner if delivery, postpartum, or breastfeeding problems

Assessment
HISTORY
- Review labor and delivery record
- Assess breastfeeding: Milk supply adequacy, nipple or breast pain, encourage exclusive breastfeeding for 6 months
- Bowels: Constipation, change in elimination pattern, hemorrhoids
- Episiotomy repair: Healed, problems, dehiscence, swelling
- Sexual relations: Resumed, problems, dryness
- Contraception: Evaluate and prescribe prn
- Bladder: Voiding problems, incontinence, Kegel exercises
- Lochia (vaginal bleeding): Resolved, clots, bleeding still
- Menses: Resumed or lactational amenorrhea
- Sleeping pattern
- Nutrition
- Psychological adaptation to newborn: Mother, family members
- Screen for symptoms of postpartum depression

PHYSICAL EXAM
- Vital signs, blood pressure
- Weight
- Urine: Screen for protein and glucose
- Breast exam: Look for mastitis, redness, tenderness, masses

- Thyroid exam: Postpartum thyroiditis not uncommon
- Pelvic exam: Episiotomy, uterus (involution should be nearly completed)
- Rectal exam: Tone, rectoceles, hemorrhoids

DIAGNOSTIC STUDIES
- Pap smear
- Hemoglobin if history of anemia

Management
- Estrogen-containing methods can safely be initiated 6 weeks to 6 months postpartum for women who are breastfeeding their infants and three weeks postpartum for women who are not breastfeeding.
- Because of a concern about hypercoagulability during the postpartum phase, many clinicians withhold hormonal contraceptives from women after childbirth, whether or not the women are breastfeeding. The World Health Organization (WHO) reviewed available evidence on this issue and suggests that the risks of estrogen-containing contraceptives may outweigh the benefits during the first three weeks postpartum. After three weeks, however, when thrombosis risk returns to normal, postpartum women who are not breastfeeding can use estrogen-containing oral contraceptives without additional restrictions.
- Since low-dose progestins are not associated with thrombosis the WHO recommends initiating progestin-only contraceptives at any point postpartum.
- Breastfeeding mothers may use progestin only contraception beginning 6 weeks postpartum.
- Continue prenatal vitamins for 3–4 months or while breastfeeding.

Follow-Up
- Routine well-woman care: Pap smear in 6–12 months
- Contraception follow-up as indicated

CASE STUDIES

Case 1. A 39-year-old sexually active woman presents with a 3-week history of white vaginal discharge, no itching, but notices a fishy odor.

HPI: Denies abdominal pain, nausea and vomiting, fever, genital lesions, lymphadenopathy, dysuria. Patient is in a monogamous relationship with same partner for 6 years.

 1. What additional history would you obtain?

Exam: Thin, white-gray vaginal discharge coating vaginal walls, cervix without inflammation or discharge, no cervical motion tenderness on bimanual examination.

 2. What might you find on examination of vaginal fluid if this woman has bacterial vaginosis?
 3. Should her partner be evaluated and treated?
 4. What is the standard treatment for nonpregnant women?
 5. What does the patient need to know regarding use of this medication?

Case 2. Jane S. comes to your office for her first prenatal visit. She has had a positive home pregnancy test. This is her third pregnancy. She reports that she has made frequent attempts to stop smoking without success.

 1. What further history do you need from Jane?
 2. What will you include in her physical assessment?
 3. What screening tests will you order?
 4. What prenatal education will she need?

Case 3. A 52-year-old woman presents with complaints of hot flashes and no menstrual period for 4–5 months. She asks if there is a blood test to determine if she has gone through menopause and would like your advice on hormone replacement therapy.

HPI: LMP 4–5 months, two periods prior to that were late and scantier than usual. Hot flashes occur daily with profuse sweating, but denies mood change or vaginal dryness. Has tried an over-the-counter herbal product without relief.

 1. What additional history would you like before advising her on treatment?
 2. What laboratory tests will you do to confirm menopause?
 3. What information will you review about hormonal treatment in menopause?
 4. What other recommendations should you provide?

REFERENCES

American Academy of Pediatrics. (2006). *The red book* (27th ed.). Elk Grove, Illinois: Author.

American College of Obstetricians and Gynecologists. (2005). ACOG practice bulletin: Clinical management guidelines for obstetrician-gynecologists: Number 61, April 2005: Human papilloma virus. *Obstetrics and Gynecology, 105*(4), 905-918.

American College of Obstetricians and Gynecologists. (2005). *Revised cervical cancer screening guidelines.* Retrieved April 3, 2008, from http://www.acog.org/from_home/publications/press_releases/nr05-04-04-1.cfm

American Society for Colposcopy and Cervical Pathology. (2006). *Cervical cancer screening consensus guidelines.* Retrieved April 3, 2008, from http://www.asccp.org/consensus.shtml

Barbosa-Cesnik, C., Schwartz, K., & Foxman, B. (2003). Lactation and mastitis. *Journal of the American Medical Association, 289*(13), 1609–1612.

Beckman, C., Ling, F., Laube, D., Smith, R., Barzansky, B., & Herbert, W. (2002). *Obstetrics and gynecology* (4th ed.). Philadelphia: Lippincott Williams & Wilkins.

Behrman, R. (2004). *Nelson's textbook of pediatrics* (17th ed.). Philadelphia: W. B. Saunders Company.

Berek, J. (2007). *Berek & Novak's gynecology* (14th ed.). Philadelphia: Lippincott Williams & Wilkins.

Bieber, E. J., Sanfilippo, J. S., & Horowitz, I. R. (2006). *Clinical gynecology.* Philadelphia: Churchill, Livingstone, Elsevier.

Bland, K., & Copeland, E. (2004) *The breast: Comprehensive management of benign and malignant disorders, volumes I & II* (3rd ed.). Philadelphia: W. B. Saunders.

Breslin, E., & Lucas, B. (2003). *Women's health nursing: Toward evidence-based practice.* Philadelphia: W. B. Saunders.

Buttaro, T. M., Trybulski, J., Bailey, P., & Sandberg-Cook, J. (2003). *Primary care: A collaborative practice.* St. Louis, MO: Mosby.

Centers for Disease Control and Prevention. (2006). Sexually transmitted diseases treatment guidelines, 2006. *MMWR: Morbidity and Mortality Weekly Reports, 55,* No. RR-11. Retrieved April 3, 2008 from http://www.cdc.gov/mmwr/PDF/rr/rr5511.pdf

Dambro, M. R. (2008). *The 5-minute clinical consult.* St. Louis, MO: Lippincott Williams & Wilkins.

Edmunds, M. W., & Mayhew, M. S. (2004). *Pharmacology for the primary care provider* (2nd ed.). St. Louis, MO: Mosby.

Gabbe, J., Steve, G., & Simpson, L. (2007) *Obstetrics: Normal and problem pregnancies* (5th ed.). Philadelphia: Churchill Livingstone.

Gilbert, D. N., Moellering, R. C., & Se, M. A. (2007). *Sanford guide to antimicrobial therapy* (37th ed.). Vienna, VA: Antimicrobial Therapy, Inc.

Hatcher, R., Trussell, J., Stewart, F., Stewart, G., Kowal, D. Guest, F., et al. (2008). *Contraceptive technology* (19th ed. rev.). New York: Ardent Media Trade, Inc.

Jernström, H., Lubinski, J., Lynch, H. T., Ghadirian, P., Neuhausen, S., Isaacs, C., et al. (2004). Breast-feeding and the risk of breast cancer in BRCA1 and BRCA2 mutation carriers. *Journal of the National Cancer Institute, 96*(14), 1094–1098. Retrieved April 3, 2008 from http://jncicancerspectrum.oupjournals.org/cgi/content/abstract/jnci;96/14/1094

Merriman, J. A., & Neff, M. J. (2007). Breast cancer screening: Authors' guide, and clinical quiz. *American Family Physician, 75*(11), 1602.

Neinstein, L., Gordon, C., & Katzman, D. (2007). *Adolescent health care: A practical guide* (5th ed.). Philadelphia: Lippincott Williams & Wilkins.

Riordan, J. (2004). *Breastfeeding and human lactation* (3rd ed.). Sudbury, MA: Jones & Bartlett.

Schroeder, B., & Sanfilippo, J. (1999). Dysmenorrhea pelvic pain in adolescents. *Pediatric Clinics of North America, 46, 559*.

Steiner, M., Haskett, R. F., & Carroll, B. L. (1980). Premenstrual tension syndrome: The development of research diagnostic criteria and new rating scale. *Acta Psychiatrica Scandinavica, 62*, 177–191.

Tierney, L. M., McPhee, S. J., & Papadakis, M. A. (2008). *Current medical diagnosis and treatment* (47th ed.). New York: McGraw-Hill Lange.

Turner-Maffei, C., O'Connor, B., Cadwell, B. A., Arnold, L., Blair, E., & Cadwell, K. (2006). *Maternal and infant assessment for breastfeeding and human lactation: A guide for the practitioner*. Sudbury, MA: Jones & Bartlett.

Uphold, C., & Graham, M.V. (2003). *Clinical guidelines in family practice* (4th ed.). Gainesville, FL: Barmarrae Books.

U.S. Preventive Services Task Force. (2006). *Guide to clinical preventive services, 2006: Recommendations of the U.S. Preventive Services Task Force* (2nd/3rd ed.). Philadelphia: Lippincott Williams & Wilkins.

Varney, H. (2004). *Varney's midwifery* (4th ed.). Sudbury, MA: Jones & Bartlett.

World Health Organization. (2004). *Medical eligibility criteria for contraceptive use* (3rd ed.). Geneva: Author. Retrieved July 29, 2008 from http://www.who.int/reproductive-health/publications/mec/mec.pdf

Male Reproductive System Disorders and Concerns

Barbara Siebert, MSN, CRNP, FNP-BC

GENERAL APPROACH

- Many complaints of the male genitourinary system are of a sensitive nature, and men are less inclined to initiate discussion or seek help for them. The nurse practitioner should take an active role in screening for such problems with an approach that is open and nonjudgmental.
- General areas for screening: Sexuality, safer sex practices, high-risk behaviors
- General history questions: Past infections (sexually transmitted diseases [STDs], urinary tract infections [UTIs], prostatitis), normal voiding patterns; current symptoms in more detail
- Exam: Assessment of the male genitalia should be part of the screening/annual physical exam, even if there are no complaints, because many male genitourinary problems are asymptomatic. Digital rectal exam (DRE) that includes palpation of the prostate gland (normal size ~2.5–3 cm) should be included starting at age 40.

Red Flags
- *Testicular torsion*: Rule out with any complaint of scrotal pain: acute onset of severe scrotal pain, in males of any age (peak ages 12–18); requires treatment within 4–12 hours surgically to preserve fertility and prevent loss of the testicle
- *Paraphimosis*: Inability of the retracted foreskin to be reduced over the glans can be a surgical emergency
- *Testicular mass*: Any mass in the testicles or attached to the testicles is cancer until proven otherwise
- *Right-sided varicoceles*: Rare and associated with obstruction of the right spermatic vein and retroperitoneal neoplasms
- *Recurrent UTIs* in men: Evaluate for prostatitis
- *Prostatic massage*: Avoid performing until acute prostatitis is ruled out or treatment is initiated to prevent hematogenous spread of infection

- *OTC medications*: Anticholinergics, parasympatholytics, and sympathomimetics precipitate or worsen urinary conditions such as benign prostatic hyperplasia; antidepressants can impact full sexual function

Contraception

Use of Condoms
- A method of pregnancy prevention used by the male to prevent the spillage of semen into the vaginal vault. A latex or polyurethane sheath applied prior to sexual intercourse/penetration that fits snugly over the entire length of the penis with a mildly constricting ring at the base to prevent slippage from the penis. The condom holds ejaculated semen after detumescence that is discarded with the condom.
- Condoms reduce risk of exposure to STDs in male-to-female or male-to-male contact.
- Approximately 21% of males use condoms as a contraceptive; more commonly used for prevention of STD transmission or exposure.
- Effectiveness averages 88% typically, up to 97% if used properly.
  FACTORS CONTRIBUTING TO UNSUCCESSFUL USE AND RESULTANT PREGNANCY
    - Allergy to latex or rubber
    - Failure to use a condom during genital foreplay when pre-ejaculate can be introduced into or near the vagina
    - Breakage or slippage of the condom during intercourse
    - Limited education about reproduction or contraception; limited access to medical care
    - Dissatisfaction with method and subsequent failure to use

  INSTRUCTION ON THE USE OF THE CONDOM
    - Apply to penis when in the erect state, prior to contact with partner's genitals as pre-ejaculate discharge near or in the vagina can contain semen adequate for fertilization.
    - Roll the condom to the base of the penis, leaving a small space at the tip to allow for collection of ejaculate and decrease pressure on the condom (decreased risk of breakage).
    - Use only water-based lubricants if needed. Spermicidal cream or jelly on the penis prior to application of the condom and penetration or used intravaginally enhances effectiveness and reduces pregnancy risk. Do not use a condom more than once.

Sterilization
- A surgical method of eliminating the transport of semen in ejaculate as a means to prevent pregnancy, which, although possibly reversible, should be considered permanent.
- An outpatient surgical procedure performed via a scrotal incision that severs and seals the vas deferens; does not require general anesthesia
- The most popular method of sterilization in the U.S.
- Approximately 12% of men are surgically sterilized via vasectomy
- Failure rate is 0.1% in the first year post-operatively
- Prior to resuming sexual intercourse, sperm counts are obtained at post-procedure follow-up to confirm success of the procedure
- Complications include potential infection and failure of sterilization

DISORDERS OF THE PROSTATE GLAND

Benign Prostatic Hyperplasia (BPH)

Description
- Nonmalignant generalized enlargement of the periurethral prostate gland related to a variety of triggers for cell growth. Believed to be under endocrine control. Enlargement mechanically obstructs urination by compressing the urethra.

Etiology
- Cause is unknown; universally seen in aging
- Hyperplasia of gland due to an abnormal increase in the number of cells in prostate tissue
- Hormonal changes: Accumulation of dihydrotestosterone (DHT) and increased estrogen in aging male seems to interact in a way that causes cell proliferation

Incidence and Demographics
- Affects approximately 50% of men by age 50 and nearly 90% of men >80 years old
- Initially asymptomatic for men in 40s, many develop urinary symptoms by age 60

Risk Factors
- Increased age
- Family member with BPH
- African American
- Diet: High fat with low fiber intake, especially vegetables
- History of sexually transmitted infections

Prevention and Screening
- No prevention other than reducing risk factors (safer sex, change in diet)
- Early screening starting in the 40s (patient history, digital rectal exam) may allow for earlier treatment, slowing of the progression of hyperplasia and possible reduction of symptoms

Assessment
HISTORY
- General: Fever, malaise, back pain, hematuria, pain with voiding indicate infection
- Obstructive symptoms: Difficulty starting/stopping stream, hesitancy, dribbling, weakening force/size of stream, sensation of full bladder after voiding, retention
- Irritative symptoms: Urgency, frequency, nocturia, urge incontinence, dysuria
- American Urological Association (AUA) Symptom Index for Benign Prostate Hypertrophy:
  - 35-point scale to assess symptom severity: Incomplete emptying, frequency, intermittency, urgency, weak stream, straining, and nocturia
  - Seven categories rated from 0 to 35 points; 0–7 mild; 8–19 moderate; 20–35 severe
  - The higher the points, the more severe the symptoms
  - Should be completed for all patients before therapy begins
- Medications, especially cold/sinus medications: Anticholinergics impair bladder contractility, sympathomimetics increase outflow resistance and worsen symptoms

- Date of last digital rectal exam (DRE), prostate-specific antigen (PSA), and results
- PMH: Explore for other conditions that may be associated with these symptoms: surgery, diabetes, neuromuscular disease (multiple sclerosis), psychogenic disorder, cardiovascular disease, and hypercalcemia

PHYSICAL EXAM

- Digital rectal exam (DRE): Intact anal sphincter tone; prostate should be nontender, firm, smooth, and rubbery; blunting or obliteration of midline median sulcus indicates BPH
- Enlargement may be symmetric, nodular, or asymmetric; any nodules should be considered possibly malignant and fully evaluated; indurated prostate requires cancer evaluation
- Abdomen: With urinary retention, possible distended bladder on percussion or palpation; costovertebral tenderness (CVAT) if renal sequelae
- Neurologic: Screening exam to note non-prostate etiology for symptoms of neurogenic or myogenic etiology, detrusor muscle impairment, compression of nerves

DIAGNOSTIC STUDIES

- Urinalysis should be negative for hematuria, glycosuria, or infection; their presence indicates secondary UTI or other problem
- Catheterization for a post-void residual (PVR) illustrates volume remaining in bladder after patient's usual void
- Serum BUN and creatinine helpful in assessing renal function; may be abnormal if urinary retention or obstruction has affected upper urinary tract, as well as with underlying renal disease
- Prostate-specific antigen (PSA) to distinguish cause (BPH or prostate cancer) of large gland; use of this test is controversial if patient is asymptomatic and results are 4–10 ng/mL; results >10 ng/mL may be cancer; PSA increases as gland enlarges, but do not assume increases are due only to gland enlargement; *increased levels may be noted 1–24 hours post-DRE, so avoid lab work during this time period*
- Advanced workup includes urinary flowmetry studies (flow rate), post-residual urine, urodynamic studies, transrectal ultrasound, intervenous pylogram (IVP), and abdominal ultrasound

Differential Diagnosis

- Diseases associated with increased urination (chronic heart failure [CHF], diabetes mellitus, hypercalcemia)
- Bladder neck contracture or cancer
- Prostate cancer
- Infectious or inflammatory disease (prostatitis, cystitis, urethritis)
- Neurologic disease
- Urethral strictures

Management

NONPHARMACOLOGIC TREATMENT

- "Watchful waiting:" Monitoring of symptoms for mild BPH with AUA scores <7
- Avoidance of bladder irritants such as coffee, alcohol, decongestants, antihistamines, anticholinergics, and tricyclic antidepressants
- Encourage frequent voiding to keep bladder volume low
- Monitor voiding; watch for signs of retention
- Limit intake of fluids in the evening, avoid large quantities in short time
- Eliminate prescription and OTC meds that may worsen symptoms
- In individuals with moderate to severe symptom presentation (>7 points on AUA scale)
  - Medical management with alpha-adrenergic antagonist or 5 alpha-reductase inhibitors;
  - Phytotherapy: With such products as saw palmetto berry, the bark of *Pygeum Africanum*, the roots of *Echinicea Purpurea*, *Hypoxis Rooperi*, pollen extract, and the leaves of trembling poplar, all still being researched
  - Surgical options for those with severe symptoms, large post-void residual, upper tract infections, or failure of medical therapy
    » Transurethral resection of the prostate (TURP)
    » Transurethral incision of the prostate (TUIP)
    » Open prostatectomy
- Minimally invasive therapy: Nonsurgical procedures to reduce the size of the prostate include the use of heat via transurethral needle ablation (TUNA) and transurethral microwave therapy (TUMT), the use of transurethral electrovaporization of the prostate (TEVP), fiber optics/laser technology, high-intensity focused ultrasound, transurethral balloon dilation of the prostate, and intraprostatic stents

PHARMACOLOGIC TREATMENT

- For mild to moderate symptoms, see Table 12–1 for primary drugs
- Less commonly used drugs include GnRH agonists, progestational antiandrogens, flutamide (Eulexin), and testolactone (Teslac)
- Saw palmetto (160 mg bid) is an alternative herbal therapy; saw palmetto decreases testosterone uptake to decrease size of gland
- Tolterodine (Detrol) to decrease bladder contractions

LENGTH OF TREATMENT

- Dependent upon type and severity of symptoms and impact on daily functioning
- Medications may be prescribed until symptoms are no longer manageable and surgery considered

Table 12–1. Pharmacologic Management of BPH

Drugs	Dosage	Comment
1α–Adrenergic Blockers		
Terazosin (Hytrin)	Progressive dosing over 1 month: 1 mg x 3 days 2 mg x 11 days 5 mg x 7 days 10 mg daily	Relaxes smooth muscle around urethra Drug of choice for smaller prostate and acute irritative symptoms Decreased smooth muscle tone in bladder neck and prostate Improvement dose-dependent, takes 4–6 weeks for maximal therapeutic effect In nonhypertensive may cause postural hypotension, dizziness, palpitations, or syncope May be beneficial for those with concomitant BPH and hypertension (HTN), can reduce number of medications needed
Doxazosin (Cardura)	1 mg qd, hs, may double every 1–2 weeks to max of 8 mg/day	Similar to terazosin
Tamsulosin HCL (Flomax)	0.4 mg qd 30 min. before meal at same time each day; may increase to 0.8 mg after 2–4 weeks	No cardiovascular side effects, postural hypotension not common May cause dizziness, abnormal ejaculation, rhinitis
5α -REDUCTASE INHIBITOR		
Finasteride (Proscar)	5 mg qd No titration needed	Blocks conversion of testosterone to DHT; gland shrinks Drug of choice for large prostate and those with contraindications or failed treatment with alpha-adrenergic medication Decreased hormonal (androgen) effect on prostate shrinks prostate size and symptoms, resulting in increased peak urinary flow rate Improvement not noted for up to 6–12 months, must be used indefinitely to sustain effect Decreased libido and ejaculate volume; erectile dysfunction Decreased PSA by up to 50%, blocking effectiveness of PSA as screening tool for CA; screen for cancer with DRE and PSA before initiating treatment

Special Considerations
- In presence of concomitant diseases (diabetes mellitus; cardiovascular or neurologic disease), particularly with aging of the patient, care should be coordinated with regard to medications, ability for self-care, and recommendations for procedural or surgical treatment.

When to Consult, Refer, Hospitalize
- Referral to a urologist is indicated for AUA index score of 8 or more, symptoms not responsive to medications, infections (epididymitis, repeat UTIs), obstruction or acute urinary retention, renal disease, or suspicion of malignancy.

Follow-Up
- Annual evaluation is indicated for asymptomatic or minor symptoms.
- Patients who opt for the "watchful waiting" strategy should be followed every 6–12 months.
- Patients on medications should be seen every 2–4 weeks until symptoms stabilize, then every 6 months.
- Those receiving surgical or procedural treatments are followed by the treating urologist/surgeon.
    - EXPECTED COURSE
        - May have prolonged course of mild or stable symptoms before advancing to stage of needing nonpharmacological treatment
    - COMPLICATIONS
        - Potentially serious sequelae: UTI, obstructive uropathy, urine retention, renal disease

Prostatitis

Description
- An inflammation and/or infection of the prostate gland traditionally categorized as acute bacterial, chronic bacterial, nonbacterial, or prostatodynia.
- New National Institutes of Health (NIH) categories of prostatitis are:
    I. Acute bacterial prostatitis
    II. Chronic bacterial prostatitis
    III. Chronic nonbacterial prostatitis/chronic pelvic pain syndrome
    IV. Asymptomatic inflammatory prostatitis

Etiology
- Various causes: Allergic, inflammatory, infectious, related to instrumentation, UTIs, STDs, prostatic abscess or stone
- Acute infectious causes: Generally Gram-negative bacilli; primarily *Escherichia. coli*; may also be *Enterobacter, Klebsiella, Proteus mirabilis, Pseudomonas aeruginosa, Staphylococcus aureus, Streptococcus faecium* and *Serratia*. Nonbacterial prostatitis causes: *Neisseria gonorrhoeae, Ureaplasma, Trichomonas vaginalis, Chlamydia trachomatis,* and *Gardnerella vaginalis.*

- Infectious causes usually occur by direct invasion from the urethra, typically UTI
- Younger men (<35 years) have an increased likelihood that the infectious organism is an STD (C. *trachomatis* or N. *gonorrhoeae*)

Incidence and Demographics
- Chronic bacterial primarily occurs in older men
- All others primarily in sexually active men ages 30–50
- Nonbacterial: Most common type, 8x greater than bacterial type, with an increased prevalence in younger males
- Acute bacterial: Least common type, occurs in younger or elderly male
- Prostatodynia: Most commonly affects ages 22–56

Risk Factors
- History of or exposure to STDs (multiple sexual partners or recent new partner)
- Age over 50: More common cause from recurrent UTI or prostatic stones
- Instrumentation of urinary tract
- Abscess elsewhere in the body
- Recurrent UTIs
- Prostatodynia may be associated with autoimmune or neuromuscular problems, stress, allergic conditions

Prevention and Screening
- Avoidance of unsafe sex decreases exposure to STDs
- Frequent voiding
- Screen with good history and DRE

Assessment (see Table 12–2)
HISTORY
- All presentations have common symptoms of dysuria related to compression of the urethra by the inflamed prostate; all are associated with some degree of pain that is variable and may be associated with intercourse, ejaculation, and defecation
- Low back pain
- Chronic bacterial prostatitis is characterized by remissions and exacerbations with recurrent UTIs
- Acute bacterial characterized by its acute onset with systemic symptoms and pattern of pain and dysuria
- Current medications (e.g., anticholinergics), other medical illness, and sexual history to assess risk of infection

PHYSICAL EXAM
- Evaluate for fever; abdominal exam to check for tenderness or distended bladder; genitalia and scrotum for urethral discharge, CVA tenderness to assess kidneys, and rectal exam
- *Warning regarding prostate examinations*: Examining the prostate is a part of this exam; however, due to exquisite tenderness and risk of bacterial spread into the bloodstream, it is to be done very gently or, in the case of suspected acute prostatitis, perhaps not at all until treatment has been initiated

• In the nonacute patient, prostatic massage *is* indicated to carry out the sequential urinalysis and culture for evaluation of prostatic secretions and as part of therapeutic treatment

Table 12-2. Clinical Presentation of Prostatitis

	Symptoms	Physical findings
Acute Bacterial	Chills, fever, malaise Dysuria, urgency, burning, frequency Hematuria Pain: pelvis, perineum, lower back, scrotum, with defecation, with intercourse	Fever Prostate very tender, boggy, warm +/- Urethral discharge
Chronic Bacterial	+/- Low-grade fever Dysuria, hesitancy Hematuria, hematospermia Pain mild: perineum, scrotal, abdominal, with ejaculation	No systemic findings Prostate may be normal, indurated, mildly tender, boggy, or irregular +/- Prostatic stones Scrotum +/- edema, erythema, and tenderness
Nonbacterial	No fever Gradual onset: dysuria, frequency, urgency Pain mild: perineum, with ejaculation Decreased libido or impotence	Urethral discharge common Prostate enlarged, boggy, and tender
Prostatodynia	No fever Dysuria, hesitancy, decreased flow, post-void dribbling Pain: perineum, back, testicle(s)	None

DIAGNOSTIC STUDIES
• Traditional sequential urinalysis and culture test for voided bladder (VB) specimens and expressed prostatic secretions (EPS; see Table 12-3)
• 2-sample method: 1) clean catch, midstream urine specimen; 2) urine specimen post prostatic massage
• Culture any penile discharge for STDs
• Blood cultures may be ordered for acute prostatitis
• Chronic prostatitis is additionally evaluated with CBC, serum BUN and creatinine, and possible IV pyelogram and/or transrectal ultrasound
• In the elderly, bladder cancer screening via urine cytology is indicated
• PSA will be elevated in prostatitis
• Urodynamic testing may be helpful in evaluating suspected prostatodynia

Table 12–3. Sequential Laboratory Tests in Prostatitis

	Specimen (Culture each sample also)	Location
VB$_1$	1st 10 mL urine	Urine from urethra
VB$_2$	Midstream urine	Urine from bladder
EPS	Urethral secretions AFTER prostatic massage	Prostatic fluid
VB$_3$	1st 10 mL urine after prostatic massage	Prostatic fluid and urine from bladder

Differential Diagnosis
- Any of the four types of prostatitis
- BPH
- Urethral stricture
- Cancer of the bladder or prostate
- Renal colic
- Other infections: abscess, epididymitis, cystitis, urethritis

Management

NONPHARMACOLOGIC TREATMENT
- Avoidance of known irritants: Caffeine, alcohol, OTC antihistamines or decongestants
- Avoidance of sex during first 2 or more weeks of acute illness
- Increase frequency of ejaculation in nonacute states
- Hydration maintenance (force fluids)
- Rest and sitz baths 20 minutes 2–3 times a day for pain prn

PHARMACOLOGIC TREATMENT
- The prostate gland is difficult to penetrate with antibiotics, therefore first-line treatment is with trimethoprim-sulfamethoxazole (Bactrim) or quinolones (Table 12–4)
- Those <35 years of age are more likely to be infected with C. *trachomatis* or N. *gonorrheae*, requiring antibiotics according to the current recommended choices of the health department or CDC (updated annually)
- NSAIDs are recommended for both anti-inflammatory effects as well as pain relief
- Stool softeners prn

Table 12–4. Diagnosis and Management of Prostatitis

Microscopic	Urine Cultures	Diagnosis	Treatment	Duration (variable recommendations)
+WBC, bacteria in VB1, few in other specimens	# bacteria VB1 > than VB2 or VB3	Urethritis	Ceftriaxone 125 mg IM x 1 or Cefixime 400 mg po x 1 or Ciprofloxacin 500 mg po x 1 **PLUS** Azithromycin 1g po x 1 or doxycycline 100 mg bid x 1	Single-dose therapy
+WBC/RBC, bacteria in VB2, possibly VB1	# bacteria VB2 > VB1 or VB3	Cystitis	Quinolone qd or bid or TMP/SMX DS bid	3–7 days if uncomplicated
+WBC, bacteria in all specimens	# bacteria EPS, VB3 > VB1 or VB2	Acute Prostatitis	< 35 yrs: ofloxacin 400 mg x 1, then 300 mg bid > 35 yrs: ciprofloxacin 500 mg bid or TMP/ SMX DS bid	At least 7 days 2–6 weeks
+ WBC, bacteria in EPS and VB3 only	Little/no growth in VB1 or VB2	Chronic Prostatitis	Ciprofloxacin 500 mg bid or Ofloxacin 300 mg bid Alternative: TMP/ SMX DS bid	3–4 months Suppressive treatment at ½ dose indefinitely, if needed
+ WBC in EPS, VB3 Nonbacterial organisms in EPS or VB3	No bacterial growth	Nonbacterial Prostatitis	Organism-specific: Chlamydia: Doxycycline 100 mg bid x 2 wks Ureaplasma: Tetracycline 500 mg bid Trichomonas: Flagyl 2.0 g x1 or 500 mg bid x 7 days	Organism-specific
No WBC, bacteria or other organisms in any specimen	No bacterial growth	Prostatodynia	NSAIDs ? Antibiotics	

Special Considerations
- Patients may have concomitant urinary symptoms and infection; recurrent UTI diagnoses warrant chronic prostatitis in the differential.
- Elderly: Increased incidence of concomitant disease in the genitourinary (GU) system indicating greater need for advanced testing and screening for BPH, prostate or bladder cancer, and UTI

When to Consult, Refer, Hospitalize
- Hospitalization is indicated for all patients who have systemic involvement for IV antibiotics and treatment of possible septicemia
- Refer to a urologist if no improvement within 48 hours of treatment
- Refer to an urologist older patients (>50 years) who are symptomatic, have recurrent prostatitis, or acute bacterial prostatitis, as BPH may be a compounding problem

Follow-Up
- For acute prostatitis, reevaluation is done within 48–72 hours, then 2–4 weeks later (1 month after completion of treatment) for urinalysis, urine, and prostatic secretion cultures to monitor treatment effectiveness and assess for signs of complications
- For chronic bacterial prostatitis, check urinalysis, culture, and sensitivity every 30 days. Sequential urine tests and EPS should be repeated 4–6 weeks after initiation of therapy
- Follow-up may be sooner as indicated based on the patient's responsiveness to treatment and changes in symptoms
  - EXPECTED COURSE
    - Prostatitis requires long-term antibiotic therapy for optimal outcomes. Nonchronic prostatitis may be resolved within 6 weeks; however, chronic prostatitis requires treatment for up to 6 months. In chronic cases treatment suppresses but does not eradicate the offending organism, hence, the recurrence of symptoms.

  - COMPLICATIONS
    - Potential for serious sequelae including development of prostatic abscess, stones, ascending UTIs, epididymitis, urinary retention, renal infection, bacteremia, progressive STD complications

Prostate Cancer

Description
- Malignant neoplasm of the prostate gland

Etiology
- Unknown cause
- 95% develop in acinar glands of prostate
- 2 types: 1) Poorly differentiated and fast-growing, and 2) androgen-dependent, well-differentiated, and slow-growing
- Metastasizes primarily to bone

Incidence and Demographics
- Second most common cause of cancer deaths in men
- Average age at diagnosis is 72 years
- About 80% of all clinically diagnosed cases of prostate cancer are men > age 65
- 69 cases per 100,000 men; CDC estimates that in the year 2005, 185,985 new cases of prostate cancer were diagnosed and 28,905 men died of it
- There is a 40% greater incidence in African-American men; they are diagnosed with prostate cancer at later stages and die of the disease at higher rates than White men

Risk Factors
- Age >60, exposure to chemical carcinogens, history of STDs
- Family history of carcinoma of the prostate; African Americans at greatest risk
- Questionable whether related to prior vasectomy or dietary fat

Prevention and Screening
- Avoid exposure to chemical carcinogens; safer sex to prevent STDs
- Annual DRE beginning at age 40–50 and DRE with PSA from age 50 is recommended for screening and early detection by some groups (AUA), although the U.S. Preventive Health Services suggest research does not support routine PSA testing due to high number of both false positives and false negatives; using the conventional PSA cut-point of 4.0 ng/dL detects a large majority of prostate cancer; however, a significant percentage of early prostate cancer (10%–20%) will be missed

Assessment
HISTORY
- Early disease is asymptomatic
- With enlargement, frequency, nocturia, dribbling develop (see BPH)
- Symptoms of urethral obstruction and bone pain occur with advanced metastatic stage
- Constitutional symptoms: Anorexia, weight loss, fatigue, weakness, back pain

PHYSICAL EXAM
- Depending on stage of the cancer, the prostate on DRE may be normal on the palpable lateral and posterior portion of the gland, or may be asymmetrical, generally firmer with hard induration, localized nodules, and obliterated median sulcus
- Lower extremity edema may develop due to lymph node metastases, pathologic fractures

DIAGNOSTIC STUDIES
- PSA levels >4 ng/mL indicate possible cancer; do not always correlate with DRE; *increased levels will be noted 1–24 hours post-DRE, so avoid lab work during this time period*
- Normal PSA in 40% of patients with cancer; PSA discredited as screening test
- CBC, urinalysis, urine culture and sensitivity for workup of urinary symptoms
- Serum alkaline phosphatase increased with late stage (metastatic) to bone

Differential Diagnosis
- BPH
- Prostatitis
- Prostatic or bladder stones
- Bladder cancer

Management
- Treatment choice is based on stage of the disease and age of patient
    NONPHARMACOLOGIC TREATMENT
    - Asymptomatic patients with life expectancy <10 years: Watchful waiting is an option
    - Treatment options if localized include watchful waiting, radical prostatectomy, and radiation therapy
    - Disseminated disease is treated with surgical or chemical castration (hormonal therapy) or chemotherapy

    PHARMACOLOGIC TREATMENT
    - Hormonal treatment: Androgen deprivation/chemical castration—flutamide (Eulexin) 250 mg po tid or leuprolide (Lupron) 1 mg SQ qd along with flutamide 7.5 mg IM monthly

    LENGTH OF TREATMENT
    - Radiation, chemotherapy treatments vary depending on staging

Special Considerations
- Concurrent with treatment of the cancer is the need for addressing the effects of the diagnosis, sequelae of the disease, and side effects of treatments. These include such things as coping with a chronic terminal illness, loss of self-image or self-esteem, transient or permanent incontinence (2%–5%), loss of libido, and impotence. Impotence occurs in 40% post-operatively and 25%–35% post-radiation, hormonal treatment may additionally result in gynecomastia, cardiovascular complications, or hot flashes.

When to Consult, Refer, Hospitalize
- All patients with PSA >10, abnormalities on DRE, and/or symptomatic are referred to specialist for advanced workup, TRUS (trans-urethral ultrasound) with biopsy, chest x-ray, bone scans.

Follow-Up
- Urologist or oncologist provides follow-up for cancer treatment
- For early stages, follow-up is initially at 3–6 month intervals for PSA and DRE; annual bone scan if indicated, Hgb and liver function tests (LFT) for monitoring status and potential progression
    EXPECTED COURSE
    - May be cured if detected and treated early; terminal if late staging

    COMPLICATIONS
    - Incontinence, erectile dysfunction, pain, pathologic fractures related to bone metastases, death

DISORDERS OF THE SCROTAL CONTENTS

Cryptochidism

Description
- Failure of one or both testicles to descend into the scrotum

Etiology
- Partial lack of or response to gonadotropic and androgenic hormones during fetal development (testes descend by 7th fetal month)
- Mechanical factors including elevated intra-abdominal pressure and retraction on the epididymis by the cremasteric muscles and gubernaculum
- May also have neural involvement
- Ectopic sites: Superficial inguinal canal (most common site), perineal (rare), femoral (rare), penile (rare), transverse or paradox descent (rare), pelvis (rare)

Incidence and Demographics
- 3%–4% full-term males, decreases to 0.8%–1.0% by 1 year of age
- 20%–30% of premature males; increased risk at lower gestation
- 6% of fathers of boys with undescended testicles had cryptorchidism; increased incidence in siblings
- 20% are nonpalpable, with 25% of those absent at surgical exploration
- Can be unilateral or bilateral

Risk Factors
- Prematurity or SGA (small for gestational age)
- Twins
- Family history

Prevention and Screening
- Careful examination during newborn exam and well-child visits: Important to document presence and position of testicle

Assessment
HISTORY
- Has parent noted both testicles in scrotum during bath or while changing diaper?
- Prematurity
- Family history of cryptorchidism

PHYSICAL EXAM
- Warm hands and the position of the patient (tailor position or sitting cross-legged, standing, or kneeling) may facilitate examination
- Examine scrotum: Testicles palpable and asymmetric size or nonpalpable; differentiate between retractile or true undescended (0.5%–1%)
- Position of testicle if palpable outside scrotum (ectopic)
- Check for hernias and hydroceles

DIAGNOSTIC STUDIES
- Various radiographic studies are utilized on an individualized basis: Selective gonadal venography, CT scan, ultrasound, MRI, and laparoscopy
- Lab studies: Urinary 17-ketosteriods, gonadotropins, and serum testosterone may help in tracing the cause
- Hormone stimulation test with HCG (human chorionic gonadotropin), questionable value
- Laparoscopic exam to locate abdominal testis: Also first and final step in surgical correction
- Chromosome analysis if bilateral (may be ambiguous genitalia)

Differential Diagnosis
- Retractile testicle
- Endocrine or chromosomal disorder
- Anorchia

Management
NONPHARMACOLOGIC TREATMENT
- Surgical correction: Orchiopexy or orchiectomy at 1 year; orchiopexy permits accessible examination to monitor for malignancy

PHARMACOLOGIC TREATMENT
- Hormone stimulation (hCG or GnRH) have variable results; may even be harmful to testes

When to Consult, Refer, Hospitalize
- Referral to a pediatric urologist at first diagnosis

Follow-Up
- Routine well-child visit schedule: Document presence of testicles, monitor for spontaneous resolution
  EXPECTED COURSE
  - 80% of retractile testicles descend by age 12 months

COMPLICATIONS
- Risks if not corrected: Testicular cancer 35–48 times more common, decreased fertility due to higher intra-abdominal temperature, cryptorchid testicle more prone to torsion, associated inguinal hernia in 25% of patients with maldescent, approximately 20% of males with unilateral undescended testis remain infertile even after an age-appropriate orchiopexy is performed

Hydrocele

Description
- A painless enlargement of the scrotum due to accumulation of clear fluid within the tunica vaginalis, surrounding the testicles. May be unilateral or bilateral.

Etiology
- True etiology is unknown
- Two types:
  - Communicating (associated with inguinal hernias): Incomplete closure of tunica vaginalis; fluid descends from the peritoneal cavity
  - Noncommunicating: Increased fluid production or decreased reabsorption within the scrotum; may be secondary to other scrotal disorders such as hernia, epididymitis, orchitis, tumors, trauma, or radiation

Incidence and Demographics
- Occur in 0.5%–1.0% of male population; approximately half coincide with a hernia
- Predominantly in childhood (up to 6% of male infants) but may occur at any age

Risk Factors
- Previous scrotal or genitourinary disorder (epididymitis, orchitis, trauma, testicular tumor)
- 50% associated with inguinal hernia
- Peritoneal dialysis

Prevention and Screening
- Prevention only by repairing inguinal hernia
- Examination of scrotum on well-child visits; periodic genital exam in adults

Assessment
HISTORY
- Sensation of heaviness and bulkiness of the scrotum
- Duration of symptoms, including presence during childhood, recent trauma or infection
- The absence of other symptoms such as fever, dysuria, pain, impotency, or altered urinary patterns aid in determining the diagnosis

PHYSICAL EXAM
- Nontender, scrotal firmness variable from soft to tense depending upon amount of fluid in the sac
- Pear-shaped, fluid-filled sac with the smaller pole superiorly, located usually behind the testicles
- May be unilateral or bilateral

DIAGNOSTIC STUDIES
- Transillumination: Transilluminates as translucent red glow with visible testicular shadow
- Doppler ultrasound is indicated if any doubt of the diagnosis, to rule out testicular torsion or cancer, particularly in a young male with sudden development and no apparent cause

Differential Diagnosis
- Varicocele
- Spermatocele
- Epididymitis
- Testicle trauma
- Hernia
- Tumor
- Cryptorchidism
- Orchitis
- Testicular torsion

Management
NONPHARMACOLOGIC TREATMENT
- Many hydroceles will resolve spontaneously during the first year of life
- Surgical correction is considered in cases of extreme size, discomfort, cosmetically bothersome, or if a hernia is present
- Drainage of the fluid is frequently followed by re-accumulation or infection, therefore not routinely done

Special Considerations
- Occurs with inguinal hernias

When to Consult, Refer, Hospitalize
- Referral to a urologist or surgeon is recommended if large
- Refer to urologist if persists past 6–8 months of age

Follow-Up
- Follow up initially every 3 months to assess for changes and determine if surgery is necessary
- Patients/parents monitor for symptoms (i.e., pain or changes in hydrocele size, contour, or weight, new symptoms)
  EXPECTED COURSE
  - Pediatric: Noncommunicating hydrocele present at birth usually resolves during first year of life
  - Adult: Hydrocele usually does not resolve on own, but may not need treatment

  COMPLICATIONS
  - For those with surgical treatment there is the potential for wound infections, hematoma, or hematocele

Spermatocele

Description
- A painless cyst in the scrotal sac containing milky fluid with sperm
- Most are small measuring <1 cm but size can be as large as 8–10 cm, which are easily mistaken for hydrocele

Etiology
- Unknown etiology
- Diverticulum in epididymis, leading to accumulation of spermatic fluid

Incidence and Demographics
- Incidence <1%

Risk Factors
- None

Prevention and Screening
- No prevention
- Periodic genital exam in adults

Assessment
HISTORY
- Often asymptomatic; often a random finding by the patient or examiner
- They may be similar to hydrocele in that the patient notes an increased bulk or weight to the scrotum and rarely can become twisted (torsion) or infected with subsequent symptoms of pain, edema, and warmth

PHYSICAL EXAM
- Spermatoceles are attached to the epididymis, located above and behind the testicle
- Palpable as round, mobile, and nontender cysts <1 cm
- There may be one or more present

DIAGNOSTIC STUDIES
- Transillumination will reveal the mass
- Ultrasound is indicated to clarify if any suspicion of cancer exists (age 18–35 with lump newly developed or sudden onset) or if thorough scrotal examination is hindered by the lump or edema

Differential Diagnosis
- Varicocele
- Hydrocele
- Tumor

Management, Special Considerations, Consultation and Follow-Up
- Same as hydrocele

Varicocele

Description
- Abnormal venous dilatation in the scrotum (varicose veins in the scrotum)

Etiology
- Etiology is unknown, however there are several theorized causes:
  - Incompetent valves in the scrotal veins
  - Increased hydrostatic pressure in the left renal vein, inferior vena cava, and internal spermatic veins
  - Increased mechanical pressure from the superior mesenteric artery
- **NOTE.** Right-sided varicoceles are rare and associated with obstruction of the right spermatic vein and retroperitoneal neoplasms.

Incidence and Demographics
- Affects 20% of the general male population
- Usually seen in older adolescents but can occur in any age group
- Almost always left-sided
- Can be associated with pathology in adult and prepubescent males

Risk Factors
- None

Prevention and Screening
- No prevention
- Monthly testicular self-exam (TSE) and periodic clinical genitalia exam in the adult male

Assessment
HISTORY
- Asymptomatic or a sense of heaviness or dull aching in the scrotum

PHYSICAL EXAM
- The characteristic presentation is a scrotum with a soft irregular mass that feels like a "bag of worms" located above and behind the testicle and epididymitis
- It is nontender, worsens in the standing position, and often improves in the reclining position
- Coughing or performing the Valsalva maneuver will accentuate the varicocele
- If only palpable during a Valsalva maneuver, it is graded I; if palpable on standing, it is graded II; and if visible on inspection alone, it is graded III
- 97% occur on the left side of the scrotum

DIAGNOSTIC STUDIES
- No testing may be needed to make the diagnosis in its classic presentation
- There are studies that are used to confirm the diagnosis, including ultrasound, thermography, echo-Doppler, and others; however, these are done when a referral to a urologist is indicated

Differential Diagnosis
- Hernia
- Epididymitis
- Hydrocele
- Spermatocele
- Tumor
- Epididymal cyst

Management

NONPHARMACOLOGIC TREATMENT
- Athletic supporters may provide increased comfort for patients with varicoceles
- Surgery to correct the blood flow may be an option depending on the grading of the varicoceles. Options include ligation, laparoscopic varicocelectomy, percutaneous varicocele occlusion, and others, and are done upon referral to an urologist or surgeon.

Special Considerations
- Right-sided varicocele is uncommon; can indicate retroperitoneal malignancy
- Sperm concentration and motility are significantly decreased in 65%–75% of patients. Infertility is often a result and can be reversed in a high percentage of patients by correction of the varicocele as soon as identified.

When to Consult, Refer, Hospitalize
- Referral is indicated for patients who have suspected infertility, a varicocele that doesn't disappear in the supine position and most importantly, if it occurs on the right side.

Follow-Up
- No firm guidelines; return if increase in pain, size, change in urinary patterns, pain with bowel movements, fever, warmth to scrotum, interference with sexual intercourse
- Early treatment and close monitoring for the younger patient (adolescents) may improve long-term fertility
- Annual exam is adequate for asymptomatic patients
- Post-procedure monitoring is indicated for recurrence of symptoms or development of complications

EXPECTED COURSE
- Variable and unpredictable
- Varicoceles have been found in 37% of patients with infertility, suggesting an association
- Not associated with sexual dysfunction or increased risk of testicular cancer

COMPLICATIONS
- Infertility
- Post-procedure complications such as wound infection

Epididymitis

Description
- An acute bacterial intrascrotal infection associated with painful enlargement of the epididymis
- Most cases of acute epididymitis are infectious and can be divided into two categories having different age distributions and causes:
  - Sexually transmitted forms typically occur in men <40 years, associated with urethritis, and result from *Chlamydia trachomatis* or *Neisseria gonorrhoeae*
  - Non-sexually transmitted forms typically occur in older men, associated with urinary tract infections and prostatitis, and caused by Gram-negative rods; the route of infection is probably via the urethra to the ejaculatory duct and then down the vas deferens to the epididymis

Etiology
- In the younger male (<35 years), STDs are the most common cause; primarily *C. trachomatis*, then *N. gonorrhoeae*
- In homosexual males practicing anal intercourse, *Escherichia coli* or *H. influenzae* is the common etiology; in heterosexual males >35, causative organisms are those associated with UTI
- Sterile epididymitis linked to vigorous physical activity (bicycle riding), trauma, and TB (rare causes)
- Gram-negative rods, *Escherichia coli*, *Pseudomonas aeruginosa*, or coliforms are common causes in men who have epididymitis that is associated with UTI (reflux of infected urine), who are over age 35, have had instrumentation, or have anatomic abnormalities

Incidence and Demographics
- The most common intrascrotal inflammation in males in the U.S.
- More than 600,000 healthcare visits/year

Risk Factors
- Exposure to STDs up to 30 days prior to onset of symptoms
- Anatomical abnormalities
- Instrumentation/surgery

Prevention and Screening
- Safe sex practices
- Antibiotics prior to instrumentation or urethral manipulation

Assessment
HISTORY
- Presents equally on the left or the right
- Testicular pain and edema that is commonly gradual in onset; symptoms may follow acute physical strain (heavy lifting), trauma, or sexual activity; associated symptoms of urethritis (pain at the tip of the penis and urethral discharge) or cystitis (irritative voiding symptoms) may occur; pain develops in the scrotum and may radiate along the spermatic cord or to the flank; on occasion, edema may double the size of the testicle in 3–4 hours

- Half of all cases present with fever, urethral discharge or voiding complaints; associated nausea and vomiting are unusual
- Explore the PMH for previous urinary symptoms or diagnoses, procedures, or instrumentation of the urinary tract, or trauma to the scrotum
- Explore the social history for information on new sexual partners, sexual practices, and use of scrotal support or protectors during sports

PHYSICAL EXAM
- Painful scrotal swelling radiating up spermatic cord, scrotal heaviness
- Epididymis is cord-like and palpable separately from the testicle; initially normal size, consistency, and position on exam, but later the two may appear as one enlarged, tender mass becoming less distinguishable with time
- Pain may be relieved by elevating the scrotum (Prehn's sign—elevation of the scrotum above the pubic symphysis improves pain from epididymitis) may be helpful but is not reliable
- Cremasteric reflex present (contraction of scrotum after light stroke to thigh) on affected side (differentiates epididymitis from testicular torsion)
- The prostate may be tender on rectal examination

DIAGNOSTIC STUDIES
- Gram stain of urethral exudate or intraurethral swab to diagnose gonococcal infection if present; culture of same specimen for N. *gonorrhoeae* and C. *trachomatis*, white cells without visible organisms on urethral smear represent nongonococcal urethritis, and C. *trachomatis* is the most likely pathogen
- Urinalysis, possible urine culture to diagnose concurrent UTI particularly in non-sexually transmitted types
- Syphilis serology; CBC shows leukocytosis
- HIV testing with counseling
- In addition, ultrasound of the scrotum or radionuclide scanning may be needed to rule out other possibilities

Differential Diagnosis
- Tumor
- Abscess
- Cyst
- Testicular torsion
- Testicular infarction
- Testicular cancer
- Mumps orchitis
- Hydrocele
- Varicocele

Management
NONPHARMACOLOGIC TREATMENT
- Bedrest
- Scrotal elevation (place a folded towel under genitals across thighs)
- Avoidance of sexual activity and physical strain until resolved

PHARMACOLOGIC TREATMENT
- Initiate treatment empirically, before culture results are available (see Table 12–5)
- Treat sexual partners if likely due to STD and contact was within last 60 days preceding symptoms

Table 12–5. Pharmacologic Treatment of Epididymitis

Indication	Medication
Age <35 with high likelihood of N. *Gonorrhoeae* **OR** C. *Trachomatis*	Ceftriaxone (Rocephin) 250 mg IM single dose **AND** Doxycycline 100 mg po bid x 10 days
Age >35 with high likelihood of enteric organisms **OR** Allergies to cephalosporins or tetracycline	Ofloxacin (Floxin) 300 mg po bid x 10 days
Fever and inflammation	Analgesics (e.g., NSAID, acetaminophen)

LENGTH OF TREATMENT
- Until fever and local inflammation have subsided, bedrest and elevation of scrotum should be maintained; antibiotic therapy should be continued for 10 days

Special Considerations
- Differentiate from other cause of acute scrotal pain, testicular torsion

When to Consult, Refer, Hospitalize
- Referral to urologist is indicated for the patient who is not improving within 3 days, or has worsening symptoms

Follow-Up
- In 72 hours to ensure that infection is resolving
  EXPECTED COURSE
  - Failure to improve within 3 days requires reevaluation of both the diagnosis and therapy
  - Swelling and tenderness that persist after completion of antimicrobial therapy should be re-evaluated, noting that swelling may take weeks to months to resolved

COMPLICATIONS
- Prompt treatment usually results in a favorable outcome; delayed or inadequate treatment may result in:
  - Epididymo-orchitis
  - Chronic pain (chronic epididymitis)
  - Abscess formation
  - Infertility (possibly up to 50% if bilateral)
  - Testicular atrophy

Testicular Torsion

Description
- Spermatic cord compression by twisting of the spermatic cord within the scrotum, resulting in compromised blood flow to the testicles. Constitutes a surgical emergency to prevent necrotic testicle.

Etiology
- Congenital anatomically abnormal free-floating testicle without fixation in the scrotum, which twists around blood supply to testicle, resulting in ischemia and potential infarction of the testicle
- May be precipitated by trauma, sudden movements that pull on the cremasteric muscle (jumping into cold water, riding bicycle), sexual activity, cold, exercise
- May occur when contents of scrotum shift in the relaxed state during sleep

Incidence and Demographics
- Most commonly occurs in those age 12–18, but can occur at any age; 1 in 4,000 in those <25 years old
- 40% occur during sleep

Risk Factors
- Age
- Paraplegics

Prevention and Screening
- No prevention except surgical correction of defect if discovered
- High index of suspicion in young male with acute scrotal pain

Assessment
HISTORY
- Typically present with sudden onset, acute, profound pain that is localized to the testicles or radiating to the groin and lower abdomen, nausea and vomiting in 50% of patients
- No dysuria, fever, or urethral discharge; no irritative voiding symptoms
- A quick history should explore precipitating events (e.g., exercise, sleep, cold exposure), current medical history and medications, sexual partners, STD exposure
- Torsion of the testicular appendage (not entire testicle) presents with less severe pain, more gradual onset of symptoms, and is not a surgical emergency

PHYSICAL EXAM
- Typically lying still, in acute distress
- Acute tenderness, edema, and erythema of the testicle, spreading to the entire scrotum
- Testicle is horizontal, elevated in the scrotum, with a negative cremasteric reflex
- Prehn's sign is negative (no relief with elevating testicle above pubic symphysis)
- Epididymis very tender, out of normal position due to twisting of spermatic cord
- If only the testicular appendage is twisted, there will be a "blue dot" sign at the superior aspect of the testicle—a small, palpable lump on superior pole of the epididymis when skin pulled taut

DIAGNOSTIC STUDIES
- Immediate surgical treatment is begun in unequivocal cases; consider risk of time lost for testing vs. preservation of testicle
- Urinalysis to quickly rule out infectious component in differentiating diagnosis
- Doppler ultrasound with color is the best; radionuclide scrotal imaging also used

Differential Diagnosis
- Epididymitis
- Torsion of testicular appendage
- Trauma
- Orchitis
- Hernia (incarcerated or strangulated)

Management
- An acute urological emergency can result in loss of the testicle
- 80% salvage rate of testicle if corrected within 4 hours; only 20% if within 12 hours
  NONPHARMACOLOGIC TREATMENT
    - Pre-operatively, elevate the scrotum, apply ice pack
    - Manual reduction followed by surgical treatment (orchidopexy)

Special Considerations
- Advise patients that both testicles will be surgically secured within the scrotum to prevent reoccurrence and that there is a risk of decreased fertility or infertility

When to Refer, Consult, Hospitalize
- NOTE. Immediate surgical consult

Follow-Up
- The surgeon follows up with the patient 1–2 weeks post-op
- Annual visits to evaluate atrophy of testicles, particularly prior to puberty
  EXPECTED COURSE
    - Potential outcomes depend on timing of treatment. The testicle may be gangrenous and removed, saved but atrophied, or minimally affected; atrophy of the twisted testicle or the unaffected testicle may occur, affecting spermatogenesis and fertility but testosterone production is unchanged

  COMPLICATIONS
    - Impaired fertility
    - Atrophy of the salvaged testicle in up to two-thirds of patients within 2–3 years

Testicular Cancer

Description
- Carcinoma of the testicles that is categorized as germinal or nongerminal

Etiology
- While the cause of testicular cancer is unknown, both congenital and acquired factors have been associated with tumor development. The strongest association has been with cryptorchid testis. Approximately 7%–10% of testicular tumors develop in patients who have a history of cryptorchidism. Seminoma is the most common form of tumor rising from this condition.

Incidence and Demographics
- Testicular cancer is rare in children, but 66% of testicular tumors in children are malignant
- 1%–2% of all male cancers, 2nd most common cancer of males age 20–34
- Germinal tumors account for 95% of all cases and are subcategorized as seminomatous (one-third to one-half) or nonseminomatous
- Leydig cell neoplasms account for 5%
- Most commonly occurs in 20–40 year age group but also in >60 and childhood

Risk Factors
- White, higher social class, rural resident, and unmarried
- Undescended testicles (cryptorchidism) or family history
- Klinefelter syndrome
- Exposure to intrapartum estrogen (diethylstilbestrol [DES])

Prevention and Screening
- Teach adolescent males to do regular TSE
- Teach adolescent males to tell parents about any abnormal findings and seek treatment
- Annual clinical screening, testicular self-exam
- Screen patients with risk factors

Assessment
HISTORY
- Frequently incidental finding on routine exam or patient notes painless swelling, sense of heaviness or thickening in scrotum or testicle
- Testicles may be tender, especially if associated with bleeding within the tumor, or if epididymitis is present concurrently
- Associated symptoms reflective of metastasis: Gynecomastia; supraclavicular lymphadenopathy; abdominal or neck mass; pain in the groin, flank, or back
- Less than 10% with seminomal tumor have symptoms of distant metastases at time of diagnosis
- Inquire about medications and past medical history, particularly relating to the associated symptoms

PHYSICAL EXAM
- Scrotal exam reveals hydrocele in up to 20% of patients with testicular cancer
- Tumors are often found on the lower pole, but can be anywhere on the testicles
- Tumors are firm, +/- tender, one or more present, on one or both testicles
- Transillumination will not reveal the normal rosy glow; there is darkness of the tumor
- Inguinal lymphadenopathy may or may not be present

DIAGNOSTIC STUDIES
- Serum alpha-fetoprotein reflects presence of nonseminomatous germ cell tumors
- Serum beta-human chorionic gonadotropin (b-hCG) positive in 70%–100% of seminomatous testicular carcinoma
- Ultrasound distinguishes between most of the differential diagnoses
- Staging determined with chest x-ray, CT scan, pedal lymphangiography

Differential Diagnosis
- Inguinal hernias
- Epididymitis
- Orchitis, hematomas
- Hydrocele
- Spermatocele

Management
- Treatment is dictated by the type of tumor, staging, and associated symptoms
  NONPHARMACOLOGIC TREATMENT
  - Seminomas: Radiation and orchiectomy
  - Nonseminomatous: Surgery, radiation, and combination chemotherapy
  - Metastasized cancer is treated with both radiation and chemotherapy

  PHARMACOLOGIC TREATMENT
  - Chemotherapy directed by the oncologist

  LENGTH OF TREATMENT
  - Directed by the oncologist

Special Considerations
- Testicular cancer in older patients most likely metastatic, usually lymphoma

When to Consult, Refer, Hospitalize
- Pediatric: All testicular masses or tumors should be referred to a pediatric urologist and oncologist
- Adult: All undiagnosed testicular masses should be referred to urologist
- Management and follow-up is directed by the oncologist

Follow-Up
  EXPECTED COURSE
  - Localized seminomatous cancer has 5-year survival rate of nearly 100%
  - Disseminated disease 5-year survival is 20%
  - Nonseminomatous germ cell tumors treated aggressively have a 5-year survival rate of 60%–90%

COMPLICATIONS
- Metastases to lung and abdomen
- Side effects of treatment (radiation, chemotherapy)
- Post-op wound infection, urinary tract infections related to instrumentation

PENILE DISORDERS

Phimosis

Description
- An inability to retract the foreskin of an uncircumcised penis that has formerly been retractable
- Paraphimosis occurs when foreskin is retracted and remains proximal to the glans, constricting the glans penis

Etiology
- Occurs when the orifice of the prepuce is too small to allow retraction of the foreskin
- Most cases occur in uncircumcised males, although excessive skin left after circumcision can become stenotic and cause phimosis
- Acquired from trauma, prior infection, or poor hygiene (retained smegma and dirt) that results in inflammation and the development of adhesions
- Can be physiologic until age 7–10 years
- Foreskin is physiologically adherent to the glans in the newborn. In the uncircumcised, male the foreskin naturally separates as the boy gets older; forcible retraction can cause scarring.
- Geriatric patients may develop phimosis with use of condom catheters

Incidence and Demographics
- Age 16 or older have 1% incidence
- Adolescence is predominant age of occurrence

Risk Factors
- Uncircumcised penis
- Poor hygiene
- Trauma
- Infection of the glans (balanitis) or prepuce (posthitis)

Prevention and Screening
- Teach parents proper care of uncircumcised penis; no need to retract until foreskin does so naturally
- Examine foreskin at routine well-child visits
- Hygiene of the genitalia with retraction of the foreskin during washing

Assessment
HISTORY
- Inability to retract foreskin when it was previously retractable
- Ballooning of the foreskin with urination
- Urinary tract infection

- Painful urination
- Patients may be asymptomatic, with phimosis discovered on examination
- When related to an infectious or inflammatory process, patient complains of irritation and tenderness of the glans, discomfort with voiding, or pain on erection
- NOTE: If severe enough, outflow of urine may be compromised, presenting as a urological emergency

PHYSICAL EXAM
- The glans is nonretractable and the prepuce is pallid, striated, and thickened
- If actively infected, there will be erythema, smegma, and/or exudate and tenderness
- In paraphimosis, there will be swelling and/or edema of the glans

DIAGNOSTIC STUDIES
- None

Differential Diagnosis
- Penile trauma
- Balanitis

Management
NONPHARMACOLOGIC TREATMENT
- Teach parents appropriate care of uncircumcised penis: gentle retraction only as far as foreskin will easily move
- Treatment of the underlying cause such as infection or inflammation with good hygiene, sitz baths, and warm compresses
- Surgical release or circumcision

PHARMACOLOGIC TREATMENT
- If concurrent infection or inflammation, treatment with topical antifungals or steroids may be sufficient to allow for retraction
- Use of a triple antibiotic ointment (Neosporin or Bacitracin or the generic brand) applied to the tip of the foreskin can act as a protective barrier to fecal contamination

LENGTH OF TREATMENT
- Topical treatment for underlying infection or inflammation for 1–2 weeks

Special Considerations
- Phimosis is normal in uncircumcised males; however, once foreskin is retractible, it is not normal for it to spontaneously adhere again.

When to Consult, Refer, Hospitalize
- Refer to urologist for surgical release or circumcision if nonresponsive to topical treatment and hygiene, urinary flow is compromised, or asymptomatic phimosis remains
- Paraphimosis can be a surgical emergency, should be referred to urologist for circumcision

Follow-Up

EXPECTED COURSE

- Resolves with treatment

COMPLICATIONS

- If there is associated infectious precipitant, complications such as meatal stenosis, UTI, or premalignant changes may occur

Erectile Dysfunction

Description

- The inability to achieve or maintain a satisfactory erection more than 25%–50% of the time (although it may be defined by patients as premature ejaculation or the loss of orgasm, emission, libido, or erections)

Etiology

- Psychological origin is likely with loss of orgasm when libido and erection are intact, and with premature ejaculation concurrent with anxiety, depression, relationship problems, new partner, or emotional disorders
- Medications such as anabolic steroids, digoxin (Lanoxin), cimetidine (Tagamet), centrally acting antihypertensives (reserpine, clonidine, methyldopa) beta-blockers and spironolactone (loss of libido), anti-depressants (MAO inhibitors, tricyclics, SSRIs)
- Lifestyle issues of alcohol, drug, and cigarette use
- A gradual loss of erections over time is indicative of organic causes
  - Hormonal and endocrine disorders of the thyroid, hypogonadism, kidney, pituitary gland or testicular function, diabetes, Addison's disease, and Cushing syndrome
  - Vascular disorders such as hypertension, arterial insufficiency, venous disease, atherosclerosis
  - Neurologic disorders, structural problems, spinal cord injury, and posttreatment of prostate disorders

Incidence and Demographics

- Widely unreported, estimated that 10% of the male population affected; 10–20 million men in the U.S.

Risk Factors

- Medication use
- Concurrent disease
- Use or abuse of alcohol, cigarettes, and drugs
- Lifestyle with high levels of stress or relationship problems

Assessment

HISTORY

- Determine the patient's perception or definition of erectile dysfunction (impotence) to clarify the problem and symptoms, the timing, circumstances, and frequency of occurrence
- Determine the nature of the patient's relationship, sexual partners, lifestyle, and stress

- Complaints include any of the following: reduced size and strength of erection, lack of ability to achieve or maintain erections adequate for intercourse, rapid loss of erection with penetration, or lack of libido
- Inquire if there are nocturnal or morning erections, as their presence reflect an intact blood supply, nervous system, and sexual apparatus and reduce the likelihood of organic cause
- Associated symptoms indicative of underlying disease: decreased body hair; gynecomastia; neuropathies; anxiety; headaches; vision changes; decreased circulation; excessive dryness or skin changes; changes in testicles' size, consistency, or shape; and changes in penis such as rash, discharge, or phimosis
- Review past medical history for other diseases, testicular infections or insults, medications (Rx, OTC, and herbal), and history of smoking, drug, alcohol use

PHYSICAL EXAM
- A complete screening physical noting general appearance, generalized anxiety or hyperactivity, vital signs for postural hypotension, dry hair, loss of secondary sex characteristics, spider angiomas, hyperpigmentation, palmar erythema, or goiter
- Chest, abdomen, and extremities for cardiac abnormalities, gynecomastia, aortic or femoral bruits, peripheral vascular deficits
- Genital examination for penile circulation, discharge, fibrosis or lesions; testicles for size, masses, varicoceles or atrophy; DRE for prostate abnormalities, sphincter tone
- Neurologic screening for cortical, brainstem, spinal or peripheral neuropathies, noting especially bulbocavernosi reflex, cremasteric reflex, pinprick or light touch to genital and perianal area, focal tenderness of spine, vision abnormalities

DIAGNOSTIC STUDIES
- Key studies to screen for underlying etiology begin with plasma glucose, prolactin, and free testosterone, CBC, urinalysis, and lipid profile
- If testicular atrophy is suspected, include luteinizing hormone and follicle-stimulating hormone
- If hypothyroidism is suspected, measure TSH
- Other tests are added depending on findings of history and physical and results of preliminary tests
- Nocturnal penile tumescence and rigidity testing
- Urologist may include duplex ultrasonography, penile angiography, nerve conduction studies, or a trial injection of prostaglandin E1, phentolamine, and papaverine intracorporeally to assess vascular integrity, noting penile response

Differential Diagnosis
- Endocrine origin:
  - Altered thyroxine
  - Testosterone
  - Prolactin
  - Insulin
  - Estrogen levels
- Neurologic origin:
  - Cortical
  - Brainstem

- Spinal cord
- Peripheral neuropathies
- Psychological:
  - Anxiety
  - Depression
  - Schizophrenia
  - Personality/relationship problems
- Vascular origin:
  - Arterial insufficiency
  - Venous insufficiency
  - Cavernosal insufficiency
- Structural:
  - Peyronie's disease
  - Microphallus
  - Hypospadias
  - Scarring
  - Trauma
- Other:
  - Medication side effects
  - Renal failure
  - Zinc deficiency

Management

NONPHARMACOLOGIC TREATMENT
- Modify lifestyle: Stress reduction techniques; stop alcohol, drugs and smoking
- Use of vacuum constriction device for those with venous disorders of the penis or nonresponsiveness to vasoactive injections
- Surgical treatment

PHARMACOLOGIC TREATMENT
- Sildenafil (Viagra): 25–50 mg 1 hour prior to desired erection (works within 30 min–4 hours). Dose variable, dependent upon concurrent disease, age; may go up to 100 mg/day. Contraindicated for patient taking nitrites; used cautiously with unstable angina and history of stroke, MI. Side effects: Headache, flushing, nasal congestion from vasodilation; abnormalities in vision (color changes, light sensitivity, blurred vision), priapism.
- Tadalafil (Cialis): 10–20 mg 30 minutes before sex; may provide longer action (up to 36 hours)
- Vardenafil (Levitra): 20 mg 1 hour before sexual activity; claims faster onset, fewer adverse effects
- Other oral agents controversial, include yohimbine, trazodone (Desyrel), gingko biloba
- Substitute or discontinue medications known to cause erectile dysfunction
  - Alternative antihypertensives include calcium channel blockers, angiotensin-converting enzyme (ACE) inhibitors, selective beta-blockers (atenolol)
  - Trial of antidepressants other than tricyclics (nortriptyline, desipramine)
  - Substitute ranitidine (Zantac) or other H2 blocker for cimetidine (Tagamet)

- Treat abnormal hormones as follows:
  - Insufficient testosterone treated with a 3-month testosterone trial (if indicated by androgen deficiency and patient does not have prostatic cancer), using testosterone injections 200 mg IM q 3 weeks or topical patches of 2.5–6 mg/day
  - Hyperprolactinemia is treated with bromocriptine (Parlodel) initially 2.5 mg bid, up to 40 mg/d
- Penile injections such as alprostadil (Caverject) first dose in office setting 1.25–2.5 mcg with repeat dose after 1 hour if no response. Patient to remain in office until detumescence completed. Partial response may have second injection in 24 hours.
- Alternatives to alprostadil are papaverine or phentolamine
- Urethral suppository of alprostadil (Muse) in various strength pellets

LENGTH OF TREATMENT
- Variable depending on treatment methods

Special Considerations
- Reasons for seeking care and etiology are age-related
- Age adolescence to 30: Concerns are often psychological or gender-related, as well as with primary organic origin
- Age 50–60 with relationship problems; most concerned about medical problems
- Age 70+ rarely seek help, most likely have physical problems
- Use of injections or oral agents require thorough patient teaching on proper use, frequency of use, side effects, and risk of priapism, and when to seek medical help, such as erection lasting >6 hours

When to Consult, Refer, Hospitalize
- Psychotherapist for individual or couples therapy, sex therapy
- Urologist, endocrinologist, cardiologist, neurologist referrals as indicated by diagnosis and requirements for further evaluation or advanced treatment

Follow-Up
- Follow-up is varied depending on diagnosis, underlying etiology, response to treatment, and need for therapy. Patients should be seen initially at shorter intervals to adjust and monitor responsiveness to treatment, then every 3 months.
  EXPECTED COURSE
  - Improvement in many patients with oral medications, vacuum devices, suppository, and penile implants; 15% spontaneously improve
  - 20% failure rate with vacuum device, 10%–30% dissatisfaction with penile implants
  - Alprostadil injections have an 85%–90% response rate, while the urethral suppository method rates are 40%–60%; oral agent sildenafil is effective for 70% of patients at maximal dose

  COMPLICATIONS
  - Variable depending on underlying etiology and treatment method side effects; these include priapism, penile bruising, hypotension, headache, flushing, nausea, side effects of testosterone (urinary retention, acne, vomiting), penile pain and irritation, and testicular pain

CASE STUDIES

Case 1. A 17-year-old male is brought to your office by his mother complaining of several days of unilateral testicular pain and swelling thought to be caused by injury while wrestling with a friend. The patient is reluctant to give more information.

    1. How can you elicit more information from this patient?
    2. What additional information would you like?

Exam: Edematous, tender hemi-scrotum with indistinguishable, tender epididymis; positive Prehn's sign; positive cremasteric reflex; no urethral discharge; temp 101°F.

    3. Can testicular torsion be ruled out?
    4. What is the most likely diagnosis?
    5. Is diagnostic testing necessary to initiate treatment?
    6. What additional intervention is needed?

Case 2. Parents bring in their 1-week-old, full-term male infant, reporting that his penis is red and swollen. He has been crying continuously since his bath several hours ago. Previously, the baby had been healthy; nursing well, gaining weight.
 HPI: Previously healthy baby has been crying for several hours.

    1. What additional history would you like?

Exam: The exam is unremarkable except for moderately edematous and reddened glans penis with retracted prepuce.

    2. What is the differential diagnosis?
    3. How would you treat this patient?
    4. What follow-up is necessary?
    5. What infant care teaching do parents need?

Case 3. A 67-year-old retired postal worker presents with a 3-month history of difficulty urinating. He denies urinary burning, hematuria, foul-smelling urine, and abdominal pain. He does complain of hesitancy, dribbling, and retention.
PMH: No history of UTIs, prostate trouble, or renal disease. Worked as mail carrier for 30 years. Has been sedentary since retirement 5 years ago. HTN identified 3 years ago, treated until about 1 year ago when he felt better so did not return for follow up. Does not smoke, drinks 3–4 beers several days a week.

    1. What additional history would you like?

Exam: BP 168/102, pulse 72 regular, afebrile. Abdomen nontender with no bladder distension, no CVA tenderness. DRE: Good sphincter tone, prostate smooth, firm, nontender with obliteration of median sulcus.

2. What diagnostic tests would you perform?
3. What does the clinician need to know regarding the indicated diagnostic test necessary for this patient?
4. Can you make a diagnosis?
5. What is your treatment plan?
6. What follow-up and screening recommendations would you give this patient?

REFERENCES

Aja, S. G., & Nayak, S. H. (2004). Sildenafil: Emerging cardiovascular indications. *Annals of Thoracic Surgery, 78*(4), 1496–1506.

Behrman, R. (2004). *Nelson's textbook of pediatrics* (17th ed.). Philadelphia: W..B. Saunders Company.

Buttaro, T. M., Trybulski, J., Bailey, P. P., & Sandberg-Cook, J. (2008) *Primary care: A collaborative practice* (3rd ed.). St. Louis, MO: Mosby.

Carson, C. C. (2004). Erectile dysfunction: Evaluation and new treatment options. *Psychosomatic Medicine, 55*(5), 664–671.

Centers for Disease Control and Prevention. (2006). Sexually transmitted diseases treatment guidelines, 2006. *MMWR: Morbidity and Mortality Weekly Report, 55*, No. RR-11. Retrieved April 3, 2008, from http://www.cdc.gov/mmwr/PDF/rr/rr5511.pdf

Chapple, C. R. (2004). Pharmacological therapy of benign prostatic hyperplasia/lower urinary tract symptoms: An overview for the practicing clinician. *British Journal Urology International, 94*(5), 738–744.

Dambro, M. R. (2008). *The 5-minute clinical consult.* St. Louis, MO: Lippincott Williams & Wilkins.

Edmunds, M. W., & Mayhew, M. S. (2004). *Pharmacology for the primary care provider* (2nd ed.). St. Louis, MO: Mosby.

Ferri, F. F. (2008). *Ferri's clinical advisor instant diagnosis and treatment.* St. Louis, MO: Mosby.

Gilbert, D. N., Moellering, R. C., & Se, M. A. (2007). *Sanford guide to antimicrobial therapy* (37th ed.). Vienna, VA: Antimicrobial Therapy, Inc.

Goroll, A., & Mulley, A. (2006) *Primary care medicine* (5th ed.). Philadelphia: Lippincott, Williams & Wilkins.

Hatcher, R., Trussell, J., Stewart, F., Stewart, G., Kowal, D., Guest, F., et al. (2008). *Contraceptive technology* (19th ed. rev.). New York: Ardent Media Trade, Inc.

Neinstein, L., Gordon, C., & Katzman, D. (2007). *Adolescent health care: A practical guide* (5th ed.). Philadelphia: Lippincott Williams & Wilkins.

Porche, D. (2005). Prostate cancer: Screening and early detection. *Journal for nurse practitioners, 1*(2), 70–71.

Porche, D. J. (2006). Men's health: Prostatitis. *Journal for Nurse Practitioners, 2*(10), 662–663.

Rosenberg, M. T. (2007). Diagnosis and management of erectile dysfunction in the primary care setting. *International Journal of Clinical Practice, 61*(7), 1198–1208.

Tanagho, E. A., & McAninch, J. W. (2008). *Smith's general urology* (17th ed.). New York: McGraw-Hill.

Tierney, L. M., McPhee, S. J., & Papadakis, A. (2007). *Current medical diagnosis and treatment* (47th ed.). New York: McGraw-Hill.

Uphold, C., & Graham, M. V. (2003). *Clinical guidelines in family practice* (4th ed.). Gainesville, FL: Barmarrae Books.

U.S. Preventive Services Task Force. (2006). Guide to clinical preventive services, *2006: Recommendations of the U.S. Preventive Services Task Force* (2nd/3rd ed.). Philadelphia: Lippincott Williams & Wilkins.

Wein, A. (2007). *Campbell-Walsh urology* (9th ed.). Philadelphia: W. B. Saunders.

Sexually Transmitted Diseases

Mary Ann Krisman-Scott, RN, PhD, FNP-BC

GENERAL APPROACH

Sexually transmitted diseases (STDs) are also known as sexually transmitted infections.

Prevention
- Counsel the adolescent or adult patient regarding sexual abstinence, the only flawless method of prevention; followed by mutual monogamy.
- Consistent use of the male latex condom is highly protective if used consistently and correctly (see Chapter 12).
- Use of female condoms and other barrier methods of contraception for women may be somewhat protective for some, but not all, STDs.
- Safer sex practices are aimed at reducing risk for patients at highest risk through partner reduction and avoidance of certain practices to reduce risk of HIV transmission (see Chapter 4).
- A quadrivalent vaccine against HPV types 6, 11, 16, 18 is recommended for females ages 9–26.

Risk Assessment
- Risk assessments and screening tests help reduce the incidence of STD and must be done on every sexually active adult and adolescent patient.
- Adolescents are at a higher risk for STDs.
- Obtain accurate, detailed history from patients to determine risk for STDs. Most people do not know they are infected with an STD and underestimate their own risk level. Ask specific questions regarding type of sexual exposure in "lay terms" in order to obtain accurate information. Maintain confidentiality by asking partners and parents to leave the room. No parental consent needed for adolescent to seek treatment for STD, the age of consent for adolescents varies by state.

- High-risk factors for STD: Current STD(s) including HIV, history of STD(s); multiple sexual partners (or a new partner); individual who exchanges sex for money or drugs; drug user or partner of drug user; homosexual or bisexual men and their partners; lack of consistent use of barrier contraceptives.

Screening

- Routine steps for all sexually active (ever) women and men.
  - Explain context: "We review this information and screen all patients because many people with infections do not have symptoms and therefore have no idea that testing might be needed. Routine review is recommended by the CDC."
  - Give prevention information and encourage wise decisions and prevention behavior
  - Review personal history for high-risk behaviors
  - Provide Pap smears annually or more frequently depending on previous Pap, history, and risk
  - Provide annual *Chlamydia* test for men and women <25 years (urine or swab)
  - Provide annual gonorrhea test if in area of high GC prevalence and age <25 years
  - If in area with high syphilis prevalence and age <25 years, or high-risk behavior, initial syphilis serology
  - Explain importance of screening because many STDs are asymptomatic
- Routine steps for high-risk women and men should include offer and encourage HIV testing, review history, and provide hepatitis B vaccination.
- Patients with known STD exposure or symptoms should be cultured from areas of exposure/penetration (e.g., anal, vaginal, oral pharyngeal, penile/urethral); culture first, then treat.
- Routine screening in pregnant women in first trimester should include syphilis serologic test, hepatitis B antigen, GC, and <25 years (high-risk); offer HIV test, Pap smear. Repeat screening for high-risk women in third trimester or at delivery: syphilis, hepatitis B antigen, GC and *Chlamydia*, bacterial vaginosis (BV).

Management

- Follow Centers for Disease Control and Prevention 2006 and 2007 updates on treatment guidelines for gonoccal infections for evaluation and management of all STDs.
- Patients who are likely not to return for follow-up, consider empiric treatment with CDC-recommended one-dose regimen when appropriate.
- Patients treated for STD should be counseled to have their sexual partners evaluated and treated.
- Sexually active patients should be counseled regarding dual protection against unintended pregnancy and STDs. The male latex condom is effective in providing dual protection if used correctly.

Red Flags

- Consult, refer, or hospitalize with unusual presentation of STD; serious complications such as pelvic inflammatory disease (PID), pregnancy, HIV infection, recurrent infection, if patient unable to tolerated oral medication, allergy to medication.
- Refer to infectious disease specialist for pregnant women with hepatitis B virus (HBV), primary cytomegalovirus (CMV), primary genital herpes, or Group B streptococcal infection, and women with syphilis and allergic to penicillin.
- STD in pediatric or adolescent population, suspect child abuse.

• If patient reports sexual assault, consult local law authorities regarding procedures for obtaining evidence. Test for *Trichomonas vaginalis*, bacterial vaginosis, yeast, *Chlamydia*, GC, HIV, hepatitis B, and syphilis. Empiric antimicrobial regimen for *Chlamydia*, gonorrhea, *Trichomonas*, and BV suggested as well as prophylactic treatment for hep B, pregnancy testing, and emergency contraception, if indicated.

INFECTIONS THAT CAUSE VAGINITIS AND CERVICITIS IN WOMEN AND URETHRITIS IN MEN

Trichomoniasis

Description
• An inflammatory process of the vagina, cervix, and vulva in women and lower genitourinary tract in men caused by a flagellate protozoan

Etiology
• Causative organism is *Trichomonas vaginalis*
• Usually sexually transmitted; *rarely* transmitted by fomites
• Men can be asymptomatic carriers

Incidence and Demographics
• Estimated 6 million women and partners infected annually

Risk Factors
• Risk factors listed under General Approach

Prevention and Screening
• Prevention listed in General Approach
• No routine screening

Assessment
HISTORY
  • Incubation period is 4–20 days with an average of 1 week

  Women
  • May be asymptomatic
  • Severe pruritus, malodorous, profuse, gray-yellow or green vaginal discharge
  • Dysuria, dyspareunia, postcoital spotting, possible menorrhagia and dysmenorrhea
  • Onset of symptoms following menses

  Men
  • Usually asymptomatic
  • Dysuria, clear penile discharge, slight penile itching

PHYSICAL EXAM
  Women
  • May have inguinal adenopathy
  • External genitalia may be irritated from scratching
  • Vulva is erythematous and edematous

- Introitus, urethra, vagina, cervix are coated with profuse malodorous, frothy, gray-yellow or green discharge
- Cervix or vagina has petechiae or strawberry patches appearance (characteristic)

Men
- Slight penile erythema with clear discharge

DIAGNOSTIC STUDIES
Women
- Saline wet mount of vaginal discharge to identify motile trichomonads
- Vaginal pH >4.5; Pap smear sometimes shows trichomonads
- Potassium hydroxide (KOH) wet mount: to rule out Candida albicans; positive whiff test (fishy odor) when KOH applied in B.V.

Men
- Microscopic exam of urine (first void in morning) positive for trichomonads

Differential Diagnosis
- Bacterial vaginosis
- Vulvovaginal candidiasis
- Gonorrhea
- Pelvic inflammatory disease (PID)
- *Chlamydia trachomatis*

Management
NONPHARMACOLOGIC TREATMENT
- Concurrent treatment of sex partners
- Patients and sex partners should avoid sex until treatment completed and asymptomatic
- Screen for other STDs
- Avoid alcohol with metronidazole and for 72 hours after due to disulfiram-like reaction (severe nausea and vomiting)

PHARMACOLOGIC TREATMENT
- First treatment choice: metronidazole (Flagyl) 2 g po as single dose or Tinadazole (Tindamax) 2 g po as a single dose
- Alternative: metronidazole (Flagyl) 500 mg po bid

LENGTH OF TREATMENT
- Single dose or 7-day regimen; if regimen fails and patient remains symptomatic, retreat with metronidazole (Flagyl) 500 mg po bid for 7 more days or Tinidzaole (Tindamax) 2 g in a single dose; if there is frequent treatment failure, treat with metronidazole (Flagyl) 2 g po daily for 3–5 days; consider culture for possible resistant stain of *T. vaginalis*

Special Considerations
- Pregnancy: Metronidazole 2 g po in a single dose.
- Allergy to metronidazole: There is no effective alternative; clotrimazole may inhibit growth of *T. vaginalis* but does not eradicate it.

When to Consult, Refer, Hospitalize
- Consult on refractory cases not responding to treatment in 2 weeks

Follow-Up
- None indicated if asymptomatic following treatment
- Evaluate the patient's sex partner
    - EXPECTED COURSE
        - Response prompt, although symptoms will return with re-infection

    - COMPLICATIONS
        - Nausea or vomiting from oral metronidazole, disulfiram-like reaction from ingestion of alcohol and metronidazole, vulvovaginal candidiasis infection following 7-day treatment course
        - The disease is associated with preterm labor and premature rupture of membranes
        - Pelvic inflammatory disease, bartholinitis, skenitis, cystitis

Gonorrhea

Description
- A sexually transmitted bacterial disease caused by *Neisseria gonorrhoeae*

Etiology
- *Neisseria gonorrhoeae* is a Gram-negative diplococci present in exudate and secretions of infected mucous secretions occurring only in humans
- Causes localized inflammatory conditions: Urethritis, epididymitis, proctitis, cervicitis, bartholinitis, pelvic inflammatory disease (salpingitis and/or endometritis), and pharyngitis of adults; vulvovaginitis of children; and conjunctivitis of the newborn and adults; presence in children almost always a result child sexual abuse
- Gonococcal bacteremia results in the disseminated systemic condition, arthritis-dermatitis syndrome sometimes associated with endocarditis or meningitis

Incidence and Demographics
- Transmission through intimate contact such as sexual intercourse; also parturition
- 60%–90% of women become infected following exposure
- Greatest incidence in sexually active 15–29-year-olds
- Approximately 15% of infected women may develop PID with possible sterility if untreated
- Most infections in men have symptoms that cause them to seek treatment before serious outcome. Many infected women do not have symptoms until complications present.
- Common sites in women are urethra, endocervix, upper genital tract, pharynx, and rectum
- Common sites in men are the urethra, epididymis, prostate, rectum, and pharynx

Risk Factors
- Risk factors listed under General Approach
- Homosexual males have 10 times greater incidence

Prevention and Screening
- Prevention methods listed under General Approach

- Screen sexually active men and women <25 years if in an area of high GC prevalence
- Screen all pregnant women at initial prenatal visit and again early in third trimester
- Prophylactic treatment to contacts of infectious patients

Assessment
HISTORY
- Incubation is short; urethritis is 2–5 days, cervicitis is 5–10 days
- Women: Often asymptomatic; dysuria, frequency, purulent urethral discharge, vaginal discharge, pelvic pain, spotting or abnormal menses; adolescent girls often have dissemination/progression within a week of menses
- Male: Could be asymptomatic; dysuria, urinary frequency, copious purulent (blood-tinged) penile discharge, testicular pain; rectal symptoms: erythematous, discharge, pain with defecation
- Both may have conjunctivitis or pharyngitis as well

PHYSICAL EXAM
- Women: Purulent discharge from cervix, inflammation of Bartholin's glands; positive cervical motion tenderness (CMT) and signs of PID if untreated
- Men: Purulent urethral discharge, signs of prostatitis or epididymitis if untreated
- Disseminated gonorrhea: Stage 1, bacteremia with chills, fever, skin lesions (petechial or pustular skin rash); endocarditis or meningitis may occur; stage 2, septic arthritis; knees, ankles, and wrists show erythema, edema, and pain

DIAGNOSTIC STUDIES
- Cervical or urethral culture for *N. gonorrhoeae* using modified Thayer-Martin media
- Nucleic acid amplification test on first-void urine in men can be used in women but is less accurate
- DNA probe (can diagnose gonorrhea and *Chlamydia*) used for men and women

Differential Diagnosis
- PID
- Nongonococcal cervicitis
- Urethritis
- Proctitis
- Nongonococcal pharyngitis
- *Chlamydia* infections
- Arthritis
- Vaginitis

Management
PHARMACOLOGIC TREATMENT
- Uncomplicated gonococcal infections (cervicitis, urethritis, rectal)
  - Ceftriaxone (Rocephin) 125 mg IM in a single dose OR
  - Cefixime (Suprax) 400 mg po in a single dose OR
  - Spectinomycin (Trobicin) 2 g IM in a single dose
- PLUS a regimen effective against possible co-infection with *C. trachomatis*
  - Azithromycin (Zithromax) 2 g po single dose OR
  - Doxycycline (Vibramycin) 100 mg po bid x 7 days

- Disseminated gonococcal infection: Ceftriaxone (Rocephin) 1 g IM or IV q 24 h
- Mild to moderate PID treated as an outpatient: Ceftriaxone (Rocephin) 250 mg IM in a single dose plus doxycycline 100 mg po bid for 14 days
- Uncomplicated gonococcal infections of the pharynx: Ceftriaxone (Rocephin) 125 mg IM in a single dose
- Gonococcal conjunctivitis: Lavage of infected eye with saline solution once; plus
  - Ceftriaxone (Rocephin) 1 g IM x 1 dose
  - Neonates: 25–50 mg/kg IM or IV x 1 dose not to exceed 125mg
  - Alternative: Spectinomycin (Trobicin) 2 g IM in single dose or ceftizoxime (Cefizox) 500 mg IM in single dose; this drug is not currently available in the United States
  - Infants with gonococcal conjunctivitis: Ceftriaxone 25–50 mg/kg IV or IM, not to exceed 125 mg in a single dose
  - Gonococcal infection in children who weigh >45 kg: Treat the same as adults
  - Gonococcal infection in children who weigh <45 kg: Ceftriaxone 125 mg IM in a single dose

LENGTH OF TREATMENT
- Uncomplicated infections: Single dose
- Disseminated infection, adults: Parenteral regimen for 24–48 hours after improvement, then switch to complete full-week therapy of cefixime 400 mg po bid or cefpodoxime 400 mg po bid
- For meningitis, 10–14 days and at least 4 weeks for endocarditis

Special Considerations
- Pregnant women should be treated with a cephalosporin; erythromycin or amoxicillin can be used for presumptive or diagnosed *Chlamydia* infection.
- Pregnant/lactating women should not be treated with quinolones or tetracycline. If pregnant woman cannot tolerate cephalosporins, treat with spectinomycin 2 g IM x 1 dose alone (not currently available in the U.S.) with effective *Chlamydia* regimen.
- All infants born with neonatal ophthalmia should be observed for gonococcal sepsis, disseminated infection.

When to Consult, Refer, Hospitalize
- Hospitalize for disseminated gonorrhea
- Hospitalize for severe PID
- Refer patients unresponsive to treatment

Follow-Up
- Retest in 1–2 months following treatment if symptomatic
  EXPECTED COURSE
  - Usually there is prompt response to therapy

  COMPLICATIONS
  - PID, sterility, salpingitis, epididymitis, prostatitis, disseminated gonococcal infection
  - Perinatal postabortal endometritis and salpingitis, acute salpingitis, increased incidence of premature rupture of membranes, preterm delivery, chorioamnionitis, neonatal sepsis, postpartum sepsis, neonatal conjunctivitis
  - May help facilitate HIV transmission

Chlamydial Infection

Description
- A sexually transmitted infection caused by *Chlamydia trachomatis*

Etiology
- *C. trachomatis* is an obligate intracellular parasite; transmission by sexual or perinatal contact.
- Infection in women may ascend from cervicitis and urethritis to salpingitis and spread vertically to cause proctitis; in men it may ascend the urogenital tract to epididymis and prostate.

Incidence and Demographics
- The most common sexually transmitted disease; prevalence is highest in persons age <25.
- 4 million cases per year, prevalence 3–4 times greater than GC
- Leading cause of infertility, ectopic pregnancy, and PID. Reportable to local health authority, case report required in most U.S. states.

Risk Factors
- Risk factors listed under General Approach
- Presence of concomitant STD, especially *N. gonorrhoeae*

Prevention and Screening
- Prevention methods listed under General Approach
- Annually screen sexually active men and women <25 years old
- When treating gonococcal infections, include treatment against possible co-infection with *C. trachomatis*
- Screening of pregnant women initially and repeat in the third trimester for high-risk women

Assessment
HISTORY
- Incubation 6–14 days
- May be asymptomatic
- Women: Increase in mucopurulent vaginal discharge, low pelvic discomfort, dysuria, urinary frequency, spotting, and possibly dyspareunia; incubation period usually 1 week
- Men: Mucopurulent urethra discharge or dysuria

PHYSICAL EXAM
- Cervix is friable, mucopurulent discharge; may have positive cervical motion tenderness, adnexal or uterine tenderness if untreated
- Occasional inguinal lymphadenopathy

DIAGNOSTIC STUDIES
- *Chlamydia* culture is definitive test but expensive
- DNA probe
- Nucleic acid amplification (PCR and LCR) in men on first-void urine, can also be used in women but less accurate

Differential Diagnosis
- PID
- Gonorrhea
- Salpingitis
- Urethritis

Management

NONPHARMACOLOGIC TREATMENT
- Sexual partners should be evaluated and treated
- Patients should abstain from sexual intercourse until they and their sex partners have completed treatment; 7 days following single dose treatment or after completion of a 7-day regimen

PHARMACOLOGIC TREATMENT
- First choice: Azithromycin (Zithromax) 1 g po single dose OR doxycycline (Vibramycin) 100 mg po bid
- Alternative choice: Erythromycin base 500 mg po qid for 7 days OR ofloxacin (Floxin) 300 mg po bid OR erythromycin ethylsuccinate 800 mg po qid

LENGTH OF TREATMENT
- Single dose of Azithromycin or 7-day course of treatment with all others

Special Considerations
- Neonatal ophthalmia and pneumonia may occur in infant born to infected mother; consult and treat with erythromycin IV
- Doxycycline, ofloxacin and erythromycin estolate contraindicated in pregnancy
- Ofloxacin contraindicated in patients <17 years
- Pregnancy: Azithromycin 1 g po in a single dose or amoxicillin 500 mg po tid
- Children 6 months to 12 years with uncomplicated genital tract infection: Erythromycin 50 mg/kg/day divided qid x 7 days

When to Consult, Refer, Hospitalize
- Consult with physician for PID in pregnant women, recurrent infection, conjunctivitis, neonatal infection.

Follow-Up
- Not necessary if symptoms resolve with treatment with doxycycline, azithromycin, or ofloxacin
- If treated with erythromycin, reculture in about 3 weeks after initial treatment may be needed if symptoms persist or re-infection suspected
- Pregnant women need repeat cultures 3 weeks after therapy completion due to high noncompliance rate, lower efficacy of erythromycin regimens

  EXPECTED COURSE
  - Prompt resolution of symptoms
  - May become re-infected if sexual partners are not treated

  COMPLICATIONS
  - PID, infertility, increased incidence of ectopic pregnancy; may help facilitate HIV transmission

Mucopurulent Cervicitis

Description
- A sexually transmitted syndrome characterized by purulent discharge visualized on the cervix or in the endocervical canal, or endocervical swab and/or sustained endocervical bleeding easily induced by gentle passage of a cotton swab through the cervical os

Etiology
- May be caused by *C. trachomatis* and *N. gonorrhoeae*; one-third of cases, agent cannot be established
- Ureaplasma (related to *Mycoplasma hominis*) may be the responsible organism

Incidence and Demographics
- Common in sexually active, especially young, women

Risk Factors
- Same as for *Chlamydia* and gonorrhea
- May be associated with frequent douching or exposure to chemical irritants

Prevention and Screening
- Prevention methods listed under General Approach
- Screening for *Chlamydia* and gonorrhea (see General Approach)

Assessment
HISTORY
- Often asymptomatic, abnormal vaginal discharge, vaginal bleeding postcoital

PHYSICAL EXAM
- Cervix has purulent or mucopurulent exudate and is friable

DIAGNOSTIC STUDIES
- DNA probe to test for gonorrhoea and *Chlamydia*
- Wet mount exam to test for *Trichomonas*
- A finding of leukorrhea (>10 WBC/high power field) on wet mount has been associated with chlamydial and gonococcal infection of the cervix
- Urine for culture and sensitivity

Differential Diagnosis
- *Gonorrhoeae*
- *Trichomonas*
- PID
- UTI
- *Chlamydia*

Management
PHARMACOLOGIC TREATMENT
- Treat according to suspicion for *Chlamydia* and/or gonorrhea; wait for test results if prevalence of both organisms is low and chance for follow-up is good
- See treatment for gonococcal and chlamydial infections

LENGTH OF TREATMENT
- Treatment for *Chlamydia* and gonorrhea single dose to 7-days per CDC guidelines

Special Considerations
- Treat pregnant women with cephalosporin, erythromycin, or amoxicillin, not with quinolones or tetracycline

When to Consult, Refer, Hospitalize
- Consult for recurrent infection

Follow-Up
- Follow-up recommended for gonorrhea or *Chlamydia* as appropriate.
- If symptoms persist, patient should refrain from sexual activity and return for evaluation.
- Sexual partners should be examined and treated for STDs.
    EXPECTED COURSE
    - Prompt response to treatment is expected

    COMPLICATIONS
    - Depending on organism, same as for gonococcal or chlamydial infections

Nongonococcal Urethritis (NGU)

Description
- Inflammation of the urethra caused by a nongonorrheal infection characterized by mucopurulent or purulent discharge and burning

Etiology
- NGU if Gram-negative intracellular organisms are not identified on Gram stain.
- C. *Trachomatis* is the major cause (23%–55%).
- Etiology of non-chlamydial NGU is unknown; however, *Ureaplasma urealyticum* and possible *Mycoplasma genitalium* may be present in as many as one-third of cases.
- Sometimes *Trichomonas vaginalis* and herpes simplex virus (HSV) cause NGU.

Incidence and Demographics
- Most common STD syndrome in males living in industrialized countries
- NGU more common than gonococcal urethritis in most areas of U.S.
- Proportion of NGU cases caused by *Chlamydia* have been declining gradually

Risk Factors
- Risk factors listed under General Approach

Prevention and Screening
- Prevention methods listed under General Approach
- Screening for gonorrhea and *Chlamydia* (see General Approach)

Assessment

HISTORY
- Patient reports urethral discharge that is purulent or mucopurulent, dysuria, urethral itching
- Recent unprotected sexual activity or new sex partner

PHYSICAL EXAM
- Urethra erythematous and positive for purulent or mucopurulent discharge

DIAGNOSTIC STUDIES
- Gram stain of urethral secretions has >5 WBCs/oil immersion field without intracellular Gram-negative diplococci
- Positive leukocyte esterase test on first-void urine, or microscopic exam of first-void urine positive for >10 WBCs/high power field
- DNA probe test for *N. gonorrhoeae* and *C. trachomatis*
- Nucleic acid amplification test for gonorrhoeae and *Chlamydia* on urine sample

Differential Diagnosis
- Gonorrhea
- UTI
- Trichomoniasis

Management

NONPHARMACOLOGIC TREATMENT
- Sexual partners should be evaluated and treated appropriately

PHARMACOLOGIC TREATMENT
- Defer treatment if no confirmation of urethritis, until results of DNA probe back
- Treat for *Chlamydia* (see Chlamydial Infection) as indicated
- Empiric treatment of symptoms for high-risk patients unlikely to return for follow-up
- Empiric treatment covers infection with gonorrhea and *Chlamydia* (refer to those entries)

LENGTH OF TREATMENT
- Treatment should be initiated immediately after diagnosis
- Single dose preferable due to better compliance, other regimens treat for 7 days

Special Considerations
- None

When to Consult, Refer, Hospitalize
- Refer when persistent or recurrent urethritis following adequate treatment

Follow-Up
- None necessary if resolves
- All sexual partners within the preceding 60 days should be referred for evaluation

EXPECTED COURSE
  • Symptoms should be alleviated soon after treatment initiated

COMPLICATIONS
  • Epididymitis, prostatitis, Reiter syndrome, may help facilitate HIV transmission

Pelvic Inflammatory Disease, Candidiasis, Bacterial Vaginosis
(See Chapter 11, Female Reproductive Disorders and Concerns)

VIRAL INFECTIONS

Genital Herpes Simplex Virus (HSV) Infection

Description
• Genital infection with primarily Type 2 herpes simplex virus and, less often, Type 1 herpes simplex virus
• HSV may present as a primary, latent, or recurrent disease

Etiology
• HSV infection transmitted through direct contact with mucous membranes and secretions
• Primary infection causes local viral replication, seeding of regional neural ganglia, and possible viremia
• Herpes viruses establish lifelong latency in neural ganglia and periodically reactivate
• Up to 50% of first episode cases of genital herpes are caused by HSV-1 but recurrences and subclinical shedding are much less frequent for genital HSV-1 infection than genital HSV-2 infection
• Many HSV-2 infected persons have not received a diagnosis of genital herpes and are unaware of transmission

Incidence and Demographics
• HSV is endemic in the U.S., with 500,000 new cases per year
• 20 million cases currently in the U.S.
• The highest frequency in 15–29 year olds
• Incidence of primary or recurrent herpes in about 10% of pregnant women
• Perinatal transmission occurs 1 in 2,000 to 1 in 10,000 live births with 60% infant mortality

Risk Factors
• Risk factors listed under General Approach

Prevention and Screening
• Prevention methods listed under General Approach; however, condoms may not block transmission of some lesions.
• Infected persons need to abstain from all sexual activity when lesions or prodromal symptoms are present.

- Sexual transmission of HSV can occur during asymptomatic periods. Asymptomatic viral shedding is more frequent in genital HSV-2 infection than genital HSV-1 infection and is most frequent during the first 12 months after acquiring HSV-2.
- Advise use of condoms during all sexual exposures; however, may not eliminate possibility of transmission.
- Patients should be informed about the risks of neonatal infection.
- No routine screening.

Assessment

HISTORY
- Genital lesions (occurring 2–14 days after exposure), which are painful papules followed by vesicles, ulceration, crusting, and healing
- First episode symptoms consist of hyperesthesias, burning, itching, dysuria, pain, and tenderness in genital area; fever, myalgia, malaise, lymphadenopathy; healing of initial lesions takes up to 21 days (average 12 days)
- Recurrent episodes usually have prodrome (unusual sensation in area before eruption of lesions), recur in same region, and length of shedding is reduced (average 7 days); healing occurs in approximately 5 days

PHYSICAL EXAM
- Examination of genital area characteristic herpetic lesions: tender vesicles on erythematous bases or ulcers in various stages of progression
- Enlarged lymph nodes in inguinal area

DIAGNOSTIC STUDIES
- Viral detection or culture from early lesion or vesicle is most sensitive and permits viral typing, which is helpful for prognostic information (HSV-1 much lower risk for symptomatic recurrent outbreaks)

Differential Diagnosis
- Syphilis
- Chancroid
- *Molluscum contagiosum*
- Folliculitis
- Trauma, burn

Management

NONPHARMACOLOGIC TREATMENT
- Cool perineal compresses, sitz baths, loose-fitting clothes to help alleviate pain
- Good handwashing and hygiene to reduce autoinoculation to other body regions

PHARMACOLOGIC TREATMENT
- Topical acyclovir is less effective than oral; use is discouraged
- First episode: Acyclovir (Zovirax) 400 mg orally tid OR acyclovir 200 mg orally 5 times/day, famciclovir (Famvir) 250 mg orally tid, valacyclovir (Valtrex) 1 g orally bid; treat 7–10 days
- Recurrent infection: Acyclovir 400 mg po tid x 5 days OR acyclovir 800 mg po bid x 5 days OR acyclovir 800 mg po tid x 2 days, famciclovir 125 mg po bid x 5 days OR famciclovir 1,000 mg po bid x 1 day

- Severe infection: Acyclovir 5–10/kg body weight IV q8h for 2–7 days or until clinical improvement; follow with oral antiviral therapy for at least 10 days
- Suppressive therapy: 6 or more outbreaks per year, consider acyclovir 400 mg orally bid or famciclovir 250 mg orally bid continuously for 12 months, then reevaluate
- Analgesics such as acetaminophen, NSAIDs, and topical astringents

LENGTH OF TREATMENT
- For first episode: 7–10 days or longer if lesions not completely healed
- For recurrent episode: 1–5 days
- Daily suppressive therapy; after one year of therapy consider discontinuation to assess rate of recurrent episodes
- For episodic recurrent infection, start treatment during prodrome or within 1 day after onset of lesions

Special Considerations
- HIV+ or immunocompromised: Acyclovir 400 mg po tid OR famciclovir 500 mg po bid x 5 days until clinically resolved, or if severe treat as for severe infection. If resistance suspected, consult with HIV specialist.
- All acyclovir-resistant strains are also resistant to valacyclovir; most are resistant to famciclovir.
- First clinical episode during pregnancy may be treated with acyclovir. Safety of acyclovir, valacyclovir, and famciclovir in pregnancy not established; benefits must outweigh risks.
- Prophylactic administration of acyclovir intrapartum for women with a history of HSV is not recommended.
- Cesarean delivery not always necessary with history of herpes, only recommended when active lesions are visible at the onset of labor.
- Signs of congenital infection may occur from birth to 4–6 weeks (vesicles around eyes, mouth, skin; respiratory distress; central nervous system [CNS] infection; sepsis).

When to Consult, Refer, Hospitalize
- Consult if pregnant, serious infection, or infections resistant to treatment
- Hospitalize if suspected encephalitis, pneumonitis, or hepatitis, or congenital infection

Follow-Up
EXPECTED COURSE
- Most symptoms reduced promptly
- Usually no follow-up indicated unless severe recurrent episodes and treatment inadequate

COMPLICATIONS
- Encephalitis, blindness, pneumonitis, hepatitis, perinatal transmission

Human Papillomavirus Infection

Description
- Infection with certain subtypes of the human papillomavirus (HPV or genital warts) causing flat, papular, or pedunculated growths on the genital mucosa
- Visible warts are known as condyloma acuminata

Etiology
- Virus enters body during sexual activity, via an epithelial defect, and infects the stratified squamous epithelium of the lower genital tract; visible genital warts are usually caused by HPV types 6 or 11
- HPV infection usually persists throughout patient's life in dormant state and becomes infectious intermittently; generally benign, may be asymptomatic or cause minor symptoms
- Highly contagious; 90%–100% of male partners of infected women become infected, mostly subclinically
- HPV infections with types 16, 18, and 31 strongly associated with cervical dysplasia
- HPV implicated in epithelial cancers, especially anorectal carcinoma, vulvar or penile cancer

Incidence and Demographics
- Increased incidence in past 2 decades
- Prevalence of infection in women ranges from 3% to 28%, depending on population
- More than 60 HPV types have been identified in humans; 20 or more infect the genital tract
- Prevalent in 15–25-year-old age group
- Most common viral STD in the U.S.

Risk Factors
- Risk factors listed under General Approach as well as early coitus and lack of barrier methods for contraception
- Growth of warts may be stimulated by oral contraceptives, pregnancy, or immunosuppression

Prevention and Screening
- Prevention methods listed under General Approach, however condoms may not eliminate risk of transmission entirely; patient with HPV still infectious even after warts are removed
- Screening of women through annual Pap smear
- A quadrivalent vaccine against HPV types 6, 11, 16 , and 18, Gardasil, is available and recommended for females aged 9–26

Assessment
HISTORY
- Usually asymptomatic or can cause palpable lesion, itching, burning, local pain, or bleeding
- Significant lesions in some individuals
- May be unknown history of contact: Incubation period from weeks to a year or longer

PHYSICAL EXAM
- Small, flesh-colored, wart-like lesions; some can become confluent as one large wart
- Some warts may be flat or difficult to visualize, others are vegetative growths
- Women: Warts seen on labia, perianal areas, vagina, cervix, or mouth
- Men: Warts seen on shaft of penis, penile meatus, scrotum, perianal areas, and mouth

DIAGNOSTIC STUDIES
- Most warts are diagnosed by visualization; can apply 3%–5% acetic acid to the vulva of woman or penis of man to reveal white coloring of lesions (called acetowhitening)
- Pap smear on women detects koilocytosis, indicative of HPV
- Should test for concomitant STDs: HIV, gonorrhea, syphilis, *Chlamydia*
- Biopsy for detection of viral DNA available but not used clinically

Differential Diagnosis
- Condyloma latum
- Neoplasm
- Granuloma inguinale
- Moles
- Herpes simplex
- Syphilis
- Folliculitis
- Skin tags
- Keratosis
- Scabetic nodules

Management
NONPHARMACOLOGIC TREATMENT
- Smoking is a co-factor for cervical cancer with HPV; encourage cessation for woman infected with HPV
- Examination of sexual partners not recommended because partner's role in re-infection is minimal
- Encourage continued use of condoms

PHARMACOLOGIC TREATMENT
- Drugs treat symptoms and may decrease size of wart; no treatment available that completely eradicates virus
- External/perianal warts
  - Patient-applied podofilox (Condylox) 0.5% solution or gel (apply bid x 3 days, then off 4 days); may repeat cycle total of 4 times **OR**
  - Imiquimod (Aldara) 5% cream: Apply q hs 3 x week; wash off after 6–10 hours; may use up to 16 weeks, may clear in 8–10 weeks
  - Provider-administered cryotherapy with liquid nitrogen, may repeat every 1–2 weeks

    – Provider-administered podophyllin 10%–25% in compound tincture of benzoin (wash off thoroughly 1–4 hours after application); repeat weekly if necessary **OR**

    – Provider-administered trichloroacetic acid (TCA) 80%–90%; apply only to warts; powder with talc or baking soda to remove untreated acid; repeat weekly if necessary

LENGTH OF TREATMENT

- Depending on the size of wart and response to treatment, could take one to several treatments

Special Considerations

- Pregnancy: Podophyllin, imiquimod, podofilox are contraindicated
- Some specialists recommend removal of visible warts during pregnancy
- HIV patients may not respond well to treatment

When to Consult, Refer, Hospitalize

- Vaginal and cervical warts: Consult with gynecologist, dysplasia must be excluded before treatment instituted
- Warts on rectal mucosa should be referred to proctologist
- Refer women with large warts (>2 cm) to gynecologist for treatment with CO_2 laser, electrodesiccation, electrocautery, cryocautery, LEEP procedure (gynecologic surgery)

Follow-Up

- Follow up during therapy; women should continue to have regular, annual Pap smears

EXPECTED COURSE

- Treatment of warts may require several visits for provider-administered treatment
- Genital warts can resolve on their own, remain unchanged, or continue to grow untreated
- Reccurrence of warts common, especially within the first 3 months following treatment

COMPLICATIONS

- Cervical dysplasia and cervical squamous cell carcinoma; invasive carcinoma of vulva and penis
- Anal squamous cell carcinoma of bi-/homosexual males
- Treatment procedures may cause scarring

OTHER STDS

Syphilis

Description
- Sexually transmitted disease affecting many organs throughout body, caused by *Treponema pallidum*
- Clinical stages include primary, secondary, early latent (up to 1 year duration), late latent, and tertiary

Etiology
- *T. pallidum*: This spirochete invades the human body by penetrating intact skin or mucous membrane during sexual contact
- Once inside body, rapidly multiplies and spreads to regional lymph nodes
- Congenital syphilis occurs from transplacental passage of organism occurring any time during gestation; can result in spontaneous abortion (second trimester), stillbirth

Incidence and Demographics
- Rate of infection declined by 84% in the U.S. between 1990 and 1997
- Despite widespread decline, the South continues to have highest syphilis rate in the nation
- Approximately 80,000 cases reported in the U.S. annually
- Congenital syphilis rate 1 in 10,000 pregnancies

Risk Factors
- Risk factors listed under General Approach

Prevention and Screening
- Prevention methods listed under General Approach
- Early diagnosis and treatment with partner notification and treatment
- Routine screening for those <25 years in high-prevalence areas; also screen those with other STD
- Pregnancy: Screening at first prenatal visit, then repeat for high-risk population at 28 weeks and delivery

Table 13-1. Stages of Acquired Syphilis

Primary	Secondary	Latent	Tertiary
Painless ulcer or chancre at site of inoculation 3–4 weeks after exposure	Rash is macular, papular, annular, or follicular (rarely pustular) and often present on palms and soles	Begins with the healing of the lesions in the secondary stage	Gummatous formation, cardiovascular or neurosyphilis
Extragenital lesions such as lips or breast may be painful	In warm moist areas, may develop broad flat lesions (condylomata lata)	Early latent <1 year (infectious)	
Primary chancre is highly infectious, heals spontaneously after 1–5 weeks and patient may not seek treatment	Rash lasts 2–6 weeks then spontaneously heals	Late latent >1 year (noninfectious)	
	Mucous patches which appear as gray erosions noted in mouth, throat, on cervix	Sometimes difficult to distinguish early latent from late latent stage due to unknown duration of symptoms	
	Generalized lymphadenopathy	Meningitis	
	Arthralgias/myalgias and "flu-like" symptoms	Cardiovascular disease, arthritis, neurologic lesions	
		Often asymptomatic	

Assessment

HISTORY AND PHYSICAL EXAM (SEE TABLE 13-1)
- Primary:
  - Incubation is approximately 3 weeks and ranges 10–90 days after exposure
  - Painless, indurated ulcer (chancre) at site of inoculation is highly infectious, heals spontaneously after 1–5 weeks and patient may not seek treatment; may be regional lymphadenopathy
  - Extragenital (lips, breast) lesions may be painful
- Secondary:
  - May occur from 6 weeks to 6 months after primary stage; most contagious
  - Rash is macular, papular, annular, or follicular and often present on palms and soles
  - Rash lasts 2–6 weeks then spontaneously heals
  - Moist, raised lesions of the skin (condyloma lata) and mucous patches in mouth, throat, on cervix
  - Generalized lymphadenopathy
  - Arthralgias/myalgias and "flu-like" symptoms
- Latent:
  - Asymptomatic, begins with the end of secondary symptoms
  - Early latent <1 year (infectious)
  - Late latent >1 year (noninfectious)

  – Difficult to distinguish early latent from late latent stage if unknown duration of symptoms
- Tertiary:
  – Gummatous formation, cardiovascular or neurosyphilis
- Congenital:
  – Asymptomatic until age 2; failure to thrive, skin rash, jaundice, rhinitis, hepatosplenomegaly

DIAGNOSTIC STUDIES
- Definitive method: Darkfield microscopy and direct fluorescent antibody tests of lesion exudate or tissue
- Serologic tests: RPR, VDRL are used for initial testing and titers, FTA-ABS, MHA-TP used to confirm diagnosis in persons with positive RPR or VDRL
- For sequential serologic tests use the same test (VDRL or RPR); titer will decrease with time and treatment
- Fourfold increase in titer indicates new infection
- Failure to achieve fourfold decrease in titer in one year indicates failed treatment
- Latent syphilis of >1 year duration, cardiovascular syphilis, and neurosyphilis: Serologic tests and lumbar puncture with tests on cerebrospinal fluid (CSF)
- Test for other STDs: HIV, gonorrhea, *Chlamydia*

Differential Diagnosis
- Genital ulcers
- Genital herpes
- Chancroid
- Neoplasm
- Lymphogranuloma venereum
- Superficial fungal infections

Management
NONPHARMACOLOGIC TREATMENT
- Abstain from sexual activity until treatment complete
- Early infection (primary, secondary, and early latent) and congenital syphilis reportable in all U.S. states

PHARMACOLOGIC TREATMENT
- Patients exposed sexually to a patient who has syphilis in any stage should be evaluated clinically and serologically and treated in the following cases:
  – People exposed within 90 days preceding diagnosis of primary, secondary, or early latent stages in a sex partner, even if seronegative
  – People exposed >90 days before the diagnosis of primary, secondary, or latent stages in a sex partner and in whom serologic test results are not available immediately and the opportunity for follow-up is uncertain
  – For purposes of partner notification and presumptive treatment of exposed sex partners, patients with unknown duration of illness and high serologic test titers (>1:32) may be considered as having early syphilis
- Patients with symptoms or history of symptoms and positive diagnostic studies, see Table 13–2

Table 13-2. Recommended Treatment of Acquired Syphilis

Stage Of Disease	Treatment Regimen
Primary, secondary, and early latent disease	Benzathine penicillin G 2.4 million units IM in single dose Penicillin-allergic patients: Doxycycline 100 mg bid x 28 days, or tetracycline 500 mg orally qid x 28 days
Late latent syphilis or syphilis of unknown duration	Benzathine penicillin G 2.4 million units IM x 3 each at 1-week intervals Penicillin-allergic patients: Doxycycline 100 mg orally bid for 4 wks, or tetracycline 500 mg orally qid x 4 wks
Tertiary disease, excluding neurosyphilis	As for late latent disease, with appropriate management of complications
Neurosyphilis	Aqueous cystamine penicillin G, 18–24 million units/day given as 3–4 million units IV every 4 hours for 10–14 days, or procaine penicillin 2–4 million units IM a day PLUS probenecid (Benemid) 500 mg orally qid, both for 10–14 days

Special Considerations
- HIV-infected persons:
  - Serologic tests and interpretation the same for HIV-infected patients
  - When clinical finding suggests syphilis, but serologic tested nonreactive or unclear, use alternate test such as biopsy of lesion, darkfield examination, or direct fluorescent antibody staining of lesion material
  - Treatment the same as HIV-negative persons
  - Neurosyphilis must be considered in differential for HIV+ patients; CSF examination should be performed on HIV-infected persons who show mental status changes, have either late latent syphilis, or syphilis of unknown duration
  - Penicillin must be used to treat; if penicillin-allergic, must be desensitized
  - Primary and secondary syphilis should have VDRL/RPR serology at 3, 6, 9, 12, and 24 months to evaluate for treatment failure; if titer increased four-fold, fails to decrease four-fold at 3 months, or symptoms persist, retreatment is indicated
- Pregnancy: Treat for appropriate stage of syphilis:
  - Some experts recommend a second dose of benzathine penicillin 2.4 mil units IM one week after initial dose for pregnant women with primary, secondary, or early latent syphilis; if penicillin allergic, desensitize patient to penicillin
  - Women treated in second trimester are at risk for premature labor and/or fetal distress
- Infants born to mothers with positive nontreponemal and treponemal test:
  - If infant was born to mother who tests positive for syphilis but adequate treatment with penicillin is not documented, the infant should be observed for congenital syphilis (into early childhood)
  - Routine physical exams for rash, hepatomegaly, lymphadenopathy, persistent rhinitis
  - Quantitative nontreponemal test on infant's blood (not cord blood)
  - Cerebrospinal fluid testing, long bone x-rays, and other testing may be indicated

- All patients may experience the Jarisch-Herxheimer reaction:
    - Upon treatment of primary or secondary syphilis, occurs due to lysis of treponemes
    - Experience fever, chills, headache, myalgias, rash
    - Treated with antihistamines and antipyretics

When to Consult, Refer, Hospitalize
- Consult with physician or refer to infectious disease specialist for pregnant women, congenital syphilis, neurosyphilis infection, or HIV+ patients
- Hospitalize for parenteral therapy and for penicillin desensitization therapy

Follow-Up
- Primary and secondary syphilis: Examine clinically and serologically at 6 or 12 months or more frequently if clinically indicated; if serologic titer (VDRL or RPR) has not declined by fourfold in 6 months after therapy, consider treatment failure.
    - Treatment failure: Reevaluate for HIV infection, provide more frequent follow-up (3 months instead of 6); if additional follow-up cannot be ensured, retreatment recommended (3 weekly IM injections of penicillin G 2.4 million units)
    - Consider CSF examination
- Latent syphilis: Serological testing at 6, 12, and 24 months; evaluate for neurosyphilis and retreat if titers increase fourfold, initial high titer (>1:32) fails to decline at least fourfold within 12–24 months, or symptomatic.

    ### EXPECTED COURSE
    - Primary stage lasts 1–5 weeks, secondary stage lasts 2–6 weeks

    ### COMPLICATIONS
    - Tertiary syphilis: Cardiovascular involvement causing aortitis, aortic insufficiency, aneurysm, and neurosyphilis; recurrent secondary symptoms possible within 1 year for 25% of cases

CASE STUDIES

Case 1. A 23-year-old sexually active male presents with a 4–5 day history of dysuria he feels is caused by a urinary tract infection.

HPI: Denies frequency, fever, flank pain, hematuria, history of urinary tract infections.

    1. What additional information will help you evaluate this patient?

Exam: Mucopurulent urethral discharge, no inguinal adenopathy, no genital lesions.

    2. What is the differential diagnosis?

    3. Should any diagnostic tests be done?

    4. What are your treatment considerations?

Case 2. A 17-year-old female comes to the family planning clinic for routine pelvic exam and contraception. She has had four sexual partners in the past year and only occasionally uses condoms. She requests an HIV test because one of her recent partners is an IV drug user.

PMH: History of 2 pregnancies with 2 abortions, no major illnesses, does not smoke, drinks two to three beers on the weekend, lives with mother and grandmother, in 11th grade, failing some classes.

    1. What additional information should you obtain?

Exam: Complete physical exam with no significant findings except flat-topped, fleshy-colored lesions on labia minora and thin yellow vaginal discharge.

    2. What screening tests should be done?

    3. What treatment should be considered today?

    4. What education and prevention topics should be discussed with this patient?

REFERENCES

American Academy of Pediatrics. (2003). *Red book 2003*. Elk Grove Village, IL: Author.

American Academy of Pediatrics. (2006). *The 2006 red book: Report of the Committee on Infectious Disease*. Elk Grove, IL: Author.

Bartlett, J. G. (2003). *Medical management of HIV infection* (2nd ed.).Cockeysville, MD: PR Graphics.

Centers for Disease Control and Prevention. (2002). Sexually transmitted diseases treatment guidelines. *MMWR: Morbidity and Mortality Weekly Report, 51* (No. RR-6), 1–78.

Centers for Disease Control and Prevention. (2006). Sexually transmitted diseases treatment guidelines. *MMWR: Morbidity and Mortality Weekly Report, 51* (No. RR-6), 1–78

Centers for Disease Control and Prevention. (2007). Updated recommended treatment regimens for gonococcal infection and associated conditions. *MMWR: Morbidity and Mortality Weekly Report*. Retrieved January 2, 2008, from http://www.cdc.gov/STD/treatment/

Gilbert, D. N., Moellering, R.C., Eliopoulus, G. M., & Sande, M. A. (2008). *The Sanford guide to antimicrobial therapy*. Hyde Park, VT: Antimicrobial Therapy, Inc.

Graham, M., & Uphold, C. (2004). *Clinical guidelines in child health*. Gainesville, FL: Barmarrae Books, Inc.

Mandell, G. L., Bennett, J. E., & Dolin, R. (2005). *Mandell, Doublas and Bennett's principles and practices of infectious diseases*. Philadelphia: Churchill Livingstone.

Neinstein, L. S. (2002.) *Adolescent health care* (4th ed.). Baltimore: Lippincott Williams & Wilkins.

Plasencia, J. M. (2000). Cutaneous warts: Diagnosis and treatment. *Primary Care, 27,* 423.

Sande, M. A., Gilbert, D. N., & Moellering, R. C. (2000). *The Sanford guide to HIV/AIDS therapy*. Hyde Park, VT: Antimicrobial Therapy, Inc.

Siberry, G., & Iannone, R. (2005). *The Harriett Lane handbook*. New York: Mosby.

Stoller, M. L., Kane, C. T., & Meng, M. K. (2008). Urology. In S. J. McPhee, M. A. Papadakis, & L. M. Tierney, Jr. (Eds.), *Current medical diagnosis and treatment* (47th ed.). New York: Lange Medical Books/McGraw-Hill.

Towers, P. M. (2000). Urinary tract infections. *Journal of the American Academy of Nurse Practitioners, 12,* 149–156.

U.S. Preventive Services Task Force. (2007). *Guide to clinical preventive services (3rd ed.): Periodic updates*. Alexandria, VA: International Medical Publishing, Inc.

Musculoskeletal Disorders

Deborah Gilbert-Palmer, EdD, FNP-BC

GENERAL APPROACH

- In infants and children, obtain history of mother's pregnancy, child's birth, and development (musculoskeletal problems comprise ~10% of childhood problems and ~25% primary care visits).
- Obtain history of problem including mechanism of injury, occupation, any sports or exercise, history of repetitive use, duration, aggravating and alleviating factors. Age is important in evaluation of any musculoskeletal findings.
- Observe gait, posture, guarding, and patient positioning; examine affected side in comparison to unaffected side.
- Provocative tests specific to area are important to rule out certain conditions.

Red Flags
- *Back pain*: Urgent referral if constant, under age 11, lasts several weeks, wakes patient at night, limitation of motion, fever, neurologic signs, weight loss, or history of malignancy.
- *Malignant bone tumors* may present as unexplained pain and swelling over a bone, decreased range of motion, night pain, pain with weight-bearing, weight loss, night sweats, pallor, malaise, and fever; have a high index of suspicion for bone metastasis in patients with previous breast, lung, or prostate cancer.
- *Osteomyelitis* may present as pain in bone, fever, difficulty bearing weight, and possible local warmth and swelling following recent trauma. Obtain a CBC, ESR, C-reactive protein and refer to orthopedist. Be aware that x-ray changes will not occur for 10–24 days after start of infection.

ARTHRITIS

Osteoarthritis (OA)

Description
- Degenerative joint disease with progressive loss of articular cartilage in movable joints, degeneration of cartilage, bone hypertrophy, formation of osteophytes and subchondral cysts, and development of subchondral sclerosis in synovial joints and vertebrae

Etiology
- Results from both mechanical and biologic events that lead to degradation of articular cartilage and subchondral bone in joint

Incidence and Demographics
- Most common form of arthritis; affects 25% of adult population; greatest prevalence in Native Americans
- Leading chronic condition among adults age >65 years; incidence increases with advancing age
- 80% of adults in U.S. have radiographic evidence by age 75 years
- Women affected more often than men

Risk Factors
- Advancing age; symptom onset typically 55–65 years
- Athletic overuse or repetitive joint use in occupation
- Joint trauma from acute injury or metabolic disease
- Obesity, heredity, congenital musculoskeletal disorders
- Metabolic disorders (e.g., gout) or endocrine disorders (e.g., hyperparathyroidism)

Prevention and Screening
- Maintain physical activity
- Maintain ideal body weight, avoid obesity
- Maintain control of metabolic and endocrine disorders

Assessment
HISTORY (TABLE 14–1)
- Gradual onset of joint pain, tenderness, and stiffness; worsens with activity and is relieved by rest
- Morning stiffness common, usually lasts <30 minutes
- Joint instability in later stages, especially with osteoarthritis of knees
- Perform review of systems for systemic symptoms to rule out other types of arthritis

PHYSICAL EXAM
- Usually localized to affected joints
- Bony hypertrophy of joint, tenderness at joint line; limited range of motion
- Common in hands: Proximal intraphalangeal (PIP) joint swelling = Bouchard's nodes; distal intraphalangeal (DIP) joint swelling = Heberden's nodes
- Coarse crepitus in joint with movement; soft tissue swelling may be present
- Joint effusion, if present, usually mild
- Cardiac and pulmonary exam as well as other body systems as indicated by history to rule out other types of arthritis

DIAGNOSTIC STUDIES
- Plain radiographs: Unequal and narrowed joint space, subchondral bony sclerosis, sharp articular margins, cysts or osteophytes
- Bone densitometry (DEXA scans), peripheral ultrasonography, quantitative computed tomography (QCT)
- No specific laboratory test; laboratory findings may be normal or show markers of systemic inflammation or autoimmune disease

Table 14–1. Differentiating Characteristics of Osteoarthritis and Rheumatoid Arthritis

Characteristics	Osteoarthritis	Rheumatoid Arthritis
Radiographic appearance	Joint space narrowing, osteophytes, subchondral bone sclerosis, subchondral cysts	Periarticular osteopenia or osteoporosis, soft tissue swelling, marginal bony erosions
Morning stiffness	Lasts <30 minutes	Lasts >1 hour before improving
Joint involvement	Usually weight-bearing (spine, hips, knees) or distal finger joints (DIP)	Multiple joints, symmetric joint involvement (esp. of hands)
Laboratory findings	ESR <20–40 mm/hr; RF negative	Positive serum RF, may have positive ANA, elevated ESR
Clinical findings	Joint pain, bony tenderness and hypertrophy, crepitus, may have some deformity; no warmth or redness	Joint deformity, muscle atrophy, soft tissue nodules (rheumatoid nodules), soft tissue swelling, warmth, redness of joints

Note. ANA = antinuclear antibody; ESR = erythrocyte sedimentation rate; RF = rheumatoid factor

Differential Diagnosis
- Rheumatoid arthritis
- Psoriatic arthritis
- Gout, pseudogout
- Septic arthritis
- Reiter's disease, lupus
- Fibromyalgia
- Tendinitis, soft tissue injury
- Osteoporosis
- Multiple myeloma

Management
- Goals are to relieve symptoms, maintain/improve function, avoid adverse effects of medication.
  NONPHARMACOLOGIC TREATMENT
    - Physical activity/therapy with supervised walking
    - Occupational therapy
    - Arthritis self-management programs and water aquatics courses
    - Ambulation aids (canes, braces, walkers)

- Weight loss programs
- Consider surgery if all other modalities fail and joint symptoms prevent normal activities

PHARMACOLOGIC TREATMENT
- Simple analgesics, available over the counter (acetaminophen, aspirin, ibuprofen, or naproxen) for pain
  - Acetaminophen 2.6–4 g/day considered first-line treatment by American College of Rheumatology due to low toxicity; extended release preparations lengthen duration
- NSAIDs indicated for failed acetaminophen trial; start with lower doses and use those with shorter half-lives in elderly patients, increase to full strength if needed, switch to different class if not effective after several weeks; beware of NSAID-induced renal insufficiency in the elderly
- Selective COX-2 inhibitors: Lower GI toxicity than other NSAIDs, still need to monitor renal function with COX-2s
- Topical analgesic creams such as capsaicin 0.025% bid to tid
- Narcotic analgesics rarely indicated; may be used short-term if necessary
- Intra-articular corticosteroid injections for joint effusion and inflammation limited to a few joints
- Hyaluronic acid injections to rebuild cartilage in a single joint
- Nutraceutical (glucosamine, chondroitin, SAM-e) may be of benefit

LENGTH OF TREATMENT
- As long as symptomatic

Special Considerations
- Presence of radiographic changes does not correlate with presence or severity of symptoms

When to Consult, Refer, Hospitalize
- Consult with physician or orthopedic specialist for intra-articular corticosteroid or hyaluronic acid injections
- Patients with functional impairment (i.e., inability to perform normal activities of daily living) and with moderate to severe pain unrelieved by other nonpharmacologic and pharmacologic therapies should be considered for joint replacement; refer to orthopedic surgeon

Follow-Up
- Follow-up appointments as needed based on pain and disability
- If on NSAIDS or acetaminophen, may need to be monitored for liver or kidney dysfunction and GI bleeding

EXPECTED COURSE
- Chronic, often progressive

COMPLICATIONS
- Joint destruction, chronic pain, limitation of mobility

Rheumatoid Arthritis (RA)

Description
- Chronic, systemic, inflammatory disease that affects mainly synovial joints in a symmetric distribution; small-joint destruction and extra-articular symptoms prominent

Etiology
- Probably autoimmune but no specific inciting factor yet identified
- Genetic, environmental factors affect progression and extent of disease
- Pathology consists of initial changes in the synovium microvasculature, swelling of endothelial cells, and synovial hyperplasia forming a pannus. Inflammatory cells invade and joint symptoms develop secondary to the inflammatory process.

Incidence and Demographics
- Worldwide incidence, involving all ethnic groups; prevalence about five times greater in females
- In children, bimodal age presentation: 2–4 years, 8–12 years
- Juvenile RA diagnosed in children <16 years old who have chronic synovial inflammation of at least one joint for 6 weeks. JRA has 3 major types:
  - *Pauciarticular* (fewer than five joints): Characterized by chronic arthritis of a few joints, usually the large weight-bearing joints, asymmetric distribution
  - *Polyarticular* (five or more joints): Resembles adult disease with chronic pain, swelling of many joints
  - *Systemic*: Associated with rash, arthritis, fever, or visceral disease

Risk Factors
- Possible genetic component, immunologically mediated; strong family history of autoimmune disorders
- Occurs in all age groups, more common with increasing age, peak onset in adults in fourth decade of life
- 5% of all cases begin in childhood

Assessment
- Early diagnosis (within first few months of symptoms) important for improved prognosis
- Important to rule out septic arthritis, typical presentation: sudden onset of pain, swelling, warmth, and redness in one large weight-bearing joint, may have fever
  HISTORY
  - Prodromal systemic symptoms: Malaise, fever, weight loss, morning stiffness lasting 30–60 minutes or more
  - Articular inflammation, swelling, pain, erythema, and warmth
  - Involvement usually symmetrical; 75% of joints involved are knees, followed by ankles and elbows
  - In children, joint pain, one or more joints affected, swelling or effusion and two of the following: limitation of range of motion, tenderness or pain in motion, warmth; usually involves large joints or hands; if systemic: fever, rash
  - Perform review of systems to identify any associated symptoms of systemic involvement; physical/emotional stress may trigger

PHYSICAL EXAM
- Edema, erythema, warmth, nodules in any joint; effervescent, pale pink salmon-colored macular rash
- Joints are tender, may feel warm to touch; bright erythema and significant palpable heat in joint usually indicative of infection
- Subcutaneous nodules over bony prominences or extensor surfaces
- Soft tissue swelling, vasculitis, palmar erythema
- As disease progresses, joint deformities become more pronounced and joint instability develops
- Systemic manifestations may be seen in the pulmonary, cardiac, hepatic, renal, vascular, hematologic systems and the eyes (dry mucous membranes, ocular problems, splenomegaly, increased lymphocytes)
- In children with systemic JRA, may have macular salmon-colored rash, splenomegaly, eye symptoms

DIAGNOSTIC STUDIES
- No single test is adequate to make diagnosis
- Positive serum rheumatoid factor (RF) in about 80% of cases; levels hard to correlate with severity of other signs; ANA increased in 20% patients; in children, RF and ANA may be positive
- Erythrocyte sedimentation rate (ESR) correlates with degree of synovial inflammation
- CRP (c-reactive protein) also may be used to monitor inflammation
- Synovial fluid shows inflammatory changes: sterile leukocytosis, increased PMN, negative culture
- CBC may show chronic, mild, normochromic or hypochromic, normocytic anemia
- Other: Eosinophilia, hypergammaglobulinemia, thrombocytosis may be present in severe disease
- X-ray shows soft tissue swelling and juxta-articular destruction

Differential Diagnosis
- Systemic lupus erythematosus (SLE)
- Seronegative spondyloarthropathy
- Psoriatic arthritis
- Septic arthritis
- Lyme disease
- Gout
- Osteoarthritis
- Lupus

Management
- Goals are early diagnosis and early, aggressive treatment to limit, prevent irreversible joint damage, maximize mobility, limit pain, halt disease progression.
  NONPHARMACOLOGIC TREATMENT
  - Rest as indicated; may require complete bedrest with acute inflammatory phase
  - Patient education (Arthritis Foundation self-help courses), physical and occupational therapy to strengthen muscles, improve joint range of motion (ROM) and function, protect joint(s)

- Regular exercise program; may use alternating heat and cold to increase comfort
- Assistive devices (canes, splints)
- Surgery to correct joint deformity if necessary

PHARMACOLOGIC TREATMENT
- Aspirin is often recommended as a first-line drug
- NSAIDs have not been shown to alter disease course, but may offer symptom relief
- COX-2s for those with risk of bleeding; COX-1 with misoprostol or proton pump inhibitors
- Biologic agents (disease-modifying anti-rheumatic drugs [DMARDs]): Tumor necrosis factor (TNF) inhibitors are new drugs that may replace methotrexate as first-line therapy
- Leflunomide (Arava), etanercept (Enbrel) and infliximab (Remicade) may cause hypersensitivity reaction, severe infections or sepsis, and autoimmunity (lupus-type syndrome)
- Work faster than methotrexate, good response in 60%
- Are extremely expensive, insurance unlikely to cover
- Hydroxychloroquine (Plaquenil): Monitor eye symptoms, neuropathy, myopathy
- Methotrexate (Mexate)
- Sulfasalazine (Azulfidine)
- Gold or gold salts
- Leflunomide, a pyrimidine synthesis inhibitor
- Minocycline: Used in mild disease
- Corticosteroids: Use short-term for severe exacerbations
- Prednisone up to 0.1 mg/kg (2.5–7.5 mg/day) po; may also be used in combination with DMARDs
- Methylprednisolone 80–60 mg IM during acute flare
- Chronic corticosteroid use decreases bone mineral density

LENGTH OF TREATMENT
- In adults, lifelong therapy is usually indicated, may have periods of remission or decreased symptoms
- In children, some have periods of long remissions

Special Considerations
- Methotrexate, hydroxychloroquine known to be detrimental to fetus; should be stopped some time prior to conception
- Pregnancy may result in remission and may allow temporary discontinuation of medications; however, exacerbations common in first 6 months postpartum. Breastfeeding not advised since antirheumatic medications secreted in breast milk.

When to Consult, Refer, Hospitalize
- Rheumatologic consultation or referral is appropriate. All children should be referred to a pediatric rheumatologist and ophthalmologist at diagnosis.

Follow-Up
- Clinical course is highly variable; until symptoms are controlled, frequent follow-up visits are indicated, then regular evaluations at 3–6 month intervals.

COMPLICATIONS
- May be severe, including carpal tunnel syndrome, pleuritis, pericarditis, vasculitis, iridocyclitis, disability, and adverse reactions from drugs; see joint deformity, hip disease

Gout

Description
- A group of metabolic diseases producing inflammatory arthritis of peripheral joints caused by deposition of uric acid or monosodium urate crystals in extracellular fluid

Etiology
- Inborn error of purine metabolism or uric acid excretion causing hyperuricemia and uric acid crystal deposition in the joint (acute gouty arthritis)
- May be primary (hereditary) or secondary (due to other conditions that cause under-excretion or overproduction of uric acid)
- Overproduction: High intake of purine-rich foods (organ meats, shellfish, peas, lentils, beans), polycythemia vera, leukemia, multiple myeloma, hemolytic anemia, psoriasis, sarcoidosis
- Under-excretion of uric acid: Reduced renal function, lactic acidosis, ketoacidosis, dehydration
- Secondary gout also associated with obesity, starvation, lead intoxication, ingestion of drugs (salicylates, diuretics, pyrazinamide, ethambutol, nicotinic acid)
- Combined overproduction/under-excretion: Alcohol abuse, glucose-6-phosphatase deficiency (G-6PD), hypoxemia

Incidence and Demographics
- Affects 2.2 million in U.S.; men affected 9 times as often as women; most common in Asians
- Rarely affects men prior to adolescence or women before menopause
- Peak incidence is fifth decade

Risk Factors
- Heredity, purine-rich diet, obesity, dehydration, starvation, alcohol ingestion

Prevention and Screening
- Correct/control underlying problem
- Avoid foods high in purines, alcohol, causative medications
- Maintain normal body weight

Assessment
HISTORY
- Sudden attack of red, hot, swollen, exquisitely tender joint is common (first metatarsal phalangeal [MTP] joint very susceptible—podagra); feeling of malaise, fever; often no apparent cause
- Foot, ankle, knee, shoulder are most common sites; wrist, elbow, fingers also may be affected

PHYSICAL EXAM
- During acute attack, joint is red, hot, swollen, exquisitely painful; low-grade fever
- Skin desquamation and pruritus during resolution of acute attack commonly seen
- Tophi (sodium urate crystals deposited in soft tissue) present in chronic tophaceous gout, usually after 2–10 years from onset of acute intermittent gout
- Joint swelling, restricted range of movement caused by chronic arthritis

DIAGNOSTIC STUDIES
- Joint aspiration: Fluid shows presence of needle-shaped crystals (negatively birefringent) on polarized light microscopy
- Serum uric acid >7.0 mg/dL supports diagnosis but is not specific; elevated ESR, elevated leukocytes
- X-ray: Normal in early disease; shows punched-out lesions in subchondral bone, usually first seen in first MTP joint ("Mickey Mouse" ears); soft tissue tophi may be seen if at least 5 mm in diameter

Differential Diagnosis
- Septic joint
- Pseudogout
- Cellulitis
- Fracture
- Rheumatoid arthritis
- Acute rheumatic fever
- Pyogenic arthritis

Management
NONPHARMACOLOGIC TREATMENT
- Dietary modification; increased fluid intake >3 liters/day
- Complete bedrest during acute attack
- Weight loss in obese patients

PHARMACOLOGIC TREATMENT
Acute attack
- First-line: NSAIDs such as naproxen at full anti-inflammatory dose; naproxen 500 mg tid po for first 2–3 days (until symptoms subside), then taper to cessation over 3–5 days; or corticosteroids depending on comorbidities, prednisone 20–40 mg po qd for 2–3 days, then taper over 10–14 days; intra-articular methylprednisolone (Depo-Medrol) one 20- to 40-mg dose; IM methylprednisolone, one 80- to 120-mg dose
- Second-line: Colchicine 0.6 mg po q 1–2 hours as soon as symptoms appear to a maximum dose of 6–8 mg or until diarrhea or abdominal cramping occurs (colchicine used for patients who are not good candidates for NSAIDs: individuals on anticoagulants, congestive heart failure, renal insufficiency). Drug has very narrow therapeutic index; maintenance dose is 0.6 mg po qd to bid

Maintenance
- Urate-lowering therapy indicated with multiple attacks, development of tophi or urate nephrolithiais, to block renal absorption of uric acid. Start allopurinol 100–150 mg qd to bid po, gradually increasing by 100 mg per week until serum uric acid is below 6 mg/dL; maximum dose of 800 mg/day. Contraindicated in patients with renal impairment
- Concurrent therapy: Use maintenance colchicine to reduce number of attacks and medications

LENGTH OF TREATMENT
- Acute symptoms treated until tolerable, then long-term therapy begun

Special Considerations
- Transplant patients (who use cyclosporine) have increased incidence
- Asymptomatic hyperuricemia with normal renal function, generally do not treat
- Slightly higher incidence in African-American males than White males
- Geriatric patients: NSAIDs less well-tolerated, dosages should be reduced

When to Consult, Refer, Hospitalize
- Consult for any complicated presentation, underlying metabolic pathology
- Refer for joint aspiration, unclear diagnosis, new/acute gout in transplant patient
- Hospitalize if intravenous administration of colchicine necessary (rare)

Follow-Up
EXPECTED COURSE
- Decrease in frequency, severity of attacks with appropriate treatment

COMPLICATIONS
- Kidney stones, renal obstruction or infection, joint destruction if under-treated

CONDITIONS OF THE BONES

Osteomyelitis

Description
- Local bone infection, usually bacterial; can be acute or chronic

Etiology
- Bacteremia with acute or subacute hematogenous spread to bone (most common form in pediatrics)
- Direct bacterial inoculation through trauma, contact infected tissue (most common in adults)
- Predominant organism *Staphylococcus aureus*

Incidence and Demographics
- Occurs in all ages, more common children <5 years old
- Males 2–4 times more than females; 5–10 cases per 10,000 children

- Increases in late summer and early fall
- Uncommon in neonatal period
- Femur and tibia most often infected, followed by humerus, calcaneus, and pelvis

Risk Factors
- General debilitating diseases (cancer, diabetes, hemodialysis); sickle cell disease; *Salmonella*
- Intravenous drug abuse
- Puncture wound: *Pseudomonas aeruginosa*

Prevention and Screening
- Careful treatment of comorbid conditions; appropriate wound care

Assessment
HISTORY
- 75% report recent trauma, 25% report recent respiratory tract infection
- Sudden onset high fever and pain in affected bone or joint; sudden refusal to bear weight or move extremity; localized warmth, swelling
- May have drainage from affected area (sinus tract develops)

PHYSICAL EXAM
- Swelling, erythema, possible abscess formation or purulent drainage; decreased ROM; fever; point tenderness over infected bone

DIAGNOSTIC STUDIES
- CBC: WBC elevated in 70% of cases
- ESR: Elevated by third day of infection
- C-reactive protein: Peaks at day 2
- Blood cultures: Positive in 50% of cases
- Bone cultures: Positive in 65% of cases; wound cultures of no benefit
- X-ray shows changes after day 10–14 of infection
- If suspicious, MRI defines area of infection, soft tissue pathology; differentiate tumor and infection
- Bone scan: Sensitive but not specific
- CT: Changes may not be evident (periosteal elevation) until after day 10

Differential Diagnosis
- Septic arthritis
- Toxic synovitis
- Cellulitis
- Sickle cell anemia
- Myositis
- Slipped capital femoral epiphysis
- Rheumatic arthritis
- Malignancy

Management
NONPHARMACOLOGIC TREATMENT
- Surgical debridement, splinting, local wound care, bedrest

PHARMACOLOGIC TREATMENT
- Intravenous antibiotics are mainstay of treatment; choice of antibiotic depends on infectious organism

LENGTH OF TREATMENT
- Antibiotic therapy for 4–6 weeks depending on organism; initially use intravenous antibiotics, may change to oral later

Special Considerations
- Culture of draining sinus tract or superficial wound does not correlate with actual infectious organism. Bone biopsy should be obtained prior to starting antibiotics.
- Geriatric patients: Constitutional symptoms (fever, elevated WBC) may be less pronounced in elderly, also presentation may be clouded by concomitant chronic illnesses.
- Pregnancy/lactation: Choice of antibiotics should be considered carefully.

When to Consult, Refer, Hospitalize
- Orthopedics referral necessary immediately
- Infectious disease consult if necessary for choice of antibiotic
- Hospitalization for central vascular catheter placement, initiation of IV antibiotics

Follow-Up
- Diagnosis and treatment plan developed by orthopedic specialist
    EXPECTED COURSE
    - Clinical improvement should be seen within 24–48 hours, then gradual resolution of drainage, pain, WBC, ESR, and fever

    COMPLICATIONS
    - Chronic osteomyelitis, need for bone and/or skin grafting, structural weakening of bone

Developmental Hip Dysplasia

Description
- Congenital displacement of the femoral head from acetabulum; ranges from subluxation to dislocation

Etiology
- Multifactorial (mechanical, physiologic, environmental, genetic)
- *Mechanical*: Breech presentation, positioning of fetal hip against mother's sacrum; tight maternal abdomen and uterine musculature causing molding and restriction of fetal movement, first born
- *Physiologic*: Ligamentous laxity due to estrogen exposure; collagen disorders
- *Environmental*: Swaddling infant with legs in extension/adduction (Navajo population); cerebral palsy
- *Genetic*: 20% have positive family history

Incidence and Demographics
- 0.5%–2% of live births
- Females more than males
- 60% involves left hip; 20% bilateral

Risk Factors
- First born, female, breech
- Positive family history

Prevention and Screening
- Avoid swaddling with legs in extension and adduction
- Check hips at birth, 2-week, 2-month, and 4-month well-baby exams

Assessment
HISTORY
- Prenatal and birth history
- Positive family history

PHYSICAL EXAM
- Limited abduction of hip; hip instability; asymmetry of thigh folds; femoral shortening on affected side
- Unequal leg lengths; unequal knee heights when supine (Galeazzi sign); limp or "duck-like" waddle

DIAGNOSTIC STUDIES
- Provocation tests: Click felt with Ortolani's maneuver; hip dislocation with Barlow's maneuver
- Ultrasound useful in neonatal period
- If older than 3–6 months may use radiographs

Differential Diagnosis
- Unstable hip in newborn period

Management
- Goal is to prevent long-term complications and pathologic changes through early diagnosis and treatment in infancy
NONPHARMACOLOGIC TREATMENT
- Birth–6 months: Pavlik harness
- 6–18 months: Pavlik harness, closed reduction with cast
- >18 months: Open reduction with casting

LENGTH OF TREATMENT
- Until corrected

Special Considerations
- About 60% of unstable hips in newborns spontaneously become normal in the first 2–4 weeks of life
- In infant >3 months, muscle tightness may mask click or dislocation
- Standard radiographs difficult to interpret before 3–6 months of age

When to Consult, Refer, Hospitalize
- At diagnosis, all children should be referred to a pediatric orthopedist for evaluation.

Follow-Up
- Followed by the orthopedic specialist
    EXPECTED COURSE
    - Most cases respond to treatment

    COMPLICATIONS
    - Osteoarthritis, pain, abnormal gait, decreased agility
    - Even with treatment, avascular necrosis of femoral head may occur

Scoliosis

Description
- Lateral curvature of the spine

Etiology
- Functional: Poor posture, leg length discrepancies, muscle spasm
- Idiopathic: Unknown cause but may be due to equilibrium dysfunction, familial causes, or asymmetrical growth

Incidence and Demographics
- 65% of all cases idiopathic
- Categorized by age
- Infantile: 0–3 years; rare in U.S.; male-to-female ratio 3:2; spontaneous resolution in 90% of cases
- Juvenile: 3–10 years; affects males/females equally; may progresses during growth spurts
- Adolescent: 5%–10% of all teens have scoliosis; progression to a significant curve (15°) occurs in <0.5%; female-to-male ratio 5–7:1; may rapidly progresses during growth spurts

Risk Factors
- 30% have positive family history; affects 20% of children with cerebral palsy
- Rapid progression during growth spurts: 12-year-old females and 14-year-old males

Prevention and Screening
- Screen during routine school age and adolescent physical exams with back fully exposed and no shoes
- Observe for asymmetry of shoulders, scapulae, and pelvis

Assessment
    HISTORY
    - Asymmetry of shoulder and or hip height; shirts or hemlines may be uneven
    - Positive family history
    - Complaints of pain

    PHYSICAL EXAM
    - Screening done with back fully exposed and without shoes
    - Observe for asymmetry of shoulders, scapulae, and hip/pelvis

- Check for leg length discrepancy, which may be present
- Bend forward at waist to 90° and slowly return to upright (Adams test)
- Assess for prominence of scapula or lateralization of spine
- 90% thoracic with right curve; left thoracic curve more likely to progress

DIAGNOSTIC STUDIES
- Routine x-rays not required for mild scoliosis
- More severe cases require x-ray entire length of spine (Cobb method)
- X-ray determines location and direction of curvature, measures degree of asymmetry, and evaluates vertebral bodies; view entire spine from C7 to S1
- Repeat x-rays to monitor progression of curve
- Consider bone age
- Scoliometer may be helpful to detect and follow smaller curves

Management
- Goal is to prevent further deformity
- Using Cobb method for evaluating degree of curvature; follow every 4–6 months in children <Tanner V
- Curves <14°: Observe, follow every 4–6 months in children <Tanner V
- Curves >15°: Refer to orthopedist to monitor for progression
- Curves >25°–30° in growing children with 5°–10° progression may need bracing to stabilize until growth is complete
- Curves > 40° in growing children require surgery with rod insertion or spinal fusion (Dormans, 2005)

Special Considerations
- Back pain uncommon in adolescents with idiopathic scoliosis so further examination warranted if pain present
- Refer to orthopedist immediately for congenital or infantile congenital scoliosis
- Scoliosis in older adults seen with deterioration of vertebral disks; often requires surgery to relieve pain, restore stability

Follow-Up
- Close follow-up essential; can be done in primary care if <15°, every 4–6 months
- Otherwise followed by the orthopedist with periodic follow-up x-rays
  EXPECTED COURSE
  - More concern with patients with large curvature at diagnosis and those with curvature before adolescent growth spurt; close follow-up essential
  - Repeat standing posterior-anterior (PA) x-ray every 6–12 months in young adolescents with mild curvature, every 3–6 months in adolescents with large curves

  COMPLICATIONS
  - Untreated scoliosis results in unacceptable cosmetic appearance and cardiopulmonary impairment
  - Spinal osteoarthritis may occur later in life

Osteoporosis

Description
- Metabolic disease with bone demineralization producing diffusely decreased bone density, diminished strength; predisposes patient to pathologic fractures, severe backache, loss of height
- Bone mineral density (BMD) at least 2.5 standard deviations (SD) below peak bone density of young adult (T score); osteopenia T score is -1.5 to -2.5 of standard deviation

Etiology
- Bone resorption by osteoclasts occurs faster than new bone matrix formation by osteoblasts and subsequent bone mineralization.
- Trabecular bone (spine, ribs, pelvis) turnover is greater than cortical bone.

Incidence and Demographics
- Approximately 20–25 million women affected; 5–6 million men in the U.S.
- White, Asian women at greater risk
- Primarily affects postmenopausal women

Risk Factors
- Inadequate calcium intake, vitamin D deficiency; excessive alcohol, protein, or caffeine intake
- Genetic predisposition: White or Asian ethnicity
- Petite frame; low weight (<127 pounds); advancing age
- Hyperthyroidism/hyperparathyroidism; rheumatoid arthritis
- Malignancy (multiple myeloma, leukemia)
- Early menopause (natural or surgical) with deficiency in estrogen/androgen
- Steroid use, Cushing syndrome
- Renal insufficiency
- Declining physical activity
- Smoking
- Sedentary lifestyle without exposure to sun

Prevention and Screening
- Balanced diet with adequate intake of calcium and vitamin D; regular weight-bearing exercise; smoking cessation; avoiding high alcohol, protein or caffeine intake; hormone replacement therapy or raloxifene (Evista) for postmenopausal women
- Estrogen replacement is the drug of choice for first-line prevention (postmenopausal)

Assessment
HISTORY
- Risk factors, fracture after age 40 (spine, hip, wrist), back pain (from vertebral fracture), osteopenia on x-ray

PHYSICAL EXAM
- No finding specific to osteoporosis; kyphosis common in elderly; loss of height

DIAGNOSTIC STUDIES
- Dual x-ray absorptiometry bone densitometry (DEXA) scan shows bone density at least 2.5 standard deviations below peak bone density, biochemical markers
- Osteopenia on x-ray (indicates loss of approximately 30% of bone mass)

Differential Diagnosis
- Endocrine disorders
- Malabsorption syndromes
- Malnutrition
- Osteomalacia
- Metastatic bone disease
- Connective tissue disorders

Management
NONPHARMACOLOGIC TREATMENT
- Prevention remains best strategy
- Regular weight-bearing exercise (20–30 minutes/day, 2–3 days /week); high-impact physical activity
- Calcium intake or supplementation (1,000–1,500 mg/day), adequate vitamin D intake (400–800 IU/day)

PHARMACOLOGIC TREATMENT
- Hormone replacement therapy for menopausal or hypogonadal women
- Selective estrogen receptor modulators (SERMs): Raloxifene (Evista) 60 mg/day po; tamoxifen (Nolvadex) 10–20 mg/day po (indicated for postmenopausal women in whom estrogen replacement therapy not indicated, e.g., breast cancer)
- Bisphosphates: Alendronate (Fosamax) 10 mg/day po, 70 mg q week; risedronate (Actonel) 5mg/day, or ibandronate (Boniva) 150 mg po q month
- Calcitonin (Miacalcin) nasal spray 200 units/day intranasal promotes osteoblastic activity

LENGTH OF TREATMENT
- Until bone density is normal

Special Considerations
- Men: Treat with calcium supplementation, vitamin D, bisphosphates, or calcitonin nasal spray
- Medications cannot be used in pregnancy

When to Consult, Refer, Hospitalize
- Refer to orthopedist for suspected fracture; hospitalize for any hip fracture

Follow-Up
- Regular follow-up for review of diet, exercise, and medications
- Repeat DEXA scan every 23 months (covered by Medicare)
  EXPECTED COURSE
  - Improvement in bone density evident 6–12 months after initiation of therapy

COMPLICATIONS
- Fracture (vertebral most common; hip has greatest mortality)

Malignant Bone Tumors

Description
- Neoplastic growth in a bone or bones

Etiology
- Malignant tumors of the bone may originate in the bone or metastasize to the bone
- In adults, most often results from seeding of another malignancy
- Metastasis from breast, lung, prostate, kidney, thyroid cancers

Incidence and Demographics
- Ewing's sarcoma most common in children, young adults
- Chondrosarcoma most common middle to late life
- Osteosarcoma most common primary bone tumor except multiple myeloma,
- Most common in children and young adults, more common in males
- In the 60–70s age group, metastatic bone cancers are more common

Risk Factors
- High doses of ionizing radiation
- Certain conditions (Paget's disease, von Recklinghausen's disease, enchondromatosis) may undergo malignant transformation

Prevention and Screening
- Early diagnosis, treatment of primary malignancy

Assessment

HISTORY (SEE TABLE 14-2)
- Unexplained pain and swelling over bone, decreased range of motion, night pain, pain with weight-bearing
- Constitutional symptoms: Weight loss, night sweats, pallor, malaise, fever

PHYSICAL EXAM
- Painful mass, swelling, limited range of motion of bone/joint
- Lymphadenopathy, hepatosplenomegaly

DIAGNOSTIC STUDIES
- X-ray may show aggressive, poorly defined lesion, irregular border, extension into soft tissue
- CT or MRI to determine extent of lesion
- Bone scan to detect metastasis
- Cytologic and pathologic examination
- CBC, liver function tests (LFTs)

Table 14-2. Malignant Bone Tumors

Malignant tumor	Typical age range, incidence	Clinical presentation	Radiographic findings
Multiple myeloma Plasma cell malignancy (most common in adults)	Incidence 3/100,000 >40 years Male/female 1.6:1	Bone pain Anemia, hypercalcemia, azotemia	Typical "punched-out" lytic lesions Diffuse osteoporosis
Osteosarcoma: 2nd most common malignant tumor in adults, most common malignant bone tumor children	Peak age 10–20 50% leg 2000–3000 per year Male/female 1.5/1	Local pain, tenderness, swelling Night pain, pain with weight-bearing Constitutional symptoms	X-ray findings: "Sunburst" pattern of radiating extensions from bone into soft tissue
Chondrosarcoma (malignant tumor of cartilage)	Middle–late adult life 90% are primary tumors; pelvis, femur, shoulder common sites Slow-growing	Acute or progressive deep pain Muscular weakness or atrophy Soft tissue mass may be palpable	Radiolucent lesions on x-ray Increased uptake on bone scan
Ewing's sarcoma: 2nd most common malignant bone tumor in children	Most common in children, young adults More common in Caucasian males	Pain, swelling, tenderness, erythema	Lytic lesion with onion skin appearance of periosteum 53% occur on extremities

Differential Diagnosis
- Benign bone tumor
- Osteomyelitis
- Metastatic disease

Management

NONPHARMACOLOGIC TREATMENT
- Surgery
- Radiation

PHARMACOLOGIC TREATMENT
- Chemotherapy

LENGTH OF TREATMENT
- Determined by oncologist

Special Considerations
- Refer for support, hospice, and pain control if necessary

When to Consult, Refer, Hospitalize
- Refer to orthopedist for any bone lesion seen on x-ray, any constitutional signs of malignancy

Follow-Up
EXPECTED COURSE
- Highly variable depending on type of tumor, patient history, tumor stage at diagnosis

COMPLICATIONS
- Loss of limb, metastases, death

CONDITIONS THAT CAUSE HIP PAIN

Toxic Synovitis

Description
- Transient synovitis
- Self-limited, unilateral inflammation of hip joint

Etiology
- Unknown cause resulting in inflammation of the synovium in the hip
- Often associated with viral infections, post vaccination, drug-mediated

Incidence and Demographics
- Most common disorder causing a limp and hip pain in children
- 2–10 years of age, average age 6; occurs more frequently in boys than girls
- Occurs more frequently in spring time

Risk Factors
- Preceding upper respiratory tract infection
- Day care attendance
- Recent antibiotic use
- Recent immunization (especially MMR)

Assessment
HISTORY
- Low-grade fever but no other systemic symptoms
- Insidious onset of pain, often complaining of vague "leg" pain or knee pain
- Antalgic limp or refusal to walk

PHYSICAL EXAM
- Well-appearing child
- Hip held in position of flexion, abduction, and external rotation, decreased internal rotation

DIAGNOSTIC STUDIES
- CBC, ESR: Usually normal or slightly elevated; ESR may be slightly elevated
- Blood culture and sensitivity to rule out infection
- Hip aspiration if septic arthritis suspected
- X-ray: Unnecessary if hip motion is full; may show capsular swelling
- Ultrasound: Can demonstrate if effusion in hip joint

Differential Diagnosis
- Septic arthritis
- Osteomyelitis
- Legg-Calvé-Perthes disease
- Slipped capital femoral epiphysis
- Juvenile rheumatoid arthritis

Management
NONPHARMACOLOGIC TREATMENT
- Bedrest for 1–3 days

PHARMACOLOGIC TREATMENT
- OTC analgesics: Acetaminophen or NSAIDS may be used for 1–2 weeks

Special Considerations
- Rule out child abuse

When to Consult, Refer, Hospitalize
- Orthopedic referral needed for hip aspiration if infection suspected
- Hospitalize for any indication of infection

Follow-Up
EXPECTED COURSE
- Improvement should occur in 24–48 hours
- If symptoms persist beyond 1 week, reevaluation important to rule out other diagnoses

COMPLICATIONS
- 2%–5% develop Legg-Calvé-Perthes disease within 1 year
- Rarely avascular necrosis of femoral head
- May experience reccurrence with subsequent viral infections

Legg-Calvé-Perthes Disease

Description
- Idiopathic juvenile avascular necrosis of femoral head

Etiology
- Unclear. Can be idiopathic or due to slipped capital femoral epiphysis, trauma, steroid use, sickle cell crisis, or congenital dislocation of hip that may cause disruption in blood flow to femoral head

Incidence and Demographics
- Children 4–8 years old; male-to-female ratio 4–5:1; low frequency among relatives
- 10% bilateral
- Increased frequency in urban areas

Risk Factors
- Low birthweight, delayed bone age, short stature
- 10% breech delivery
- 17% with previous trauma
- History of steroid use, sickle cell disease, congenital hip dislocation
- Older parents, from large families of lower socioeconomic status

Prevention and Screening
- If child is obese, weight reduction may reduce risk of developing in other hip.

Assessment
HISTORY
- Either subtle or sudden onset of limp, may be intermittent in early stages
- Sudden onset of groin, thigh, or knee pain
- Pain worse in morning and after activity

PHYSICAL EXAM
- Presents with painful or painless limp
- Resists internal rotation and abduction
- Leg kept in position of flexion and external rotation
- May have atrophy of quadriceps muscles

DIAGNOSTIC STUDIES
- X-ray AP and frog leg views
- Early x-ray may be negative or show widening of joint space
- Later x-ray with increased density, decreased femoral head size, and flattening of femoral head
- Ultrasound may show joint effusion early

Differential Diagnosis
- Septic arthritis
- Trauma
- Slipped capital femoral epiphysis
- Neoplasia
- Hemophilia
- JRA
- Acute/chronic infection

Management
NONPHARMACOLOGIC TREATMENT
- Bedrest initially, followed by limited activities
- Physical therapy to maintain range of motion; may need crutches initially
- Containment of the femoral epiphysis with cast, brace, or orthosis

PHARMACOLOGIC TREATMENT
• OTC NSAIDs for pain relief

Special Considerations
• Pain often referred to knee

When to Consult, Refer, Hospitalize
• All suspected cases require orthopedic consult

Follow-Up
EXPECTED COURSE
• Related to degree of femoral head involvement and age at onset; symptoms slowly resolve over 12–18 months
• Children <6 years old with better prognosis; children >8 years old have increased risk of degenerative arthritis in adulthood and may need hip replacement

COMPLICATIONS
• Hip replacement may be needed

Slipped Capital Femoral Epiphysis (SCFE)

Description
• Anterior displacement of femoral neck of femur from the capital femoral epiphysis, sudden or gradual dislocation of the head of the femur from its neck and shaft at the proximal epiphyseal plate

Etiology
• True etiology unclear, likely a combination of factors
• Mechanical factors (motor vehicle accident, fall from height, abuse)
• Endocrine (hypothyroidism, pituitary disorders)
• Genetic
• Inflammatory

Incidence and Demographics
• Most common adolescent hip disorder; male-to-female ratio 2:1; 2 cases per 100,000
• Peak age 12 years for girls, 14 years for boys
• 30% present with bilateral involvement
• 5% of cases with positive parental history of SCFE

Risk Factors
• Obesity
• Increased height
• African American
• Sedentary lifestyle

Assessment
HISTORY
• Pain in hip, infrequently referred pain to medial aspect of knee
• Severe pain in acute displacement
• Insidious dull pain in gradual displacement

PHYSICAL EXAM
- Presents with limp or inability to walk; walks with foot turned outward
- Local tenderness over hip
- Decreased flexion, abduction, and internal rotation
- Muscle atrophy and leg length shortening

DIAGNOSTIC STUDIES
- AP, lateral and frog-leg x-rays diagnostic: Femoral head resembles ice cream falling off cone
- Early slippage may be missed on x-ray, if suspicious order bone scan

Differential Diagnosis
- Toxic synovitis
- Legg-Calvé-Perthes disease
- Osteochondritis dissecans
- Chondrolysis
- Tumor
- Muscle strain
- Osteomyelitis
- Juvenile rheumatoid arthritis

Management
- Goals to prevent increased slippage and maintain hip function
  NONPHARMACOLOGIC TREATMENT
  - Early disease: Surgical placement of pin through femoral head and growth plate; rapid recovery with excellent prognosis
  - Late disease: Reconstructive surgery; poor outcome due to degenerative arthritis and need for early hip replacement

Special Considerations
- Prognosis is good if diagnosed early; avoid delay in diagnosis.

When to Consult, Refer, Hospitalize
- Emergency referral to orthopedist for surgical repair

Follow-Up
EXPECTED COURSE
- Depends on how quickly it is picked up
- Anatomic position must be maintained postoperatively
- In children <10 years old, monitor for bilateral slip

COMPLICATIONS
- Avascular necrosis of femoral head
- May have slight but persistent leg length shortening
- Chondrolysis more common in African-American children

CONDITIONS THAT CAUSE KNEE PAIN

Osgood-Schlatter's Disease

Description
- Overuse syndrome causing traction apophysitis of tibial tubercle

Etiology
- Repetitive microtrauma causing partial avulsion of patellar tendon insertion site on tibia (tibial apophysis)

Incidence and Demographics
- Boys 11–18 years old; girls 10–16 years old; more common in boys
- 30% bilateral

Risk Factors
- Physically active adolescents

Prevention and Screening
- Avoid overuse
- Adequate stretching with exercise

Assessment
HISTORY
- Pain below knee that begins during or after activity and is relieved by rest

PHYSICAL EXAM
- Local tenderness and swelling over tibial tubercle
- Resisted knee extension worsens pain

DIAGNOSTIC STUDIES
- Plain x-ray shows characteristic fragmentation of tibial tubercle; also to rule out other conditions if diagnosis uncertain
- May show soft-tissue swelling and thickening of patellar tendon

Differential Diagnosis
- Osteogenic sarcoma
- Patellar tendinitis

Management
NONPHARMACOLOGIC TREATMENT
- Avoid activities that cause pain
- Ice for 20 minutes after exercise
- Quadriceps strengthening exercises qid
- If pain interferes with school and sleep, consider knee immobilization

Special Considerations
- Recurrence rate 60%

When to Consult, Refer, Hospitalize
- Consult and or refer if not improving with conservative treatment after 4 weeks

Follow-Up
- At 2–4 week intervals
  EXPECTED COURSE
  - Usually self-limited
  - Resolves when tubercle fuses to diaphysis

  COMPLICATIONS
  - 5%–10% of cases become chronic and may require surgical resection of ossicle

Knee Injury

Description
- Damage to the knee or its supporting structures caused by trauma

Etiology
- Direct or indirect force to the knee
- Common in sports that require rapid changes in direction, acceleration/deceleration; knee injuries common in outpatient setting
- Often tear of ligaments or cartilage in knee
- May be fracture of the patella; children's ligaments and tendons are relatively stronger than bones, therefore children are at increased fracture risk

Incidence and Demographics
- Common in all ages, especially adults
- Meniscus injuries more common in adults than children

Risk Factors
- Participation in contact, running sport
- Poor conditioning
- Osteoarthritis
- Poorly fitting footwear, especially if associated with falls

Prevention and Screening
- Proper training, protective gear

Assessment
- See Tables 14–3 and 14–4

Table 14–3. Summary of Common Knee Injuries

Injury	Demographics	History	Physical
Fracture	Any age	Trauma Steroid use, osteoporosis Sudden swelling, pain, worse with weight-bearing	Effusion (hemarthrosis) Bony tenderness/pain to palpation Decreased ROM Difficulty bearing weight
Medial collateral ligament (MCL) injury	Adolescents and adults Contact sports	Sudden valgus stress to knee May have heard or felt "pop" Medial knee pain Localized swelling 1–4 hours	Tenderness to palpation Varying degree of joint laxity Small effusion
Lateral collateral ligament (LCL) injury	Adolescents and adults Contact sports	Direct blow to medial aspect of knee (varus stress) Similar to MCL injury but lateral	Tenderness over LCL Varying degree of joint laxity Small, if any, effusion
Anterior cruciate ligament (ACL) injury	Adolescents and adults Athletes	Pain and almost immediate swelling after sudden turning, deceleration, jumping May have heard or felt a "pop" Weight-bearing difficult due to feelings of instability	Effusion (hemarthrosis) Pain/tenderness in posterolateral joint Positive provocation tests (anterior drawer, Lachman's)
Posterior cruciate ligament (PCL) injury	Athletes Gymnasts	Forced hyperextension of knee Direct blow to anterior proximal tibia while knee is flexed and foot is planted	Mild to moderate effusion Positive posterior drawer, Godfrey's tests
Meniscus tear	Adolescents, adults Athletes Elderly with OA of knee	Pain, especially with twisting of knee (getting in and out of vehicles) Locking, catching or giving way Harder to descend stairs than climb them	Swelling Tenderness over tibial medial or lateral joint line Positive McMurray's test
Quadriceps rupture	Athletes Elderly with concomitant diseases (diabetes, peripheral vascular disease)	Often, fall on extended knee that forces joint into flexion Inability to straighten knee	Swelling Sometimes, palpable defect just superior to patella Inability to extend knee against resistance

Table 14–4. Clinically Relevant Provocative Tests of the Knee

Test Name	How to Perform Test
Valgus stress (tests MCL)	With patient's knee in 20°–30° of flexion, the examiner stabilizes the leg with one hand while applying inward-directed pressure to the joint. Test is repeated with knee in full extension.
Varus stress (tests LCL)	As above but stress at joint is directed from medial to lateral direction.
Anterior drawer (tests ACL)	With patient supine, his/her knee is flexed to 90° while examiner stabilizes patient's tibia (usually by sitting on foot/ankle). Examiner grasps proximal posterior tibia, pulling it forward. Anterior movement (translation) of tibia greater than uninvolved side is positive test.
Posterior drawer (tests PCL)	Patient and examiner in same position as for anterior drawer, but examiner pushes tibia posteriorly.
Lachman's test (more accurate than anterior drawer)	With patient supine, his/her knee is flexed to 30°. Using one hand, examiner stabilizes patient's distal femur while using other hand to pull proximal tibia anteriorly.
McMurray's test (for meniscus injury)	Patient's knee maximally flexed, then internally rotated; as leg is passively extended, examiner simultaneously externally rotates leg while palpating tibial joint line. Repeat with leg externally rotated, internally rotating while extending. Positive test is palpable click or tibial joint line pain.

DIAGNOSTIC STUDIES

- Joint aspiration: Diagnostic and therapeutic (presence of fat globules seen with fracture; removal of effusion can improve ROM, increase patient comfort)
- X-ray: Diagnose fracture, osteoarthritis
- CT: Evaluate extent of fracture depression (if any), position of fracture fragments
- MRI: Differentiate ligamentous, cartilaginous injuries

Differential Diagnosis

- Worsening osteoarthritis
- Septic joint
- Gout
- Tumor

Management

NONPHARMACOLOGIC TREATMENT

- Fracture: Immobilization, no weight-bearing, surgical repair sometimes necessary
- Grade I, II collateral ligament sprains: Hinged knee brace; surgery usually not required
- Grade III sprains involve complete tearing of ligament: Surgery usually required
- Cruciate ligament sprains: Bracing, physical therapy, surgical reconstruction may be necessary
- Meniscus tears: Arthroscopic repair (preferred treatment)
- Physical therapy for improving ROM, strength

PHARMACOLOGIC TREATMENT
- NSAIDs for 1–2 weeks regularly for inflammation and pain
- Analgesics , including narcotic medications for short-term pain management (up to 7–10 days)

Special Considerations
- Active younger patients may require functional bracing to return to sports

When to Consult, Refer, Hospitalize
- Consult for grade II, III sprains
- Refer immediately for suspected fracture, inability to flex or extend joint, hemarthrosis, suspected septic joint or tumor

Follow-Up
- Follow up in 1–2 weeks and at 2–4-week intervals until resolved
  EXPECTED COURSE
  - Except for fractures, meniscus tears, complete ligamentous disruption, most knee injuries will heal in 4–8 weeks

  COMPLICATIONS
  - Deformity, accelerated degenerative changes of joint, stiffness, or instability

CONDITIONS THAT CAUSE ANKLE PAIN

Ankle Sprain

Description
- Stretching and/or tearing of ligaments around the ankle
- Standard grading indicates extent of damage
  - Grade I: Stretching but no tearing of ligament; no joint instability (local tenderness, minimal edema, full ROM, can bear weight, discomfort)
  - Grade II: Partial (incomplete) tearing of ligament; some joint instability but definite end-point to laxity (immediate pain, localized edema, ecchymoses, pain on weight-bearing, reduced ROM)
  - Grade III: Complete ligamentous tearing; joint unstable with no definite endpoint to ligamentous stressing (acute pain with injury, significant edema of foot and ankle, profound and continuing development of ecchymoses, cannot bear weight, ankle ROM restricted)

Etiology
- Usually a forced inversion, affects lateral ankle, most common; or eversion injury affects medial ankle, second most common type

Incidence and Demographics
- Most common musculoskeletal injury
- Occurs at rate of 1 per 10,000 persons per day; males more often affected

Risk Factors
- Sports requiring sudden turns, jumping; foot in supinated, plantar flexed position

Prevention and Screening
- Conditioning exercises for sports, avoidance of high-heeled shoes, ankle-strengthening exercises

Assessment
HISTORY
- Sudden, forced inversion or eversion of foot, often in plantar flexed position
- Sudden onset of pain, rapid onset of swelling; often with inability to initially bear weight on affected ankle
- Bruising may develop within 2–4 days
- Sensation of pop, snap, locking of joint

PHYSICAL EXAM
- Edema, ecchymosis, tenderness over injured ligaments; pain aggravated by repeating motion that caused original injury
- Talar tilt test used to assess stability of calcaneofibular ligament (heel is grasped and supinated)
- Anterior drawer sign used to assess anterior talofibular ligament (while holding the lower leg steady, the heel is grasped and pulled forward)

DIAGNOSTIC STUDIES
- X-rays not indicated in adult population unless at least one of the following (Ottawa rule):
  - Unable to bear weight right after injury or when examined
  - Tenderness over posterior edge of distal 6 cm of the medial or lateral malleolus
  - Tenderness over tarsal navicular or fifth metatarsal
- If x-rays necessary, AP, lateral, and mortise views should be ordered

Differential Diagnosis
- Syndesmosis injury
- Fracture
- Tendon rupture

Management
NONPHARMACOLOGIC TREATMENT
- Remember the mnemonic, all grades respond to RICE protocol:
  - R: Rest (non weight-bearing)
  - I: Ice (20 minutes qid until swelling has resolved)
  - C: Compression (elastic bandage)
  - E: Elevation for 48–72 hours
- Splinting, weight-bearing as tolerated, ankle ROM and strengthening exercises
- Grade III injuries may require casting, surgery

PHARMACOLOGIC TREATMENT
- NSAIDs or OTC analgesics

LENGTH OF TREATMENT
- Most Grade I or II sprains heal in 6–8 weeks

Special Considerations
- Medial ankle sprains require greater force to cause injury; may have other associated injury
- Geriatric patients: Older patients may require longer healing time

When to Consult, Refer, Hospitalize
- Consult for any degree of ankle instability; refer for positive anterior drawer or talar tilt test, or for suggestion of syndesmosis injury

Follow-Up
- Follow up in 1–2 weeks if not improving after initial diagnosis
    EXPECTED COURSE
    - Most uncomplicated sprains show improvement in 3–4 weeks, heal within 6–8 weeks

    COMPLICATIONS
    - Syndesmosis injury, peroneal tendinitis, recurrent injury, chronic instability, avascular necrosis

Sever's Disease

Description
- Inflammatory condition causing a calcaneal apophysitis

Etiology
- Traction-induced microtrauma at the insertion of the Achilles tendon on the calcaneus, causing inflammation

Incidence and Demographics
- 8–13-year-olds
- Athletes

Risk Factors
- Accelerated growth
- Tight heel cords
- Soccer players or runners

Assessment
    HISTORY
    - Heel pain with activity
    - Bilateral or unilateral

    PHYSICAL EXAM
    - Tenderness at insertion of the Achilles tendon on the calcaneus

DIAGNOSTIC STUDIES
  • X-rays may show partial fragmentation and increased density of the os calcis

Differential Diagnosis
• Bone cyst
• Stress fracture
• Strain

Management
NONPHARMACOLOGIC TREATMENT
  • Activity modification
  • Stretching, ice
  • Heel cups

PHARMACOLOGIC TREATMENT
  • NSAIDs

LENGTH OF TREATMENT
  • Until resolved, 4–6 weeks

Special Considerations
• May need to modify activity, exercise, or shoes until improved

When to Consult, Refer, Hospitalize
• Achilles tendon rupture or not improving with treatment

Follow-Up
• In 2 weeks to make sure it is resolving
  EXPECTED COURSE
    • Improvement in 2–4 weeks with activity modification

  COMPLICATIONS
    • Rupture of the Achilles tendon

CONDITONS THAT CAUSE SHOULDER PAIN

Fractured Clavicle

Description
• Fracture of clavicle; most frequently fractured bone during delivery

Etiology
• Birth trauma due to delivery of shoulder in vertex position and extended arms in breech delivery
• Fall on out-stretched arm or on clavicle

Incidence and Demographics
• 3.5% of births

- 80% middle third of clavicle
- Occurs in all ages, more common in children; in adults usually occurs after a fall

Risk Factors
- Large fetus, shoulder dystocia
- Breech position
- Fall on outstretched arm

Prevention and Screening
- Methods to reduce birth trauma
- Check for fractures at birth and 2-week well-child visits

Assessment
HISTORY
- Difficult delivery or characteristic injury
- Pain, displacement, or bump on clavicle

PHYSICAL EXAM
- Newborn or patient may not move arm on affected side (Erb's palsy)
- Absent Moro reflex on affected side in newborn

DIAGNOSTIC STUDIES
- X-rays not usually done in newborns
- X-rays done if history of fall or trauma

Differential Diagnosis
- Fractured humerus
- Brachial nerve palsy

Management
- Prognosis is excellent even with no treatment if fracture is not displaced
- Callus formation occurs in 1–2 weeks
  NONPHARMACOLOGICAL TREATMENT
  - Consider immobilization of arm and shoulder on affected side, figure eight sling or clavicular strap

  PHARMACOLOGIC TREATMENT
  - Analgesics as needed

  LENGTH OF TREATMENT
  - Until healed (4–6 weeks)

Special Considerations
- Check in babies with history of breech or difficult delivery, large size, mothers with gestational diabetes

When to Consult, Refer, Hospitalize
- Refer to orthopedist for any symptoms of neurovascular injury

Follow-Up
- Follow up if not improving in 3–4 weeks
  EXPECTED COURSE
    - Heals in 3–4 weeks in children
    - Heals in 6 weeks in adults

  COMPLICATIONS
    - 10% of infants will also have concomitant brachial plexus injuries
    - Permanent bump at site of callus formation in adults; rare in children <10 years
    - Neurovascular injury

OTHER SHOULDER INJURIES AND CONDITIONS

Description
- Pain in the shoulder girdle

Etiology
- Traumatic, arthritic, infectious, or degenerative conditions (Table 14–5)

Table 14-5. Common Causes of Acute and Chronic Shoulder Pain

Acute Conditions	Chronic Conditions
Trauma: Fracture (proximal humerus, greater tuberosity, clavicle, scapula)	Inflammatory conditions: Bursitis (subacromial and subdeltoid)
Rotator cuff strain, tear	Bicipital, rotator cuff tendinitis
Dislocation (anterior most common)	Impingement syndrome
Acromioclavicular separation ("separated shoulder")	Degenerative conditions: Osteoarthritis
Sternoclavicular injury	Subacromial spurring
	Other: Chronic instability
	Adhesive capsulitis (frozen shoulder)

Incidence and Demographics
- Acute injuries tend to occur in adolescents and younger adults; chronic shoulder pain and fracture due to falls more often are found in older adults

Risk Factors
- Repetitive overhead activity (occupational, recreational)
- Rheumatoid or osteoarthritis
- Previous shoulder injury

Prevention and Screening
- Injury prevention

Assessment

- See Table 14–6

  DIAGNOSTIC STUDIES
  - Plain x-ray: Useful for evaluating fracture, AC separation, presence of osteophytes, calcific tendinitis
  - MRI: Can show tendinitis, rotator cuff tear, ligamentous or cartilage injury
  - Arthrogram: Still used to identify extent of rotator cuff tear

Differential Diagnosis

- Septic joint
- Gout
- Complex regional pain syndrome
- Chondroclavicular disease
- Acromegaly

Table 14-6. Assessment of Shoulder Injuries

Condition	History	Physical findngs
Fracture	Fall directly onto shoulder or outstretched arm Localized pain, swelling Decreased ROM Often, no bruising evident for first few days after injury	Patient holds arm close to body Point tenderness Varying degree of bony deformity (usually most pronounced with clavicle fracture) Decreased ROM
Rotator cuff tear	Age usually >40 years Pain may radiate into deltoid area May have felt "pop" or "something give" in shoulder Inability to raise arm overhead Weakness or inability to externally rotate arm Inability to sleep on affected side	Weakness or inability to externally rotate shoulder Limited abduction, forward flexion of shoulder Inability to maintain resisted abduction at 90°
Dislocation	Direct blow to shoulder or trying to avoid fall by grabbing onto something; shoulder in abducted, externally rotated position Sensation of shoulder slipping out of joint "Popping" or clicking of joint May note swelling	Positive apprehension test: shoulder abducted to 90° and elbow flexed to 90°; shoulder then passively externally rotated; resistance by patient is a positive test Palpable clicking with ROM Deformity may be visible
Separated shoulder	Usually, direct blow or fall onto top of shoulder Pain, especially with adduction of arm Swelling Deformity depends on severity of injury	Tenderness over acromioclavicular (AC) joint Pain with adduction (across chest) Varying degree of AC deformity (more deformity with more severe injury) Bruising may be present

Table 14–6. Assessment of Shoulder Injuries (cont.)

Condition	History	Physical findngs
Inflammatory conditions	Progressive pain with certain activities (usually overhead) that may progress to constant pain Pain often worse with lifting, pushing objects away Difficulty lying on affected side	Tenderness over inflamed tendon(s)—palpated in bicipital groove May have weak abduction Painful arc (i.e., pain at 70°–120° of abduction)
Adhesive capsulitis	Middle-aged women more likely to be afflicted May or may not have history of trauma Progressive loss of motion Pain varies from minimal to severe	Marked restriction in active and passive ROM Pain over anterior joint, rotator cuff Patient often uses scapular muscles to "increase" abduction

Management

NONPHARMACOLOGIC TREATMENT
- Initially, short period of rest/immobilization (no more than 14 days) then begin passive ROM exercises; progress to active, resistive exercises as healing continues
- Surgical intervention indicated for complete rotator cuff tear, displaced fracture
- Manipulation under anesthesia may be necessary for severe adhesive capsulitis
- Physical therapy to maintain, improve ROM, strengthen muscles

PHARMACOLOGIC TREATMENT
- NSAIDs, other analgesics
- Local corticosteroid injection

LENGTH OF TREATMENT
- As long as symptomatic

When to Consult, Refer, Hospitalize
- Refer for any fracture, suspected rotator cuff tear, rheumatoid arthritis, AC separation with deformity, dislocation or chronic instability, adhesive capsulitis, corticosteroid injection

Follow-Up
- Follow-up visits are variable depending on condition and severity, may be 2–4 week intervals.

EXPECTED COURSE
- Varies according to pathology
- Tendinitis symptoms should improve within 3–4 weeks of conservative therapy but may not resolve for 6 or more weeks; follow-up in 3–4 weeks if no improvement
- AC separation (mild) should be re-evaluated in 2–3 weeks; resolution usually in about 6 weeks
- Osteoarthritis: Reevaluate 4–6 weeks after starting treatment

COMPLICATIONS
- Permanently decreased ROM, muscular weakness

CONDITIONS THAT CAUSE ELBOW PAIN

Epicondylitis

Description
- Inflammation of the lateral or medial epicondyle
- Lateral epicondylitis ("tennis elbow"): Involves extensor tendons of forearm; common
- Medial epicondylitis ("golfer's elbow"): Involves flexor tendons of forearm; less common

Etiology
- Overuse syndrome caused by damage to tendons, progressing to periostitis at origin on epicondyle
- Stress on tendons; may be due to repetitive motions, poor technique when playing racquet or throwing sports; most common in middle age

Risk Factors
- Weak shoulder and wrist muscles (extensors and/or flexors)
- Repetitive motion of forearm with wrist extended or flexed against resistance

Prevention and Screening
- Strengthening of shoulder muscles, wrist extensors, and flexors
- For sports, appropriate-sized grips on racquets, proper body mechanics when throwing

Assessment
HISTORY
- Pain on affected side of elbow that progresses down forearm, occasionally into wrist
- Difficulty lifting objects, even a cup of liquid
- Numbness and tingling are NOT usually associated

PHYSICAL EXAM
- Lateral or medial epicondyle is tender to palpation
- Lateral epicondylitis: Pain upon grasping a weighted cup or resisted wrist extension
- Medial epicondylitis: Pain with pronation, flex wrist against resistance, or squeezing hard rubber ball

DIAGNOSTIC STUDIES
- None

Differential Diagnosis
- Carpal tunnel syndrome
- Ulnar nerve entrapment
- Septic arthritis
- Elbow fracture
- Collateral ligament injury

Management
NONPHARMACOLOGIC TREATMENT
- Rest, ice
- Avoid activities that exacerbate pain
- Compression with counterforce bands—tennis elbow band
- Physical therapy, including ultrasound, stretching exercises after pain subsides
- Recalcitrant cases may require surgery (Bosworth procedure)

PHARMACOLOGIC TREATMENT
- NSAIDs
- Triamcinolone corticosteroid injection if not improving with rest and NSAIDs

LENGTH OF TREATMENT
- Symptoms should resolve in 3 months with conservative treatment or maximum of 3 injections at 6-week intervals

Special Considerations
- More than 3 corticosteroid injections unlikely to improve chance of remission but is more likely to cause adverse effects (tendon weakening, subcutaneous fat necrosis, hypopigmentation of skin)

When to Consult, Refer, Hospitalize
- Refer to orthopedist if no improvement after 3 months of conservative treatment

Follow-Up
- Provide patient education about removing underlying cause of the problem to avoid recurrence
  #### EXPECTED COURSE
  - Noticeable improvement should occur within 6 weeks of treatment

  #### COMPLICATIONS
  - Not common but chronic, untreated epicondylitis can progress to epicondylar spur formation and damage to collateral ligament

Subluxation of Radial Head

Description
- Subluxation of the annular ligament into the radio humeral joint; also known as "nursemaid's elbow"

Etiology
- Sudden longitudinal pull on hand with elbow extended and forearm pronated
- Ligament becomes trapped when radius recoils

Incidence and Demographics
- Most common elbow injury in 2–4-year-olds
- Peak incidence 1–3-year-olds

Prevention
- Avoid pulling on child's arm, swinging child by hands, or lifting by one hand.
- Screening: No routine screening; with presenting symptoms only.

Assessment

HISTORY
- Report of child's arm being suddenly and vigorously pulled immediately followed by crying and refusal to move arm
- May have heard or felt a "click"

PHYSICAL EXAM
- Child holds arm close to body in a flexed, pronated position
- Flexion and extension normal; limited supination
- No swelling, deformity, point tenderness, warmth, or erythema noted

DIAGNOSTIC STUDIES
- X-ray if reduction unsuccessful

Differential Diagnosis
- Fracture
- Sprain/strain

Management

NONPHARMACOLOGICAL TREATMENT
- Reduce subluxation by gentle supination with arm in 90° flexion
- "Click" usually heard or felt with immediate pain relief

Special Considerations
- Observe child after reduction to ensure use of arm
- Have child grasp a sticker with affected hand

When to Consult, Refer, Hospitalize
- Refer to orthopedist if closed reduction unsuccessful or recurrent

Follow-Up

EXPECTED COURSE
- Full use returns in 30 minutes

COMPLICATIONS
- Can be recurrent in some children

CONDITONS THAT CAUSE WRIST PAIN

Ligament and Tendon Injuries

Description
- Acute or chronic pain in the wrist due to inflammation of soft tissue

Etiology
- Trauma (radiocarpal sprain), developmental (ganglion cyst), overuse (De Quervain's tenosynovitis, tendinitis)

Incidence and Demographics
- Common problem that affects all ages, sexes, races

Risk Factors
- Repetitive use of hands, wrists
- Injury to wrist
- Osteoarthritis

Prevention and Screening
- Wear protective wrist guards with sports
- Proper positioning of computer, keyboard, or other equipment
- Avoid overuse

Assessment (Table 14–7)

Table 14–7. Common Causes of Wrist Pain

Condition	History	Physical Findings
Radiocarpal sprain	Trauma: Usually forced hyperextension or flexion Pain with movement Decreased ROM	Varying degree of swelling Numbness/tingling are unusual more than a day or two after injury Pain with active and passive ROM Tenderness over radiocarpal joint but no point bony tenderness
Ganglion cyst	Usually no history of trauma May have repetitive use of hands/wrists Progressive localized swelling that tends to fluctuate in size depending on activity Usually nonpainful	Most common on dorsum of wrist but also seen on volar surface Encapsulated, slightly fluctuant, mobile lesion Pain may occur with compression of mass
De Quervain's Tenosynovitis	Insidious onset of burning, aching pain over radial aspect of wrist and base of thumb Common in nursing mothers (due to holding infant with thumb extended); pain often worse with grasping movements	Pain with passive, active thumb extension May have visible thickening of tendon Positive Finklestein's test: pain with ulnar deviation of clenched fist (with thumb tucked inside fist)

DIAGNOSTIC STUDIES
- Clinical examination usually sufficient to diagnose these problems
- X-rays should be obtained if any suggestion of fracture
- MRI can be used to differentiate ganglion cyst from other soft tissue masses, look for more serious wrist injury (triangular fibrocartilage tear)

Differential Diagnosis
- Nerve entrapment
- Fracture
- Gout
- Rheumatoid arthritis
- Osteoarthritis

Management
NONPHARMACOLOGIC TREATMENT
- Splinting, moist heat, aspiration of ganglion (fairly high recurrence rate)
- Surgical release of tendon sheath, surgical excision of ganglion

PHARMACOLOGIC TREATMENT
- NSAIDs
- Corticosteroid injection into first dorsal tendon sheath for de Quervain's

Special Considerations
- Women more often affected by de Quervain's, ganglion cysts

When to Consult, Refer, Hospitalize
- Consult with orthopedist for wrist condition that doesn't improve within 3–4 weeks of conservative treatment; refer for corticosteroid injection, any suspicion of fracture

Follow-Up
- If not improving in expected timeline
  EXPECTED COURSE
  - Most wrist pain resolve in 4–6 weeks; ganglion cysts tend to recur

  COMPLICATIONS
  - Less but chronic wrist pain can occur

OTHER MUSCULOSKELETAL CONDITIONS AND INJURIES

Fractures

Description
- Complete or incomplete chip or break in bone

Etiology
- Usually some type of trauma, but tumor, osteoporosis, osteomyelitis, osteomalacia can also cause bone to break

Incidence and Demographics
- Common in children due to activity, and in advancing age
- White women over age 60 have a higher incidence of fracture than men
- Vertebral fractures are most frequent, followed by wrist fracture

Risk Factors
- Trauma, falls
- Neoplasms
- Osteoporosis, osteomyelitis
- Smoking, malnutrition (vitamin D deficiency), malabsorption, chronic steroid use
- Renal osteodystrophy
- Osteogenesis imperfecta

Prevention and Screening
- Maximize bone density during adolescence/young adulthood
- Weight-bearing physical activity
- Adequate dietary intake of calcium and vitamin D
- Avoidance of smoking, excessive alcohol intake

Assessment
HISTORY
- Pain is predominant symptom (fall, direct or indirect violence are also common)
- Pain worse with movement
- Swelling occurs rapidly, may be associated with bruising, variable degree of deformity or asymmetry

PHYSICAL EXAM
- Point tenderness over bone; muscle weakness/pain with movement; deformity

DIAGNOSTIC STUDIES
- X-ray: Most cost-effective; usually adequate for showing fracture
- Bone scan: Useful for identifying occult/stress fracture
- CT: For evaluating degree of displacement, compression of fracture
- MRI: Identifying lesions that may affect bone
- Laboratory studies not usually indicated

Differential Diagnosis

- Sprain
- Hematoma
- Abscess
- Tumor

Management

NONPHARMACOLOGIC TREATMENT

- Immobilization by splinting or casting of extremity
- Monitor and maintain neurovascular integrity
- Surgery may be necessary for open reduction and internal fixation if fracture is displaced

PHARMACOLOGIC TREATMENT

- Analgesics, narcotic analgesia common
- NSAIDs after first 24 hours (immediate administration may increase hematoma formation due to platelet inhibition)

LENGTH OF TREATMENT

- Primary care treatment is immobilization and referral to orthopedic surgeon
- Most simple fractures heal in 4–6 weeks; longer immobilization should be expected in presence of displaced fractures, chronic disease (diabetes, cardiovascular disease), smoking, malignancy

Special Considerations

- In geriatric patients, consider x-ray even if no trauma to rule out compression fracture or tumor
- Consider stress fracture if persistent bony tenderness and negative initial x-ray
- Epiphyseal fractures (Salter I–V) in children may disrupt growth of the bone

When to Consult, Refer, Hospitalize

- Refer all compound, displaced, or compression fractures immediately
- Consult with orthopedist to determine need for specialty care
- Need to hospitalize determined by orthopedist

Follow-Up

- In 4–6 weeks if improving, sooner if pain persists
  ### EXPECTED COURSE
  - Fracture healing should occur in 4–6 weeks; if casted, persistent but gradually decreasing swelling and improving strength may take another 4–6 weeks to resolve

  ### COMPLICATIONS
  - Persistent deformity, arthritis, compression neuropathy, fibrous union

Stress Fracture

Description
- Fracture resulting from indirect trauma to a bone, creating a very fine fracture line that cannot easily be seen on x-ray

Etiology
- Microtrauma to a normal bone that exceeds that bone's capability for repair
- Fracture of a bone without trauma

Incidence and Demographics
- More common in runners, athletes who participate in jumping activities, military recruits
- Metatarsal stress fractures most common but tibial shaft, calcaneus, patella, pubic ramus, pars interarticularis also affected

Risk Factors
- Training errors (sudden increase in intensity or duration)
- Overuse
- Metabolic disorders

Prevention and Screening
- Proper training, wear appropriate footwear, use good body mechanics

Assessment
HISTORY
- Insidious onset of pain intensified by running, jogging; pain may persist for 2–3 weeks before patient seeks treatment

PHYSICAL EXAM
- Mild erythema, diffuse swelling, and point tenderness over fracture site

DIAGNOSTIC STUDIES
- Bone scan most useful for early diagnosis since x-ray changes not usually apparent for 3–4 weeks

Differential Diagnosis
- Sprain
- Infection

Management
NONPHARMACOLOGIC TREATMENT
- Limit physical activity
- Correct underlying biomechanical problem

PHARMACOLOGIC TREATMENT
- NSAIDs
- Narcotic analgesics rarely necessary

LENGTH OF TREATMENT
- 4–6 weeks

Special Considerations
- Consider in athletes, postmenopausal women with persistent bone pain without trauma

When to Consult, Refer, Hospitalize
- Consult or refer to orthopedist if any question about diagnosis, treatment

Follow-Up
- In 4–6 weeks, sooner if not improving
- Stress fractures can progress to complete fractures
    EXPECTED COURSE
    - Once treated, normal activities usually can be resumed in 4–6 weeks

    COMPLICATIONS
    - Left untreated, can progress to full fracture

Muscle Strain

Description
- Over stretching or partial tearing of muscle fibers; graded I–III
    - Grade I: Stretching, tearing of muscle fibers but fascia remains intact, no loss of muscle function; movement strong and painful
    - Grade II: Tearing of muscle fibers resulting in significant hemorrhage, mild loss of muscle strength; movement is fairly strong and painful
    - Grade III: Rupture of muscle, damage to fascia; movement is weak and pain-free

Etiology
- Excessive stress placed on any muscle resulting in over-stretching of fibers and resultant tearing and inflammation

Incidence and Demographics
- Common problem, many instances self-treated

Risk Factors
- Contact sports, running
- Lifting or moving heavy objects

Prevention and Screening
- Appropriate stretching, warm-up exercises prior to participating in running, sports; proper body mechanics

Assessment
    HISTORY
    - Sudden onset of muscle pain associated with activity; bruising, swelling, and loss of function may occur with more severe injury
    - Gradually increasing muscle pain may occur with repetitive use of specific muscle/group

PHYSICAL EXAM
- Localized tenderness, swelling, ecchymosis; pain with resisted muscle contraction and passive stretching of muscle; weakness with more severe injury

DIAGNOSTIC STUDIES
- MRI may be useful to identify extent of muscle involvement but usually not necessary

Differential Diagnosis
- Tendinitis
- Tumor

Management

NONPHARMACOLOGIC TREATMENT
- Rest, ice, compression (if an extremity), elevation; physical therapy to regain strength, mobility

PHARMACOLOGIC TREATMENT
- NSAIDs are mainstay of treatment
- Narcotic analgesics may be necessary for first 2–3 days

LENGTH OF TREATMENT
- 10–14 days

Special Considerations
- More active patients should not return to contact sports until they are pain-free

When to Consult, Refer, Hospitalize
- Consult with orthopedist for grade III injuries; refer for any injury involving muscle weakness

Follow-Up
- In 2 weeks if not improving

EXPECTED COURSE
- Varies with degree of injury
- Mild strains resolve in 2–3 weeks; severe injuries may require >8 weeks of treatment

COMPLICATIONS
- Permanent deformity, loss of strength

Bursitis

Description
- Inflammation or infection of synovial membrane of the bursal sac overlying bony prominences
- Common sites are shoulder (subacromial or subdeltoid), elbow (olecranon), hip (trochanteric), knee (prepatellar, pes anserine, suprapatellar), heel (retrocalcaneal)

Etiology
- Trauma, overuse causing pressure and irritation of bursa lining
- Bacterial infection may cause inflammation

Incidence
- No accurate incidence available in research literature. Estimated to account for up to 0.4% of all primary care visits.

Demographics
- Most commonly seen in athletes or as an overuse injury

Risk Factors
- Chronic pressure on bursa (kneeling, resting point of elbow on hard surface, overhead activity)
- Rheumatoid, gouty, or inflammatory arthritis
- Bakers' cyst
- Chronic or acute overuse particularly in middle age or elderly

Prevention and Screening
- Avoidance of activities that apply pressure to bursae
- Use of appropriate protective/padded equipment

Assessment
HISTORY
- Sudden or gradual onset of localized painful swelling
- Increased pain and discomfort with activity

PHYSICAL EXAM
- Localized fluctuant swelling (swelling over greater trochanter difficult to evaluate), sometimes warm and/or painful to touch
- No loss of ROM
- If erythema or warmth, consider septic bursitis

DIAGNOSTIC STUDIES
- None needed unless redness or warmth
- If redness or warmth, fluid aspiration analysis to evaluate for infection or gout; CBC

Differential Diagnosis
- Septic joint
- Gout
- Joint effusion
- Trauma
- Rheumatoid arthritis
- Cellulitis

Management

NONPHARMACOLOGIC TREATMENT
- RICE protocol
- Aspiration of bursal sac to reduce pain from pressure

PHARMACOLOGIC TREATMENT
- If septic bursitis, oral antibiotics, often dicloxacillin (Dynapen) or cephalexin (Keftab)
- NSAIDs (ibuprofen, sodium naproxen)
- Local corticosteroid injection: Not performed unless infection is ruled out
- Retrocalcaneal injection not recommended due to risk of Achilles tendon rupture

LENGTH OF TREATMENT
- NSAIDs for 1–3 weeks until swelling subsides

Special Considerations
- Surgical drainage/removal may be necessary if infection does not respond to antibiotics, local aspiration.

When to Consult, Refer, Hospitalize
- Refer to physician for bursa aspiration as necessary
- Consult with physician for local skin infection, marked cellulitis, or signs of systemic illness associated with bursitis for parenteral antibiotics, possible hospitalization

Follow-Up
- Provide patient education about need for rest for area

EXPECTED COURSE
- Symptoms usually improve within 2–3 days of aspirating/injecting bursa (if not infected)
- If infected, localized erythema should improve within 3–5 days

COMPLICATIONS
- Chronic bursitis

Carpal Tunnel Syndrome (CTS)

Description
- Entrapment neuropathy of median nerve at the wrist

Etiology
- Multiple causes, including any process that encroaches on the carpal tunnel, compressing the median nerve, or causes enlargement of median nerve
- Mnemonic for causes is PRAGMATIC: pregnancy, rheumatoid arthritis, growth hormone abnormalities, metabolic disorders, alcoholism, tumors, idiopathic, connective tissue disorders
  - Work/hobby repetitive flexion and extension of wrist: Computer typist, cashiers, sorters, musicians, hairdressers, use of vibrating tools, painters
  - History of trauma to wrist: Fracture, dislocations

Incidence and Demographics
- Affects approximately 1% of U.S. population
- Women affected more often than men; onset ages 30–50 years, incidence increases with age
- More common in people using forceful, repetitive wrist and hand movements or use of vibratory tools

Risk Factors
- Repetitive wrist flexion/extension movement; collagen vascular disease, history Colles' fracture

Prevention and Screening
- Proper ergonomics for wrist
- Treatment of underlying problem

Assessment
HISTORY
- Initially burning or aching pain, numbness, tingling that wakes patient at night and resolves after shaking the affected hand ("wake-and-shake")
- As disorder progresses, symptoms affect thumb, index and middle finger, may radiate into arm

PHYSICAL EXAM
- Tinel's sign: Positive if symptoms are reproduced by tapping the median nerve at the wrist
- Phalen's sign: Positive if pain within 60 seconds of bilateral wrist flexion with hands held in opposition (clinically, may be more useful than Tinel's)
- Carpal compression test: Positive if numbness and tingling develop with direct pressure over carpal tunnel
- Painless thenar muscle wasting is late finding; usually no visible abnormality; pain exacerbated by extreme volar flexion
- May have decreased grip strength, decreased sensation of first three digits

DIAGNOSTIC STUDIES
- Electromyography/nerve conduction studies—EMG/NCS
- Electromyography/nerve conduction velocity (EMG/NCV) studies are standard
- Mild to moderate symptoms should be present for 6 months for EMG/NCV studies to be accurate
- Plain x-rays if any history of trauma to rule out fracture
- If secondary cause suspected, order appropriate test, e.g., TSH, RF, HbgA1c

Differential Diagnosis
- Cervical radiculopathy (C6, C7)
- Brachial plexopathy
- Carpal navicular fracture

Management

NONPHARMACOLOGIC TREATMENT
- Splinting (cock-up wrist splint at night) to relieve compression on nerve, elevate extremity
- Ergonomic modification of work, hobby
- Surgical release if conservative methods fail

PHARMACOLOGIC TREATMENT
- NSAIDs in standard doses, on daily basis
- Acetaminophen up to 4,000 mg/day in divided doses po
- Corticosteroid injection into carpal tunnel (not nerve)

LENGTH OF TREATMENT
- Depends on severity of symptoms
- Generally, allow 6 weeks from onset of symptoms before obtaining EMG/NCS

Special Considerations
- Pregnancy: Increase incidence likely due to fluid retention
- Lactation: May be aggravated by wrist flexion while holding nursing infant

When to Consult, Refer, Hospitalize
- Consult with orthopedist or neurologist if patient's symptoms not improved with splinting, NSAIDs
- Consider referral for corticosteroid injection

Follow-Up

EXPECTED COURSE
- Mild cases usually respond to conservative measures
- Patient may require surgical release of nerve if burning, numbness, tingling persist or increase; loss of grip/pinch strength is persistent; or evidence of muscle atrophy

COMPLICATIONS
- Irreversible nerve damage, thenar muscle atrophy

Low Back Pain (LBP) and Herniated Nucleus Pulposus (HNP)

Description
- Common problem; goal is to rule out serious causes
  - LBP: Pain in lower lumbar, lumbosacral, or sacroiliac area that may radiate down one or both buttocks/legs
  - HNP: Rupture of an intervertebral disc with herniation of nucleus pulposus into spinal canal; disk compresses spinal cord or irritates associated nerve root
  - *Spondylolysis* is an acquired condition with a bony defect of the pars interarticularis usually at L5–S1
  - *Spondylolisthesis* is slip of the vertebral body in an adjacent vertebrae with a bilateral pars defect at a single vertebral level
  - Sciatica refers to pain and paresthesias extending down the leg in a dermatomal pattern

Etiology
- LBP: Ligamentous (sprain) or muscular problems (strain), osteoarthritis, other diseases (fibromyalgia, osteoporosis, osteomyelitis), tumor
- HNP: Trauma, degenerative spine disease, spinal stenosis
- Spondylolysis and spondylolisthesis develops in children doing vigorous athletic activity
- Spondylolisthesis can occur in adults with degenerative changes of the facet joints without spondylolysis of the pars
- Sciatica most common cause is herniated disk at L4–5, L5–S1

Incidence and Demographics
- Estimated that 80% of adults in U.S. have an episode of back pain, 10% HNP
- Most common at 20–40 years old, working adults
- Back pain not common in children
- Spondylolysis occurs in 5% pre-adolescent children, 12% in divers/gymnasts

Risk Factors
- Physical deconditioning, weak paraspinal or abdominal muscles
- Poor body mechanics/poor posture
- Occupational strain, heavy lifting
- Obesity, arthritis
- Mechanical disorders, e.g., scoliosis, leg length discrepancy, kyphosis
- Tobacco use

Prevention and Screening
- Regular exercise program
- Maintain ideal body weight
- Proper body mechanics

Assessment
HISTORY (TABLE 14–8)
- Assess carefully: Duration of symptoms, any known precipitant, any associated symptoms
- Symptoms suggestions more serious problem: Bilateral leg weakness, bowel/bladder incontinence, saddle paresthesia, pain unrelieved by rest, pain worse at night, pain worsens with rest
- Symptoms suggesting strain: Pain, stiffness associated with identified activity; worsens with activity, improves with rest
- Ask if bowel or bladder dysfunction or saddle numbness or paresthesia—indicates cauda equina syndrome, a neurologic emergency
- Children: Ask if trauma, recent infection, athletics, inflammatory disease, or malignancy
- Adults and geriatric patients: Ask about occupation, sports, leisure activities, underlying medical problems
- Exclude urgent medical conditions with mnemonic MICE (metastatic, infection, compression fracture, cauda equina syndrome) or referred pain from pelvic, abdominal pathology
- HNP is associated with pain radiating to buttock, leg, or foot

Table 14-8. Differentiating Low Back Pain

Clinical Problem	History	Physical Examination
Low back pain	Pain in back, buttocks, and/or thigh Onset after exertion and with movement No history of trauma, infection, malignancy Pain relieved by lying supine	Paravertebral tenderness, muscle spasm Loss of normal lumbar lordosis common No neurologic deficit
Herniated nucleus pulposus	Initially, back pain severe Chronic herniation usually results in leg pain greater than back pain Often, + history of trauma, forced flexion Central herniation results in bilateral leg weakness, bowel/bladder dysfunction	L5–S1 (most common): pain in posterior thigh, posterior/lateral calf, heel; weak plantar flexion of foot; diminished ankle reflex L4–5: pain in lateral thigh, anterior calf and dorsum of foot; weak dorsiflexion of foot L3–4: pain in anterior and lateral thigh, medial calf, and foot; weak quadriceps; diminished patellar reflex
Spinal stenosis	Gradual onset bilateral pain, neurogenic claudication: leg pain, paresthesias, weakness with walking, standing May have bowel and bladder dysfunction Usually relieved when flexes spine or rests	X-ray: Osteophytes Weakness: Foot, ankle Diminished reflexes: Ankle, knee May have atrophy in leg muscles
Spondylosis and spondylolisthesis	Vigorous athletic activity as child Positive family history Low back pain, may radiate into buttocks	Lumbosacral tenderness Accentuation of pain with hyperextension of spine, one leg raised off ground, flexed 90° at knee and hip
Low back pain in children	More common in adolescence Red flag if: constant, under age 11, last several weeks, wakes child at night, limitation of motion, fever, neurologic signs	If spinal tenderness, fever, neurologic or systemic symptoms, x-ray and labs indicated

PHYSICAL EXAM
- Note gait, check for ability to walk on heels and toes
- Palpate spinal column, note abnormal curvature
- Perform ROM extension, flexion, hyperextension, lateral bend, rotation
- Palpate paraspinal muscle tenderness, spasm
- Check deep tendon reflexes bilaterally: Knee, Achilles, Babinski
- Check strength, vibratory and proprioceptive sensation bilaterally
- Check weakness in dorsiflexion (ankle and great toe)

- Check light touch sensation of medial, dorsal, and lateral foot, peroneal area
- With the patient on his/her back, raise one leg with knee absolutely straight, until pain is experienced in the thigh, buttock and calf; record angle at which pain occurs; a normal (pain-free) value would be 70°–90°, higher in people with lax ligaments
- Then perform sciatic stretch test: dorsiflex foot at point of discomfort; test is positive if more pain results
- Flexing the knee will relieve the buttock pain but this is restored by pressing on the lateral popliteal nerve
- Severe root irritation is indicated when straight raising of the leg on the unaffected side produces pain on the affected side

DIAGNOSTIC STUDIES
- X-ray studies usually not necessary unless history of trauma, suspicion of systemic or structural changes
- Order diagnostic imaging and testing when severe or progressive neurologic deficits are present or serious underlying conditions are suspected
- MRI: Most useful for identifying HNP, diskitis, tumors
- CT: May help identify cord impingement (especially laterally), good for examination of osseous areas
- Bone scan: Helpful for identifying metabolically active processes such as tumor, occult fracture, infection, abscess
- Serum studies usually not helpful but ESR elevated in infection; HLA-B27 elevated in ankylosing spondylitis

Differential Diagnosis
- Spinal disorders:
  - Herniated disk
  - Spondylolisthesis
  - Spinal stenosis
- Metabolic disorders:
  - Osteoporosis
  - Osteomalacia
  - Paget's disease
- Rheumatologic disorders:
  - Rheumatoid arthritis
  - Reiter syndrome
  - Psoriatic arthritis
  - Ankylosing spondylitis
- Tumor:
  - Benign
  - Malignant
  - Metastatic
- Infection:
  - Bacterial
  - Tuberculous
- Miscellaneous:
  - Peptic ulcer
  - Sickle-cell disease

– Pancreatic disease
– Renal stones
– Tumor
– Infection
– Peptic ulcer
– Abdominal aortic aneurysm
– Ovarian cysts, tumors

Management
- Most LBP responds to conservative treatment within 4–6 weeks; in the absence of acute neurological deficit, 80% or more of patients with HNP also respond to conservative treatment.

    ### NONPHARMACOLOGIC TREATMENT
    - Short course of bedrest (1–2 days) then activity as tolerated; encourage patient to remain active
    - Chiropractic manipulation may be helpful if no radiculopathy
    - Patient education for proper body mechanics, back strengthening
    - Physical therapy to learn muscle conditioning exercises, proper body mechanics
    - Behavioral management

    ### PHARMACOLOGIC TREATMENT
    - NSAIDs or acetaminophen are first-line treatment
    - Muscle relaxants may be helpful for first 48–72 hours if low back strain with spasm in those who fail to respond to NSAIDs
    - Narcotic analgesics rarely necessary

    ### LENGTH OF TREATMENT
    - Most episodes resolve within 4–6 weeks of conservative treatment

Special Considerations
- In jobs requiring heavy lifting or exertion, incidence is somewhat greater for women.
- Pregnancy: LBP common, as is sciatica; symptoms frequently resolve after delivery.

When to Consult, Refer, Hospitalize
- Refer to neurosurgeon or orthopedist for patients who do not respond to 4 weeks of conservative treatment, spinal instability, expanding pain that worsens at night, signs of infection, neurologic deficit, cauda equina syndrome
- Hospitalize for abscess, tumor, signs suggestive of abdominal aneurysm

Follow-Up
- If patient in severe pain, reevaluate in 24–48 hours
- Provide patient education about body mechanics, conservative therapy, use of medications and their side effects

    ### EXPECTED COURSE
    - Remitting and recurring symptoms are common; most LBP resolves in 4–6 weeks with conservative care; 90% resolves within 2 months

COMPLICATIONS
- Without neurologic deficit, few complications if diagnosed and treated, though recurrence is common

Fibromyalgia

Description
- Musculoskeletal syndrome characterized by generalized nonarticular pain, diffuse aching, stiffness, and fatigue with multiple tender points

Etiology
- Unknown
- Possible triggers are viral infections, stress, immunologic abnormalities, depression, heightened perception of physiologic stimuli

Incidence and Demographics
- Affects 2% of population
- Peak incidence at ages 20–40 years; 75% female

Risk Factor
- Unknown. Possible genetic predisposition.
- May be associated with rheumatoid arthritis, Lyme disease, osteoarthritis, sleep apnea, metastatic carcinoma, hypothyroidism
- Associated with sedentary childhood although not sure if some problem produces more sedentary child or a sedentary child is more likely to develop fibromyalgia

Assessment
HISTORY
- Diffuse/widespread myalgia pain and tender points
- Muscle weakness; stiffness after prolonged sitting or sleeping
- Fatigue disproportionate to exertion; nonrestorative sleep
- Headache, atypical chest pain, irritable bowel symptoms

PHYSICAL EXAM
- Normal examination except for pain at trigger points; see diagnostic criteria below (Box 14–1)

DIAGNOSTIC STUDIES
- No specific serum, radiographic, biopsy, radionucleotide abnormalities are present

Box 14–1. Classification of Fibromyalgia (American College of Rheumatology)

History of widespread pain

Description: Pain is considered widespread when all of the following are present: pain in the left side of the body, pain in the right side of the body, pain above the waist, and pain below the waist. In addition, axial skeletal pain (cervical spine, anterior chest, thoracic spine, or low back) must be present. In this description, shoulder and buttock pain is considered as pain for each involved side. "Low back" pain is considered lower segment pain.

Pain in 11 of 18 tender point sites on digital palpation

Description: pain on digital palpation, must be present in at least 11 of the following 18 tender point sites:

Occiput: bilateral, at the suboccipital muscle insertions

Low cervical: bilateral, at the anterior aspects of the intertransverse spaces at C5–C7

Trapezius: bilateral, at the midpoint of the upper border

Supraspinatus: bilateral, at origins, above the scapula spine near the medial border

Second rib: bilateral, at the second costochondral junctions, just lateral to the junctions on upper surfaces

Lateral epicondyle: bilateral, 2 cm distal to the epicondyles

Gluteal: bilateral, in upper outer quadrants of buttocks in anterior fold of muscle

Greater trochanter: bilateral, posterior to the trochanteric prominence

Knee: bilateral, at the medial fat pad proximal to the joint line

Adapted from *Primer on the rheumatic diseases* (12th ed.) by J. H. Klippel, 2001, Atlanta: The Arthritis Foundation.

Differential Diagnosis
- Rheumatoid arthritis
- Hypothyroidism
- Myofascial pain syndrome
- Infections: HIV, hepatitis, Lyme disease
- Chronic fatigue syndrome
- Polymyalgia rheumatica
- SLE
- Psychiatric disorder
- Multiple sclerosis

Management

NONPHARMACOLOGIC TREATMENT
- Behavior modification and patient education
- Gradual reconditioning program (low-impact aerobics, walking, swimming), biofeedback, heat, massage

PHARMACOLOGIC TREATMENT
- Cyclobenzaprine (Flexeril) 5–40 mg every night po
- Amitriptyline (Elavil) 10–150 mg every night po; if not tolerated, zolpidem (Ambien) 5–10 mg every night or an SSRI in low doses
- Tramadol (Ultram) 50–100mg q 4–6 h prn may be helpful for pain
- Lyrica: Approved by FDA for fibromyalgia; initially 75 mg bid, max 45ø mg daily. Requires tapering if discontinued

- Selective serotonin reuptake inhibitors—fluoxetine
- Corticosteroids and opioids are ineffective

LENGTH OF TREATMENT
- Chronic, may require years of medication

Special Considerations
- Psychogenic factors need consideration

When to Consult, Refer, Hospitalize
- Hospitalization generally not indicated
- Patient-involved therapy seems to have better prognosis
- Consult or refer if differential diagnoses cannot be excluded or if there is suggestion of psychiatric component; rheumatology referral to assist with evaluation and management plan

Follow-Up
EXPECTED COURSE
- Only 5% have complete remission

COMPLICATIONS
- Chronic pain, lack of "cure" may initiate depression

CASE STUDIES

Case 1. 13-year-old White male presents with pain in right hip that has worsened over the past 2 weeks.
HPI: Prefers to play video games, does not play sports, denies trauma.
PMH: PETs at age 5, >100% for weight on growth chart

    1. What other history would you like?
    2. What type of examination should be done?

Exam: Patient has local tenderness over hip with decreased flexion, abduction, and internal rotation.

    3. What diagnostic tests should be ordered?
    4. What is the diagnosis and plan for management?

Case 2. 34-year-old man with complaint of left elbow pain for the last 2 weeks.
HPI: Played in two golf tournaments 2 weeks ago. Denies trauma. C/o dull ache in elbow joint that radiates down forearm. Denies numbness or tingling.
PMH: Overweight, history of "borderline hypertension."

    1. What other history would you like?
    2. What should be done on physical exam?

Exam: Medial epicondyle is tender to palpation, + pain with pronation, flexing wrist against resistance, or squeezing hard rubber ball.

    3. What diagnostic tests should be ordered?
    4. What is the diagnosis and plan for management?

Case 3. A 15-year-old girl presents with complaint of right knee pain during and after exercise.
HPI: Pain in anterior right knee area, just below knee joint during and after exercise. Denies trauma, plays basketball on her high school team, currently practicing nightly for an upcoming tournament.
PMH: Well, no history of serious illness, accidents, or medical problems.

    1. What other history would you like?
    2. What type of examination should be done?

Exam: No fever; no redness, edema, warmth, or effusion; ROM/ligaments all intact; bony tenderness, slight swelling at tibial tubercle on right.

    3. What diagnostic tests should be ordered?
    4. What is the diagnosis and plan for management?

REFERENCES

American College of Rheumatology Subcommittee on Rheumatoid Arthritis Guidelines. (2002). Guidelines for the management of rheumatoid arthritis. *Arthritis & Rheumatism, 46,* 328–346.

Bennet, R. (2004). Fibromyalgia: Present to future. *Current Pain and Headache Reports, 8*(50), 379–384.

Burns, C. E., Brady, M. A., & Dunn, A. M. (2004) *Pediatric primary care: A handbook for nurse practitioners* (3rd ed.). St. Louis, MO: Elsevier.

Carr, A. (2004). *Orthopedics in primary care* (2nd ed.). Philadelphia: Butterworth-Heinemann Medical.

Chou, R., Qaseem, A., Snow, V., Casey, D., Cross, T., Shekelle, P., et al. (2007). Diagnosis and treatment of low back pain: A joint clinical practice guideline from the American College of Physicians and the American Pain Society. *Annals of Internal Medicine, 147,* 478–491. Retrieved February 15, 2008, from http://www.annals.org/cgi/reprint/147/7/478.pdf

Crowther, C. L. (2003). *Primary orthopedic care* (2nd ed.). St Louis, MO: Mosby.

Dormans, J. P. (2005). *Pediatric orthopaedics: Core knowledge in orthopaedics.* Elsevier: Philadelphia.

Edmunds, M. W., & Mayhew, M. S. (2004). *Pharmacology for the primary care provider* (2nd ed.). St Louis, MO: Mosby.

Eggebeen, A. T. (2007). Gout: An update. *American Academy of Family Physicians, 76*(6), 801–808.

Goroll, A. H., & Mulley, A. G. (2006). *Primary care medicine: Office evaluation and management of the adult patient.* Philadelphia: Lippincott Williams & Wilkins.

Griffin, L. Y., & Green, W. (2005). *Essentials of musculoskeletal care* (3rd ed.). Rosemont, IL: American Association of Orthopedic Surgeons.

Klippel, J. H. (2001). *Primer on the rheumatic diseases* (12th ed.). Atlanta: The Arthritis Foundation.

Lattavo, K. (2007). Osteoarthritis and rheumatoid arthritis: Can you tell the difference? *Med-Surg Matters, 16*(5), 6–10.

Nonsurgical treatment is effective for carpal tunnel syndrome. (2004). *Journal of Family Practice, 53*(9), 685.

Uphold, C., & Graham, M. (2003). *Clinical guidelines in family practice* (4th ed.). Gainesville, FL: Barmarrae, Inc.

U.S. Preventive Services Task Force. (2007). *Guide to clinical preventive services, 2007.* Retrieved February 4, 2008, from http://www.ahrq.gov/clinic/pocketgd.htm

Wright, W. (2008). Management of mild to moderate osteoarthritis: Effective intervention by the nurse practitioner. *Journal for Nurse Practitioners, 4*(1), 25–34.

Wynne, A., Woo, T., & Olyael, A. (2007). *Pharmacotherapeutics for nurse practitioner prescribers.* Philadelphia: F.A. Davis.

Neurological Disorders

Deborah Gilbert-Palmer, EdD, FNP-BC

GENERAL APPROACH

For All

- Neurological problems range from chronic to acute to lethal.
- A screening neurological exam should be done on all patients with symptoms suspicious for a neurologic disorder and would include: Mental status (level of consciousness, orientation, memory, cognitive function, language), motor function (body position, involuntary movement, muscle tone, strength), sensory function (light touch, pain, position sense), reflexes (deep tendon reflexes [DTRs], abdominal, Babinski), cerebellar function (gait, rapid alternating movements, point-to-point movements, Romberg), cranial nerves (I–XII, motor and sensory components).
- Abnormalities should be further evaluated with additional assessment techniques and/or referred to a neurologic specialist and for diagnostic testing. Additional assessment includes techniques such as the Mini Mental Status Examination (MMSE), discriminating sensory testing (stereognosis, two-point discrimination), and meningeal irritability testing.

Children

- The nervous system is more difficult to examine in the infant and younger child because it is less mature. Special attention is paid to head circumference and fontanelles, general appearance and positioning, primitive reflexes, and developmental milestones.

- Knowledge of normal childhood developmental milestones and the patient's previous behavioral history is important to the diagnosis.
- Early recognition of problems is of utmost importance to future development and prevention of disability.
- Birth history of the patient, including gestational age, type of birth, complications, Apgar scores, incidence of trauma, congenital anomalies, birthweight, perinatal illness or drug use is important.
- Also consider a cardiac or metabolic etiology or an adverse medication reaction in the differential diagnosis whenever a neurological problem is suspected.
- Neurological "soft signs" (clumsiness, hyperkinesis, language disturbances, developmental delays, mirroring movements, echolalia, short attention spans) are more difficult to assess and diagnose but must be considered in the neurological evaluation.
- In infants and toddlers, fontanels can provide information regarding increasing intracranial pressure (IICP) as well as hydration status and clues to development.

Older Adults

- 20% decrease in blood flow to the brain with changes in autoregulation; contributes to risk of orthostatic hypotension.
- No changes in thinking, behavior, or intellectual function, although response time and processing of information is slower.
- Greater incidence of sensory deficits with aging and chronic illness (decreased hearing, decreased visual acuity, decreased position sense) may contribute to or mimic neurologic problems.
- Consider cardiac or metabolic etiology, or adverse medication reactions particularly for global complaints such as syncope, weakness, or change in cognition without focal (unilateral) neurological symptoms; also consider dementia, delirium, or depression.

Red Flags

For All

- Refer to a neurologist if unusual presentation or no response to adequate trial of standard therapy.

Children

- Obtain timely consultation and referral for the following:
  - Any sudden loss of function or developmental milestone
  - Retention of normal newborn reflexes past the sixth month of life
  - A bulging fontanel, widening of suture lines, sunset eyes, frontal bossing, or head circumference growth inconsistent with percentiles in the newborn
  - Headache associated with early morning vomiting or awakening from sleep
  - Sudden onset of vomiting after head injury—IMMEDIATE REFERRAL
  - Nuchal rigidity with fever—IMMEDIATE REFERRAL

Adults/Older Adults

- Focal findings suggest a space-occupying lesion of the brain or spinal cord, or a peripheral compressive neuropathy; refer to neurologist or neurosurgeon.
- Acute or sudden onset of symptoms such as headache, unilateral weakness, aphasia, visual changes or change in level of consciousness require immediate consult, referral, or hospitalization, as do deficits resulting from head or spinal trauma.

GENERAL NEUROLOGIC AND NEUROSURGICAL DISORDERS

Spina Bifida Occulta

Description
- A midline defect of the vertebral bodies without protrusion of the spinal cord or meninges
- Is occasionally accompanied by a dermoid sinus, which may have a hairy tuft, discoloration of the skin, or a lipoma
- Usually found at L5 and S1
- Is more benign than other variants of spina bifida (meningocele and myelomeningocele) and, with a normal physical and neuro exam, requires no treatment unless other symptoms occur

Etiology
- Is a neural tube defect (NTD) resulting from failure of the neural tube to close during the third and fourth week of fetal development
- Neural tube defects include anencephaly, encephalocele, myelomeningocele, and occult spinal dysraphism

Incidence and Demographics
- Incidence for all NTDs is 1 per 1,000 live births

Risk Factors
- Poor prenatal care
- Folic acid deficiency, maternal
- Previous delivery of an infant with NTD (2%–4%)

Prevention and Screening
- Addition of folic acid to the diets of women of child-bearing age, starting in adolescence
- Alpha-fetoprotein screen prenatally at 16–18 weeks gestation

Assessment
HISTORY
- History of pregnancy, birth, and delivery as well as prenatal care and maternal risk factors, especially nutrition and folic acid deficiency, gestational diabetes, maternal use of anticonvulsants or alcohol, maternal hyperthermia during days 20–28 of gestation
- Patient history of back pain, bowel or bladder dysfunction, decreased motor strength or coordination
- Past history of meningitis or recurrent episodes of meningitis

PHYSICAL EXAM
- Neurological exam for strength, coordination, and reflexes, especially in the lower extremities
- Gait evaluation
- Back examination for small sinus tract in the lower midline region along the vertebrae, and skin integrity at the site

- Scoliosis
- Head circumference
- Presence of other dysmorphic features
- Rectal exam to assess sphincter tone

DIAGNOSTIC STUDIES
- Spinal x-ray will show a defect in the closure of the posterior vertebral arches and laminae, typically involving L5 and S1
- Ultrasound in the newborn period
- MRI to rule out tethered cord, if having motor symptoms or back pain, or other brain abnormalities
- Urodynamic studies to assess bladder function, if affected

Differential Diagnosis
- Spina bifida occulta complicated by tethered cord
- Syringomyelia, or diastematomyelia
- Dermal sinus tract
- Lipoma or other tumor
- Cysts
- Sacral agenesis

Management
NONPHARMACOLOGIC TREATMENT
- Usually no treatment, unless complications develop or associated defects become apparent
- Surgical release is required for tethered cord

PHARMACOLOGIC TREATMENT
- None

Special Considerations
- Spina bifida occulta may be an incidental finding on x-ray in many children who have no dermal sinus.

When to Consult, Refer, Hospitalize
- With a normal physical and neurological exam, no referrals are necessary.
- If a dermal sinus is found in the newborn or new symptoms (foot weakness, bowel or bladder dysfunction) develop in an older child, further evaluation is required; consult with a physician.
- Referral to a pediatric neurosurgeon is only necessary with associated defects, e.g., tethered cord.

Follow-Up
- Patients with this deformity should have routine health assessments and immunizations.
- Special attention to the back evaluation, history of infections, bowel and bladder function, and lower limb motor strength at each assessment.

Tourette Syndrome/Tics

Description
- Tourette syndrome is a lifelong chronic condition, which has four components, not all of which need to be present in each case. They include: motor tics, vocal tics, obsessive-compulsive behavior, and attention-deficit hyperactivity disorder.
  - Tics are sudden, rapid, recurrent, purposeless, nonrhythmic, stereotyped movements or vocalizations.
  - Tics increase in intensity and frequency during any form of physical or mental stress.
  - Tics tend to be unnoticed by the patient and even disappear when asleep.
  - Tics develop over time from simple to complex.
  - Tics begin midline and progress.
- Tourette syndrome differs from simple tic disorder in that tics are present for >1 year during which time no more than 3 consecutive months pass without tics.

Etiology
- Exact etiology unknown.
- Suspected to be an abnormality along the circuits connecting the brain's cortex and subcortex, which leads to failure of the filtering mechanism along a neural pathway. This allows an interfering impulse to trigger an urge or tension in the muscle group to respond.

Incidence and Demographics
- 24% of all children experience tics; most are minor and do not lead to a clinical diagnosis
- Lifetime prevalence of 5–10 per 10,000 (0.05%–0.1%)
- Motor tics typically present around age 6 or 7, the most common being eye blinking
- Phonic tics present around 8 or 9, usually as coughing, sniffing, or clearing the throat
- Complex vocal tics include echolalia (repeating what is said by another, or what is heard); palilalia (repetition of words and sounds made by the patient); and coprolalia (use of obscene language, but involuntarily so)

Risk Factors
- Genetic predisposition
- Low birthweight
- Maternal stress during pregnancy
- Obstetrical complications (e.g., use of forceps, vacuum delivery)
- Maternal use of coffee, cigarettes, or alcohol during pregnancy
- Androgenic hormones
- Autoimmune mechanisms/pediatric autoimmune neuropsychiatric disorders associated with streptococcal infections (PANDAS)
- Overuse of amphetamines

Assessment
HISTORY
- Medical and developmental history of the child
- Family history, including tics and other developmental and behavioral disorders
- Psychosocial adaptation

- Environmental supports and stresses
- Prior diagnosis of comorbid conditions, including attention-deficit hyperactivity disorder (ADHD) and use of amphetamines
- The child's impression of the tics, presence of aura, etc.
- Recent history of sore throat or throat infection, head trauma, or use of medications or drugs

PHYSICAL EXAM
- The child may need to be observed from another room, via videotaping, etc., as the tics wax and wane
- Assess for comorbid conditions through general physical and screening neurologic exam

DIAGNOSTIC STUDIES
- None unless to rule out comorbid conditions
- Head CT if onset of tics associated with head injury
- Throat culture and ASO titer, if recent history of sore throat, prior to onset of tics
- Urine or serum drug toxicology screen, if history indicates
- Serum copper level if history of family hepatic and neurological diseases

Differential Diagnosis
- Sydenham's chorea
- Drug-induced movements
- Wilson's disease
- Head injury
- Seizures
- Metal poisoning

Management

NONPHARMACOLOGIC TREATMENT
- Behavioral therapy and biofeedback
- Family support and counseling
- Individual Educational Plans, including classroom modifications

PHARMACOLOGIC TREATMENT
- Stimulants: Dextroamphetamine (Dexedrine) or methylphenidate (Ritalin) to treat comorbid ADHD
- Alpha-2 adrenergic agonists: Clonidine (Catapres) to treat tics alone or with comorbid ADHD
- Neuroleptic agents used to treat tics alone include risperidone (Risperdal), haloperidol (Haldol), pimozide (Orap), and fluphenazine (Prolixin)

LENGTH OF TREATMENT
- True Tourette syndrome is a lifelong condition, requiring constant treatment

Special Considerations
- For best outcome, have multimodal management plan, including the patient, family, and school.

When to Consult, Refer, Hospitalize
- Consult with a physician for use of drug therapy when behavioral strategies are not working.
- Refer to neurologist if tics are hard to control or if the diagnosis is not clear.

Follow-Up
- Biannually to evaluate control of tics, school performance, need for further intervention
  EXPECTED COURSE
    - At least one-third of children outgrow tics by adulthood, and another one-third have less severe tics by that time

  COMPLICATIONS
    - Social problems

Down Syndrome

Description
- A congenital syndrome consisting of mental retardation and multiple physical abnormalities, including hypotonia, flat facies, up-slanting palpebral fissures, and small ears
- The defects are caused by trisomy of chromosome 21

Etiology
- 95%–97% due to chromosomal nondisjunction in the maternal DNA
- 1% with trisomy 21 mosaicism occurring after conception; are generally less severely affected
- Down syndrome is associated with many conditions, the most common of which are:
  - Mental retardation (100%)
  - Infant hypotonia
  - Hearing loss (60%–90%)
  - Visual problems: refractive error (70%), strabismus (50%), nystagmus (35%), cataracts (3%)
  - Obesity (50%)
  - Congenital heart disease (40%)
  - Hypothyroidism (10%–20%)
  - Atlanto-occipital and atlanto-axial subluxation (15%)
  - Gastrointestinal obstructions and atresias (12%)
  - Seizures (6%–10%)
  - Genitourinary problems, including hypospadias, cryptorchidism
  - Blood dyscrasias, including leukemia, anemia
  - Retinoblastoma and testicular germ cell tumors

Incidence and Demographics
- Incidence 1/600–800 live births
- Incidence increases with advancing maternal age with incidence being 1:100 by maternal age of 40–44
- Is the most recognized and frequent chromosomal syndrome in humans

Risk Factors
- Advanced maternal age
- Previous history of Down syndrome in sibling

Prevention and Screening
- Prenatal genetic testing via amniocentesis or chorionic villus sampling

Assessment

HISTORY
- History of previous infant in family with Down syndrome
- Review of genetic testing report

PHYSICAL EXAM
- General: Hypotonia with an open mouth and protruding tongue
- Head: Brachycephaly with flattened occiput, microcephaly, false fontanel
- Eyes: Up-slanting palpebral fissures, inner epicanthal folds, Brushfield spots, strabismus, nystagmus
- Ears: Small, prominent, low-set ears, with over-folding of the upper helix; small ear canals
- Nose: Small, flat nasal bridge
- Tongue: Protruding tongue, which appears large for mouth
- Mouth: High-arched or abnormal palate
- Teeth: May have missing, irregular, or hypoplastic teeth
- Neck: Excessive skin at the nape (infants), short appearance
- Lungs: Assess for signs of infections or congestive heart failure
- Heart: Assess for murmur, arrhythmia as cardiac defects common
- Abdomen: In neonate, observe for distention, which could indicate obstruction or atresia
- Genital: Straight pubic hair, small penis, cryptorchidism (adolescents)
- Extremities: Hand is broad with short metacarpals and phalanges; short fifth finger with clinodactyly; simian crease; wide gap between the second and third toes; hyper flexible joints
- Skin: Fine, soft, sparse hair, hyperkeratotic dry skin; may be cyanotic

DIAGNOSTIC STUDIES
- CBC as newborn
- ECG and echocardiogram within first month of life to detect associated cardiac defects
- Auditory brainstem response testing within the first 6 months of life
- Lateral cervical spine x-ray to rule out atlantoaxial instability by school age
- Diagnosis is confirmed by karyotype testing, usually in utero or neonatal period

Differential Diagnosis
- Other genetic or chromosomal syndromes

Management

NONPHARMACOLOGIC TREATMENT
- Many infants require surgical repair of associated heart defects
- Parents need ongoing emotional support
- Genetic testing and counseling within family

PHARMACOLOGIC TREATMENT
  • Specific to associated problems

LENGTH OF TREATMENT
  • Down syndrome requires lifetime surveillance for management of the associated disabilities and emergence of new problems

Special Considerations
• Parents need ongoing support, both emotional and financial; parents should apply for Supplemental Security benefits (SSI) for the child

When to Consult, Refer, Hospitalize
• Almost always identified at birth and immediate referrals made for unstable newborn
• Otherwise, consult with a physician or specialist for infant or child entering the health care system
• If stable, referrals as follows:
  – Cardiac consult within first month of life
  – Ophthalmology consult by age 6 months and then every 1–2 years
  – Audiologic evaluation, in first 3 years, than every 2 years; may need ENT referral to visualize tympanic membranes (TMs), due to small canals
  – Orthopedic evaluation, as needed
  – Endocrine consult, if thyroid screening abnormal
  – Early language and learning intervention may prove helpful

Follow-Up
• Patients need routine health examinations, as well as routine immunizations, in the newborn period and at least every 2 years through childhood and adolescents
• Encourage physical activity and review diet to prevent obesity
  COMPLICATIONS
    • Wide variety of complications due to associated abnormalities, including recurrent otitis media, constipation, airway problems, joint problems
    • Emergencies in the newborn period include intestinal obstruction and cardiac disease

Cerebral Palsy

Description
• A group of nonprogressive disorders resulting from the malfunction of the motor centers and pathways of the brain; a major cause of disability of children
• There are varying degrees and clinical manifestations of cerebral palsy
• Symptoms generally include paralysis, weakness, incoordination, or ataxia

Etiology
Prenatal factors (most common)
• Infection, such as rubella, toxoplasmosis, herpes simplex, and cytomegalovirus
• Maternal anoxia, anemia, placental infarcts, abruptio placenta
• Prenatal cerebral hemorrhage, maternal bleeding, maternal toxemia, Rh or ABO incompatibility

- Prenatal anoxia, twisting or kinking of the cord
- Genetic factors
- Miscellaneous: Toxins, drugs

Perinatal factors
- Anoxia from any cause including anesthetic and analgesic drugs administered during labor, prolonged labor, placenta previa or abruptio placenta, respiratory obstruction, cerebral trauma during delivery, complications of birth
- "Small for date" babies, including prematurity and intrauterine growth retardation
  - Hyperbilirubinemia
  - Hemolytic disorders
  - Respiratory distress
  - Infections
  - Serum chemistry disturbances (hypoglycemia, hypocalcemia)

Postnatal factors
- Head trauma
- Infections, including meningitis, encephalitis, and brain abscesses
- Vascular accidents
- Anoxia
- Neoplastic and late neurodevelopmental defects

Incidence and Demographics
- Cerebral palsy occurs in approximately 2 per 1,000 live births

Risk Factors
- Young or advanced maternal age
- Lack of prenatal care
- Birth trauma or anoxia
- Maternal infection

Prevention and Screening
- Prenatal care including the provision of prenatal vitamins
- Prenatal screening for maternal illness and infection
- Management of maternal toxemia of pregnancy
- Developmental screening for well-babies
- Immunization programs for well-babies

Assessment
HISTORY
- A thorough history, including prenatal, perinatal, and postnatal risk factors
- Attention to birth trauma, prematurity, low birthweight, Apgar scores
- History of infant activity, feeding, crying, growth

PHYSICAL EXAM
- Early signs:
  - Asymmetric movements, hypertonia, scissoring of the lower extremities
  - Listlessness or irritability

- Poor sucking with tongue thrust
- Excessive, high-pitched, or feeble cry
- Long, thin infants who are slow to gain weight
- Poor head control
- Late signs:
  - Failure to follow normal pattern of motor development; delayed gross motor development is a universal manifestation of cerebral palsy
  - Persistence of infantile reflexes
  - Weakness
  - Preference for one hand before the infant is 12–15 months old
  - Abnormal postures
  - Delayed or defective speech
  - Evidence of mental retardation
- General health:
  - Functional assessment, including ability to perform normal daily activities
  - Developmental assessment; use Denver II developmental or other screening tool
  - Ability to protect airway: Gag reflex, swallowing
  - Nutritional status: Growth, or weight loss
  - Neuromuscular function and mobility: Range of motion, spasticity, coordination

DIAGNOSTIC STUDIES
- Computed tomography (CT) scan or magnetic resonance imaging (MRI) to rule out tumor
- Laboratory testing to include CBC, urinalysis, chemistry panel, toxicology screen to rule out other disorders
- Psychological testing to determine cognitive functioning in an older child
- Gait analysis
- EEG, if seizures suspected

Differential Diagnosis
- Tumors and neoplasms
- Meningitis, encephalitis
- Metabolic diseases
- Connective tissue disorders

Management
NONPHARMACOLOGIC TREATMENT
- Orthopedic management of scoliosis, contractures, dislocations
- Selective surgical dorsal rhizotomy in an attempt to decrease spasticity
- Enrollment in a child development program
- Physical, speech, and occupational therapy
- Assistive devices, such as braces, joint supports, walkers to assist with movement and prevent contractures
- Biofeedback (limited success)
- Family and individual counseling can be integral components of the management plan

PHARMACOLOGIC TREATMENT
- Administration of antispasticity medications, such as dantrolene (Dantrium) or diazepam (Valium)
- Administration of antireflux medications, metoclopramide (Reglan) or bethanechol (Duvoid)
- Administration of seizure medications, as needed
- Injection of botulism toxin (Botox), can relax muscles up to 3–6 months
- May need stool softeners to help prevent constipation due to immobility

Special Considerations
- The best outcomes require a multimodal management plan, which includes the patient; family; neurology; orthopedics; nutritionist; the school, physical, and occupational therapists.
- Parents need frequent support.
- Patients need to receive routine immunizations as scheduled.

When to Consult, Refer, Hospitalize
- Refer all cases to a pediatric neurologist; patient should be followed by a multi-disciplinary team.
- Hospitalization is usually for amelioration of orthopedic problems.

Follow-Up
- Routine health assessments and immunizations, biannual individual education plan (IEP)

COMPLICATIONS
- Scoliosis, seizures, ADHD, behavioral problems

Fragile X Syndrome

Description
- Congenital syndrome characterized by mental retardation or developmental delay, characteristic physical features, and abnormal behavioral patterns

Etiology
- The genetic defect is a discontinuous site on the long arm of the X chromosome

Incidence and Demographics
- Frequency is estimated at 1/2,500 to 1/1,250 in males and 1/5,000 to 1/1,650 in females
- The most common hereditary cause of mental retardation

Risk Factors
- Family history of the syndrome

Prevention and Screening
- Genetic testing and carrier detection for siblings and relatives of identified cases

Assessment

HISTORY

- Family history of mental retardation or fragile X syndrome
- Developmental history, speech or language delay
- Behavioral problems, such as hyperactivity, aversion of gaze, manneristic behavior, hand mannerisms or stereotypies, and perseverative speech
- School performance problems
- History of visual or hearing difficulties, motor or joint instability, and/or seizures

PHYSICAL EXAM

- Appearance: Prominent forehead; a long, thin face and a prominent jaw that appears late in childhood; large, protuberant, and slightly dysmorphic ears
- Strabismus, nystagmus, or ptosis
- Evaluate heart sounds for murmurs or clicks with associated mitral valve prolapse
- Musculoskeletal exam for flat feet, scoliosis, or loose joints; in infants, hypotonia
- Genitourinary exam for macroorchidism, inguinal hernias

DIAGNOSTIC STUDIES

- Echocardiogram to assess for mitral valve prolapse
- EEG if there is history of seizures or staring episodes

Differential Diagnosis

- Mental retardation
- Klinefelter syndrome
- Autism

Management

NONPHARMACOLOGIC TREATMENT

- Behavioral, developmental, IQ testing
- Speech/language therapy as needed
- Orthotics for flat feet if a gait disturbance is present
- Corrective lenses or corrective surgery for strabismus
- Inguinal hernia repair
- Early intervention programs for education and learning

PHARMACOLOGIC TREATMENT

- Medications used only to treat symptoms of associated problems, such as hyperactivity or depression

Special Considerations

- Special classroom arrangements or learning situations
- Adolescents will need special counseling regarding sexuality and birth control
- Patients may have trouble adjusting to social situations due to behavioral issues and may suffer from depression due to failure to fit in

When to Consult, Refer, Hospitalize
- Refer all suspected cases to pediatric neurologist or developmental specialist
- Refer to other specialties for associated problems (ophthalmology, orthopedics, psychology)
- Refer family for genetic counseling

Follow-Up
- Routine health assessments and immunizations according to the recommended schedule
  - EXPECTED COURSE
    - Life into adulthood with interdisciplinary support of the family, usually in group home situation

  - COMPLICATIONS
    - School failure
    - Behavioral dysfunction can be a significant component of fragile X

Headache: Tension, Migraine, Cluster

Description
- Head pain may be a symptom of underlying disease or pathology or the disease process itself (cluster headache, migraine). Head pain arises from extracranial structures (muscles, skin, scalp arteries), or from the posterior fossa, the dura, intracranial arteries, and cranial nerves at the base of the brain.
- Brain tissue itself is not sensitive to pain.
- Tension, migraine, and cluster are primary headaches.
- Unusual for new-onset primary headache syndromes to occur after age 50.
- Secondary headaches are a symptom of an underlying disorder.
- A sudden and severe headache is significant and warrants immediate attention.
- The pattern of a headache may suggest the etiology such as acute recurrent headaches. A chronic nonprogressive pattern might suggest postconcussion syndrome. A chronic progressive headache is more concerning and would possibly indicate a brain tumor or other serious etiology.
- Tension headaches are described as squeezing band-like pain, onset usually gradual and lasts days to years, is present when awaking, and may be associated with anxiety or depression, no aura or associated neurological symptoms.
- Medication overuse headache (MOH), previously referred to as analgesic rebound headache, is a chronic headache that can develop from the frequent use of headache medications, including OTC analgesic, triptans, ergotamine, caffeine, opiates, or benzodiazepines.
- Cluster headaches have unilateral, excruciating pain lasting 20 minutes to 2 hours with several attacks a day for 4–8 weeks, followed by a cluster-free interval for 6 months to years; or chronic form with little cluster-free interval.
- Migraines may be preceded by a prodromal or "warning" feeling; then some have an aura of visual or somatosensory disturbance immediately prior to headache; the headache may be unilateral or bilateral, lasting hours to several days, associated with photophobia, phonophobia, and nausea and vomiting.
  - Migraines are recurrent, throbbing headaches of vascular origin
  - The majority of primary pediatric headaches are migraines, MOH, and tension

- Classified as migraines without aura (80%) or migraines with aura (focal neurologic dysfunction begins and ends prior to onset of headache)
- Migraine variants include ophthalmoplegic migraine; hemiplegic migraine; basilar migraine (vertigo, dysarthria, ataxia, tinnitus); persistent migraine; transformed migraine (chronic)

Etiology
- Tension headache:
  - Essentially unknown cause
  - Studies have not supported "muscle tension" or increased muscle contractions
  - Depression, anxiety, or stress may play a role
- Migraines:
  - Believed to be caused by a genetically linked vascular disruption (constriction and dilation of extracranial and intracranial blood vessels), possibly triggered by neurochemical disruption
- Cluster:
  - Unknown, may be related to cyclic neurochemical imbalances causing an inflammatory response; tend to be seasonal, occurring in spring or fall
- Secondary headaches:
  - Are most common in the elderly, often due to disease outside the central nervous system (CNS)
  - Causes include subarachnoid hemorrhage, head trauma, brain tumors, giant cell (temporal) arteritis, meningitis, encephalitis, cervical arthritis, visual acuity problems, fever, sinusitis, intoxication (drugs, chemicals, carbon monoxide), hypothyroidism

Incidence and Demographics
- 18 million outpatient visits a year are for headache.
- Incidence declines in 6th–10th decades.
- Tension
  - 70%–90% of adults experience tension-type headache at some time
  - 5:4 ratio of women to men; 40% have family history
- Migraines:
  - Prevalence 16%–45% women, 10%–21% men
  - Most common during ages of 30–45, unusual to begin after age 50; unmask earlier incidence of undiagnosed migraine via focused history; rule out other causes
  - Migraine occurs in 3%–5% of children before puberty, and increases to 10%–20% during the second decade of life
  - Female-to-male ratio is equal in childhood and rises to 2:1 after puberty
  - There is a strong genetic component; family history supports the diagnosis in the child
- Cluster:
  - Rare, much more frequent in men >30

Risk Factors
- Age, sex, stress, alcohol, caffeine (for all)
- Migraine triggers: Menstruation; foods such as chocolate and aged cheese; caffeine and nicotine or withdrawal; alcohol; sunlight; too much or too little sleep; missing meals; emotional stress or relief of stress; medications, including estrogen and vasodilators

Prevention and Screening
- Due to the many causes of headache, there is no primary prevention
- Avoid identified individual triggers
- Keeping a headache diary helps in the identification of triggers and also in the administration of prophylactic medications

Assessment

HISTORY
- Evaluate every headache for chronology (most important item); location, duration quality; associated activity (exertion, sleep tension, relaxation); timing of menstrual cycle; presence of associated symptoms (focal neurological deficits, vomiting, fever); presence of triggers
- Recent falls or head injuries, trauma, previous and current medical and nonpharmacologic management, diagnostic testing and referrals
- Activities using the trapezius muscles, such as wearing heavy backpacks
- Suspect tension headaches with gradual onset over months to years, with episodes lasting days without neurological symptoms; may be associated with anxiety, depression and stress
- Suspect migraine with history of aura and neurologic symptoms that resolve, then actual headache accompanied by photophobia and/or nausea and vomiting; usually follows same pattern and precipitating events each episode
- Suspect tension headache with constant, gradual onset, daily headaches; generalized, bilateral; common around occiput, lasts for several hours, vague symptoms, no focal neurological deficits
- Suspect cluster headaches by cyclic nature of attacks
- Headache described as the "first" or "worst" of the patient's life should be evaluated to rule out potentially serious etiology
- Functional history: Headache interferes with work, school, functional activities of daily living (ADLs) and instrumental ADLs; headaches that do not interfere with ADLs tend to be tension type
- History of sudden onset, change in character, associated neurologic symptoms, fever, neck pain, rash or weight loss suggests a serious headache and potential emergency; brain tumor usually causes additional symptoms within 6 months of headache onset
- Family history of headache
- If patient is febrile, consider meningitis, brain abscesses or other infection, encephalitis, sinusitis
- Review of systems:
  - Neurological: Aura, paresthesias, paralysis, vertigo, mood, sleep changes
  - Visual symptoms: Photophobia, diplopia, scotoma, tearing
  - Any ear, nose, or throat symptoms: May indicate sinusitis
  - Gastrointestinal: Nausea, vomiting, diarrhea, constipation
  - Constitutional symptoms: Fever, chills, weight changes, appetite changes
- Also see brain tumor, stroke, meningitis for pertinent history of these secondary causes of headache

PHYSICAL EXAM

- Screening neurological exam is usually normal with primary headaches; neurologic deficits suggest a secondary cause such as subarachnoid hemorrhage (SAH), cerebrovascular accident (CVA), tumor, or subdural hematoma
- Funduscopic exam to rule out papilledema (signals increased intracranial pressure)
- Muscle tone, reflexes, gait, sensation, coordination, and strength for any abnormality
- Auscultate for bruits, a sign of cerebrovascular disease
- Measure head circumference, and check the fontanels and sutures in the young child
- Cervical and suboccipital tenderness, range of motion (decreased in cervical arthritis)
- Temporal artery tenderness and visual changes, particularly in patients >50 years old, suggests giant cell arteritis
- Focused physical exam, including vital signs, to rule out secondary causes or infectious process
- Rash over facial distribution of cranial nerve V with corresponding pain indicates herpes zoster
- Examine the teeth for obvious cavities; include an assessment of jaw movement
- ENT exam for signs of infection of the pharynx or sinuses

DIAGNOSTIC STUDIES

- History consistent with primary headache with normal physical exam usually does not require further diagnostic evaluation
- Tension headaches with stress or psychogenic component, consider psychological testing
- CBC if chronic anemia or infection is suspected
- Consider brain CT if:
  - Significant new type headache of few weeks in duration
  - New headache in patient over 50
- Immediate CT if:
  - Sudden, severe headache
  - Progressive headache
  - Headache with exertion, straining, sexual activity, or coughing
  - Change in mental state, persistent focal neurologic deficits, or fever
- Lumbar puncture (if there is a negative CT but SAH suspected, or to rule out meningitis)
- Erythrocyte sedimentation rate (ESR) to rule out giant cell arteritis in those over 50
- Sinus CT or x-rays if sinusitis without response to adequate antibiotics, recurrent sinus pain, vague symptoms without definite physical findings
- Cervical spine x-rays or MRI if cervical arthritis or radiculopathy is suspected
- Other diagnostic testing as directed by history and physical exam to rule out infectious, metabolic, or autoimmune process
- Evaluate for cardiovascular disease with ECG and risk factors before prescribing 5-HT agonists ("triptans") or dihydroergotamine (DHE 45 or Migranal)
- Electroencephalogram is not useful in screening or diagnosing headaches

Differential Diagnosis
- Subarachnoid or intracranial hemorrhage/cerebral aneurysm
- Brain tumor
- Giant cell arteritis
- Subdural hematoma
- Post-traumatic headache
- Meningitis
- Encephalitis
- Brain abscess
- Hydrocephalus
- Sinusitis or other referred pain from ear, eyes, teeth, or temperomandibular joint (TMJ)
- Viral syndrome
- Drug-induced, caffeine withdrawal, or intoxication
- Depression and anxiety
- Post-concussive syndrome
- Stress
- Cervical radiculopathy
- Trigeminal neuralgia
- Pseudotumor cerebri or benign intracranial hypertension (cause unknown)

Management

NONPHARMACOLOGIC TREATMENT
- Tension:
  - Relaxation techniques, biofeedback, stress reduction
  - Physical therapy: TENS, massage, ultrasound
  - Headache logs
- Migraine and cluster:
  - Avoid food and drugs that trigger attacks
  - Rest and periods of exercise
  - During attack rest in quiet, dark room with head elevated, use cold compresses
  - 100% oxygen inhaled for 10–15 minutes

PHARMACOLOGIC TREATMENT

Abortive therapy
- Tension:
  - Analgesics: Acetaminophen 650–1,000 mg qid as needed, or NSAIDs
  - Under age 10, acetaminophen 15 mg/kg/dose q4h, or ibuprofen 10 mg/kg/dose q6h
  - Children under 10 with headaches more than once per week may benefit from daily prophylactic therapy with cyproheptadine (Periactin) 0.2–0.4 mg/kg/d in 2–3 divided doses, starting with 4 mg at bedtime
  - Older children can be managed with analgesics to control pain, including acetaminophen and ibuprofen
  - Avoid opioids including butalbital (Fiorinal and Fioricet) due to risk of habituation as well rebound phenomenon
  - If headache occurs more than once per week, preventive medications for adults and children include amitriptyline (Elavil) and/or propranolol (Inderal)

- Migraines and cluster headaches: Treatment very individualized:
  - Analgesics: Acetaminophen, aspirin, or NSAIDs, often in combination with caffeine taken as soon as possible at onset; avoid opioids for reasons noted above
  - 5-HT agonists ("triptans") if nonnarcotic analgesics ineffective
  - Sumatriptan (Imitrex)—oral: 25 mg taken as soon as possible at onset, 25–100 mg every 2 hours up to 300 mg in 24 hours in adults; in children, maximum oral dose is 0.6 mg/kg
  - Injection: 6 mg SC adults; in children, maximum dose 0.6 mg/kg.; may be repeated once after 1 h
  - Following initial injection, 25–50 mg tablets q2h up to 200 mg orally in 24 hours
  - Intranasal: Single dose of 5, 10, or 20 mg administered in one nostril, may repeat once after 2 hours, not to exceed 40 mg in 24 hours in adults; dosage based on body weight in children
  - Other 5-HT agonists include zolmitriptan (Zomig), naratriptan (Amerge), rizatriptan (Maxalt)
  - Ergotamine derivatives: Cafergot: 2 tablets taken as soon as possible at onset, may repeat at 30-minute intervals, do not exceed 6 tablets per day, 10 tablets per week; not recommended in children
  - Injectable triptans at migraine doses more effective than oral agents for individual attacks (NOTE: First dose of injectable preparations should be given under medical supervision and, possibly, accompanied by monitoring with ECG)
  - Injectable or inhaled ergotamines and triptans are contraindicated in those with history of uncontrolled hypertension, Prinzmetal's angina, myocardial infarction, or symptomatic ischemic heart disease
  - Sumatriptan should not be used in conjunction with any vasoconstrictor medication, nor should it be used within 2 weeks of taking a monoamine oxidase inhibitor
- Treat nausea or vomiting in adults and children with metoclopramide (Reglan) or phenothiazine 15–20 minutes before oral medication
  - Prophylactic treatment for two or more migraine attacks per month that produce impairment lasting three or more days per month: Daily NSAIDs, beta-blockers, calcium channel blockers, tricyclic antidepressants (limited experience with SSRIs, especially in children; see Table 15–1)
  - Topiramate, lithium carbonate, methysergide, and valproate can also be effective; however, before initiating valproate, baseline liver enzyme levels must be drawn and then monitored thereafter approximately every 3–6 months
  - Generally, prophylactic agent(s) should be tried for a minimum of 2–3 months before switching to another drug
  - Neurology referral for headaches unresponsive to treatment or prophylaxis

PHARMACOLOGIC TREATMENT

Preventive therapy

- U.S. Headache Consortium Guidelines based on clinical efficacy, significant adverse events, safety profile, and clinical experience of the participants:

- Group 1. Medications with proven high efficacy and mild-to-moderate adverse events
- Group 2. Medications with lower efficacy (i.e., limited number of studies or studies reporting conflicting results) or efficacy suggesting only "modest" improvement, and mild-to-moderate adverse events
- Secondary headaches:
  - Manage and treat the underlying cause
  - Avoid opioids if level of consciousness needs to be monitored
  - Acetaminophen for pain and fever if not contraindicated

Table 15-1. Pharmacologic Treatment: Preventive Therapy for Migraine

Group	Medication	Usual Daily Adult Dose	Usual Daily Peds Dose	Side Effects
1	Divalproex Na (Depakote)	Usual dose for age >16: start with 250 mg bid; usual max 1 g/day	20–40 mg/kg	GI upset, liver disease, thrombocytopenia. Therefore need to monitor closely
	Sodium Valproate	800–1,500 mg/day	—	Alopecia, rash, abdominal pain, constipation, diarrhea, pancreatitis
1	Propranolol	160–240 mg/day in divided doses	< 35 kg: 10–20 mg po tid > 35 kg: 20–40 mg po tid	Heart block, Raynaud's, SLE, fatigue, dizziness, constipation, hypotension
1	Timolol (Blocadren)	10–30 mg/day divided qd–bid	—	Heart block, Raynauds, fatigue, dizziness, nightmares, hypotension
1	Amitriptyline (indicated for relief of symptoms of depression only)	50–100 mg/day	—	HTN, syncope, QT prolongation, seizures, extrapyramidal symptoms, leucopenia, drowsiness, dizziness, dry mouth
2	Guanfacine (Tenex)	0.5–1 mg/day	—	Hypotension, alopecia, dermatitis, constipation, loss of appetite, xerostomia
2	Gabapentin	900–2,400 mg/day	—	Peripheral edema, myalgia, ataxia, dizziness, mood swings, fatigue

Table 15–1. Pharmacologic Treatment: Preventive Therapy for Migraine (cont.)

Group	Medication	Usual Daily Adult Dose	Usual Daily Peds Dose	Side Effects
2	Fluoxetine	20mg qod–40 mg/day	—	Insomnia, fatigue, tremor, stomach pain, rash, sweating, xerostomia
2	Atenolol	100 mg/day	—	Arrhythmia, diarrhea, dizziness, fatigue, insomnia
2	Verapamil	240 mg/day	—	Edema, hypotension, constipation, nausea, dizziness
2	NSAIDS: Aspirin Flurbiprofen Ketoprofen Naproxen sodium	325 mg/day 200 mg/day 150 mg/day 1,100 mg/day	—	Gastritis, occult GI bleed, tinnitus, indigestion, nausea, vomiting
2	Ergotamine + caffeine + butalbital + belladonna	2 caps a day for 3 days before, during, and 2 days after menses	—	Pruritus, nausea, vomiting, muscle weakness, parasthesia, visual disturbances
2	Estradiol Gel	1.5 mg/day for 7 days	—	Edema, pruritus, weight gain, nausea, amenorrhea, break-through bleeding
2	Feverfew	50–82 mg/day	—	Eczema, edema, nausea, abdominal pain, diarrhea, tachycardia
2	Magnesium	400–600 mg/day	—	Blurred vision, diarrhea, HTN, increased bleeding times
2	Vitamin B2	400 mg/day	—	Rare adverse events

Note. HTN = hypertension

LENGTH OF TREATMENT
- Treat acute attacks until headache resolves or maximum daily dose is reached; narcotics can be used to treat intractable pain
- Prophylaxis: Primary headache syndromes tend to decrease or resolve in late middle age or after menopause; attempt to wean periodically

Special Considerations
- Consider cardiovascular, gastrointestinal, renal, and hepatic disease when prescribing therapy in geriatric patients
- Increased risk of GI bleed, renal failure, edema and elevated blood pressure (BP) with NSAIDS in elderly
- There are no randomized control studies for migraine treatment in the elderly
- Headaches are common in the first trimester of pregnancy
- Migraines usually do not become worse during pregnancy
- Counsel women of childbearing age regarding headache management and pregnancy
  - Ergotamine derivatives are strong uterine stimulants
  - Ergotamine is secreted in breast milk and may cause vomiting and diarrhea in infants

When to Consult, Refer, Hospitalize
- Consult with physician as needed, if narcotic analgesics needed
- Refer to neurologist if unable to manage symptoms using typical therapy or if patient develops symptoms of increased intracranial pressure (ICP), or if tumor, aneurysm, or AVM suspected
- Refer to neurologist if patient is experiencing multiple headaches/week, and/or is taking multiple doses of medication without benefit (e.g., rebound headaches due to medication effects)
- Refer to emergency department (ED) for severe unresponsive migraine or cluster headache with vomiting and need for IV hydration; or sudden, severe headache; or headache with change in level of consciousness
- Refer to surgeon or ophthalmologist for temporal artery biopsy if temporal arteritis suspected
- Refer to psychologist or therapist for relaxation therapy or psychotherapy, or when depression suspected that does not respond to trial of antidepressants
- Refer to interdisciplinary pain center for chronic, intractable pain, interfering with daily life

Follow-Up
- Routine annual health assessments
- Weekly to monthly when adjusting or changing medications
  EXPECTED COURSE
  - Tension headaches can be lifelong
  - Migraines get better in more than two-thirds of all children, but the prognosis of remission diminishes after age 18
  - In adults, migraines and cluster headaches usually resolve during middle age, or following completion of menopause

  COMPLICATIONS
  - Unrecognized or mistreated serious headaches from secondary causes
  - Lost wages and productivity, and troubled relationships from chronic pain

Brain Tumors

Description
- Primary brain tumors are abnormal growth of cells arising from structures within the cranium
- Classified by cell of origin (Table 15–2) and include gliomas, meningioma (rare in children), acoustic neuroma, ependymoma, craniopharyngioma, pediatric ganglioma (benign, may be accompanied by seizures)
- May be malignant or benign
- Secondary brain tumors most often metastasize from the lung, breast, kidney, or gastrointestinal tract

Etiology
- The exact cause of brain tumors is unknown
- Gliomas of the supporting glial tissues account for 46% of all central nervous system tumors
  - Grades I, II (astrocytomas), III, IV (glioblastoma multiforme)
  - Grade III and IV are more invasive, faster-growing, and have a poor prognosis
- Meningiomas develop from the covering of the brain
  - Rarely malignant, usually cure is possible with complete excision, except for meningiomas of the posterior fossa where complete excision is difficult
- Presenting signs and symptoms depend on the location and size of the tumor

Incidence and Demographics
- Second most common cause of cancer in children
- Occur in all age groups, but peak in the interval between age 5 and 9 years
- Estimated incidence in children is 2.5 to 3/100, 000
- Incidence of primary brain tumor is 8/100,000 in the U.S.
- Benign primary tumors (meningiomas) 10/100,000
- Malignant primary tumors (astrocytomas and glioblastoma multiforme) 5/100,000
  - Greatest incidence in 60–70-year-olds; second most common cause of cancer in children; 20% of all malignant neoplasms; make up 50%–60% of all childhood brain tumors

Table 15-2. Primary Brain Tumors

Tumor	Structure	Treatment and Prognosis
Astrocytoma (Grade I, II glioma)	Glial tissue	Total excision usually not possible May respond to radiation Variable prognosis
Glioblastoma multiforme (Grade III, IV glioma)	Glial tissues	Total excision not possible, recur Radiation and chemotherapy may slow growth Poor prognosis
Oligodendroglioma	Cerebral hemispheres	Slow-growing Successful surgical treatment
Ependymoma	Glioma usually of the fourth ventricle	Presents with signs of IIP Shunt, surgical resection if possible Radiation therapy

Table 15–2. Primary Brain Tumors (cont.)

Tumor	Structure	Treatment and Prognosis
Craniopharyngioma	Sella tunica Depresses optic chiasm	Surgical resection usually incomplete Bitemporal visual field cuts Endocrine dysfunction
Meningioma	Dura or arachnoid mater	Surgical excision, difficult to completely remove posterior fossa tumors Cure with complete resection
Acoustic neuroma	Nerve sheath Vestibular branch of 8th cranial nerve at the cerebellopontine angle	Excision usually good outcome May have residual ipsilateral hearing loss, imbalance, facial weakness or numbness
Primary cerebral lymphoma	Reticuloendothelial system in immunocompromised patients	Shunt Prognosis depends on CD4 count

Risk Factors
- Previous radiation therapy
- Neurofibromatosis
- Meningiomas increase with age
- Primary cerebral lymphoma associated with AIDS

Assessment
- Classic triad: Morning headache, vomiting, papilledema
    HISTORY
    - Focused, complete neuro history including weakness, slurred speech or word-finding difficulty, visual changes including diplopia or field cuts, hearing loss, cognitive changes, drowsiness, seizures, headache
    - Children: Changes in behavior or school performance; PMH, including birth history, recent illness or trauma; growth and development history, including delays; family history of neurological disease or neurofibromatosis
    - Tumors are suspected in patients with progressive deficits
    - The deficit may suggest the location of the tumor (Table 15–3)
    - In children, presence of new-onset headache, especially for 1 week or intermittent for 1 month
    - Headache associated with tumor is dull and aching and increases over weeks
    - Headaches are usually secondary to hydrocephalus or posterior fossa tumors stretching pain-sensitive structures
    - New onset seizures at any age suggests a tumor, possibly temporal lobe
    - Review of systems include HEENT for loss of sense of smell or visual field cuts suggest pituitary adenoma or craniopharyngioma; with unilateral hearing loss consider acoustic neuroma
    - History of vomiting without nausea with deficits or headache in the morning suggest increased intracranial pressure
    - Assess for symptoms of Cushing syndrome (see Chapter 17) if pituitary adenoma suspected

PHYSICAL EXAM
- Attention to head circumference and fontanels in young children
- Complete neurological exam may reveal focal cranial nerve or motor deficits
- Other systems as indicated by history, including eye exam, eye movements, papilledema and, in children, skin for signs of neurocutaneous disease
- If pituitary adenoma suspected, will need complete endocrine assessment; elevated blood pressure may be present
- Metastatic brain tumor: If primary tumor site unknown, will need to evaluate for lung, breast, kidney, or colon cancer
- Gait abnormalities, incoordination, cranial nerve paralysis, optic atrophy, loss of visual fields, nystagmus, focal motor weakness and sensory abnormalities, hyperreflexia

DIAGNOSTIC STUDIES
- CT used as fast screening exam but MRI gives better results
- Magnetic resonance imaging for suspected posterior fossa lesions and intrasellar lesions
- Angiography of intrasellar lesion with normal hormone levels to differentiate pituitary adenoma from an aneurysm
- Pituitary adenoma: ACTH, thyroid function tests, serum glucose and electrolytes, prolactin
- Metastatic brain tumors: Chest x-ray, mammogram, colonoscopy as appropriate to locate primary tumor if unknown
- Open biopsy of the tumor
- EEGs are not helpful unless seizures are a presenting symptoms
- Skull x-rays many demonstrate nonspecific findings associated with increased ICP

Differential Diagnosis
- Subdural hematoma
- Arteriovenous malformation, aneurysm
- Cerebrovascular accident
- Hydrocephalus
- Pseudotumor cerebri
- Epilepsy
- Primary headache syndrome
- Abscess
- Hamartoma (causing a brain gliosis)
- Neurofibromatosis with neuromas (when indicated by history)
- Viral infections

Management
- Surgery, radiation, chemotherapy as indicated
- Side effects of radiation therapy are hair loss and otitis externa
- Patients must be monitored for panhypopituitarism, if radiation to the pituitary gland
- Side effects of chemotherapy are myelosuppression and infection, hair loss, and weight loss from nausea/vomiting
- Patients and parents need continuous emotional support during therapy

LENGTH OF TREATMENT
- Radiation therapy: 6 weeks
- Chemotherapy: 1–2 years

Special Considerations
- Patients who receive large-field radiation to the cerebrum are at high risk for cognitive deficits
- All patients receiving radiation are at increased risk for recurrent tumors
- Malignant brain tumors: Those <45 live 3 times longer than those >65
- Prognosis decreases with lower premorbid function based on the Karnofsky Performance Rating
- Coordinate obstetrical and oncology care for pregnant or lactating patients

When to Consult, Refer, Hospitalize
- Consult with physician if unsure of symptoms or diagnosis
- Refer to pediatric neurologist (for children and adolescents) or a neurologist (for adults and elders) for further evaluation and treatment
- Refer to social services, home health services, and counseling as needed

Follow-Up
- Patient will be followed closely by neurology/surgery/oncology team
  COMPLICATIONS
  - Persistent neurologic deficits, seizures, increased intracranial pressure and death; refer to Table 15–3

Table 15–3. Location and Signs and Symptoms of Intracranial Lesions

Location	Signs and Symptoms
Frontal lobe	Intellectual and cognitive decline
	Personality change
	Contralateral grasp reflex
	Expressive aphasia
	Focal motor seizures, contralateral weakness
	Anosmia
Temporal lobe	Seizures (may be partial without loss of consciousness)
	Emotional and behavioral change
	Auditory hallucinations
	Visual field cuts
	Receptive aphasia
Parietal lobe	Contralateral sensory loss
	Loss of tactile discrimination (astereognosis)
	Contralateral field cuts
	Alexia, agraphia, apraxia, acalculia
	Right–left confusion
Occipital	Homonymous hemianopsia
	Visual agnosia
	Cortical blindness

Table 15-3. Location and Signs and Symptoms of Intracranial Lesions (cont.)

Location	Signs and Symptoms
Cerebellum and brain stem	Ataxia and incoordination
	Cranial nerve palsies
	Nystagmus
	Motor and sensory deficits (unilateral or bilateral)
	Increased intracranial pressure

Trigeminal Neuralgia

Description
- A pain syndrome, also called *tic douloureux*, consists of paroxysmal lancinating pain of the face, usually unilateral; originates near mouth and shoots to nose, eye, or ear
- Can also occur in multiple sclerosis

Etiology
- Compression of the 5th cranial nerve root usually by vascular structure or malformation

Incidence and Demographics
- Most common in middle age to older women

Risk Factors
- Triggers for pain are touch, movement, cold air, chewing

Prevention and Screening
- None identified

Assessment
HISTORY
- Focused history if chief complaint of facial pain beginning near the side of the mouth, shooting up to ipsilateral eye, ear, or nostril
- Establish time frame, description of episode, any triggers and pain management; initially episodes are separated by months of pain-free time
- Review of systems to identify any neurologic deficits such as weakness, numbness, diplopia, or other symptoms of a space-occupying lesion
- Any ear, nose, throat, or dental symptoms indicating sinusitis, dental abscess, or otitis
- History of 5th cranial nerve herpes zoster, or multiple sclerosis

PHYSICAL EXAM
- Examine head, eyes, ears, nose, throat, mouth, neck, and cranial nerves
- Neurologic exam if cranial nerve abnormalities
- No physical findings with classic trigeminal neuralgia except possibly poor dental hygiene or lack of shaving or makeup on affected side

DIAGNOSTIC STUDIES
- CT or MRI indicated if neurologic deficits present to rule out space-occupying lesion
- ESR if temporal (giant cell) arteritis suspected

Differential Diagnosis
- 5th cranial nerve tumor
- Post herpetic neuralgia
- Temporal arteritis
- Multiple sclerosis, particularly in the young or with bilateral pain
- Herpes zoster, pain may present before vesicular rash
- Sinusitis, otitis, dental abscess, TMJ

Management
NONPHARMACOLOGIC TREATMENT
- Avoid triggers
- Surgical decompression, radiofrequency rhizotomy, gamma radiosurgery in severe cases

PHARMACOLOGIC TREATMENT
- Carbamazepine (Tegretol) 100 mg bid, increase by 100–200 mg every 2–3 days up to 1,200 mg daily in divided doses; use lowest effective dose
- Phenytoin (Dilantin) 300–600 mg/day
- Gabapentin (Neurontin) 100 mg tid; titrate up to 1,800 mg divided/day
- Baclofen (Lioresal) 10–20 mg tid or qid, alone or in combination with carbamazepine

LENGTH OF TREATMENT
- Attempt to decrease or discontinue dose every 3 months; decrease one drug at a time

Special Considerations
- CNS side effects: Start with lowest possible dose of medications for elderly, titrate up slowly
- Adjust gabapentin dose for renal insufficiency

When to Consult, Refer, Hospitalize
- Refer to neurosurgeon for surgical decompression if intractable pain with adequate trials of medication, or unable to tolerate medications
- Surgery is inappropriate for trigeminal neuralgia secondary to multiple sclerosis

Follow-Up
- Follow every 3 months
- Monitor CBC and liver function if on anticonvulsant medication
   COMPLICATIONS
   - Generally none

Bell's Palsy

Description
- An acute unilateral paralysis or paresis of the face in a pattern consistent with peripheral nerve dysfunction without a detectable cause. Usually due to lower motor neuron facial weakness due to inflammation of the 7th cranial nerve.
- Most patients have sudden onset of a unilateral facial droop, accompanied by drooling (especially in young children) and failure to completely close the affected eye; may also have discomfort behind ear or of jaw, change in hearing, loss of taste; pain is usually transient.
- The paralysis may be difficult to assess when the patient is at rest but evident with crying or talking.

Etiology
- Unknown, although reactivation of herpes simplex virus has been implicated.
- Cases are often preceded by an upper respiratory infection, Lyme disease.
- There is an acute inflammatory response causing swelling of the facial nerve and entrapment in the foramen of the temporal bone.
- Paresis typically progresses over 7–10 days, most patients fully recover in 6 months.

Incidence and Demographics
- 20–30 per 100,000 individuals a year; peak incidence is 10–40 years; no gender or race predilection
- 10% have a familial association

Risk Factors
- Trauma, diabetes mellitus, hypothyroidism, AIDS, Lyme disease, syphilis, sarcoidosis, viral infection
- Pregnancy, due to increased intravascular volume particularly during the third trimester, increases the risk for facial nerve edema and subsequent compression

Assessment
HISTORY
- In the newborn, history of birth trauma
- Abrupt onset facial paresis, face feels "pulled to side"
- Most important to establish time frame; sudden onset over hours to a few days suggests Bell's palsy, progressive weakness over weeks indicates a tumor or other space-occupying lesion
- Past medical history including any recent upper respiratory infection, otitis, facial trauma, and history of chronic illness including diabetes, thyroid disease, multiple sclerosis, sarcoidosis, and HIV
- Review of systems of neuro and HEENT including facial movements; visual changes, pain, or tearing; altered hearing or otalgia; altered taste; skin rash or possible tick bite

PHYSICAL EXAM
- Vital signs, noting any increase in blood pressure or temperature
- Complete HEENT exam for decreased tone, signs of infection, lesions, or rashes
- Screening neuro exam including all cranial nerves, paying attention to eye movement, jaw strength, symmetry of the face, hearing

- Bell's palsy indicated by complete unilateral peripheral 7th nerve paresis or paralysis, with flattening of the forehead furrows, inability to raise eyebrow, inability to complete close the ipsilateral eye, flattening of the nasolabial fold, inability to puff out cheek, drooping of the mouth, inability to smile or frown; rest of cranial nerves and neuro exam is usually normal
- A central 7th nerve palsy, or only drooping of the mouth, indicating damage only to the lower branch of the facial nerve, indicates an upper motor neuron lesion (stroke or tumor)
- Inspect eye for corneal abrasion, tearing
- Inspect ear canal and TM for otitis or vesicular lesions, indicate cephalic herpes zoster
- Palpate parotid glands for masses
- Check for lymphadenopathy and thyroid enlargement
- Inspect skin for rash, particularly target lesion or erythema migrans of Lyme disease (although rash may not still be present)

DIAGNOSTIC STUDIES
- No testing usually necessary unless diagnosis in question
- EMG and nerve conduction studies 5–10 days after onset of symptoms if complete paralysis or no improvement, to guide prognosis and treatment; if more than 90% neural degeneration, surgical decompression may be indicated
- X-ray if temporal bone fracture suspected
- CT scan or MRI if tumor or space-occupying lesion suspected; also images facial nerve and temporal bone
- Complete blood count, chemistry panel, thyroid function tests, syphilis testing, HIV serology if indicated by history to rule out associated chronic diseases
- ESR if temporal (giant cell) arteritis suspected
- Lumbar puncture if meningitis suspected
- Lyme titer if exposure to ticks or a rash suggestive of Lyme disease
- VDRL and/or HIV screen if history warrants
- Audiology testing if hearing affected >1 week or acoustic neuroma suspected
- EMG testing is occasionally used to predict prognosis and progression of disease (usually is done if symptoms last longer than 6–12 months)

Differential Diagnosis
- Tumor
- Stroke or transient ischemic attack (TIA)
- Herpes zoster
- Temporal bone fracture or other trauma
- Giant cell arteritis
- Lyme disease
- HIV
- Guillain-Barré syndrome (typically symmetric bilateral weakness)
- Neurofibromatosis
- Möbius syndrome
- Infections (otitis media, mastoiditis, meningitis, mumps, rubella, syphilis)
- Parotid gland obstruction or mass
- Multiple sclerosis or other demyelinating conditions
- Diabetic neuropathy

- Hypothyroidism
- Pregnancy
- Sarcoidosis

Management
NONPHARMACOLOGIC TREATMENT
- Protect eye, artificial tears during the day, lubricant ointment and patch eye at bedtime
- No evidence that surgical decompression improves outcomes
- Physical therapy, including heat, electrical stimulation, or massage, may be beneficial

PHARMACOLOGIC TREATMENT
- Medical treatment of Bell's palsy remains controversial
- One study of prednisone and acyclovir demonstrated a statistically significant reduction in nerve degeneration compared to prednisone and placebo
- Prednisone in children: 2 mg/kg/day for 1 week, with a slow taper and discontinue by day 14; in adults and elders: 60–80 mg/day divided for 3–5 days, then taper over 10 days
- Acyclovir 400 mg 5 times/day for 10 days if there is evidence that herpes virus is the causative agent
- Artificial tears to keep affected eye moist during daytime and ointment at night

LENGTH OF TREATMENT
- Eye protection until patient can close and protect eye
- Steroid and antiviral therapy for 10–14 days

Special Considerations
- Incomplete recovery is associated with increased age.
- Poor prognosis is associated with complete paralysis, pain, or hyperacusis at presentation; these characteristics, combined with increased age and comorbidity, should guide decision to treat with steroids and antiviral agents.

When to Consult, Refer, Hospitalize
- Refer to ophthalmologist if corneal abrasion or significant prolonged decreased lacrimation
- Refer to neurologist if other deficits present, recurrent paresis, or paresis lasting >6 months
- In patients >6 years, refer to plastic surgeon for persistent cosmetic disfigurement

Follow-Up
- At 1-week intervals to ensure eye protection and recovery
  ### EXPECTED COURSE
  - Most have spontaneous recovery in 2–3 weeks
  - 15% may have residual weakness for several months and some have permanent weakness

COMPLICATIONS
- Incomplete recovery or recurrent paresis or paralysis
- Corneal abrasion
- Recurrent episodes

Stroke and Transient Ischemic Attack

Description
- Strokes are ischemic or hemorrhagic.
- Ischemic stroke or "brain attack" is an interruption in blood flow to the brain causing neuronal death or infarction. Hemorrhage accounts for less than 10% of strokes; the bleed may be intraparenchymal or subarachnoid.
- Transient ischemic attack (TIA) is a temporary interruption in cerebral vascular blood flow; the deficit lasts less than 24 hours. There is no infarcted tissue.

Etiology
- Ischemic strokes:
  - Lack of blood flow to brain due to hypoxia, decreased cardiac output, thrombus, or embolus
- Thrombotic stroke:
  - Caused by progressive accumulation of atherosclerotic plaque that occludes an intracranial vessel
  - Most common in the posterior cerebral circulation
- Embolic stroke:
  - Caused by atherosclerotic debris from the heart, aorta, or carotids that flow into the internal carotids and occlude the smaller vessels of the cerebral circulation
  - Usually affects the anterior cerebral circulation
- Lacunar infarcts:
  - Less than 5 mm; occur in the internal capsule, basal ganglia, or thalamus
  - Due to slow, progressive occlusion of the penetrating arterioles
- TIAs; may be thrombotic, embolic, or lacunar in nature.
- Hemorrhagic stroke:
  - Intracerebral hemorrhage: Spontaneous bleeding into parenchyma from microaneurysm of perforating vessels, most commonly occurs in the basal ganglia; due to hypertension, hematological disorders, or anticoagulation therapy
- Subarachnoid hemorrhage:
  - Bleeding from a ruptured aneurysm in the Circle of Willis or arteriovenous malformation

Incidence and Demographics
- Acute stroke afflicts 600,000 Americans per year; incidence increases with age.
- One-fourth will die, making stroke the third leading cause of death.
- 50% of the survivors will have some disability, 15%–30% will require nursing home placement.

Risk Factors
- Previous cerebrovascular disease, stroke or TIA; 20%–40% of ischemic strokes are preceded by TIA within days to months
- Aging

- Traditional risks for vascular disease: Hypertension, diabetes, hyperlipidemia, smoking
- Traditional risks for emboli: Atrial fibrillation, cardiomyopathy, coronary artery disease

Prevention and Screening
- Management of hypertension; screening for hypertension is recommended at least every 2 years in the normotensive, treatment is recommended per Joint National Commission 6 guidelines
- Screening for asymptomatic carotid stenosis by auscultation of carotid bruits or carotid ultrasound remains controversial with insufficient evidence to recommend for or against
- High-risk patients over age 60 with other risk factors for vascular disease, that have access to vascular surgery with morbidity and mortality rates of less than 3%, may benefit from screening and subsequent endarterectomy
- Antiplatelet therapy with aspirin, ticlopidine (Ticlid), or clopidogrel (Plavix) may decrease the risk of stroke in those with asymptomatic carotid artery stenosis
- Anticoagulation is recommended for patients with atrial fibrillation, particularly those with additional risk factors
- Evidence suggests improved glycemic control may decrease microvascular events in type 2 diabetes
- Decreasing serum lipids may delay progression of carotid atherosclerosis and decrease cerebrovascular events
- All patients will benefit from diet and exercise counseling and smoking cessation

Assessment
  HISTORY
- Onset, duration, and progression of symptoms most important in determining etiology and management
- Resolution of symptoms in minutes to hours is suggestive of a TIA
- Onset during sleep with progression suggests thrombotic stroke
- Sudden onset with activity suggests embolic or hemorrhagic stroke
- Detailed description of symptoms or deficits including visual changes, aphasia, motor weakness, paresthesias may give clue to location of stroke or lesion
- Review of systems: Headache, seizure, loss of consciousness, syncope, vertigo, vomiting, cardiac symptoms:
  - Lack of headache excludes hemorrhagic stroke
  - Vomiting is associated with increased intracranial pressure, usually due to hemorrhage
  - Loss of consciousness is associated with hemorrhage or posterior circulation thrombosis
  - Syncope more often related to cardiac etiology than stroke
  - Vertigo suggests vestibular disease, but may occur with vertebrobasilar insufficiency
- Past medical history: Cardiac disease; peripheral vascular disease; diabetes; IV drug abuse; previous neurologic conditions such as seizure, head trauma, dementia, brain tumors gives clues to etiology and possible differential diagnosis
- Review all medications, particularly those that can alter level of consciousness or cause bleeding

PHYSICAL EXAM
- Complete neurologic exam including level of consciousness, cognitive ability (apraxia, agnosia, aphasia, agraphia), motor and sensory function (contralateral deficits), cranial nerve exam including funduscopic and visual deficits, reflexes (hyperreflexia or Babinski on affected side)
- Cardiovascular exam: Hypertension, orthostatic changes, atrial fibrillation, heart murmurs, carotid bruits, abdominal bruit from aneurysm
- Signs of carotid TIA: Weakness of contralateral arm, leg, or face, individually or in combination; numbness or paraesthesia may occur alone or in combination with motor deficit; dysphagia; monocular visual loss; carotid bruit; TRS may be hyperreflexic during attack; atherosclerotic changes on funduscopic exam; signs and symptoms disappear as attack resolves
- Signs of vertebrobasilar TIA: Vertigo, ataxia, diplopia, dysarthria, dimness or blurry vision, perioral numbness, weakness or sensory complaints on one or both sides of the body, drop attacks with bilateral leg weakness
- Lacunar infarction: Contralateral pure motor or sensory deficit, ipsilateral ataxia, dysarthria, with complete symptom resolution over 1–2 months
- Cerebral infarction: Deficit depends on vessel so any variety of focal neurological deficits may develop
- Cerebellar infarction: Vertigo, ataxia, nystagmus, nausea/vomiting
- Hemorrhagic CVA: Typically associated with hypertension, sudden onset, symptoms usually present during activity, initial loss of or impaired consciousness, rapidly evolving hemiplegia or paresis

DIAGNOSTIC STUDIES
- CT scan; MRI if posterior circulation involved
- Lumbar puncture if CT negative for hemorrhage and subarachnoid hemorrhage suspected
- Carotid duplex for evaluation of symptomatic carotid stenosis, if patient surgical candidate for endarterectomy; carotid studies are useless for evaluation of posterior circulation
- Angiography remains the "gold standard" for assessing carotid stenosis, as well as identifying aneurysms, AVM, and vasculitis
- Electrocardiogram, chest radiograph, echocardiogram
- Transesophageal echocardiogram if intraventricular thrombus or patent foramen ovale is suspected
- Holter monitor to rule out paroxysmal arrhythmias
- CBC, ESR, coagulation studies, RPR, chemistry panel, and lipid profile to evaluate cause

Differential Diagnosis
- TIA, thrombotic, embolic or lacunar stroke
- Subarachnoid or intracerebral hemorrhage
- Cerebral aneurysm or AVM
- Intracranial tumor
- Seizure
- Migraine with aura
- Encephalopathy

- Intoxication
- Hypoglycemia
- Multiple sclerosis
- Syncope
- Vertigo
- Postural hypotension

Management
NONPHARMACOLOGIC TREATMENT
- Educate patients at risk and families about "brain attack," need for same immediate response as heart attack
- Diet and exercise counseling for primary and secondary prevention; smoking cessation
- Carotid endarterectomy for surgical candidates with carotid stenosis over 70%
- Care post-stroke is largely supportive: Physical therapy, occupational therapy, speech therapy
- Emotional support of patient and family

PHARMACOLOGIC TREATMENT
- Tissue plasminogen activator (TPA) must be administered in a hospital within 3 hours of onset of symptoms of ischemic stroke; contraindicated in hemorrhagic stroke; patients awaking with focal deficits are not appropriate for TPA because duration of deficits is unknown
- Medical management in the post-acute phase involves anticoagulation or antiplatelet agents, and treatment of underlying heart disease, hypertension, diabetes and hyperlipidemia
  - Aspirin 325 mg each day
  - Ticlopidine (Ticlid) 250 mg bid, reduce dose to qd for renal patients, monitor for neutropenia, check CBC every 2 weeks for 3 months, then every 3 months
  - Clopidogrel (Plavix) 75 mg each day, does not cause neutropenia, but has been more effective at preventing peripheral vascular disease than stroke
  - Warfarin (Coumadin): Used for patients with symptoms on antiplatelet medication or those with atrial fibrillation or prosthetic heart valves; dose is individualized due to small therapeutic window and interactions with food and other medications; International Normalized Ratio (INR) is stabilized at 2–3 for atrial fibrillation or antiplatelet failure and 2.5–3.5 for prosthetic valve

LENGTH OF TREATMENT
- As long as antiplatelet or anticoagulation is not contraindicated (increase risk of GI or intracerebral bleeding)

Special Considerations
- Men are at greater risk than women, although more women die of stroke because of age and population dynamics.

- Increased risk with age and poorer prognosis, increased incidence of infection, myocardial infarction, renal failure, and delirium. Consider patient's risk of falls, ability to manage a complex medication regime, and INR monitoring when initiating warfarin therapy.
- Do not discount stroke in young people, may be hemorrhagic stroke secondary to AVM or embolic stroke secondary to unidentified patent foramen ovale (right-to-left shunt).

When to Consult, Refer, Hospitalize
- Send all patients with sudden onset of focal neurologic deficit to emergency facility; if TIA, may need urgent work up and treatment to prevent stroke; if diagnosed as stroke and of less than 3 hours duration, may start TPA therapy
- Send patients to emergency facility with sudden severe headache, decreasing level of consciousness, vomiting, or focal neurological deficits
- Consult with physician or neurologist for evaluation and management of patient with history of TIA or previous stroke

Follow-Up
- Patients with risk for cerebrovascular disease should monitored every 3–6 months for symptoms of TIA, hypertension, and counseled regarding stroke prophylaxis, diet, exercise, and smoking cessation

    EXPECTED COURSE
    - Variable; most stroke recovery occurs early, the longer deficits last, the less likely they are to resolve although improvement may be seen for 6 months
    - 27% of stroke patients die within 1 year, and 53% within 5 years
    - Physical therapy improves functional recovery
    - Older age, coma, and early acute CT changes are associated with poor prognosis

    COMPLICATIONS
    - Intracerebral hemorrhage from TPA therapy
    - Myocardial infarction, infection, renal failure
    - Falls, depression, dementia
    - Intracerebral bleed or GI bleed from anticoagulation

Alzheimer's Disease (AD)/Multi-Infarct Dementia (MID)

Description
- Dementia: Impairment of global intellectual and cognitive function characterized by memory loss, aphasia, agnosia, and apraxia with preservation of level of consciousness
- MID and Alzheimer's disease make up the majority of progressive, irreversible dementias
- MID: Dementing process caused by strokes characterized by step-wise decline
- AD: Gradual onset and progressive decline without focal neurological deficits
    - 1st stage of AD manifested by short-term memory impairment. Activities of daily living become increasingly challenging. Social, occupational, and cognitive impairment manifest themselves.
    - 2nd stage of AD characterized by increasing loss of social and cognitive ability, with concomitant increasing behavioral changes. These can range from agitation and restlessness to outright combativeness. Eventually, the patient no longer recognizes friends and loved ones.

– 3rd and last stage of AD brings the disease full cycle, as cognitive disability is eventually followed by physical decline

Etiology

- AD: Not fully understood
- More neuritic plaques and neurofibrillary tangles are found on autopsy as compared to nondemented patients
- Three genes on different chromosomes have been identified in families with history of AD, although all cases may not be inherited
- MID: Multiple lacunar infarcts

Incidence and Demographics

- Affects 5%–10% of those >65 and increases with age
- AD and related dementias affect 2–4 million Americans
- Often misdiagnosed or unrecognized, especially in early stages
- AD: 50%–60% of all dementias; MID: 10%–20% of all dementias

Risk Factors

- AD: Down syndrome
- Familial or inherited
- MID: Hypertension, previous stroke, TIA

Prevention and Screening

- Routine screening is not recommended because there is no definitive treatment, and it is difficult to recognize early dementia.
- Those >65 should have cognitive and functional evaluation at least every 3 years.
- Be aware of early symptoms to facilitate early assessment and recognition and rule out age-related memory changes, unidentified conditions, or reversible forms of dementia (Table 15–4).
- Interpretation: Positive findings in any of these areas generally indicate the need for further assessment for the presence of dementia.

Assessment

HISTORY

- Detailed history of present illness, including time frame and progression, any associated neurological symptoms such as amaurosis fugax, aphasia, unilateral weakness
- Past medical history: Hypertension, strokes, head trauma
- Psychiatric history: Depression, anxiety, schizophrenia
- Social history: Present living situation, marital status, occupation, education, alcohol, tobacco, illicit drug use
- Medications including over-the-counter, supplements, and home remedies
- Initial and periodic functional history and assessment
- Validate history with family member and/or caregiver but also be aware of potential for self-serving motives; informants may exaggerate or deny symptoms

Table 15-4. Guide for Recognition and Initial Assessment of Dementia

Does the person have increased difficulty with any of the activities listed?

Learning and retaining new information	Is repetitive; has trouble remembering recent conversations, events, appointments; frequently misplaces objects
Handling complex tasks	Has trouble following a complex train of thought or performing tasks that require many steps such as balancing a checkbook or cooking a meal
Reasoning ability	Is unable to respond with a reasonable plan to problems at home or work, such as knowing what to do if the bathroom is flooded; shows uncharacteristic disregard for rules of social conduct
Special ability and orientation	Has trouble driving, organizing objects around the house, finding way around familiar places
Language	Has increasing difficulty with finding the words to express what he or she wants to say and with following conversations
Behavior	Appears more passive and less responsive; is more irritable than usual; is more suspicious than usual; misinterprets visual or auditory stimuli

PHYSICAL EXAM

- Assess level of consciousness along a continuum from alert, to drowsy, to stupor, to coma
- Perform complete mental status evaluation using instrument such as Folstein Mini-Mental State Examination (MMSE), the Short Portable Mental Status Questionnaire, or Blessed Dementia Rating Scale; test results are not diagnostic, but serve as baseline for assessing trends in cognitive impairment
    - Generally, a score of <26 on the MMSE (which tests orientation, registration, attention and calculation, recall and language) indicates cognitive impairment, but this is only a crude indicator of functioning
- Complete neurologic exam with attention to focal neurologic deficits, which may indicate MID or other neurologic problem
    - MID: Focal motor weakness or impaired sensation, reflex asymmetry, positive Babinski
- Assess for sensory impairments (hearing, vision) that masquerade as or worsen dementia
- Pulmonary and cardiac exams (murmurs, arrhythmias, heart enlargement, orthostatic hypotension)
- Any evidence of infectious processes
- Signs of physical and mental abuse

DIAGNOSTIC STUDIES

- CBC, chemistry profile, thyroid function tests, B12 level, folate level to rule out causes of delirium and reversible dementia; syphilis, HIV, and drug toxicity if indicated by history
- CT for early dementia of <2 years in duration may show atrophy, infarcts, or unexpected lesions
- Other testing based on presentation

- Neuropsychological testing is recommended under certain circumstances: to differentiate depression, stroke, or delirium in unusual presentations; identify areas of preserved cognitive function to develop a care plan

Differential Diagnosis

- Delirium
- Other dementias: Lewey bodies dementia, Pick's disease
- Depression and anxiety
- Normal pressure hydrocephalus
- Tumor
- Hearing loss
- B12 and folate deficiency
- Parkinson's disease
- Trauma—consider subdural hematoma, falls (whether witnessed or not)
- Alcohol intoxication
- Infectious process: chronic infection, AIDS, tertiary syphilis
- Cardiovascular or cerebrovascular accidents
- Medications: polypharmacy, interactions

Management

- Foremost, rule out or treat any conditions that may contribute to cognitive impairment
- Discontinue all unnecessary medications, especially sedatives and hypnotics
- MID: Nonpharmacologic and pharmacologic reduction of stroke risks (see management of TIA and stroke)

    NONPHARMACOLOGIC TREATMENT
    - Explain memory/cognition status assessment results to the patient, putting them within the context of overall patient status
    - Educate patient and family about the illness, treatment, community resources
    - Assist with long-term planning including financial, legal, and advance directives
    - Assess home and driving safety
    - Behavior therapy identifies causes of problem behaviors, and changes the environment to reduce the behavior
    - Recreational, art, and pet therapy create pleasurable experiences for the patient
    - Reminiscence therapy
    - Incontinence care; supportive care

    PHARMACOLOGIC TREATMENT
    - Cognitive symptoms:
        - Cholinesterase inhibitors such as donepezil (Aricept) 5 mg, may increase to 10 mg qd
        - Common side effects are headache, nausea, diarrhea
        - LFT monitoring not required as was with tacrine (Cognex), an earlier cholinesterase inhibitor
    - Psychosis and agitation:
        - Haloperidol (Haldol) 0.5–3 mg at bedtime or up divided during day
        - Risperidone (Risperdal) 0.5–3 mg bid
        - Lorazepam (Ativan) 0.5–4 mg a day in divided doses as needed for anxiety

- Depression:
  - Paroxetine (Paxil) HCl 10–40 mg/day
  - Sertraline (Zoloft) HCl 25–200 mg/day
  - Nortriptyline (Pamelor) 10–50 mg/day for the elderly, may be divided or given at bedtime
- Sleep disturbances:
  - Zolpidem (Ambien) 5–10 mg at bedtime
  - Trazodone (Desyrel) 25–75 mg at bedtime

LENGTH OF TREATMENT
- Cholinesterase inhibitors: May be initiated for mild to moderate Alzheimer's disease and discontinued when significant cognitive decline is noted; ineffective for MID
- Use other medications PRN; if needed regularly, use lowest effective dose and attempt to wean periodically

Special Considerations
- Consider language and education level when administering and interpreting mental status tests
- Integrate cultural beliefs into the management of minority patients with dementia

When to Consult, Refer, Hospitalize
- Consult with physician for diagnosis and long-term treatment planning
- Refer to neurologist for unusual presentation
- Refer to psychiatrist if unable to differentiate from depression; intractable behaviors
- Utilize social worker and multidisciplinary services for long-term care planning
- Hospitalize with deteriorating conditions such as exacerbation of chronic heart failure (CHF), chronic obstructive pulmonary disease (COPD), dehydration, pneumonia, or injury. Be aware that demented patients are likely to become more confused and delirious, and fall when hospitalized.

Follow-Up
- Generally follow up every 60 days
  ### EXPECTED COURSE
  - AD: Slowly progressive
  - MID: Stepwise with gradual deterioration; associated with new focal deficits and decline with each additional stroke

  ### COMPLICATIONS
  - Depression and suicide
  - Complications usually related to comorbidity or complications due to immobility with severe end-stage dementia

Delirium

Description
- Acute disorder of attention with onset of hours to days, characterized by confusion, disorientation, and fluctuation over the course of a day

Etiology
- Functional disorder of the brain caused by organic factors
- Any number of factors can cause delirium: polypharmacy, infections, metabolic and electrolyte abnormalities, dehydration, nutritional deficiencies, cardiopulmonary disease, urinary retention, fecal impaction, trauma, anesthesia, environmental change

Incidence and Demographics
- 10%–40% of hospitalized patients >65 years old

Risk Factors
- Age, dementia, frailty, visual impairment, presence of many other chronic diseases

Prevention and Screening
- Eliminate unnecessary medications
- Adequate hydration, nutrition, and oxygenation
- Correct visual and auditory deficits
- Continuity of care and environment

Assessment
HISTORY
- Detailed history of present illness, including cognition, time frame, and progression
- Comprehensive review of systems to identify underlying etiology
- Functional history and assessment
- Validate history with family member and/or caregiver

PHYSICAL EXAM
- Complete neurologic exam with attention to level of consciousness, focal neurologic deficits
- Hearing and visual impairments
- Pulmonary and cardiac exams (murmurs, arrhythmias, heart enlargement)
- Any evidence of infectious processes
- Signs of trauma
- Evaluate for orthostatic hypotension, urinary retention, and fecal impaction
- Folstein Mini-Mental State Examination
- Geriatric Depression Scale

DIAGNOSTIC STUDIES
- CBC, chemistry profile, thyroid function tests, B12 level, folate level to identify a reversible cause for cognitive impairment or etiology of delirium
- Computed tomography to identify infarcts, space-occupying lesions
- Syphilis, HIV, and drug toxicity if indicated by history

- Urinalysis if urinary tract infection suspected
- Arterial oxygen or pulse oximetry if hypoxemia is considered
- ECG and chest x-ray identify cardiopulmonary cause
- EEG to rule out seizure disorder
- Lumbar puncture for suspected encephalopathy or meningitis

Differential Diagnosis
- Dementia
- Depression
- See etiologies above

Management
- Identify and treat underlying cause
  ### NONPHARMACOLOGIC TREATMENT
  - Continuity of care
  - Minimize environmental stimuli
  - Provide eyeglasses or hearing aids
  - Clocks and calendars to maintain orientation
  - Maintain hydration, nutrition, oxygenation
  - Adequate bowel and bladder regimen

  ### PHARMACOLOGIC TREATMENT
  - Haloperidol (Haldol) 0.5 mg po or IM q 2–6 h for agitation

  ### LENGTH OF TREATMENT
  - Depends on etiology, often continue therapy until baseline cognitive function returns

Special Considerations
- Highest incidence in hospitalized elderly

When to Consult, Refer, Hospitalize
- Consult physician for any primary care patient with suspected delirium
- Hospitalize unless underlying etiology such as urinary tract infection (UTI) without sepsis can be managed at home with supervision to ensure patient safety, adequate hydration, and prescribed treatment

Follow-Up
- Regularly to monitor for recurrence
  ### EXPECTED COURSE
  - Usually reversible

  ### COMPLICATIONS
  - Injury due to falls
  - Associated with increased morbidity and mortality

Parkinson's Disease

Description
- Neurodegenerative disease characterized by slow movement (bradykinesia), rigidity, flexed posture, loss of postural reflex, freezing, and resting tremor

Etiology
- Unknown, although genetics, endogenous toxins, and exogenous toxins have been implicated.
- In Parkinson's disease, destruction of the substantia nigra and nigrostriatal tract occur resulting in damage to dopaminergic neurons, leaving active unopposed acetylcholine neurons intact.
- Imbalance of dopamine and acetylcholine result in loss of refinement of voluntary movement.
- Parkinson's that is reversible can occur in patients receiving metoclopramide, neuroleptic agents, or reserpine.

Incidence and Demographics
- Prevalence 350 per 100,000 in U.S. with 50,000 new cases per year
- Greater in men than women at a 3:2 ratio; usual onset during ages 45–65
- Less prevalent in Africans and African Americans than in Asians, Europeans, and White Americans
- Affects 1% of those age >50

Risk Factors
- Age, heredity
- Possible environmental factors

Prevention and Screening
- None, although older patients may benefit from periodic assessment of mobility, cognitive, and functional status

Assessment
HISTORY
- Focused detailed history of chief complaint, including time frame and progression, aggravating and alleviating factors such as stress or rest; interview family, patient, and caregiver
- Complete review of neurologic symptoms including weakness, paresthesia, tremor, diplopia, aphasia, mood, and cognitive changes
- Past medical history including neurological disorders, exposure to environmental toxins, illicit drugs
- Family history of Parkinson's disease, other movement disorders or dementia
- Medications including over-the-counter anticholinergics, antihistamines, decongestants, or cough and cold preparations that worsen condition
- Functional assessment: Difficulty with functional and instrumental ADLs, mobility including stair-climbing (patients with progressive supranuclear palsy will have problem descending stairs) and rising from chair
- Falls and injuries

- Review of systems for associated autonomic dysfunction, including perspiration, incontinence, constipation, and postural hypotension
- Assess for depression and mental status, may use Geriatric Depression Scale and MMSE or other tools

PHYSICAL EXAM
- General: Manner, affect, dress and hygiene, speech may be soft and monotone
- Cranial nerve exam: Normal in Parkinson's, 4th cranial nerve palsy with progressive supranuclear palsy
- Motor exam: No weakness but has cogwheel rigidity (rigidity to passive movement)
  - Bradykinesia: Slowness of voluntary movement and difficulty initiating movement, difficulty rising from chair, shuffling gait, problems with turns and stopping movement
  - Tremor: Slow (4–6 cycles per second) resting tremor present in one limb, limbs on one side, four limbs, or may be absent in 20% of Parkinson's patients; tremor may be obvious at rest and exaggerated with stress; some tremor of mouth and lips
  - Tremor may increase with emotional stress, and decrease with voluntary activity
- Gait and posture: Stooped posture with knees and hips flexed, hands held in front, close to body
- "Masked facies": Fixed facial expression, drooling, wide palpebral fissures, soft voice
- Meyerson's sign: Repetitive tapping on the bridge of the nose produces sustained blink response
- Incoordination of rapid alternating movements; decreased automatic movement, decreased blinking
- Deep tendon reflexes are unaffected
- General examination: Seborrhea
- Vital signs: Orthostatic hypotension

DIAGNOSTIC STUDIES
- Consider head CT if diagnosis not clear and stroke or space-occupying lesion is suspected

Differential Diagnosis
- Benign essential tremor
- Progressive supranuclear palsy
- Depression
- Dementia
- Cerebrovascular disease
- Brain tumor
- Adverse effects of anticholinergic medications, particularly antipsychotics
- Drug-induced Parkinson's
- Carbon monoxide poisoning
- Normal pressure hydrocephalus
- Huntington's disease
- Creutzfeldt-Jakob disease

Management

- There is no cure for Parkinson's. Current therapy is aimed at managing symptoms to preserve independence and mobility.
- The Hoehn and Young Scale can be helpful for staging the disease and guiding pharmacological and supportive therapy.
  - Stage I: Unilateral involvement
  - Stage II: Bilateral involvement but no postural abnormalities
  - Stage III: Bilateral involvement with mild postural instability, the patient leads an independent life
  - Stage IV: Bilateral involvement with postural instability, the patient requires substantial help
  - Stage V: Severe, fully developed disease, the patient is restricted to bed and chair

    NONPHARMACOLOGIC TREATMENT
    - Patient and family education regarding progressive nature of disease and complex pharmacologic treatments
    - Nutritional counseling regarding low-protein diet and dietary management of constipation
    - Compression stockings for postural hypotension
    - Physical, occupational, speech therapy with appropriate assistive devices for ambulation and ADLs
    - Fall precautions and home safety evaluation; install rails, raised toilet seats, tub chairs
    - Encourage walking, social activities, and interaction
    - Emotional support
    - Deep brain stimulation
    - Surgical interventions—unilateral stereotaxic thalamotomy or pallidotomy, implantable high-frequency thalamic stimulation to suppress resting tremor for difficult-to-control cases

    PHARMACOLOGIC TREATMENT (SEE TABLE 15–5)
    - Dopamine precursor:
      - 25 mg carbidopa/100 mg levodopa tid–qid; or 10 mg carbidopa/100 mg levodopa tid–qid, titrate up by 1 tablet every 2–7 days as needed and tolerated, not to exceed 200 mg carbidopa and 800 mg levodopa a day
      - "On-off" phenomenon occurs in 40%–50% of patients after 2–3 years, patients will experience inconsistent effect from the same dose
      - "Wearing-off" symptoms appear before next dose is due
      - Use lowest doses possible, consider addition of dopamine agonists
    - Dopamine agonists:
      - Pramipexole (Mirapex) 0.125 mg tid, titrate up to 1.5 mg tid over 7 weeks
      - Ropinirole (Requip) 0.25 mg tid, titrate up weekly by 1.5 mg a day to a total dose of 24 mg a day; maintenance dose is 3–24 mg a day; discontinue slowly over 1 week
    - MAO-B Inhibitor:
      - Selegiline (Eldepryl) 5 mg bid (at low doses is a selective MAO inhibitor and can be safely administered with levodopa)
      - Nonselective MAO inhibitors are contraindicated in combination with levodopa; their use can precipitate hyperpyrexia and hypertensive crisis and must be discontinued at least 14 days before initiating levodopa

- Anticholinergic agent:
  - Benztropine (Cogentin) 1–2 mg qd
- Catechol O-methyltransferase (COMT) inhibitor:
  - Tolcapone (Tasmar) 100–200 mg 3 tid

Table 15–5. Treatment Algorithm for Parkinson's Disease

Stage or Problem	Therapeutic Alternatives
Mild Disease (Stage I and II)	Selegiline for neuro protection
	Anticholinergics if tremor predominant
	Amantadine (best for rigidity and bradykinesia)
	Group support, exercise, education, nutrition
Functionally impaired (Stage III) Age <60 years	Tremor predominant: anticholinergics
	Functional disability: sustained-release carbidopa/levodopa (lowest dose possible); dopamine agonist
Age >60 years	Sustained-release carbidopa/levodopa
Stage IV or V	Immediate-release carbidopa/levodopa
	Dopamine agonists
Poor symptom control	Increase carbidopa/levodopa dose
	Add or increase dopamine agonist dose
	Add COMT inhibitor
Suboptimal peak response	Begin combination dopaminergic therapy
	Add levodopa to dopamine agonist
	Add dopamine agonist to levodopa
	Increase dose of levodopa/carbidopa or dopamine agonist
	Add COMT inhibitor as levodopa adjunct, switch dopamine agonists
Wearing off	Begin combination of dopaminergic therapy
	Add levodopa to dopamine agonist
	Add dopamine agonist to levodopa
	Increase frequency of levodopa dosing
	Increase dose of levodopa/carbidopa (sustained or immediate release)
	Add COMT inhibitor and decrease levodopa dose
	Change to sustained-release carbidopa/levodopa
	Add liquid levodopa/carbidopa
	Add selegiline if not already taking
On-off	Begin combination dopaminergic therapy
	Add levodopa to dopamine agonist
	Add dopamine agonist to levodopa
	Add COMT inhibitor
	Modify distribution of dietary protein
Freezing	Increase or decrease carbidopa/levodopa dose
	Add dopamine agonist
	Increase or decrease dopamine agonist dose
	Discontinue selegiline
	Gait modification, assistance device

Table 15–5. Treatment Algorithm for Parkinson's Disease (cont.)

Stage or Problem	Therapeutic Alternatives
No "on" time	Manipulate time and dose of levodopa
	Add COMT inhibitor
	Avoid dietary protein
	Increase GI transit time

Adapted from "Antiparkinson agents" by L. R. Young, 2004, in M. W. Edmunds & M. S. Mayhew (Eds.), *Pharmacology for the primary care provider* (2nd ed., p. 512), St. Louis, MO: Mosby.

LENGTH OF TREATMENT
- Medication combinations and dosages must be individualized, and adjusted during the course of the disease; disease is lifelong and progressive

Special Considerations
- Prescribe Parkinson's medications with caution in the elderly, particularly those with comorbidity of heart, renal, or liver disease
- Avoid anticholinergics in the elderly, tend to be poorly tolerated, have increased risk of side effects including confusion, agitation, arrhythmias, urinary retention
- Differentiate Parkinson's disease from essential tremor which may occur at any age from childhood but increases with age and affects the distal upper extremities and head; may be familial
  - If mild, reassurance may be only intervention needed
  - May be treated with beta-adrenergic blockers such as propranolol (Inderal) and metoprolol (Lopressor); primidone (Mysoline); benzodiazepines
  - May be disabling; refer for possible neurosurgery

When to Consult, Refer, Hospitalize
- Refer to neurologist for confirmation of diagnosis and guidance with medical management
- Neurosurgical consultation for those with severe symptoms refractory to medications, or unable to tolerate medications

Follow-Up
- Every 3 months, as well as any time a change is made in medication and/or therapy regimens
- Episodic office visit if symptoms worsen
- Annual health assessment and physical examination
  EXPECTED COURSE
  - Progressive; 30% develop coexisting dementia with poorer prognosis

  COMPLICATIONS
  - Related to immobility and falls; hip fractures are common, pneumonia may occur in Stage 5
  - Aspiration of food
  - Depression and social isolation occur

Multiple Sclerosis (MS)

Description
- Progressive neurodegenerative disease characterized by demyelination and inflammation of the neuronal sheath in the brain and spinal cord that produces episodic neurologic symptoms such as sensory abnormalities, visual disturbances, sphincter disturbances, and weakness with or without spasticity

Etiology
- Autoimmune disease, possible causes may be genetic, viral, immunologic or environmental; strong association with HLA-DR2 antigen

Incidence and Demographics
- Incidence 250,000–300,000 per year in the U.S.
- Prevalence is higher in temperate zones, ranging from only 5–10/100,000 in tropical zones to 50–175/100,000 in cooler environments
- Women-to-men ratio 2–3:1, estrogen and progesterone may be implicated as symptoms often develop during the menstrual cycle and after pregnancy
- Age of onset 15–55 years; greatest incidence in young adults <55 years
- Late onset of MS in the 6th–7th decade usually severe and rapidly progressive

Risk Factors
- Familial 1%–3% increased risk in first-degree relatives (15 times greater than general population)
- Climate or place of residence, established by residence in the first 15 years of life
- Urban dwelling, upper socioeconomic status; Western European descent

Assessment
HISTORY
- Neurological history: Paresthesias, weakness and spasticity, ataxia fatigue, visual changes, vestibular disturbances, trigeminal neuralgia, optic neuritis, bowel and bladder dysfunction
- Time frame with exacerbations and remission
- Past medical history for differential diagnosis: Systemic lupus erythematosus, Lyme disease, cerebral and spinal tumors, HIV, seizures, peripheral neuropathy, head or spinal trauma
- Triggers may be infection, trauma, pregnancy

PHYSICAL EXAM
- Complete neurologic exam:
  - Cranial nerve deficits
  - Optic neuritis: Decreased visual acuity, abnormal pupillary response, hyperemia and edema of optic disk
  - Internuclear ophthalmoplegia: Cranial nerve 6 palsy or weakness of the medial rectus muscle with lateral gaze, nystagmus
  - Decreased strength, increased tone, clonus, positive Babinski; weakness, numbness, tingling or unsteadiness in a limb; disequilibrium; urinary urgency, hesitancy, incontinence

– Decreased proprioception and vibratory sensation, positive Romberg; pyramidal, sensory, or cerebellar deficits in some or all limbs
– Lhermitte's sign: An electrical sensation down the back into the legs is produced with neck flexion

DIAGNOSTIC STUDIES
- MRI may visualize characteristic multiple lesions of demyelinated areas with reactive gliosis
- Cerebrospinal fluid analysis for lymphocytosis, immunoglobulins, and oligoclonal bands
- Visual, auditory, and sensory evoked potentials

Differential Diagnosis
- Stroke
- Cerebral or spinal tumors
- Ischemic optic neuropathy
- Systemic lupus erythematosus
- Lyme disease
- Peripheral neuropathy
- Seizure disorder
- AIDS
- Intoxication
- Amyotrophic lateral sclerosis

Management
- Aimed at delaying progress, managing chronic symptoms, and treating acute exacerbations

NONPHARMACOLOGIC TREATMENT
- Physical and occupational therapy
- Mental health services for assistance with coping strategies

PHARMACOLOGIC TREATMENT
- Complex, treatment regimen *must* be coordinated with a neurologist
- Immunosuppressive therapy may arrest progression
  – Interferon beta (Avonex) 30 mcg IM once a week
  – Glatiramer acetate (Copaxone) 20 mg SQ qd
  – Azathioprine (Imuran) unlabeled use
- Acute exacerbations: Prednisone 60–80 mg/day for 1 week, taper over 2–3 weeks
- Spasticity: Baclofen (Lioresal) 40–80 mg a day in divided doses, start with 5 mg tid and titrate up every 3 days
  – Clonazepam (Klonopin) unlabeled use
- Fatigue
  – Amantadine (Symmetrel) 100 mg bid
  – Consider tricyclic antidepressants or selective serotonin reuptake inhibitors
  – Treat underlying spastic bladder, depression

LENGTH OF TREATMENT
- Use corticosteroids only for acute exacerbations, not for maintenance
- Antibodies may develop to interferon
- Stop interferon if progression of disabilities continues after 6 months of treatment

Special Considerations
- New onset or exacerbations with menstrual cycle and postpartum
- Family planning and fertility should be discussed with women of childbearing age, menses may be irregular and fertility impaired due to demyelination but pregnancy not contraindicated
- Oral contraceptives are not contraindicated except with impaired mobility
- Consult with obstetrician regarding medications for pregnancy and lactation

When to Consult, Refer, Hospitalize
- Refer all patients with suspected MS to neurologist for confirmation of diagnosis and development of management plan
- Ophthalmology referral
- Continence specialist or urologist for bladder dysfunction
- Mental health referral for coping or depression

Follow-Up
- Followed closely by neurology; primary care for routine health visits
  EXPECTED COURSE
    - Progressive with exacerbations and remissions

  COMPLICATIONS
    - Hydronephrosis and renal failure secondary to urinary retention
    - Falls
    - Depression

Vertigo

Description
- Sensation of motion of the body or environment when there is no movement
- Not a disorder, but a symptom of an underlying condition

Etiology
- Peripheral vestibular dysfunction:
  - Benign positional vertigo: Believed to be caused by free-floating debris in the semicircular canal
  - Occurs with change in position with a delay between movement and symptoms; symptoms will fatigue or disappear with repeated movement
  - Labyrinthitis: Infection of the inner ear, most likely viral, often follows an upper respiratory infection
  - Ménière's disease: Swelling of the endolymphatic system of the inner ear; may be caused by syphilis or head trauma, or viral

- Traumatic vertigo is due to labyrinth concussion or basilar skull fracture
- Central vestibular dysfunction is due to vertebrobasilar insufficiency, acoustic neuroma, or compression of the 8th cranial nerve by blood vessel loops similar to trigeminal neuralgia

Incidence and Demographics
- Benign positional vertigo most common in those over 60
- Labyrinthitis: Affects any age, usually after upper respiratory infection
- Ménière's occurs at 40–70 years
- Central lesions are less common

Risk Factors
- Age: Increasing incidence with increasing age
- Upper respiratory infection
- Trauma

Assessment
HISTORY
- Detailed description of sensation without using terms dizzy and vertigo, include time frame, duration, association with movement, alleviating and precipitating factors
    - Vertigo is associated with a sensation of movement
    - Dizziness or lightheadedness associated with presyncope due to cardiac cause
    - Imbalance or gait instability is associated with cerebellar disease or peripheral neuropathy
- Associated symptoms of hearing loss, tinnitus, nausea, vomiting with Ménière's
- History of upper respiratory infection or trauma
- Time frame:
    - Positional vertigo and vertebrobasilar insufficiency occur in seconds
    - Ménière's, vestibular migraine occur over hours
    - Labyrinthitis, traumatic vertigo, and vestibular neuritis occur over days
    - Acoustic neuroma, multiple sclerosis, cerebellar disease occur over months, progressive

PHYSICAL EXAM
- Screening neurologic exam with attention to cranial nerves
- Sustained nystagmus is indicative of vertigo but may be central or peripheral
- Facial palsy may or may not be present with acoustic neuroma
- Assess gait and balance
- Dix-Hallpike maneuver: Lay patient flat with head to one side hanging over edge of table, sit patient up quickly with head held to side, repeat with other ear down; reproduction of symptoms and nystagmus are positive for positional vertigo; Nystagmus that is purely vertical and not fatigueable with subsequent trials may be due to central vestibular dysfunction
- Otologic exam

DIAGNOSTIC STUDIES
- MRI if central lesion suspected
- Audiogram to evaluate sustained hearing loss, which may occur with Ménière's
- Depending on clinical findings and suspected underlying etiology may consider CBC, chemistry panel, lipid panel, thyroid function studies, ESR, RPR

Differential Diagnosis

- Benign positional vertigo
- Labyrinthitis
- Ménière's disease
- Cerumen impaction
- Otitis media or externa
- Sinusitis
- Vertebrobasilar insufficiency
- Vestibular migraine
- Acoustic neuroma
- Presyncope with probable cardiac etiology
- Multiple sclerosis
- Cerebellar disease
- Peripheral neuropathy

Management

NONPHARMACOLOGIC TREATMENT
- Remove cerumen if present
- Rest in quiet, darkened room
- Safety precautions to change positions slowly, may need walker for support
- Bland diet with small portions, fluids if nausea and vomiting present
- Ménière's disease: Low-sodium diet
- Benign positional vertigo: Vestibular rehabilitation to reduce symptoms

PHARMACOLOGIC TREATMENT
- Meclizine (Antivert) 25–100 mg in divided doses may reduce vertigo
- Hydrochlorothiazide 25–50 mg or triamterene 50 mg a day for Ménière's
- Antibiotics may be helpful in labyrinthitis if bacterial infection suspected

LENGTH OF TREATMENT
- Taper and stop meclizine when symptoms resolve, generally within 1–2 weeks; do not use prophylactically or as maintenance

Special Considerations

- Elderly are more sensitive to antihistamines, so use only if necessary for severe debilitating symptoms; may cause drowsiness, confusion, anticholinergic symptoms.

When to Consult, Refer, Hospitalize

- Hospitalize for dehydration and inability to take oral rehydration secondary to severe nausea and vomiting
- Neurosurgical referral for acoustic neuroma or other space-occupying lesions

- Neurology referral if focal neurologic deficits, severe headaches, seizures, or other suggestions of central nervous system problem, or symptoms do not resolve with treatment

Follow-Up
- Follow up as needed for recurrence or worsening symptoms
    ### EXPECTED COURSE
    - Benign positional vertigo episodes last several days; may reoccur
    - Labyrinthitis resolves in several days
    - Ménière's may have multiple episodes with remissions

    ### COMPLICATIONS
    - Hearing loss with Ménière's
    - Falls
    - Dehydration with associated nausea and vomiting

Meningitis

Description
- Central nervous system infection of the covering of the brain and spinal cord by any infectious agent including bacteria, virus, mycobacteria, spirochetes, fungi, protozoa, and parasites

Etiology
- Caused by virulent infectious organism in a susceptible host; local host defenses are overcome
- Bacteria causing meningitis varies by the age of the patient:
    - <1 month: Group B streptococci, E. coli, Listeria monocytogenes
    - 4–6 weeks: H. influenzae type b, E. coli, S. pneumoniae, Group B streptococci
    - 6 weeks–6 years: S. pneumoniae, N. meningitides, H. influenzae type b
    - > 6 years: S. pneumoniae, N. meningitides
- Viral meningitis can be caused by any of over 70 different strains of viruses; most common are the enteroviruses (85%) and herpes simplex. Less serious and resolves spontaneously
- Most common fungal causes are Candida sp., Aspergillus, Cryptococcus neoformans
- Candidal meningitis occurs mostly in ill premature infants and immunocompromised patients, but 30% of all patients with fungal meningitis have no underlying immunodeficiency
- Aseptic meningitis can be caused by Borrelia burgdorferi (Lyme disease) or Treponema pallidum (syphilis)
- Meningitis can also be caused by tuberculosis
- H. influenzae, N. meningitides, and S. pneumoniae cause 80% of bacterial meningitis in adults, older persons
- S. aureus, S. pneumoniae and Gram-negative bacilli are common causes of postsurgical or posttraumatic meningitis
- Possible Gram-negative bacilli in geriatric patients

Incidence and Demographics
- In children, 80% of bacterial meningitis occurs before 24 months of age
- Incidence approximately 1/100,000 persons a year
- More prevalent in lower socioeconomic groups, crowded housing, urban areas
- Three times more prevalent in college students residing on campus than those living off campus and the general population

Risk Factors
- Poverty and lack of childhood immunizations
- Crowded living conditions
- Immunodeficiency
- College students living in campus housing and soldiers in barracks
- Infectious disease close to meninges: pneumonia, pharyngitis, otitis media, sinusitis, endocarditis
- Penetrating head trauma
- Syphilis infection
- Lyme disease

Prevention and Screening
- Routine administration of the *H. influenzae* type b (HIB) vaccine has significantly reduced the incidence of meningitis
- Administration of the Prevnar vaccine
- Adolescents planning to attend college and reside in dormitories should receive meningococcal vaccine
- Post-exposure prophylaxis for bacterial meningitis with oral rifampin (Rifadin) for household and day care contacts, and those with direct exposure to oral secretions (kissing) of infected patient
  - *H. influenzae:* Rifampin 20 mg/kg/dose qd for 4 days
  - *N. meningitides:* Rifampin 10 mg/kg/dose bid for 2 days
- The American Academy of Pediatrics recommends prophylaxis to day care or nursery school contacts if two or more index cases occur in a unit within 60 days of each other

Assessment
HISTORY
- Rapid onset within 24–36 hours
- Progressive, severe headache accompanied by neck and back pain with flexion
- Neurologic symptoms: Drowsiness, irritability, confusion, photophobia, hearing loss, focal neurologic deficits, seizures, nuchal rigidity, photophobia
- Associated symptoms: Fever, nausea, vomiting, rash
- In infants, complaints of sleep disturbances, irritability, or vomiting
- Recent history of respiratory infection, head trauma, invasive neurosurgical procedures, or dental procedures
- Past medical history: Meningitis, polio, immunodeficiency
- Social history: Living in crowded environment, IV drug use, foreign travel
- Environmental exposure to bird or pigeon droppings (fungal) or tick bite (Lyme)
- Medications: Immunosuppressants

PHYSICAL EXAM
- General: Fever, tachycardia, hypotension, rash
- Assess fontanels in infants for bulging, hydration status
- Complete neurologic exam: Decreased level of consciousness (drowsiness or agitation), papilledema, cranial nerve III, IV, VI, VII and/or VIII deficits, focal motor deficits, seizure, mental status
- Meningeal irritation: Nuchal rigidity, positive Brudzinski's sign (adduction and flexion of legs with neck flexion), positive Kernig's sign (after flexing thighs, extension is met with resistance and pain in hamstring muscles)
- Complete physical exam for sites of primary infections:
  - Head trauma or surgery, dental abscess or caries, otitis media, sinusitis, pneumonia, pancreatitis, genital lesions, skin rashes

DIAGNOSTIC STUDIES
- Cerebrospinal fluid analysis, culture (diagnosis usually made on Gram stain): Gold standard diagnosis
  - Viral infection: Some lymphocytes, normal glucose, moderately high protein content, normal or mildly elevated opening pressure
  - Bacterial infection: Increased lymphocytes, decreased glucose, high-protein content, markedly elevated opening pressure
- Brain CT prior to lumbar puncture (LP) if space-occupying lesion (brain abscess, subdural empyema, tumor, subdural hematoma) suspected with papilledema and/or focal neurologic findings; LP is contraindicated with increased intracranial pressure
- CBC, platelet count, PT/PTT, electrolytes, BUN, creatinine, glucose, arterial blood gases (as indicated), blood cultures
- Chest and/or sinus x-ray if exam indicates source of infection

Differential Diagnosis
- Bacterial meningitis
- Aseptic meningitis
- Encephalitis (herpes, rabies)
- Brain abscess
- Noninfectious meningeal irritation (sarcoidosis, systemic lupus erythematosus, cancer, medications and chemical irritants)
- Bacterial sinusitis or mastoiditis
- Vertebral osteomyelitis
- Amebic meningoencephalitis

Management
NONPHARMACOLOGIC TREATMENT
- Medical emergency; immediate transport to hospital for IV antibiotics and supportive care
- Assurance of adequate airway, cardiac function, fluid support
- Educate family, significant others regarding illness, treatment, and prognosis
- Inform family and contacts of post-exposure prophylaxis

PHARMACOLOGIC TREATMENT
- IV antimicrobials in acute care setting, usually cefotaxime, ceftriaxone, or vancomycin
- Acyclovir has been used in the neonate with viral meningitis
- Administration of dexamethasone before or with antibiotics appears to reduce the incidence of sensorineural hearing loss without increasing mortality or complications

LENGTH OF TREATMENT
- *H. influenzae* and *N. meningitidis*: 7 days
- *S. pneumoniae*: 10–14 days
- Gram-negative bacteria: 21 days

Special Considerations
- Antibiotics given in doses smaller than usually used to treat meningitis for the 3–4 days before lumbar puncture will not significantly alter the cerebrospinal fluid (CSF) findings
- Rifampin contraindicated for post-exposure prophylaxis in pregnant patients
- Rifampin secreted in breast milk

When to Consult, Refer, Hospitalize
- Medical emergency; immediately transfer all suspected meningitis cases to an acute care facility
- Most patients with viral meningitis can be managed at home, if stable, after physician consultation

Follow-Up
- Patients should be seen in follow-up a few days after hospital discharge
- Parents and patients should be instructed to follow up if any new neurological sequelae present, include hearing and vision problems

EXPECTED COURSE
- 90% survival with early diagnosis, treatment, and supportive care

COMPLICATIONS
- Mortality rate is more than 50% in those who are not diagnosed early and referred; 10% for those who receive prompt diagnosis, appropriate IV antibiotics, and supportive care; mortality of bacterial meningitis in neonate is 10–20%; in infants/children is 3%–10%
- Complications of meningitis include seizures (2%–8%), hearing defects (10%), mental retardation (10%), visual abnormalities (3%–7%), language delay (15%), motor abnormalities (3%–7%), inappropriate ADH secretion (SIADH), sixth cranial nerve palsy; occurrence of sequelae is estimated at 25%–50% of meningitis survivors

SEIZURES AND EPILEPSY

General Information

- A seizure is a transient sudden, paroxysmal electrical discharge of a group of neurons in the brain that causes an alteration in neurological function.
- May involve abnormal motor activity, sensory symptoms, a change in the level of alertness, an alteration in autonomic function, or a combination of these.
- A seizure is not a diagnosis, but rather a clinical symptom of an underlying neurological dysfunction.
- Seizures classified by etiology: Genetic (25%), symptomatic (50%), and idiopathic (25%).
- Neonatal seizures are rarely idiopathic and immediate attention must be paid to identifying the underlying disorder.
- Febrile seizures occur in infants and children as a result of fever, not underlying neurologic disorder.
- Epilepsy, or recurrent, spontaneous seizures unrelated to fever, may occur in children and adults.
- Rolandic epilepsy, associated with a typical EEG pattern, is the most common type in children.
- Infantile spasms are myoclonic seizures occurring in the first year of life, usually in clusters, associated with a typical EEG pattern.

Neonatal Seizures

Description

- Seizures in a newborn almost always reflect significant nervous system pathology.
- Seizures in this age group may present in several ways:
  - Focal-rhythmic twitching of muscle groups, including the face
  - Multifocal clonic: Similar to focal, but involving multiple muscle groups
  - Tonic: Rigid posturing of the extremities and trunk
  - Myoclonic: Focal or generalized jerking of the extremities, that generally involve the distal parts of the body
  - Subtle: Chewing motions, excessive salivation, or autonomic changes such as apnea, blinking, nystagmus, pedaling motions, and skin color changes

Etiology

- Time of onset and characteristics of seizure may suggest most probable cause.
- Rarely idiopathic; typical causes of neonatal seizures include trauma from birth or from congenital malformations, including hypoxia, intracranial hemorrhage, infection, drug withdrawal, metabolic disorders, inborn errors of metabolism, neurocutaneous disorders, pyridoxine dependency, and cerebral dysgenesis.
- Focal seizures may be caused by metabolic disturbances and do not necessarily imply a focal lesion.

Incidence and Demographics

- Thought to occur in 0.5% of all term infants and 20% of preterm infants.

Risk Factors
- Complicated labor or delivery, prematurity
- Infants of diabetic mothers
- Family history of metabolic disorder associated with seizures; maternal drug use

Prevention and Screening
- Neonatal seizures are not preventable, but the incidence of prematurity and birth trauma may be decreased with good prenatal care and maternal education.

Assessment

HISTORY
- Prenatal and perinatal history including maternal risk factors and complications of pregnancy, labor, and delivery
- Family history of seizure disorders or metabolic disease, congenital syndromes
- Exact description of the event, movements, or reactions that has triggered the concern

PHYSICAL EXAM
- Complete physical, focus on dysmorphic features, atypical, or rhythmic movements
- Assess growth, vital signs
- Neurological exam, presence/absence of newborn reflexes, head size/shape
- Eye exam to look for chorioretinitis (inflammation that destroys superficial tissue areas visible on funduscopic exam, and that causes a well-defined but irregular area of white sclera that has smaller areas of dark pigment); or coloboma (a developmental abnormality in which a moderate-to-large sized area of sclera with well-demarcated borders is seen below the disc)
- Any unusual skin pigmentation or body odors for metabolic disorder
- Presence of hepatosplenomegaly, signs of drug withdrawal

DIAGNOSTIC STUDIES
- Laboratory testing to include CBC, electrolytes, calcium, magnesium, pH, sodium bicarbonate, bilirubin, BUN, and ammonia
- Urinalysis and urine toxicology screen
- Lumbar puncture, if presence or suspicion of infection or intracranial hemorrhage
- Neuroimaging to rule out brain injury or mass
- Chromosomal analysis if presence of dysmorphic features
- Metabolic screen, including amino acids, lactate, and urine organic acids
- TORCH Screen
- Drug screen
- EEG: Changes may not always be present

Differential Diagnosis
- Jitteriness
- Gastroesophageal reflux disease (GERD)
- Apnea
- Benign idiopathic neonatal convulsions: "Fifth-day fits"
- Benign familial neonatal convulsions: Days 2–4 of life, with familial history

Management
- Treatment is guided by correcting the underlying abnormality
  NONPHARMACOLOGIC TREATMENT
  - Ensure adequate ventilation and perfusion

  PHARMACOLOGIC TREATMENT
  - For metabolic disorders: calcium gluconate, magnesium sulfate, and/or pyridoxine
  - Antibiotics if infection is present
  - Seizure management includes the use of phenobarbital, phenytoin, or lorazepam

  LENGTH OF TREATMENT
  - Duration of therapy is based on the underlying etiology

When to Consult, Refer, Hospitalize
- Any newborn with suspected seizures should receive prompt evaluation and admission for work-up.
- Infant with history of neonatal seizures should be followed in conjunction with a physician and a neurologist.

Follow-Up
- Infants should be followed by neurology at regular intervals until seizure-free and off medications; follow-up may be extended if neurological sequela ensue
  - Infants need routine health assessments to monitor growth and development and should receive routine immunizations
  - Infants with cognitive or motor deficits should be referred to an early intervention program
  EXPECTED COURSE
  - Highly individual; child may develop normally following seizure period

  COMPLICATIONS
  - Mortality rate is approximately 15%, but is much higher in preterm infants
  - Mental retardation and motor deficits are more common sequelae, occurring in about 29% of affected infants
  - Prognosis is dependent upon the underlying etiology, with cerebral dysgenesis having the worst outcomes
  - The likelihood of recurrent seizures is 15%–20% overall

Febrile Seizures

Description
- A seizure event in infancy or early childhood, associated with fever, but without evidence of intracranial infection or defined cause
- Febrile seizures have been classified as:
  - Simple: Isolated, brief, generalized seizure lasting <15 minutes
  - Complex: Prolonged (>10 minutes), multiple seizures within a 24-hour period, or focal in nature

Etiology
- Febrile seizures are caused or brought on by a fever.
- The most common causes are normal childhood illnesses, such as tonsillitis, upper respiratory infections, and otitis media.
- Genetic predisposition: Occurred in approximately 10% of parents; 20% chance occurrence in sibling.

Incidence and Demographics
- Occur in approximately 2%–4% of all children; more common in males
- Usual onset in the second year of life but can occur at any time from 6 months to 5 years of age
- Usually occurs within the first 24 hours of fever
- Approximately 30% of children will experience one or more recurrences
- Risk of recurrence is related to the age of the child, family history, and complexity of the first seizure

Risk Factors
- Very high fever, >38.8°C (101.8°F)
- Family history of febrile seizures
- Neonatal discharge from hospital >28 days
- Delayed development
- Day care attendance (increased rate of febrile illness)
- Low serum sodium

Prevention and Screening
- Subsequent febrile seizures may be prevented by early and adequate fever control

Assessment
HISTORY
- Family history of febrile seizures
- Complete description of the seizure, duration, recovery, motor involvement, etc.
- Any history of recent illness or exposure to illness, onset of headaches, vomiting, or unusual symptoms
- Recent trauma, medication exposure
- Prenatal/perinatal history, including developmental history
- Exposure to toxins (e.g., lead)

PHYSICAL EXAM
- Document presence of fever
- Complete physical exam: Identify underlying illness or infection requiring treatment
- Complete neurological exam, including level of consciousness, presence of meningismus, or a tense bulging fontanel; obtain head circumference
- Signs of physical abuse
- Neurocutaneous skin lesions

DIAGNOSTIC STUDIES
- Lumbar puncture: If suspicion of meningitis or for children <18 months with first seizure
- Routine lab studies are not indicated, unless no source of fever can be elicited on physical examination
- EEG is not warranted
- MRI limited to children with focal seizures
- Serum lead level, if indicated

Differential Diagnosis
- Meningitis or encephalitis
- Anoxia
- Trauma
- Stroke or hemorrhage
- Metabolic encephalopathy
- Neurodegenerative disorder
- Neurocutaneous syndromes
- Brain tumor
- Lead poisoning or other toxins
- Epilepsy

Management
NONPHARMACOLOGIC TREATMENT
- Because febrile seizures are very frightening to the parents, parental reassurance and education are vitally important
- An active search for the underlying cause of the fever and appropriate treatment with each incidence

PHARMACOLOGIC TREATMENT
- Vigorous control of fevers by antipyretics and sponging with tepid water
  - Acetaminophen 10–15 mg/kg per dose either orally or per rectum
  - Ibuprofen 10 mg/kg per dose orally
- Prophylaxis is controversial, but may be used; consider if 3–5 febrile seizures in 1 year
  - Diazepam orally or rectally to prevent recurrences only during a febrile illness (1 mg/kg/day divided into three doses over the first 3 days of illness or 0.5 mg/kg rectally at onset of seizure)
  - Phenobarbital has had limited results
  - Side effects of prophylaxis include ataxia, behavior problems, and lethargy

LENGTH OF TREATMENT
- During febrile episodes

Special Considerations
- Seizure(s) occurring late in the course of a febrile illness raise serious concerns about meningitis or encephalitis
- Relieving parental anxiety should be the focus of management

- Small risk of developing epilepsy later in life if:
  - Abnormal development before the seizure
  - Family history of afebrile seizures
  - Complex first febrile seizure

When to Consult, Refer, Hospitalize
- Due to parental anxiety, the first febrile seizure may be evaluated at the emergency department
- Consult with physician; however, no referrals or consultations are necessary in simple febrile seizures
- Consult or refer to neurologist if seizures become more focal or complex
- If the seizure is generalized, lasts longer than 20 minutes, is focal, or the suspected disease process is complex, the child should be hospitalized
- Continued seizures past age 6 are not compatible with febrile seizures and require a neurology referral

Follow-Up
- Patients with febrile seizures should receive the routine childhood immunizations and health assessments at regular intervals
  - EXPECTED COURSE
    - Full return of function following resolution of fever; child will outgrow

  - COMPLICATIONS
    - Permanent cognitive and/or motor damage can occur if febrile seizures are not treated in a timely and effective manner
    - Lacerated tongue, broken teeth, bones, etc., can occur if the child's seizure is not safely contained

Rolandic Epilepsy of Childhood

Description
- Benign partial epilepsy of childhood with centrotemporal or rolandic spikes (EPEC) is the most common variant of epilepsy seen in children of school age. It is a syndrome consisting of unilateral tonic-clonic contractions of the face, paresthesias of the tongue and cheek, and occasional clonic seizures of the ipsilateral upper extremity.

Etiology
- The etiology of most seizures is unknown
- Seizures are typically focal (e.g., twitching of the mouth)

Incidence and Demographics
- The prevalence of epilepsy in the pediatric population is 4–6 per 1,000 cases; male-to-female ratio of 3:2
- Rolandic epilepsy occurs at 2–14 years, with the peak incidence at age 9–10 years; majority resolve or "outgrow" by age 16 years
- Approximately 75% occur during sleep but can occur during daytime with average of fewer than four episodes per year in most cases

Risk Factors
- History of previous seizures (febrile or afebrile)
- Recent withdrawal of anticonvulsant medications
- History of remote neurological insult such as head trauma
- Family history of seizures

Assessment

HISTORY
- Complete description of the seizures, including duration, aura, signs of infection, motor involvement, timing or stimulus
- Family history of seizure disorders or previous history in this child
- History of any head trauma or insult
- Any recent use of medications or drugs
- Health history of the patient
- Any recent onset of headaches, weakness or sensory deficits

PHYSICAL EXAM
- Physical exam with attention to screening neurological exam (usually normal)
- Parents may need to videorecord an event for the provider to view
- Signs of systemic infection; signs of physical abuse
- Skin evaluation for neurocutaneous disorders

DIAGNOSTIC STUDIES
- EEG, either routine or 24-hour recording: Characteristic spike focus in the centrotemporal or rolandic area with normal background activity
- CT/MRI to rule out intracranial abnormality, especially if anticonvulsant therapy is not effective

Differential Diagnosis
- Night terrors
- Complex partial seizures
- Simple partial seizures
- Tics
- Migraine
- Breath-holding spells

Management

NONPHARMACOLOGIC TREATMENT
- Occasional seizures require no therapy, just careful monitoring

PHARMACOLOGIC TREATMENT
- Carbamazepine (Tegretol) initial dose 10 mg/kg/day, increasing to 20–30 mg/kg/day as maintenance
- Phenytoin (Dilantin) 5–10 mg/kg/day in 3 divided doses
- Valproate (Depakene) 15–30 mg/kg/day in 2–3 divided doses

LENGTH OF TREATMENT
  • If seizure-free for at least 2 years with a normal EEG, consider weaning from medication over 4–6 months and supervise closely
  • Higher risk for seizure recurrence in children with developmental delay, age >12 years at onset, neonatal seizures, and multiple seizures before control attained

Special Considerations
• In children with poor seizure control despite appropriate medication, consider drug compliance, growth spurts, and possible other epileptic etiologies
• Persons with seizures should not swim alone or play sports that are conducive to head injuries (e.g., football, lacrosse)

When to Consult, Refer, Hospitalize
• If epilepsy is suspected, the patient should be referred and managed by a pediatric neurologist
• Patients with rolandic epilepsy rarely need hospitalization

Follow-Up
• At least annual follow-up with pediatric neurologist
• Routine health maintenance follow-up
  EXPECTED COURSE
    • Most remit by adolescence (nearly 100%)

  COMPLICATIONS
    • Essentially none, as response to anticonvulsant agents is excellent

Seizures and Epilepsy in Adults/Older Adults

Description
• A transient alteration in behavior, function, and/or consciousness that results from an abnormal electrical discharge of neurons in the brain
• Epilepsy refers to chronic recurrent seizures
• Most older adults have partial seizures that may quickly generalize to tonic-clonic
• The International League Against Epilepsy has classified seizures based on clinical presentation and EEG findings (Table 15–6)

Etiology
• A seizure is a symptom of an underlying disorder; most frequent cause of repetitive seizures is failure to take antiseizure medications.
• Cause is unknown for most epilepsy, including primary epilepsy, but is believed to be related to abnormalities of neurotransmission.
• Patients with primary epilepsy can continue to have seizures into old age.
• Secondary epilepsy is due to injury to cerebral cortex.
• Most new-onset epilepsy in elderly is secondary due to tumors, hematomas, or stroke.
• Space-occupying lesions, stroke, metabolic disorders, and alcohol withdrawal also can cause seizures.
• Vascular disease is the most common cause of onset > age 60.

Incidence and Demographics
- 10% of Americans will have a seizure at some time during their lives; 1%–2% have epilepsy.
- New-onset epilepsy is highest among those <20 years of age.

Risk Factors
- Intracranial lesions, head trauma, hypoglycemia, chronic illness that predisposes metabolic abnormality; medications that lower seizure threshold (e.g., selective serotonin reuptake inhibitors, certain atypical antidepressants, ciprofloxacin, metronidazole, theophylline)
- Certain triggers: Sleep deprivation, menses, flashing lights/television; emotional stress, fever, hormonal imbalance
- Alcohol intoxication or alcohol withdrawal

Prevention and Screening
- Head trauma prevention: Seatbelt use, bicycle and motorcycle helmets
- Fall prevention for the elderly; home safety counseling

Assessment
HISTORY
- Interview witness to seizure if possible; this information is most important in making diagnosis
- Detailed history of event; include description of seizure activity, loss of consciousness, duration, incontinence, possible triggers
- Prodromal symptoms such as aura, confusion, or focal neurological symptoms
- Postictal state: Antegrade amnesia, level of consciousness
- Prior seizure history including type, frequency, duration
- Seizure medications: Any changes, missed doses, levels
- Past medical history: Previous intracranial lesions or trauma, diabetes, HIV, stroke, migraines, dementia, psychiatric illness
- Medications: Ciprofloxacin (Cipro), metronidazole (Flagyl), theophylline, stimulants, antipsychotics can lower seizure threshold
- Diuretic, antihypertensives, diabetes medicines can cause metabolic disturbances that can cause seizure
- Family history of seizure

PHYSICAL EXAM
- Assess for head trauma
- Screening neurologic exam may be normal even with structural lesions
- Focal deficits may be worse immediately after seizure
- Evaluate cardiovascular and pulmonary status
- Blood pressure and pulse will be elevated during and immediately after a seizure

DIAGNOSTIC STUDIES
- First-time seizure: Metabolic panel, toxicology if appropriate
- Brain CT scan even with a metabolic etiology because the metabolic abnormality could lower the seizure threshold in the presence of a structural lesion

- EEG for first time patient has seizure with identified etiology but need not be repeated
- EEG for first time seizure without etiology, may determine seizure type and guide treatment and prognosis; if seizures continue and EEG nondiagnostic may consider closed-circuit video EEG
- Lumbar puncture if new neurologic findings are not explained by imaging, or if fever or continued unexplained headache are present

Differential Diagnosis

Causes for seizure
- Head trauma
- Brain tumor
- Stroke
- Metabolic disorders
- Alcohol withdrawal
- Withdrawal from some medications can also cause seizure

Disorders that may appear to be seizures
- Syncope
- Transient ischemic attack
- Pseudo-seizures
- Panic attacks or psychosis
- Drug intoxication
- Migraine
- Multiple sclerosis
- Postural hypotension

Table 15–6. Seizure Classification and Recommended Medication

Seizure Type	Description	Medication
Simple partial	Focal motor or sensory symptoms, reflects area of brain affected; no change in consciousness	Phenytoin, carbamazepine valproic acid, phenobarbital
Complex partial	Characterized by an aura, followed by impaired consciousness with automatisms, usually originating from temporal lobe	Carbamazepine, phenytoin, phenobarbital, valproic acid
Secondarily generalized	Simple or complex partial seizures that progress to generalized tonic-clonic seizures	Phenytoin, carbamazepine, phenobarbital, valproic acid
Generalized tonic-clonic	Formerly "grand mal," sudden loss of consciousness with tonic-clonic motor activity, postictal state of confusion, drowsiness, and headache	Phenytoin, carbamazepine, phenobarbital, valproic acid
Absence	Formerly "petit mal," brief (<30 seconds) episodes of unresponsiveness characterized by staring, blinking, or facial twitching	Ethosuximide, valproic acid, clonazepam

Management

NONPHARMACOLOGIC TREATMENT

- Educate patient and family about seizure disorder and cause
- Educate them about safety management, including using any aura period to prepare for seizure
- Stress the importance of keeping an extra supply of medication readily available at all times
- First episodes of seizures without known cause do not have to be treated with anticonvulsants
- Educate family about acute seizure management; to protect patient from injury, place on left side to maintain airway if possible
- Patients with known recurrent seizures do not need to go to emergency department for every seizure, only if seizure lasts more than 2 minutes or breathing is impaired (aspiration)
- Advise regarding state driving regulations
- Advise regarding swimming alone or operating dangerous equipment
- Teach about side effects and toxic effects of medications, not to discontinue seizure medicines abruptly, may precipitate seizure
- Discuss seizure triggers: Sleep deprivation, alcohol, menses, stress, low-grade fever, and infection
- Wear medic alert bracelet

PHARMACOLOGIC TREATMENT

- Anticonvulsants first initiated by a neurologist: Phenytoin (Dilantin), phenobarbital (Luminal), carbamazepine (Tegretol), and valproic acid (Depakene) are first-line choices (Table 15–6)
- 40%–50% of patients can be maintained seizure-free on a single agent
- Phenytoin initially 100 mg three times a day, maintenance dose 300–600 mg/day divided
- Phenobarbital 60–100 mg/day
- Carbamazepine initially 200 mg twice a day, increase by <200 mg/day in divided doses 3–4 times a day up to 1200 mg
- Valproic acid initially 15 mg/kg/day, increase at 1-week intervals by 5–10 mg/kg/day until seizures are controlled or side effects prevent further increase in dose, maximum dose 60 mg/kg/day, divide totally daily doses over 250 mg.; before initiating, baseline liver enzyme levels (specifically ALT and AST) must be drawn and then monitored thereafter approximately every 3–6 months, to determine safe serum levels

LENGTH OF TREATMENT

- Consider discontinuing seizure medications in those without seizures for more than 2 years
- Obtain an EEG before stopping medication
- 40% will have a reoccurrence, most within the first year
- Must consider the risk factors of seizure recurrence and medications for each individual patient, consult with neurologist

Special Considerations
- First-time seizures in patients >50, must consider an underlying intracranial lesion or metabolic etiology.
- Anticonvulsants are metabolized in the liver and involve the cytochrome P450 enzyme system; care must be used when administering these medications with any other medications.
- Patients must be counseled about the signs and symptoms of liver disease, including nausea and vomiting that seem protracted, abdominal pain, anorexia, fatigue, and dark urine/stools.
- Lower, less frequent doses may be needed for those with hepatic and renal dysfunction.
- All anticonvulsants have been associated with increased birth defects.
- Babies of epileptic mothers have 2–3 times the normal risk of birth defects.
- Must counsel all women of child-bearing age regarding risks of medications during pregnancy.
- Seizures may increase, decrease, or remain the same during pregnancy.
- Neurologist should be consulted before pregnancy for medical management.
- Anticonvulsants except valproic acid alter the effectiveness of birth control pills.
- Some anticonvulsants are excreted in breast milk and may have serious adverse effects for the nursing infant.
- There is no evidence that prophylactic anticonvulsant therapy prevents epilepsy following head trauma or brain surgery, therefore not necessary to maintain these patients on long-term anticonvulsants.
- Educate patients about specifics of state laws limiting driving for seizure patients.

When to Consult, Refer, Hospitalize
- Referral to neurologist for first-time seizures, when considering discontinuing therapy, seizures refractory to adequate trials of monotherapy, pregnancy
- Neurosurgeon for stereotaxic procedures for intractable seizures
- Status epilepticus is a medical emergency defined as two or more seizures without complete recovery or a seizure lasting >30 minutes; the primary care provider witnessing a seizure lasting >2 minutes must activate 911, and be prepared to initiate emergency procedures. IV access and administration of IV benzodiazepines (Lorazepam) should be initiated as protocols permit

Follow-Up
- Most patients should be seen every 3 months by their primary care provider and at least annually by their neurologist; more frequent visits are needed if medications or seizures change.
- Anticonvulsants have small therapeutic ranges; levels should be drawn when adjusting therapy, and with change in seizure frequency.
- Liver enzymes must be monitored.
  - EXPECTED COURSE
    - Variable, one seizure to intractable seizures

  - COMPLICATIONS
    - Status epilepticus, airway obstruction, injury during seizure activity

CASE STUDIES

Case 1. 49-year-old African-American female presents with new onset headache over the past 2 months.

HPI: She states that prior to these episodes, she never thought of herself as a "headachey" person. She relates that the headaches are "nearly always" occipital, and are often accompanied by pain so severe that it feels like the top of her head will come off. When questioned, it is clear that she is both photophobic and phonophobic and also experiences lightheadedness associated with the headache.

PMH: Healthy female; perimenopausal. Medications: Monthly Advil for menstrual cramps. Has tried Excedrin migraine with these headaches to no avail.

1. What other history is needed?
2. What type of physical exam would you do?
3. What screening tests would you do?
4. What is the most likely diagnosis?
5. How would you manage this patient?

Case 2. A 3-year-old Asian male comes in for follow-up after management in the emergency department for multiple febrile seizures.

PMH: No prior history of virus-induced high fevers associated with seizing. No medications except over-the-counter acetaminophen liquid for fevers.

1. What other history do you want to obtain?
2. What physical examination would you perform?
3. What further diagnostic tests would you want to order?
4. How will you initially manage this patient?

Case 3. A 78-year-old male presents with his wife and daughter complaining of an episode over the weekend of sudden-onset right-sided weakness that completely resolved in about 2 hours. He did not seek medical attention at the time because it resolved.

PMH: Smoker, 64 year pack-a-day history. Mild hypertension diagnosed in 1985. Was told he had elevated lipids "a few years back" but refused to take medication or change his lifestyle at that time. Has not been back to see a provider since.

Medication: Hydrochlorothiazide 50 mg/day "for a year or so," 1985–1986. Occasional acetaminophen.

1. What other history is important?
2. What systems will you examine?
3. What is the most likely diagnosis?
4. What is your plan?

REFERENCES

Agency for Health Care Policy and Research. (1996). *Early Alzheimer's disease: Recognition and assessment. Guideline 19.* Washington, DC: U.S. Department of Health and Human Services.

American Academy of Pediatrics. (1999). Health supervision for children with Fragile X syndrome. *Policy Reference Guide of the American Academy of Pediatrics.* Elk Grove, IL: Author.

American Academy of Pediatrics. (1999). Health supervision of children with neurofibromatosis. *Policy Reference Guide of the American Academy of Pediatrics* (12th ed.). Elk Grove, IL: Author.

American Academy of Pediatrics. (2001). Health supervision for children with Down syndrome. *Pediatrics, 107*(2), 442–449.

American Academy of Pediatrics, Pickering, L. K. (Ed.). (2006). *Red book: 2006 report of the Committee on Infectious Disease* (26th ed.). Elk Grove, IL: Author.

Berman, S. (2003). *Pediatric decision making* (4th ed.). Philadelphia: Mosby.

Burke, M. M., & Laramie, J. A. (2003). *Primary care of the older adult.* Philadelphia: Elsevier Health Sciences.

Buttaro, T. M., Bailey, P. P., & Trybulski, J. (2007). Primary care: *A collaborative practice.* Philadelphia: Elsevier Health Sciences.

Coombs, J. B., & Davis, R. L. (2000). A synopsis of the American Academy of Pediatrics practice parameter on the management of closed head injury in children. *Pediatrics in Review, 21*(12), 413–415.

Downey, D. (2008). Pharmacologic management of Alzheimer disease. *Journal of Neuroscience Nursing. 40*(1), 55–59.

Edmunds, M. W., & Mayhew, M. S. (2004). *Pharmacology for the primary care provider* (2nd ed.). St. Louis, MO: Elsevier Mosby.

Freeman, J. M. (2003). What every pediatrician should know about the ketogenic diet. *Contemporary Pediatrics, 20*(5), 13–127.

Graham, M. V., & Uphold, C. (Eds.). (2003). *Clinical guidelines in child health.* Gainesville, FL: Barmarrae Books.

Hay, W. W., Levin, M. J., & Sondheimer, J. M. (2006). *Current pediatric diagnosis and treatment.* New York: Lange Medica Book/McGraw Hill.

Hill, A. (2000). Neonatal seizures. *Pediatrics in Review, 21*(4), 117–121.

Hilton, G. (1997). Seizure disorders in adults: Evaluation and management of new onset seizures. *The Nurse Practitioner, 22*(9), 42–59.

Hirtz, D. G. (1997). Febrile seizures. *Pediatrics in Review, 18*(1), 5–9.

Holmes, G. L. (2004). *"Confusion" in a 9-year-old: An interactive case study on epilepsy.* Medscape. Retrieved September 9, 2004, from www.medscape.com/viewprogram/3087_pnt

Hopkins, A., & Appleton, R. (1996). *Epilepsy: The facts.* New York: Oxford University Press.

Hudson, G. T., & Dixon, D. (2003) Autism challenges in diagnoses and treatment. *Clinician Reviews, 13*(70), 46–51.

Kaufman, B. A. (2004). Neural tube defects. *Pediatric Clinics of North America, 51*(3), 389–419.

Kliegman, R., Behramn, R. E., & Jenson, H. (Eds). (2007) *Nelson's textbook of pediatrics* (17th ed.). Philadelphia: Elsevier Health Sciences.

Labuguen, R. H. (2006). Initial evaluation of vertigo. *American Family Physician, 73*(2), 244–251.

Leira, E. C., & Adams, H. P. (1999). Management of acute ischemic stroke. *Clinics in Geriatric Medicine, 15*(4), 701–720.

McPhee, S. J., Tierney, L. M., & Papadakis, M. A. (2007). *Current medical diagnosis & treatment.* New York: McGraw-Hill.

Millar, J. S. (2006). Evaluation and treatment of febrile seizures. *American Family Physician, 73*(10), 1761–1764.

Moloney, M. F., Matthews, K. B., Scharbo-Dehaan, M., & Strickland, O. L. (2000). Caring for the woman with migraine headaches. *The Nurse Practitioner, 25*(2), 17–36.

Ramadan, N. M., Silberstein, S. D., Freitag, F. G., Gilbert, T. T., & Frishberg, B.M. (2000). *Evidence-based guidelines for migraine headache in the primary care setting: Pharmacological management for prevention of migraine.* Retrieved February 14, 2008, from http://www.aan.com/professionals/practice/pdfs/gl0090.pdf

Rau, J. D. (2003). Is it autism? *Contemporary Pediatrics, 20*(4), 54–82.

Reimschisel, T. (2003). Breaking the cycle of medication overuse headache. *Contemporary Pediatrics, 20*(10), 101–116.

Robertson, J., & Shilkofski, N. (2005). *The Harriet Lane handbook.* Philadelphia: Elsevier Health Sciences.

Rossi, A., Biancheri, R., Cama, A., Piatelli, G., Ravegnani, M., & Tortori-Donati, P. (2004). Imaging in spine and spinal cord malformations. *European Journal of Radiology, 50*(2), 177–200.

Schwartz, M. W., Bell, N. M. & Bingham, P. M. (2005). *The 5 minute pediatric consult.* Philadelphia: Lippincott Williams & Wilkins.

Simms, M. D., & Rschum, R. L. (2000). Preschool children who have atypical patterns of development. *Pediatrics in Review, 21*(5), 147–158.

Swain, S. E. (1996). Multiple sclerosis primary health care implications. *The Nurse Practitioner, 21*(7), 40–54.

Tapper, V. J. (1997). Pathophysiology, assessment, and treatment of Parkinson's disease. *The Nurse Practitioner, 22*(7), 76–95.

Uphold, C. R., & Graham, M. V. (2003). *Clinical guidelines in family practice* (4th ed). Los Angeles: Barmarrae Books.

U.S. Preventive Services Task Force. *Guide to clinical preventive services, 2007.* Retrieved February 4, 2008, from http://www.ahrq.gov/clinic/pocketgd.htm.

Young, L. R. (2004). Antiparkinson agents. In M. W. Edmunds & M. S. Mayhew (Eds.), *Pharmacology for the primary care provider* (2nd ed., pp. 502–515). St. Louis, MO: Mosby.

Zinner, S. H. (2000). Tourette disorder. *Pediatrics in Review, 21*(11), 372–383.

Hematologic Disorders

Elizabeth Petit de Mange, PhD, MSN, BSN, NP-C, RN

GENERAL APPROACH

- Most common anemia in all age groups is iron deficiency anemia.
- Do not assume that anemia in patient with chronic inflammatory disease is "anemia of chronic disease."
- Do not begin treatment for B12 deficiency without assessing and treating folate deficiency.
- *Physiologic anemia* of the newborn occurs at 10–12 weeks due to rapid growth, increase in blood volume, and shortened red cell survival time; hemoglobin (Hgb) level may reach a low of 10 g/dL in full-term infants; this is followed by a gradual increase in red blood cells (RBCs), with correspondingly slower hemoglobin rise; healthy term infants do not require therapy.
- Hematopoiesis is slowed in the elderly when the presence and number of progenitor cells decline; 60% of all anemias are seen in people over age 65.

Definitions

- *Anemia*: Hematocrit (Hct) <36% for females, <40% for males; or Hgb <12 for females, <13.5 for males, or a red blood cell count <4.0 x 106/microliter for females and <4.5 x 106/microliter for men. In children note that specific values defining anemia vary depending on age.
- *Mean corpuscular (cell) volume* (MCV): Represents the size of the RBC and is calculated from the hemoglobin, hematocrit, or RBC count. Used in differentiation of types of anemia.
- *Ferritin*: Represents iron storage in the serum. May be elevated during infection or chronic inflammation and decreased in iron deficiency.

- Hypochromic: Erythrocytes containing decreased level of Hgb, causing the cells to appear "paler" on smear
- Hyperchromic: Erythrocytes containing increased level of Hgb, causing cells to appear "darker" on smear
- Macrocytic anemia: Decreased Hct/Hgb/RBC with associated MCV >100
- Megaloblastic anemia: Anemia characterized by a large, nucleated, embryonic type of cell that is a precursor of erythrocytes in an abnormal erythropoietic process seen almost exclusively in pernicious anemia
- Microcytic anemia: Decreased Hct/Hgb/RBC with associated MCV <80
- Normocytic anemia: Decreased Hct/Hgb/RBC with associated MCV 80–100
- RDW: Red blood cell distribution width, a statistical index of the variation in red cell widths
- Total iron binding capacity (TIBC): Amount of iron in serum plus amount of transferrin available in serum. (Transferrin is a transport protein, which regulates iron absorption.) Decreased in anemia of chronic disease.

Red Flags
- Blood values helpful in identifying anemias can be found in Table 16–1.
- Anemia in the presence of splenomegaly requires further diagnostic evaluation.
- Anemia of prematurity manifests at 4–8 weeks of age and is more severe than physiologic anemia.
  - Influencing factors include birthweight, perinatal complications, blood transfusion history, and presence of vitamin E deficiency. Nadir Hgb values reach 6 g/dL
  - Asymptomatic, growing preterm infants require no therapy; however, signs of hypoxia (apneic episodes, tachycardia, irritability, poor feeding) indicate need for evaluation and more aggressive intervention
- Hemolytic anemia during the newborn period is due to physiologically immature liver incapable of rapidly conjugating bilirubin created by normally rapid turnover of relatively excessive RBC.
  - Hemolysis in the neonate is accompanied by reticulocytosis, nucleated RBC, and sometimes spherocytosis on peripheral blood smear
  - Most common cause of hemolytic anemia in the newborn is ABO incompatibility with hyperbilirubinemia/jaundice, usually within 24 hours of birth
  - All cases of suspected hemolytic anemia in the newborn should be evaluated in the hospital
- Multiple myeloma is a malignant disease of the plasma cells with peak incidence during the 7th decade. It may present with bone pain of the back, chest or extremities; weakness and fatigue; pathologic fractures; abnormal bleeding; palpable liver and spleen; Bence-Jones protein in the urine; elevated creatinine and calcium; increased sedimentation rate. Refer for bone marrow biopsy.
- Hodgkin's lymphoma is a malignant disease with lymphoreticular proliferation and presence of Reed-Sternberg cells; there is a bimodal age distribution: 15–34 (peak at 20) and >50 (peak at 70) with male-to-female ratio of 8:1.
  - Presents with persistent fever, night sweats, persistent dry cough, unexplained pruritus, substernal discomfort, persistent painless lymphadenopathy, weight loss >10%, anorexia, immediate pain after alcohol ingestion; increased incidence in those with AIDS
  - Diagnostic tests may show mediastinal adenopathy on chest x-ray, elevated erythrocyte sedimentation rate (ESR), increased serum alkaline phosphatase and lactate dehydrogenase (LDH), lymphocytopenia, mild leukocytosis, thrombocytosis, Reed-Sternberg cells on smear

– Refer suspected cases to hematologist for diagnosis and management with chemotherapy and radiation; prognosis is good depending on classification at diagnosis

- *Non-Hodgkin's lymphoma* is a malignant disease of the lymphoreticular system differentiated from Hodgkin's lymphoma by absence of giant Reed-Sternberg cells; increased incidence in those with AIDS.
  – Presents similar to Hodgkin's lymphoma; prognosis not as good
  – Refer all suspected cases to hematologist for diagnosis and management
- *Deficiency of coagulant factor VIII (Hemophilia A) or factor IX (Hemophilia B)* is rare and presents in males during first few years of life as excessive bruising, bleeding after circumcision, bleeding hours or days after injury, hematuria, hemorrhage or hematoma after minor injury. Laboratory results include normal platelet count, partial thromboplastin time (PTT) greatly prolonged, factor VIII low in hemophilia A, factor IX low in hemoglobin-B. Refer to hematologist for management.

Table 16-1. Blood Values Helpful in Differentiating Anemias

Anemia	MCV	Appearance of red cell
Iron deficiency	<80 fl	Normocytic or microcytic, hypochromic
Folate deficiency	>100 fl	Macrocytic, hyperchromic
Vitamin B12	>100 fl	Macrocytic, hyperchromic
Chronic disease	Normal	Normochromic, normocytic or microcytic
Sideroblastic	<80 fl	Hypochromic
Sickle cell	<80 fl	Sickle cells, normochromic
G6PD	Normal	Heinz bodies, bite cells, blister cells
Thalassemia	<80 fl	Microcytic
Drug-induced	Normal	Normocytic, normochromic
Aplastic	Normal	Normocytic, normochromic
Post-hemorrhagic	Normal	Normocytic, normochromic

Note. MCH = mean corpuscular hemoglobin; MCHC = mean corpuscular hemoglobin concentration; RBC = red blood cells; TIBC = total iron binding capacity; fl = femtoliter (10–15 Liter); pg = pictogram (10–12 g); ng = nanogram (10–9 g); µl= microliter (10-6)

Table 16-2. Normal Ranges for RBC Studies

Test	Females	Males
Hematocrit	36%–48%	40–53%
Hemoglobin	12–16 g/dL	13.5–17.7 g/dL
RBC (106/µl)	4.0–5.4	4.5–6.0
MCV	80–100 fl	80–100 fl
MCH	26–34 pg	26–34 pg
MCHC	31–37% g/dL	31–37% g/dL
Reticulocyte Count	0.5–1.5% of RBC	0.5–1.5% of RBC
Serum Iron	50–170 mcg/dL	65–175 mcg/dL
TIBC	250–450 mcg/dL	250–450 mcg/dL
Ferritin	10–120 ng/mL (avg. 55)	20–250 ng/mL (avg. 125)

NORMOCYTIC ANEMIAS

Anemia of Chronic Disease

Description
- A mild hypoproliferative anemia associated with chronic disease, infections, and malignancies that has persisted for >1–2 months. Probably a consequence of long-term disease with inflammatory process.
- Diagnosis of exclusion from active blood loss or production abnormalities associated with iron or folate intake.

Etiology
- The pathophysiology of anemia of chronic disease is not well understood but may be due to decreased RBC life span, erythropoietin reduction, and problems of iron transfer.
- Occurs as a result of renal disease, liver disease, endocrine disorders, rheumatoid arthritis, infections, and some forms of cancer.

Incidence and Demographics
- The second most common anemia in the world; incidence parallels the rate of chronic inflammatory disease
- The most common anemia in older adults

Risk Factors
- Chronic diseases: Renal, liver, endocrine disease; rheumatoid arthritis; infection; and some cancers

Prevention and Screening
- Attention to good nutrition
- CBC screening for those with chronic disease

Assessment
HISTORY
- Chronic disease
- Fatigue, dyspnea on exertion, irritability, listlessness, easy fatigability

PHYSICAL EXAM
- Perform a complete physical exam for signs of the underlying disease
- Signs of anemia, depending on severity: Pallor, tachycardia, tachypnea on exertion

DIAGNOSTIC STUDIES (TABLE 16–2)
- CBC, reticulocyte count, iron studies (serum iron, TIBC, ferritin); studies pertinent to underlying disorder; repeat iron studies important for diagnosis and management
- Characteristic labs: Hgb usually 8–12 g/dL, Hct 25%–35%, MCV 75–85 as Hgb falls <10, often low serum iron and TIBC, and normal or increased ferritin (TIBC is increased and ferritin decreased in iron deficiency), serum erythropoietin normal, but not generally assessed

Differential Diagnosis
- Iron deficiency anemia
- Multifactorial anemia
- Chronic renal insufficiency
- Liver disease (usually alcohol-related)
- Post-hemorrhagic anemia
- Endocrine disorders: hypothyroidism
- AIDS
- Aplastic anemia

Management

NONPHARMACOLOGIC TREATMENT
- Treat underlying disease
- Ensure appropriate nutrition
- Transfusion only in severe, symptomatic cases

PHARMACOLOGIC TREATMENT
- Recombinant erythropoietin (Epogen, Procrit) in selected patients

LENGTH OF TREATMENT
- Treatment required as long as underlying disease and anemia persist

Special Considerations
- A similar profile as iron deficiency may eventually develop with patient becoming mildly microcytic and hypochromic as Hgb falls <10 g/dL.
- Patients with AIDS often have anemia of chronic disease. As disease progresses, pancytopenia may occur due to marrow damage. At that point, checking serum erythropoietin level may help determine if patient will benefit from recombinant erythropoietin injections.
- Anemia of renal disease relates to severity of renal failure, due to decreased erythropoietin production, may benefit from erythropoietin.
- In patients with diabetes mellitus, anemia is frequently severe early in the disease process.

When to Consult, Refer, Hospitalize
- Refer if diagnosis is questionable
- Refer to confirm underlying cause (e.g., rheumatologist for collagen/vascular problem, oncologist for cancer, nephrologist for renal disease, infectious disease specialist for infections)

Follow-Up
- Frequent monitoring of blood pressure, CBC, iron studies with recombinant erythropoietin therapy

  EXPECTED COURSE
  - Anemia will improve or worsen as the underlying disease improves or progress
  - Patient often can tolerate fairly low Hct and Hgb, as low as 30/10, as they develop gradually

COMPLICATIONS
- Possible exacerbation of cardiopulmonary disease, particularly in the elderly (anemia results in less oxygen delivered to tissues, heart rate and cardiac output increase to compensate, heart may begin to fail)

Aplastic Anemia

Description
- Aplastic anemia is characterized by intrinsic bone marrow dysfunction or failure; pluripotent stem cell expression is impaired so pancytopenia with hypercellularity of the bone marrow is seen.
- Intrinsic marrow dysfunction produces defective RBC synthesis; produces anemia, neutropenia, thrombocytopenia, pancytopenia.

Etiology
- Autoimmune suppression of hematopoiesis is most common cause, but may be precipitated by viral illness, autoimmune suppression, drug or chemical exposure, tumor, radiation, or inherited disorder.
- Inherited: Fanconi's anemia, Schwachman-Diamond syndrome

Incidence and Demographics
- Not common in U.S.
- 50% idiopathic; 20% drug or chemical exposure (chloramphenicol—rare); 10% viral

Risk Factors
- Family history, some medications (anticonvulsants, antibiotics, gold), radiation, exposure to some toxic chemicals such as insecticides, herbicides, organic solvents, paint removers and others.

Prevention and Screening
- Most cases cannot be prevented.
- There are no general screening methods recommended.
- Individuals should avoid contact exposure to certain chemicals such as insecticides, herbicides, organic solvents, paint removers, and other toxic chemicals. This is especially important if you already have had aplastic anemia caused by toxic chemicals. Recurrent exposure may increase your risk of a reccurrence of the disease.
- Individuals who have had exposure to toxic chemicals or have had aplastic anemia in the past should have regular physical examinations.
- Individuals should report the following signs and symptoms early: fever, fatigue, weight loss, weakness, sore throat, dyspnea, palpitations, and bleeding.

Assessment
HISTORY
- Insidious onset of fever, fatigue, weight loss, weakness, sore throat, dyspnea, palpitations
- Bleeding problems such as menorrhagia, rectal bleed, epistaxis
- History of potential sources of exposure to toxic agents: Medications, chemical exposure at work, hobbies, etc.
- History of associated anomalies: Kidney, hypospadias, short stature

PHYSICAL EXAM
- General: Pallor, petechiae, bruises
- Thorough physical for tumors, signs of infection, signs of bleeding
  - Cardiac exam: Systolic ejection murmur may be present
  - Eyes: Retinal flame hemorrhage
  - Rectal: Occult or rectal bleeding

DIAGNOSTIC STUDIES
- Pancytopenia is pathognomonic
- Severe anemia, decreased reticulocytes
- CBC with differential, peripheral smear, bleeding studies, TIBC, urinalysis, bone marrow, liver function, CT of thymus as indicated
- Lab results: Normochromic, normocytic anemia; TIBC normal; hematuria
- Bone marrow shows hypoplasia, fatty infiltration

Differential Diagnosis
- Leukemia
- Hypersplenism
- Systemic lupus erythematosus (SLE)
- Myelodysplasia
- Sepsis

Management
NONPHARMACOLOGIC TREATMENT
- Education and supportive care
- A well-balanced diet decreases risk of infection
- Manage underlying cause
- Perform human leukocyte antigen (HLA) testing on patients and immediate families for inherited conditions

PHARMACOLOGIC TREATMENT
- Immunosuppression therapy, oxygen
- All cases: RBC and platelet transfusions, parenteral antibiotics for infection due to severe neutropenia
- Severe cases: Bone marrow transplant is considered (may be age-dependent)

LENGTH OF TREATMENT
- Lifelong treatment may be required unless effective bone marrow transplant is curative

Special Considerations
- Must avoid further exposure to etiologic agents

When to Consult, Refer, Hospitalize
- Refer immediately to hematologist when diagnosis is suspected; work with hematologist throughout therapy

Follow-Up
EXPECTED COURSE
   • Often favorable outcome depending on age and treatment response
   • Untreated cases are fatal; successful bone marrow transplant is curative

COMPLICATIONS
   • Infection, leukemia, heart failure, hemorrhage

HYPOCHROMIC ANEMIAS

Iron Deficiency Anemia

Description
   • Microcytic, hypochromic anemia due to decreased iron stores, poor iron utilization, or poor iron reutilization

Etiology
   • Hemorrhage, occult malignancy, increased need (pregnancy and growth spurts), impaired absorption, inadequate dietary intake

Incidence and Demographics
   • Prevalent in all ages and populations in the U.S.
   • Seen in 7%–10% of adult population; 10%–20% of infants and toddlers; 15%–45% of pregnant women; 20% women overall
   • More common in women than men because of menstruation, pregnancy

Risk Factors
   • Low iron stores; occurs in premature and low birthweight infants and when Hgb is lower than normal at birth (e.g., hemorrhage and/or smaller of twins).
   • Increased need for iron: Demands for iron higher than normal such as low birthweight infants experiencing rapid catch-up growth or the normal rapid growth of infancy and adolescence, pregnancy and lactation, athlete.
   • Insufficient intake of iron from low dietary intake, poor bioavailability of the dietary iron, or malabsorption. Low intake is the most common etiologic factor seen in infants, toddlers, teens, elderly, institutionalization.
   • Increased loss of iron, due to disease process including Meckel's diverticulum, peptic ulcer disease, polyps, hemangiomas, parasitic infections, or cow's milk enteropathy. Losses may also occur from menorrhagia, chronic use of NSAIDS, uncommonly recurrent epistaxis, and possibly strenuous exercise.
   • Conditions such as achlorhydria, gastric surgery, celiac disease, pica that cause impaired absorption.
   • Conditions such as neoplasm, duodenal/gastric ulcers, diverticulosis, ulcerative colitis.
   • Repeated blood donations.

Prevention and Screening
- Encourage breastfeeding of all infants for the first 12 months of life; after 1 year of age, limit cow and soy milk consumption to <24 ounces/day. Adequate diet; consume orange juice with meals to enhance iron absorption.
- Dietary supplements if patient has risk factors.
- Selective screening for at-risk populations such as some elderly and menstruating women.

Assessment

HISTORY
- Preterm and low birthweight (LBW) infants
- Initially asymptomatic; insidious onset of gradually progressing fatigue, dyspnea on exertion, irritable, listless, easy fatigability, dysphagia, postural hypotension
- Possible palpitations, shortness of breath, impaired muscular performance
- Diet history: Low in iron, pica, drug/chemical exposure
- Family history of iron deficiency anemia
- Review of systems (ROS) for blood loss, symptoms of gastrointestinal problems, neoplasms

PHYSICAL EXAM
- Obtain height, weight for infants and children and plot on growth chart
- Observe for pallor or chlorosis (peculiar greenish pallor)
- Angular stomatitis, ulcerations or fissure of the mouth
- Ozena: chronic atrophy of the nasal mucosa
- Dry skin and mucous membranes
- Koilonychia: thinning and flattening of the nails and then spooning
- Auscultate heart for systolic flow murmurs
- Splenomegaly
- Brittle hair, tachycardia, tachypnea

DIAGNOSTIC STUDIES
- CBC with differential and smear, TIBC, serum iron, ferritin, special tests to determine underlying bleed
- Laboratory findings (see Table 16–3): Hgb <12 g/dL in adults and older children, variable in younger children; serum ferritin level <10 nanograms/mL in women and <20 nanograms/mL in men; low Hct; "pencil cells" on smear, MCV and MCH decrease, RDW >15, increased TIBC >400 mcg/dL, low serum iron <30 mcg/dL; transferrin saturation <15%; MCV <80 mcg/dL; reticulocyte count elevated in cases of blood loss, decreased in iron deficiency; increased platelet count >400,000; bone marrow absent for iron staining
- Bone marrow aspiration if severe, questionable diagnosis, or resistant to treatment

Table 16–3. Comparison of Differential Laboratory Findings in Microcytic Anemias

Laboratory Finding	Thalassemia Trait	Lead Poisoning	Iron Deficiency	Anemia of Chronic Disease
Hgb	Decreased	Decreased	Decreased	Decreased
MCV	Decreased	Decreased	Decreased	Normal
Ferritin	Normal	Normal	Decreased	Increased
FEP (free erythrocyte porphyrins)	Normal	Very High	High	Mild Increase

Differential Diagnosis
- Thalassemia
- G6PD deficiency
- Infection
- Cancer
- Chronic diseases
- Lead poisoning
- Hypothyroidism
- Renal failure

Management
NONPHARMACOLOGIC TREATMENT
- Diagnose and treat underlying cause
- Normal dietary intake meets only daily losses, not therapeutic; RDA iron = 10 mg/day for men and up to 15 mg/day for women and children; must increase iron intake
- No dairy product or antacid within 2 hours of oral iron
- Symptomatic care on treatment side effects (constipation, nausea, cramps, diarrhea)

PHARMACOLOGIC TREATMENT
- Oral iron supplements: Up to 300 mg of elemental iron divided 3–4 times a day for adolescents and adults
  - 325 mg of ferrous sulfate contains 65 mg of elemental iron
  - Liquid preparation 2–3 mg/kg/day for children
  - Oral iron therapy is safer and less costly than IM or IV iron
  - Reduce dose to decrease GI side effects; no real benefit to more expensive preparations
  - Vitamin C will help increase absorption; meals will decrease absorption by up to 50%
  - Parenteral iron if poor absorption or inability to tolerate oral iron
  - Blood transfusion is not recommended for iron supplementation

LENGTH OF TREATMENT
- Treat until deficiency corrected; expect to see improvement within 4 weeks; return to baseline blood levels in 8 weeks; continue therapy 3–6 months to replace iron stores

Special Considerations
- If unresponsive to therapy, reevaluate underlying cause and compliance

When to Consult, Refer, Hospitalize
- Refer to hematologist if patient is not responsive to treatment or underlying cause cannot be determined

Follow-Up
- Follow-up recommended after 1 month and every 6 months if stable until resolved
  EXPECTED COURSE
  - Cure expected; increase in Hgb of 1 g/week expected
  - Prolonged course of treatment may be required because of noncompliance

  COMPLICATIONS
  - May have unidentified underlying source of bleeding
  - Growth delay, learning difficulty, heart failure (late, untreated)

MEGALOBLASTIC ANEMIAS

Vitamin B12 Deficiency

Description
- A megaloblastic anemia in which MCV is >100 resulting from a deficiency of intrinsic factor, which leads to inadequate vitamin B12 absorption (<200 picograms/mL) and impaired red blood cell synthesis

Etiology
- Pernicious anemia: Caused by congenital enzyme deficiency so B12 cannot be absorbed; overgrowth of intestinal organisms, autoimmune reaction involving gastric parietal cells, gastrectomy
- Malabsorption: GI parasites, GI surgery, Crohn's, chronic alcoholism, strict vegetarians (rare)
- Elderly stomach is less acidic, B12 needs acid to be absorbed

Incidence and Demographics
- Onset at age 50–60; median age at diagnosis = 60
- Women slightly > men

Risk Factors
- Age (common presents around age 60), family history of pernicious anemia
- Chronic alcoholism
- GI surgery, Crohn's disease, immunologic diseases

Prevention and Screening
- Adequate dietary intake—meat and dairy products
- Routine screening for B12 level in dementia and malnutrition

Assessment

HISTORY

- Insidious onset of peripheral numbness, personality changes, memory loss, anorexia, diarrhea, glossitis, distal paresthesias, ataxia
- Assess for risk factors, underlying causes
- Should be considered in differential diagnosis of dementia

PHYSICAL EXAM

- Characteristic beefy red, shiny tongue
- Abdominal tenderness, organomegaly, tachycardia, tachypnea, pallor, hepatosplenomegaly
- Neurologic signs: Numbness, sensory ataxia, limb weakness, spasticity, changes in deep tendon reflexes, decreased vibratory sense, impaired proprioception, impaired fine motor movement, positive Romberg test, progressive mental status impairment

DIAGNOSTIC STUDIES

- CBC with differential, peripheral smear, LDH and serum B12 levels; consider Schilling test with and without intrinsic factor to test B12 absorption; consider bone marrow aspiration
- Laboratory results: Serum B 12 levels <200 picograms/mL; Hct decreased; MCV markedly elevated; decreased reticulocyte count; WBC and platelet count reduced, elevated LDH
- On smear: A large, nucleated, embryonic type of cell that is a precursor of erythrocytes in an abnormal erythropoietic process
- Schilling's test documents decreased oral B12 absorption

Differential Diagnosis

- Folic acid deficiency
- Myelodysplasia
- Liver dysfunction
- Side effects of medications
- Alcoholism
- Bleeding/hemorrhage
- Hypothyroidism

Management

NONPHARMACOLOGIC TREATMENT

- Education and supportive therapy; maintain balanced diet, good health and hygiene

PHARMACOLOGIC TREATMENT

- Initial: 800–1,000 mcg of vitamin B12 IM daily for 4–8 weeks
- Maintenance: 100–1,000 mcg monthly
- Oral cobalamin 1,000 mcg daily is alternative replacement
- May require iron supplementation for the first month of therapy during rapid regeneration of RBCs

LENGTH OF TREATMENT

- Lifelong

Special Considerations
- If patient presents with abnormal neurologic signs, the symptoms might be irreversible
- Might have hypokalemia in first week of treatment
- Do not begin treatment for B12 deficiency without assessing for and treating folate deficiency also
- Check serum B12 levels in patients with distal polyneuropathies (even if no anemia or macrocytosis seen)
- Oral B-complex vitamin only valuable when B12 deficiency is nutritional

When to Consult, Refer, Hospitalize
- Refer as needed for underlying cause; refer for follow up endoscopy q 5 years to rule out malignancy

Follow-Up
> EXPECTED COURSE
>> - Response rapid; good prognosis if treatment within 6 months of neurological signs

> COMPLICATIONS
>> - Stomach cancer
>> - Permanent central nervous system (CNS) signs/symptoms

Folic Acid Deficiency

Description
- Anemia as a result of inadequate folic acid present for DNA synthesis and RBC maturation. Lack of folic acid (folate) causes macrocytic, normochromic, and megaloblastic anemia.
- Also associated with increased incidence of embryonic neural tube defects.

Etiology
- Folic acid–deficient diet, malabsorption syndromes, or increased demand for folic acid (pregnancy)

Incidence and Demographics
- All races and age groups
- Most common at ages 60–70 years

Risk Factors
- Pregnancy, elderly, alcoholics
- Malnourished or malabsorption syndromes; hemodialysis patients
- Medications that interfere with folic acid absorption (e.g., trimethoprim, phenytoin, oral birth control pills, phenobarbital, sulfamethoxazole/trimethoprim, sulfasalazine)

Prevention and Screening
- Adequate intake of folic acid: 400 mcg for pregnant women, 200 mcg for all others

Assessment

HISTORY
- Indigestion, constipation, diarrhea, anorexia, lethargy
- Fatigue, weakness, headache, dizziness, dyspnea on exertion, depression, apathy

PHYSICAL EXAM
- Pallor, atrophic glossitis (red, shiny tongue), stomatitis
- Change in mental status, confusion but no focal neurologic deficits
- Tachycardia, wide pulse pressure, heart murmur
- Peripheral neuropathy

DIAGNOSTIC STUDIES
- CBC, RBC folate more reliable for diagnosis than serum folate; serum B12, TIBC, LDH, RDW
- Laboratory results: Serum folate <3 nanograms/mL, RBC folate <150 nanograms/mL, Hct decreased, Hgb normal, RDW elevated, TIBC normal, LDH and MCV elevated >100 mcg/mL; MCHC normal, Schilling test normal, serum B12 normal

Differential Diagnosis
- Vitamin B12 efficiency
- Myelodysplastic syndromes
- Pernicious anemia
- Hypothyroidism

Management

NONPHARMACOLOGIC TREATMENT
- Education and supportive therapy; good oral hygiene
- Folate rich diet: Green leafy vegetables, red beans, wheat bran, fish, bananas, asparagus
- Need for frequent rest

PHARMACOLOGIC TREATMENT
- Folic acid replacement 400 mcg for pregnant women, 200 mcg for all others
  - Prescription supplements usually contain 1 mg folic acid, but be aware that supplementation of greater than 400 mcg may mask B12 deficiency

LENGTH OF TREATMENT
- Treat until anemia corrected, usually about 2 months until folic acid stores replenished
- Duration of treatment depends on elimination of underlying cause

Special Considerations
- Folate body stores can be depleted in about 4 months
- Women on birth control who are potentially child-bearing should routinely take folic acid preparations to decrease incidence of embryonic neural tube defects

When to Consult, Refer, Hospitalize
- Not usually needed; refer patients that do not improve with therapy

Follow-Up
- In 2 months and periodically thereafter
    EXPECTED COURSE
    - Good prognosis

    COMPLICATIONS
    - Failure to thrive
    - Neural tube defects of infants born to deficient women

Hemolytic Anemias

Hemolytic conditions produce anemias in which accelerated RBC destruction occurs as a result of an intrinsic genetic RBC defect as seen in hemoglobinopathies (sickle cell and thalassemia), in metabolic enzyme deficiencies (G6PD), or in cytoskeleton disorders (spherocytosis or elliptocytosis). The intrinsic destruction could also be acquired as seen in paroxysmal nocturnal hemoglobinuria or alcoholic cirrhosis. Extrinsic causes of hemolysis include antibody-mediated processes such as autoimmune reactions, drug-related reactions, transfusion reactions, and reactions to infections.

Important Features
- Peripheral blood smear shows spherocytosis and may be hyperchromic
- Coombs test will be positive in immune hemolysis
- An elevated reticulocyte count in the patient with anemia is the most useful indicator of hemolysis
- Other laboratory findings include increased unconjugated bilirubin (indirect), decreased heptoglobin, possible increase in LDH, increased urine hemoglobin, increased urine bilirubin. Hemosiderin is a delayed sign and may represent chronic hemolysis.
- Bone marrow shows normoblastic erythroid hyperplasia
- The most common and clinically observed hemolytic anemias are discussed here

Sickle Cell Anemia/Trait

Description
- Sickle cell disease (SSD) is a group of hemoglobin disorders characterized by production of hemoglobin S (HbS); the most common of which is sickle cell anemia (HbSS). Other common genotypes are sickle-cell C (HbSC) and sickle beta-thalassemia (HbS beta-thalassemia). Severe hemolytic anemia may be produced in which abnormal hemoglobin (due to DNA point mutation in the B-globin chain) leads to chronic hemolytic anemia, with recurrent painful crises in individuals who are homozygous for hemoglobin S.
- Sickle cell disorders are characterized by chronic hemolytic anemia.

Etiology
- Hemoglobin S readily deforms the RBC into a sickle shape, the sickle cells hemolyze, and clusters of sickle cells occlude small blood vessels
- Autosomal recessive gene (hemoglobin S gene from each parent)
- Sickle cell trait (Hgb AS) is seen when one normal Hgb gene and one sickle hemoglobin-producing gene are inherited from the parents; this will not cause sickle cell disease.

Incidence and Demographics

- Sickle cell anemia present in about 1 in 400–500 African Americans; 8%–10% of African Americans carry hemoglobin S gene
- No gender predominance; onset in first year of life

Risk Factors

- Factors that precipitate sickle cell crisis:
  - Deoxygenation of Hgb molecule, as in high altitude
  - Infection
  - Dehydration
  - Overexertion/stress
  - Exposure to extreme temperatures, hot or cold

Prevention and Screening

- Screening for sickle cell trait and genetic counseling for couples at risk; prenatal diagnosis via chorionic villus sampling or amniocentesis
- Universal newborn screening
- Good health maintenance with anticipatory guidance for potential complications
- All regular immunizations as well as pneumococcal and influenza (yearly) vaccinations
- Recognition and avoidance of known pain-precipitating factors

Assessment

HISTORY

- Hemolytic anemia starting in first year of life
- Family history of sickle cell anemia or trait
- Sickle cell trait may be asymptomatic unless provoked by exertion at high altitudes
- Sickle cell anemia: Acute, sudden, excruciating episodes with pain in long bones, back, chest, abdomen; priapism; chronic leg ulcers; delayed puberty

PHYSICAL EXAM

- May include chronically ill appearance, jaundice
- Splenomegaly (primarily in children)
- Hot, tender, swollen joints
- Retinopathy
- Cardiomegaly (laterally displaced point of maximum impulse (PMI), systolic murmur
- Chronic lower leg ulcers, blood loss

DIAGNOSTIC STUDIES

- Hgb electrophoresis: Definitive diagnostic test
- CBC: Classic findings (by age 1 year) include Hct in the 20s, reticulocyte count in the 20s, normal MCV, slightly elevated WBC count, and elevated platelet count
- Peripheral blood smear: Fragmented cells, long crescent-shaped irreversible sickled cells, target cells, Howell-Jolly bodies, and occasional nucleated red blood cells

- Elevated LDH and indirect bilirubin during increased hemolysis
- Laboratory results: Hgb decreased, MCV might be elevated slightly, chronic neutrophilia, increased platelet count, erythrocytes with classic sickle shape on peripheral smear, Hgb S predominates

Differential Diagnosis

- Other hemoglobinopathies (e.g., hemoglobin C, D, or E)
- Compound hemoglobinopathies (e.g., hemoglobin SC disease, hemoglobin S beta thalassemia)

Management

NONPHARMACOLOGIC TREATMENT

- Hydration, nonpharmacologic pain modalities, patient and family education and supportive care, genetic counseling

PHARMACOLOGIC TREATMENT

- Do not give iron (increases Hgb S production)
- Manage pain (often narcotic analgesia will be needed)
- Folic acid 1–2 mg po daily
- Oxygen for hypoxia
- Consider transfusion

LENGTH OF TREATMENT

- Lifelong

Special Considerations

- In some patients, hydroxyurea 500–750 mg daily may decrease number of painful crises (long-term safety unknown)
- Individuals have different patterns of crisis
- Crises might increase during pregnancy

When to Consult, Refer, Hospitalize

- Refer all suspected cases to a hematologist; hospitalize for acute episodes of sickling
- Consult with physician for specialized care in the primary care setting
- Any temperature of >38.5° Celsius (101.3°F) must be considered a medical emergency and hospitalized immediately

Follow-Up

EXPECTED COURSE

- Number of crises decrease in young adulthood but complications increase
- Life expectancy is 60 years

COMPLICATIONS

- Anemia, bone infarct, cerebrovascular accident (CVA), cardiac enlargement, priapism, retinopathy, acute chest syndrome, infections, gallstones, hemosiderosis (secondary to multiple transfusions), increased fetal loss during pregnancy, and sepsis

Thalassemia

Description
- A group of hereditary disorders with hypochromic microcytic anemia because of gene deletion or point mutation; causes abnormal synthesis of alpha and beta globin chains resulting in abnormal hemoglobin synthesis and displacement of hemoglobin A1 with abnormal types—microcytosis is out of proportion to the degree of anemia.

Etiology
- Autosomal recessive genetic disorder producing defective hemoglobinization of red blood cells. Normal adult hemoglobin, Hgb A, has four chains or globins, two alpha and two beta. Delta and gamma chains are similar to beta and are found in Hemoglobin A2 (two gamma, two delta chains), and Hemoglobin F (fetal Hgb, two delta and two gamma chains). Hemoglobin cannot be formed without the α chains; unaffected individuals have 4 copies of gene for α globin.
- *Alpha thalassemia* is a result of a gene deletion where not enough alpha chains can be synthesized.
- *Beta thalassemia* results when point mutation causes decreased or no synthesis of beta chains.
- *Thalassemia major* (beta) occurs when unbalanced hemoglobin chain synthesis results in severe anemia (usually presents in infants or young children).
- *Thalassemia intermedia* is a more minor form of beta thalassemia; may or may not need transfusions.
- *Thalassemia trait* (alpha or beta) is a milder form of anemia, not requiring aggressive therapy.

Incidence and Demographics
- Alpha thalassemia: People originating from Southeast Asia, China, occasionally Africa
- Beta thalassemia: People originating from the Mediterranean, also, less commonly, Asia and Africa; about 1,000 patients with severe thalassemia in the U.S.
- Trait present in 3%–5% of at-risk populations

Risk Factors
- One or both parents with any combination of alpha and/or beta thalassemia syndromes

Prevention and Screening
- Screening of prospective parents at risk (ideally prior to pregnancy), genetic counseling
- Prenatal diagnosis (fetal blood sampling or chorionic villus sampling) if desired

Assessment
HISTORY
- Alpha trait (one of four alpha genes affected) usually asymptomatic; alpha-thalassemia minor (two of four alpha genes affected) and beta-thalassemia (heterozygous form) are mild forms, usually asymptomatic; beta-thalassemia major (Cooley's anemia—both genes affected)—easy fatigueability, palpitations, shortness of breath with exertion, headaches
- Family or personal history of lifelong anemia
- Infants and children with thalassemia major will have symptoms of severe and chronic anemia: Pallor, shortness of breath, lethargy

- Children and adults with thalassemia trait may present with history of unresponsive anemia or signs of iron toxicity

PHYSICAL EXAM
- Normal exam in thalassemia minor syndromes
- Pallor and enlarged spleen in alpha thalassemia with one alpha globin gene (also called hemoglobin H disease)
- Multiple abnormalities in thalassemia major (homozygous beta thalassemia) starting in infancy: bony deformities, jaundice, enlarged spleen, and enlarged liver

DIAGNOSTIC STUDIES (SEE TABLE 16-4)
- CBC with attention to RBC morphology and hemoglobin electrophoresis, iron studies
- Laboratory results: Microcytic, hypochromic, acanthocytes, target cells, serum iron and TIBC normal to increased, serum ferritin >100

Table 16-4. Diagnostic Studies Used in Thalassemia

Diagnostic Studies	Findings
Alpha Thalassemia Trait	Hematocrit 28%–40%
	Very low MCV (60–75 mcg/mL)
	Reticulocyte count normal
	Iron parameters normal
	Mild anemia; significant microcytosis
Alpha Thalassemia Minor and Beta Thalassemia Minor	Hematocrit 28%–40%
	MCV 55–75 mcg/mL
	Reticulocyte count normal or slightly elevated
	Iron parameters normal
	Hemoglobin electrophoresis shows elevation HgB A2 to 4%–8% and occasional Hgb F to 1%–5%
Beta Thalassemia Major	Hematocrit 10%
	MCV <75 mcg/mL
	Peripheral blood smear: severe poikilocytoses, hypochromia, basophilic stippling, and nucleated red blood cells; virtually no Hgb A present; major hemoglobin present in Hgb F
Hemoglobin H Disease	Hematocrit 22%–32%
	MCV <7 mcg/mL
	Peripheral blood smear markedly abnormal: hypochromia, microcytosis, poikilocytosis
	Reticulocyte count elevated
	Hemoglobin electrophoresis shows HgbH as 10%–40% of Hgb

Differential Diagnosis
- Iron deficiency anemia
- Combined hemoglobinopathies

Management

- No treatment needed for beta thalassemia minor or alpha thalassemia trait
  NONPHARMACOLOGIC TREATMENT
    - Severe thalassemia major: Regular transfusions; bone marrow transplants in children; splenectomy if needed; patient and family education and supportive care

  PHARMACOLOGIC TREATMENT
    - Folic acid supplementation
    - Iron chelation therapy with deferoxamine (Desferal)
    - Appropriate immunizations (especially if splenectomy contemplated)
    - Avoid iron supplements and iron-fortified foods; avoid oxidative drugs (e.g., sulfonamides)

  LENGTH OF TREATMENT
    - Lifelong

Special Considerations

- Support for family as coping with guilt is a major problem for parents

When to Consult, Refer, Hospitalize

- Consult or refer when diagnosis is in question; refer all patients with thalassemia major or intermedia to hematologist, hospitalize for complications. Refer all patients with severe disease to specialty clinic experienced in iron chelation and transfusions.

Follow-Up

- Follow-up depends on severity of disease
  EXPECTED COURSE
    - Thalassemia minor: Benign
    - Thalassemia intermedia: Patients have chronic hemolytic anemia but will generally only need transfusions when under stress; live into adulthood
    - Children with thalassemia major die in their teens or even younger unless they receive regular transfusions and iron chelation therapy; with compliance, live well into adulthood

  COMPLICATIONS
    - Limited growth and bony deformities; iron overload (due to frequent transfusions), which can cause cirrhosis, diabetes, cardiac dysfunction (including arrhythmia); failure of sexual maturation; decreased life expectancy

Glucose-6-Phosphate Dehydrogenase (G6PD) Deficiency

Description
- An anemia of red blood cell destruction (hemolysis), occurring suddenly and episodically when red blood cells are under oxidative stress from acute illness or certain medications

Etiology
- Most common form of G6PD deficiency is an X-linked, recessive hereditary enzyme defect.
- The lack of enzyme leaves RBCs vulnerable to attack, causing hemolysis.
- G6PD can result in neonatal hyperbilirubinemia.

Incidence and Demographics
- Seen in African Americans and those of Mediterranean descent
- 7%–15% of African-American males affected
- Mediterranean variant is less common but poses a more severe deficiency of G6PD

Risk Factors
- Episode of hemolysis may be provoked by infection; oxidant drugs, such as certain antibiotics (e.g., dapsone, nalidixic acid, nitrofurantoin, sulfonamides), antimalarials (e.g., primaquine, quinine), phenazopyridine, doxorubicin, quinidine, and others; ingestion of fava beans

Prevention and Screening
- Immunizations (influenza, pneumococcal pneumonia, hepatitis B) and measures to avoid infections
- Avoid known oxidant drugs
- Family and genetic counseling as indicated
- Avoid specific drugs list in Box 16-1, stress, and fava beans

Assessment
HISTORY
- Family history, medication history for oxidative drugs
- May be no history of anemia or anemia is mild so patient may only be symptomatic of the underlying infection

PHYSICAL EXAM
- Signs of mild anemia, signs of underlying infection
- Splenomegaly may be present

Box 16-1. Substances for People with G6PD Deficiency to Avoid

Analgesics	Antimalarials	Other
Aspirin	Primaquine	Vitamin K (OK in the newborn)
Phenacetin	Chloroquine	Probenecid
	Quinacrine	Dimercaprol (BAL)
	Pamaquine	Fava beans
		Mothballs (naphthalene)
		Henna
Antibiotics	**Antihelminths**	**Illness**
Sulfonamides	B Naphthol	Diabetic ketoacidosis
Chloramphenicol	Stibophen	Hepatitis
Dapsone	Niridazole	Other
Nitrofurans (Macrodantin)		
Nalidixic acid		

Adapted from *Essence of office pediatrics* (p. 161) by J. Stockman & J. Lohr, 2001, Philadelphia: W. B. Saunders.

DIAGNOSTIC STUDIES
- CBC, reticulocytes, indirect bilirubin, G6PD
- In infants, direct and indirect Coombs test should be done to exclude autoimmune hemolytic anemia
- Usual laboratory results: CBC normal between episodes along with Heinz bodies and low level of G6PD; during episodes of hemolysis there is increased reticulocytes, increased indirect bilirubin, decreased RBC, decreased Hgb, decreased Hct

Differential Diagnosis
- Suspect Mediterranean variant if anemia is severe
- Iron deficiency anemia
- Combined anemias, (e.g., G6PD deficiency and sickle cell anemia)
- Acute hemolytic transfusion reactions (Coombs +)

Management
- Supportive
- Find and eliminate anemia trigger

Special Considerations
- Anemic episodes are self-limiting

When to Consult, Refer, Hospitalize
- Refer severe variants with exacerbations; refer patients with combined anemias

Follow-Up
- For exacerbations
  EXPECTED COURSE
  - There is usually a spontaneous resolution of the anemia as older RBCs with minimal enzyme activity are destroyed and then replaced with new RBCs that have enough (even though reduced) enzyme activity

  COMPLICATIONS
  - Generally none
  - Possible severe hemolytic anemia and death with the Mediterranean variant

Immune Hemolysis

Description
- Red cell destruction occurs as a result of the binding of antibodies or complement components to the erythrocyte membrane. This may occur as a result of autoimmunization, alloimmunization, or drug reactions.
- Warm-reacting antibodies hemolyze optimally at 37°C
- Cold-reacting antibodies hemolyze optimally at 30°C

Etiology
- IgM (cold) and IgG (warm) antibodies induce red cell destruction after binding with antigens on the RBC wall. This binding causes a complement cascade resulting in defective RBCs, which are prematurely removed and destroyed by hepatic macrophages.

Incidence and Demographics
- Seen in all races and in all age groups
- Warm agglutinin disease associated with neoplastic or collagen vascular disorder in 40% of the cases
- Cold agglutinin disease seen in patients with lymphoproliferative disorders, infectious diseases (Epstein-Barr virus [EBV], cytomegalovirus [CMV]), and in the elderly, and is usually a diagnosis of exclusion

Risk Factors
- Systemic lupus erythematosus, rheumatoid arthritis
- Adenocarcinoma of the stomach, ovarian teratoma, chronic lymphocytic leukemia

Prevention and Screening
- Screening of prospective parents at risk (ideally prior to pregnancy), genetic counseling

Assessment
  HISTORY
  - Family or personal history of any of the above states
  - Acute episodes may present with dizziness, exertional dyspnea, palpitations, and fatigue

PHYSICAL EXAM
- In warm agglutinin disease, chronic effects are mild and may present with jaundice and/or splenomegaly; acute episodes may present with pallor in addition to above symptoms
- In cold agglutinin disease secondary to infections, symptoms are short-lived and mild in most cases. In disease associated with neoplastic or idiopathic disorders, exposure to cold may lead to severe acrocyanosis and Raynaud's-type reactions worsened by cold

DIAGNOSTIC STUDIES
- CBC with attention to RBC morphology; spherocytosis dramatically increased
- In cold agglutinin disease, blood clots at times upon being removed from the vein, distorting the red cell count, MCV, and hematocrit. The serum haptoglobin is decreased and LDH is increased

Differential Diagnosis
- Thalassemia
- Sickle cell disease
- Paroxysmal nocturnal hemoglobinuria
- Hypersplenism

Management
- Warm agglutinin disease:
  - Glucocorticoids
  - Splenectomy
  - Immunosuppressive drugs: Cyclophosphamide, azathioprine
  - Transfusion
- Cold agglutinin disease:
  - Identify underlying cause
  - Chlorambucil (Leukeran) 2–4 mg, up to 10 mg daily
  - Advise to move to a warmer climate
  - Avoid transfusions, but when needed, infuse warmed, well-matched products

Special Considerations
- None

When to Consult, Refer, Hospitalize
- Consult with physician or refer to hematologist for acute episodes

Follow-Up
EXPECTED COURSE
- Warm agglutinin disease is usually chronic so prognosis is affected by the underlying disease
- If cold agglutinin disease related to an infectious syndrome, complete cure occurs when the infection is cleared
- Otherwise, course is similar to warm agglutinin disease

COMPLICATIONS
- Major cause of death related to a thromboembolic event

OTHER PROBLEMS OF IRON AND RED BLOOD CELLS

Hemochromatosis

Description
- An autosomal recessive inherited disorder resulting in an excess of iron stores in the liver, pancreas, heart, kidneys, adrenals, testes, and pituitary gland as hemosiderin

Etiology
- This disorder results in inefficient erythropoiesis
- It is the most common iron storage and genetic liver disease in the U.S.

Incidence and Demographics
- 3/1,000 in the U.S.
- Seen in men more than women
- Presentation seen during person's middle years

Risk Factors
- Alcohol ingestion, iron supplementation, chronic transfusions, ingestion of large amounts of vitamin C
- Type 2 diabetes, B-thalassemia

Prevention and Screening
- Genetic counseling
- Screening of family members of patient with hereditary hemochromatosis

Assessment
HISTORY
- Often asymptomatic
- Weakness, dyspnea on exertion, lassitude, weight loss
- Loss of libido, impotence, testicular atrophy, amenorrhea
- Slate- or brown-colored skin, alopecia
- Abdominal pain

PHYSICAL EXAM
- Hepatosplenomegaly, ascites, cardiomyopathy, peripheral edema, arthropathy
- Changes in skin pigmentation: Slate gray or brown

DIAGNOSTIC STUDIES
- Liver biopsy is the diagnostic gold standard
- Laboratory results: Blood glucose elevated, AST increased, serum albumin decreased, FSH and LH decreased, serum ferritin >300 units/L for men and >120 units/L for women, transferrin saturation high, urinary iron present

Differential Diagnosis
- Cirrhosis
- Excessive iron ingestion
- Repeated transfusions

Management
NONPHARMACOLOGIC TREATMENT
- Regular diet; avoid iron-fortified foods and iron supplements, increase tea intake (chelates iron), restrict vitamin C to small amounts between meals
- Phlebotomy of 500 mL initially 1–2x/week until mild anemia, then 4–6x/year maintenance

PHARMACOLOGIC TREATMENT
- Use iron-chelating agent only if phlebotomy is not feasible or diagnosis is secondary hematochromatosis

LENGTH OF TREATMENT
- Treat initially until patient is iron deficient (mild anemia), then lifelong maintenance therapy

Special Considerations
- Menstruation delays onset of symptoms in women
- Problem uncommon in people with African or Asian heritage

When to Consult, Refer, Hospitalize
- Refer to hematologist to confirm initial diagnosis and consult throughout therapy; hematology office or infusion center for phlebotomy.

Follow-Up
EXPECTED COURSE
- Usually normal life expectancy, but if more than 18 months needed to achieve mild anemia, life expectancy is decreased

COMPLICATIONS
- Cirrhosis, type 1 diabetes, hepatocellular carcinoma, arthritis, cardiomyopathy

Polycythemia Vera

Description
- Chronic, acquired myeloproliferative disorder showing overproduction of red blood cell mass resulting in an elevation in hematocrit and red blood cell mass (males Hct >51%, females Hct >48%)

Etiology
- As a primary disorder is a hematologic malignancy with excessive erythroid, myeloid, and megakaryocytic elements in the bone marrow
- Secondary causes are lung disease, heart disease, kidney disease, and possible other malignancies

Incidence and Demographics
- Prevalence = 1–3/100,000
- Most common in newborn or age >60

Risk Factors
- Moore prevalent in people with Ashkenazi Jewish ancestry
- Smoking
- Age >60 years

Prevention and Screening
- Cannot prevent onset
- No routine screening currently recommended
- Often found as a result of blood studies performed for other reasons
- Advise patients to seek medical attention for onset of: Headache; dizziness; blurred vision; tinnitus; vertigo; spontaneous bruising; menorrhagia; peripheral cyanosis; epistaxis; upper GI bleed; pruritus, especially after bathing; rib and sternal bone pain/ tenderness; sweating; weight loss; fatigue

Assessment
HISTORY
- May be no symptoms in early stages or vague symptoms
- Headache, dizziness, blurred vision, tinnitus, vertigo
- Spontaneous bruising, menorrhagia, peripheral cyanosis, epistaxis, upper GI bleed
- Pruritus, especially after bathing
- Rib and sternal bone pain/tenderness
- Sweating, weight loss, fatigue

PHYSICAL EXAM
- Plethora (reddish flush of skin) on face, hands, feet
- Elevated systolic blood pressure, epistaxis, distended retinal veins
- Hepatosplenomegaly
- Do complete exam to look for underlying cause

DIAGNOSTIC STUDIES
- CBC with differential, serum B12, chemistries, indirect bilirubin, bone marrow aspiration, CT for underlying malignancy
- Laboratory results: Increased Hgb and Hct, thrombocytosis, leukocytosis, increased leukocyte alkaline phosphatase, increased serum vitamin B12, indirect bilirubin elevated

Differential Diagnosis
- Secondary polycythemia
- Secondary erythrocytosis
- Spurious polycythemia
- Hemoglobinopathy

Management
NONPHARMACOLOGIC TREATMENT
- Phlebotomy to remove 500 cc weekly until hematocrit 45%; patient/family education and support

PHARMACOLOGIC TREATMENT
- Medications for hyperacidity, pruritus, uric acid reduction as needed
- Hydroxyurea may be used, a myelosuppressive agent

LENGTH OF TREATMENT
- Lifelong

Special Considerations
- Phlebotomy worsens iron deficiency but iron supplement not recommended
- Benign polycythemia caused by high-altitude dwelling

When to Consult, Refer, Hospitalize
- Refer to hematologist for management

Follow-up
EXPECTED COURSE
- Survival with treatment = up to 10 years; without = 6–18 months

COMPLICATIONS
- Vascular thrombosis, leukemia, hemorrhage, peptic ulcer, gout

WHITE BLOOD CELL (WBC)–RELATED PROBLEMS

Leukemia

Description
- The leukemias are a collection of disorders that produce a variety of bone marrow and white blood cell abnormalities that may be quickly fatal or may remain asymptomatic for years.
- Types include:
  - Malignant proliferation of immature lymphocytes (acute lymphocytic leukemia—ALL) or myeloid cells (acute myeloid leukemia—AML or acute nonlymphocytic leukemia—ANLL)
  - Proliferation of mature-appearing neoplastic lymphocytes (chronic lymphocytic leukemia—CLL) or immature granulocytes (chronic myeloid leukemia—CML)
  - Rarely: Proliferation of mature B cells with prominent projections (hairy cell leukemia)

Etiology
- Unknown malignancy that affects the bone marrow and other organs; may be due to exposure to chemicals and/or ionizing radiation, genetic factors (chromosomal abnormalities), viral agents
- Commonly see elevated WBC, abnormal WBCs on blood smear, bone marrow failure, and involvement of other organs

Incidence and Demographics

- ALL: Most common childhood malignancy with peak incidence at 4 years of age, most common in Caucasians and boys, higher incidence in industrialized countries; adult ALL approximately 100 cases/year in U.S.
- AML or ANLL: 50% of cases under age 50
- CLL: Most common form of adult leukemia in Western countries, occurring during middle age and in the elderly
- CML: Middle age
- Hairy cell leukemia: Rare, disease of old age

Risk Factors

- Several immunodeficiency states have an associated risk for lymphoma and leukemia in children (Wiskott-Aldrich, X-linked agammaglobulinemia, severe combined immune deficiency, and ataxia telangiectasia)
- Chemical and/or radiation exposure
- Chromosomal abnormalities
- Cigarette smoking
- Some types increase with age

Prevention and Screening

- Currently there is no standard screening process to detect early stages of leukemia.
- There is no way to prevent leukemia, but an individual can make lifestyle changes to lower risk.
- Educate patients to report new onset of symptoms early.
- Patients with family history of leukemia should have regular physical examinations.
- Patients who have been treated with chemotherapy for other types of cancers should have regular physical examinations.
- Avoid exposure to chemicals such as benzene.
- Quit smoking or don't start.

Assessment

HISTORY
- General: Fever, malaise, weakness, bruising, bleeding weight loss
- ALL: Joint pain, limping, anorexia, infection
- AML: Sternal tenderness
- CLL: Might be asymptomatic, dyspnea on exertion
- CML: Might be asymptomatic, night sweats, blurred vision, anorexia, respiratory distress, sternal tenderness

PHYSICAL EXAM
- Lymphadenopathy, confirmation of symptoms
- ALL: Generalized lymphadenopathy, hepatosplenomegaly, petechiae and purpura
- AML: Mouth sores, occasional lymphadenopathy
- CLL: Hepatosplenomegaly, lymphadenopathy, sustained absolute lymphocytosis, bone marrow + lymphocytes
- CML: Splenomegaly, priapism, Philadelphia chromosome in bone marrow

DIAGNOSTIC STUDIES
- CBC with differential and platelet, peripheral smear, chemistries, reticulocyte count, bone marrow aspiration
- Laboratory results: Decreased RBC, neutrophils, platelets, reticulocyte count; elevated LDH and uric acid
- Consider chest x-ray, ultrasound or CT scan, coagulation profile
- ALL: Peripheral blood lymphoblasts
- CLL: Sustained absolute lymphocytosis, bone marrow + lymphocytes
- CML: Philadelphia chromosome in bone marrow

Differential Diagnosis
- Aplastic anemia
- Viral diseases
- Mononucleosis
- Pertussis
- Paroxysmal nocturnal hemoglobinuria
- Gaucher's disease
- Myelodysplasia syndromes

Management
NONPHARMACOLOGIC TREATMENT
- Good diet, compliance with treatment, management of side effects, chronic effects of diagnosis
- Avoid activities that might cause injury; avoid medications that affect platelets (e.g., aspirin)
- Bone marrow transplantation

PHARMACOLOGIC TREATMENT
- Chemotherapy, infection prevention medications
- Hospitalization required for induction of chemotherapy
- Interferon treatment for CML

LENGTH OF TREATMENT
- Goal is remission

Special Considerations
- Children with ALL may benefit from referral to specialty center involved in clinical trials.
- Patients with leukemia are prone to other infections.

When to Consult, Refer, Hospitalize
- Refer to hematologist upon suspicion of diagnosis and will be followed by hematologist throughout therapy

Follow-up
EXPECTED COURSE
- ALL: Remission rate is very good
- AML: Remission rate is 60%–80%
- CLL: Depends on stage at diagnosis; median survival about 9 years

- CML: Usually transforms into the acute phase within 2 years, then poor survival rate
- Patients who have undergone stem cell transplantation have a 10-year survival rate of 70%

COMPLICATIONS
- Infections, bleeding, side effects of chemotherapy and/or radiation, relapses

COAGULATION DISORDERS

Idiopathic Thrombocytopenia Purpura (ITP)

Description
- An autoimmune disorder characterized by accelerated, spleen-mediated platelet destruction, resulting in a decreased platelet count (<100,000/mL) that predisposes the patient to a decreased ability for primary clotting. May be acute (with spontaneous resolution within 2 months after an acute infection—usually children) or chronic (persists >6 months without identifiable cause—usually adults). IgG autoantibody binds to platelets, splenic macrophages bind to antibody-tagged platelets and destroy them.

Etiology
- Unknown, perhaps autoimmune response after viral illness

Incidence and Demographics
- Predominantly occurs in pediatric population; uncommon in geriatric population
- Slight seasonal peaks in winter and spring
- Adult female-to-male ratio = 3:1; most common acquired platelet disorder of childhood

Risk Factors
- No genetic predispositions described
- Acute infection (usually viral, e.g., varicella, EBV, CMV), HIV, cardiopulmonary bypass, hypersplenism, preeclampsia
- Exposure to drugs with antiplatelet effects (aspirin, seizure medications, heparin)
- History of autoimmune diseases (rheumatoid or collagen vascular symptoms, thyroid disease, hemolytic anemia)

Prevention and Screening
- None

Assessment
HISTORY
- Insidious onset in otherwise well person
- Prolonged purpura, bruising tendency, gingival bleeding, menorrhagia, epistaxis, petcchiae
- History of acute viral illness

PHYSICAL EXAM
- Nonpalpable spleen is essential criterion
- Signs of GI bleeding, dysmorphic features

DIAGNOSTIC STUDIES
- Often diagnosed on routine CBC with differential and platelets; also get peripheral smear; consider HIV, liver function, CT abdomen, stool guaiac as needed
- Laboratory results: Platelets decreased, normal RBC and WBC morphology

Differential Diagnosis
- Viral infection
- SLE
- Bone marrow disorders
- AIDS
- Drug-induced
- Hemolytic-uremic syndrome
- Liver disease
- Congenital thrombocytopenia (e.g., Fanconi syndrome)
- Sepsis

Management

NONPHARMACOLOGIC TREATMENT
- Education and supportive care
- Avoid medications that increase bleeding risk
- Decrease activities that might cause bruising, injury
- Monitor patient for platelet count, associated symptoms

PHARMACOLOGIC TREATMENT
- Acute: Prednisone 1–2 mg/kg qd for 4 weeks, then taper
- Chronic: 60 mg/day for 4–6 weeks, then taper
- Severe: IV gamma globulin (IVGG) 0.4 g/kg/day for 3–5 days or high dose parenteral glucocorticoids
- Platelet transfusion ONLY during life–threatening hemorrhage
- Splenectomy if platelets <30,000 after 6 weeks of pharmacologic treatment (splenectomy response not good if IVGG response poor)

LENGTH OF TREATMENT
- Until remission

Special Considerations
- Focus: Bleeding, exclusion of other diagnoses

When to Consult, Refer, Hospitalize
- Any febrile child with thrombocytopenia and petechiae (with or without elevated PT and PTT) should be hospitalized and treated for presumed sepsis.
- Refer all suspected cases to hematologist; refer to surgeon for splenectomy.

Follow-Up

EXPECTED COURSE
- Acute = 80%–85% remission, 15% become chronic; chronic = 20% spontaneous remission

COMPLICATIONS
- Cerebral hemorrhage (1% mortality); other blood loss, pneumococcal infection

CASE STUDIES

Case 1. L. O. is a 9-month-old Hispanic male brought to the clinic by his mother for a routine well-child check-up. His mother states all is going well. L.O. lives at home with his mother, father, and his maternal grandmother, who cares for him while his parents are at work. He is eating table food and drinking cow's milk.

PMH: UTD on immunizations; no illnesses requiring antibiotics. Current medications: none.

Exam: This is a very plump male infant who is interactive with his mother and the examiner. His vital signs are WNL. His weight is in the 95th percentile for his age whereas his height is in the 50th percentile. In your office setting you perform a Hgb which is 9g.

1. What additional history would you like?
2. What type of anemia is most likely in this case?
3. What is the most likely cause of L.O.'s anemia?
4. What corrective actions might you recommend at this time?

Case 2. B.C. is a 48-year-old White female who presents to your clinic complaining of feeling tired all the time. She works full time and cares for her elderly mother in the home. B.C. reports "getting plenty of sleep and eating well." She finds little time for exercise and "doesn't have the energy to even go for a walk." ROS: Pertinent only for heavy bleeding during her periods which she states began about 8 months ago. B.C. reports having to stay close to home and using a hand towel to supplement peri-pads.

PMH: Denies any hospitalizations or surgeries. Anemia during pregnancy. LMP: 1 week prior to clinic visit. Otherwise healthy; does not smoke or drink alcohol.

1. What type of physical exam would you do?
2. At this point what might you include in your differential diagnosis?
3. What diagnostic studies would you order?

Test Results: Hgb: 10g; RBC: 3.6; MCV: 72; TSH: 1.56 (normal)

4. What would your recommendations be for B.C. at this point?

Case 3. B.W., an 85-year-old African-American male, is brought to clinic by his daughter for evaluation of possible dementia. She is worried that he cannot care for himself as evidenced by the fact that he forgets his car at church some Sundays and walks home, and by his apparent weight loss. She is concerned that he cannot prepare his own meals anymore.

PMH: Hypertension—controlled; bladder irritability responsive to medication. NKDA; currently taking Vasotec 5 mg qd, Ditropan 5 mg qd

SH: B.W. lives alone in his own home one block from his church. There is a gentleman who lives on his block who assists him with paying his bills, going for doctor's appointments, and getting medication refills. B.W. reports being able to fix his own meals and denies feeling hungry.

ROS: Denies SOB, CP, anorexia, but admits he has lost some weight. Denies bowel changes. Does have some trouble remembering things but has always been able to find his car because the only time he drives is to church.

1. What would you include in your differential diagnosis at this time?

Exam: Alert, well-dressed 85-year-old African-American male who looks younger than his stated age. His vital signs are WNL. He scores 27 on the MMSE. CN II–XII are intact. He is able to ambulate without assistance. Romberg's intact, no evidence of ataxia. No lymphadenopathy. Lungs are clear without adventitious breath sounds. Heart: Regular rate and rhythm without murmur or gallop. Abd: no distention, bowel sounds positive. No palpable masses. No hepatosplenomegaly or CVAT. Genital exam WNL. Rectal exam: Normal size prostate, enlarged without nodules. Stool is brown and heme negative.

2. What diagnostic studies would you order at this time?
3. B.W. comes to see you 1 week later and has the following laboratory results: Hgb: 9 g; Hct: 27.2%; MCV=72; reported as hypochromic; all other parameters are WNL. He has lost two more pounds, despite the fact that his daughter has been cooking for him and encouraging him to eat. His FOBT are all positive. What type of anemia does this man most likely have and what would be the next step in your diagnostic work-up of this gentleman?

REFERENCES

Andreoli, T. E. (Ed.). (2007). *Cecil essentials of medicine* (7th ed.). Philadelphia: W. B. Saunders Elsevier.

Beghe, C., Wilson, A., & Ershler, W. B. (2004). Prevalence and outcomes of anemia in geriatrics: A systematic review of the literature. *American Journal of Medicine, 116*(Suppl 7A), 3S–10S.

Fauci, A.S., Braunwald E., Kaspar, D.L., Hauser, S. L., Longon, D. L., Jameson, J. L., et al. (Ed). (2007). *Harrison's principles of internal medicine* (17th ed.). New York: McGraw-Hill.

Dambro, M. R. (2006). *The 5 minute clinical consult.* St. Louis, MO: Lippincott Williams & Wilkins.

Dodd, J., Dare, M., & Middleton, P. (2004). Treatment for women with postpartum iron deficiency anemia. *Cochrane Database of Systematic Reviews, 18*(4), CD004222. Retrieved July 7, 2008, from http://mrw.interscience.wiley.com/cochrane/clsysrev/articles/CD004222/frame.html

Ferri, F. F. (2008). *Ferri's clinical advisor 2008* (11th ed.). St. Louis, MO: Elsevier Mosby.

Frank, J. E. (2005). Diagnosis and management of G6PD deficiency. *American Family Physician, 72*, 1277–1282. Retrieved July 7, 2008, from http://www.aafp.org/afp/20051001/1277.html

Goolsby, M. J., & Grubbs, L. (2006). *Advanced assessment: Interpreting findings and formulating differential diagnoses.* Philadelphia: F. A. Davis.

Hebbar, A. K., Gibson, M. V., & D'Epiro, P. (2006). Recognizing and managing anemia of chronic disease. *Patient Care for the Nurse Practitioner, 40*(11), 36–40.

Hoffman, P. C. (2006). Immune hemolytic anemias. *Hematology: American Society of Hematology Education Program, 13*(8). Retrieved March 15, 2008, from http://asheducationbook.hematologylibrary.org/cgi/content/full/2006/1/13

Hurley, G. (2007). Anemia: Overview and management. *Primary Health Care, 17*(6), 25–30.

Killip, S., Bennet, J. M., & Chambers, M. D. (2007). Iron deficiency anemia. *American Family Physician, 75*(5), 619–621, 671–678, 756.

Kleigman, R. M., Marcdante, K J., Jensen, H. B., & Behrman, R. E. (2006). *Nelson essentials of pediatrics* (5th ed.). Philadelphia: Elsevier Saunders.

Kulkarni, P., & Cortez, J. (2007). Anemia. *Clinical Pediatrics, 46*(5), 462–465.

Kumar, V. (2007). Pernicious anemia. *Medical Laboratory Observer, 39*(2), 28, 30–31.

McPhee, S. J., Papdakis, M. A., & Tierney, L. M. (Eds.). (2008). *Current medical diagnosis and treatment* (47th ed.). New York: Lange Medical Books/McGraw-Hill.

Murray, C. K., Chinevere, T. D., Grant, E., Johnson, G. A. Duelm, F., & Hospenthal, D. L. (2006). Prevalence of glucose 6-phosphate dehydrogenase deficiency in Army personnel. *Military Medicine, 171*(9), 905–907.

Novak, B. (2007). The benefits of folic acid. *Nurse Prescribing, 5*(5), 215–220.

Rakel, R. E., & Bope, E. T. (2006). *Conn's current therapy.* Philadelphia: Saunders Elsevier.

Rund, D., & Rachmilewitz, E. (2005). Medical progress: β-thalassemia. *New England Journal of Medicine, 353*(11), 1135–1146, 1193–1196.

Stockman, J., & Lohr, J. (2001). *Essence of office pediatrics.* Philadelphia: W. B. Saunders.

Endocrine Disorders

Shirlee Drayton-Brooks, PhD, FNP-BC, APRN-BC

GENERAL APPROACH

- A defect in one aspect of the endocrine regulatory systems can cause systemic consequences, morbidity, and death.
- Endocrine disorders generally manifest in one of four ways:
  - Excess hormone (e.g., Cushing syndrome, excess cortisol secretion)
  - Deficit hormone (e.g., diabetes mellitus [DM] type 1, insulin secretion is low or absent)
  - Abnormal response of end organ to the hormone (pseudohypoparathroidism)
  - Gland enlargement (e.g., pituitary adenoma)
- Endocrine diseases may be associated with a deficiency or hypersecretion of hormones that affect target organs.
  - There are basically three types of hormone: steroids such as cortisol (adrenal cortex), estrogen, progesterone (ovaries) and testosterone (testes); amino acids, tyrosine such as thyroxine (thyroid), catecholamines (adrenal medulla); and proteins, peptides such as insulin (pancreas)
  - Regulation of hormone secretion is through negative feedback system
  - Patients of all ages may need to carry or wear MedicAlert or similar identification for many endocrine disorders
- The FNP must consider normal physiologic changes occurring with growth, development, and aging when managing various endocrine diagnoses across the life span.

Red Flags

- *Type 1 diabetics* may present with *acute ketoacidosis*: nausea, fatigue, abdominal pain, thirst, hunger, polyuria progressing to vomiting, confusion, lethargy, hypotension, fruity breath odor.
- *Type 2 diabetics* may present with *hyperglycemic, hyperosmolar, nonketotic syndrome (HHNKS)*, characterized confusion and lethargy, blood glucose >600 mg/dL, minimal ketosis, serum osmolality >340, and profound dehydration.
- *Hypoglycemia* may present as initial headache, hunger, difficulty problem-solving, sweating, shakiness, tremor, anxiety, irritability, behavior change; progresses to coma and seizures without treatment.
- *Thyroid nodules* are common but <10% of solitary nodules are malignant. Risk factors for malignancy include family history of thyroid cancer or multiple endocrine metaplastic type 2 carcinoma; male gender; extremes in age (<15 and >70); exposure to radiation of head, neck, or chest; single nodule.
- *Acute adrenal insufficiency* or Addisonian crisis may present as severe abdominal pain, nausea and vomiting, hypotension, hypoglycemia, and shock; is precipitated by surgery, infection, exacerbation of comorbid illness, sudden withdrawal of long-term glucocorticoid replacement.
- *Pituitary adenoma* may present as headache with visual changes, amenorrhea, or galactorrhea; obtain a prolactin level and MRI of the brain or CT with attention to the sella turcica.

DISORDERS OF THE PANCREAS

Diabetes Mellitus Type 1

Description

- Some genetically predisposed individuals develop autoimmune beta cell destruction in response to some environmental trigger. A syndrome produced by disorders in metabolism of carbohydrate, protein, and fat due to absolute lack of insulin resulting in hyperglycemia. Without insulin, therapy ketoacidosis occurs rapidly. Formerly called insulin-dependent diabetes mellitus (IDDM), juvenile-onset.

Etiology

- Destruction of beta cells in pancreatic islets and absolute deficiency and/or failure to produce insulin related to autoimmune response or environmental trigger (e.g.., virus)
- Human leukocyte antigens HLA, HLA-DR3, or HLA-DR4, associated with type 1
- May be triggered in susceptive individuals by viruses, toxic chemical agents, or cytotoxins
- Genetic susceptibility influenced by environmental factors
- Hyperglycemia results from inability of glucose to enter cell for utilization as energy
- Ketoacidosis results from the utilization of free fatty acids for energy

Incidence and Demographics

- Type 1 accounts for 10%–12% of all diabetes cases in U.S.
- Generally occurs in puberty between ages 8–14
- Highest prevalence in Scandinavia where 20% of diabetics are type 1; Japan and China <1%
- Can develop in adulthood but rarely occurs after 30 years of age; very rare in elderly
- Idiopathic etiology most common in individuals of Asian or African descent

Risk Factors
- First-degree relative with type 1 diabetes mellitus; other autoimmune disorders

Prevention and Screening
- No prevention and no routine screening in childhood

Assessment

HISTORY
- Acute onset of polyuria, polydipsia, polyphagia, weight loss, blurred vision, fatigue, abdominal pain, nausea/vomiting, vaginal itching/infections, unhealed wounds, skin infections/rashes, dehydration, hypoglycemic or ketotic episodes
- Nightmares, night sweats, or headache may indicate nocturnal hypoglycemia in both children and adults
- History provided by parent including frequent diaper changes, bed-wetting, listlessness or fatigue, frequent sick days from school or daycare, changes in school performance or behavior
- Pediatric patients: Birthweight and history of complications at birth, health status at birth
- Family history of diabetes

PHYSICAL EXAM
- Exam may be normal or patient may be ill-looking with fruity odor to breath
- Weight loss, thin (children and adults) or failure to thrive (infants), signs of dehydration, orthostatic hypotension
- Presence of skin infections, oral or vaginal candidiasis (more common in Type 2)
- Diabetic ketoacidosis: Dehydration, labored breathing, confusion/disorientation, lethargy
- Signs of complications:
  - Delayed sexual maturation (adolescents)
  - Late disease: Ophthalmic changes: microaneurysm with soft and hard exudates, deep retinal hemorrhages, neovascularization, cataracts, glaucoma; peripheral vascular insufficiency; diminished deep tendon reflex
  - Possible cardiovascular changes occurring in late disease: Postural hypotension, resting tachycardia, "silent" myocardial infarctions
  - Possible peripheral vascular changes occurring in late disease: Cool extremities due to decreased circulation, decreased pulses, edema, delayed capillary refill
  - Possible neurological changes occurring in late disease: Diminished pain sensation, proprioception, vibration, light touch, absent lower extremity reflexes, dysfunction in extraocular movements, weakness, ataxic gait, paresthesias, may have change in level of consciousness

DIAGNOSTIC STUDIES
- Random glucose level >200 mg/dL plus symptoms of polyuria, polydipsia, and weight loss OR subsequent day fasting plasma glucose (FPG) >126 mg/dL
- FPG > 126 mg/dL on two occasions
- FPG > 110 mg/dL and <126 mg/dL is diagnostic of "prediabetes"

- Oral glucose tolerance test (OGTT) no longer recommended for routine clinical use except in screening for gestational diabetes
- May consider serum C peptide or insulin level (decreased)
- Glucose and ketones in urine
- Baseline diagnostic studies: BUN, serum creatinine, urinalysis, urine microalbumin, and fasting lipid profile; glycosylated hemoglobin (HbA1c) (5.5%–7% good control)
- ECG and chest x-ray for coronary and pulmonary pathology in adults
- Elevated BUN and creatinine if dehydrated; hypertriglyceridemia: triglyceride levels >150 mg/dL
- Thyroid-stimulating hormone (TSH) level

Differential Diagnosis

- Diabetes mellitus type 2
- Diabetes insipidus
- Pancreatitis or pancreatic disease
- Pheochromocytoma
- Cushing syndrome
- Acromegaly
- Liver disease
- Salicylate poisoning
- Glucosuria w/o hyperglycemia in renal tubular disease or benign renal glucosuria
- Secondary effects of oral contraceptives, corticosteroids, thiazides, phenytoin, nicotinic acid
- Severe stress from trauma, burns or infection
- Urinary tract infection (UTI)

Management

NONPHARMACOLOGIC TREATMENT

- Patient education: Basic pathophysiology, cause, general management and long-term complications of Type 1 diabetes, administration of insulin, medications
- Short- and long-term goals of treatment: Whole blood glucose average 80–120 mg/dL preprandially and 100–140 mg/dL bedtime; HbA1c goal <7%
- Lifestyle modifications—diet, exercise, smoking cessation (if appropriate), avoid alcohol
- Medical nutrition therapy prescribed by a registered dietician, following American Diabetes Association (ADA) guidelines; constant reinforcement by all providers
- General guidelines for adults: 10%–20% calories from protein, <10% from saturated fats, <10% from polyunsaturated fats, and 50%–70% from carbohydrates and monounsaturated fats; cholesterol 300 mg per day, fiber to 25–35 g/1,000 calories
- General guidelines for children: Consistent timing and amount of meals (three meals and three snacks). However, for those on fast-acting insulin (such as NovoLog) and insulin glargine, or using fast-acting insulin in an insulin pump, exact timing and amount of meals not as critical. A well-balanced, healthy diet is recommended, with dosing adjusted to number

of carbohydrate consumed at any meal and adjustments made for high or low blood sugar. Diet should include 15% of calories from protein, 30% of calories from fats, 55% of calories from carbohydrates.
  – Daily exercise regimen for adults and physical activity for children
- Use a multidisciplinary approach to help work with the patient and the family, including the patient, parents (if appropriate), primary care provider, endocrinologist, nurse educator, and dietician
  – Teach patient/parent recognition and management of episodes of hypoglycemia due to inadequate oral intake, increased exercise without adequate increase in caloric intake, or excess insulin
  – Self/parental glucose monitoring education: tid, before meals and bedtime; check for urine ketones if blood glucose is >300 mg/dL, during illness, stress, pregnancy, or symptoms of ketosis such as nausea, vomiting, or abdominal pain; keep self-monitoring blood glucose (SMBG) log
- Establish a foot care plan
- Establish a dental care plan
- Annual eye examination
- Teach patient/parent how to modify therapy if he/she is ill. "Sick day guidelines" require continuing usual dose of insulin, frequent SMBG and adjustment of insulin if necessary, check urine for ketones if SMBG >300 mg/dL, increase intake of fluids.
- Referral to local support groups and American Diabetes Association
- MedicAlert or similar identification bracelet or necklace
- Inform school, work, and/or friends of condition
- Pneumococcal vaccine and annual influenza vaccines

PHARMACOLOGIC TREATMENT
- Insulin therapy: See Table 17–1
  – Individual presenting with ketones must be started on insulin. Goal of therapy is to maintain blood sugar as follows:
    » Fasting 90–130 mg/dL
    » 1 hour postprandial <180 mg/dL
    » 2 hours postprandial <150 mg/dL
- Insulin therapy options:
  – (1) Give daily doses of short- or ultra–short-acting insulin prior to meals based on carbohydrate counting; 1 unit of insulin per 10–15 grams (initially, adjust ratio up or down to individual as needed) of carbohydrate content; and a dose of long-acting insulin (ultralente) prebreakfast and predinner with daily dose equal to 0.5 x weight in kg/2, split evenly between prebreakfast and predinner
  – (2) Daily doses of short- or ultra–short-acting insulin prior to meals based on carbohydrate counting; 1 unit of insulin per 10–15 grams of carbohydrate content (initially, adjust to each individual as needed) and a single dose of insulin glargine (Lantus) at nighttime = to 0.5 x weight in kg/2
  – (3) Combine short- or ultra–short- and intermediate-acting (NPH) insulin as follows:
    » Premeal short- or ultra–short-acting insulin based on carbohydrate counting as described above

» NPH total daily dose = 0.5 x weight in kg/2
» One half NPH given at nighttime
» Remaining NPH divided evenly among the three meals and administered premeal with short- or ultra–short-acting preparations
- Pediatric insulin initiation: Refer to endocrinologist
  - Preschoolers: FPG range 90–140 mg/dL and postprandially 90–200 mg/dL
  - School-aged: FPG range 80–120 mg/dL and postprandially 80–180 mg/dL
- Insulin doses in general can be divided into 2–4 injections per day or continuous subcutaneous insulin infusion (insulin pump) once stabilized; typical regimen for children and adults is two injections per day; adolescents may require three injections per day
- Adjust insulin doses according to glucose monitoring
- Honeymoon period or remission phase after diagnosis may last from several months to 2 years
- Insulin glargine (Lantus) is a long-acting preparation designed for once a day administration at bedtime; it cannot be mixed with other types of insulin

Special Considerations
- Puberty: Initially, increased caloric need, followed by a decrease to 35 calories/kg of ideal body weight as growth is completed; pubertal growth spurt will require insulin adjustment (1.25–1.5 units/kg/day)
- Co-management with pediatrician or pediatric endocrinologist

Table 17–1. Comparison of Insulin Products

Product	Onset (Hr)	Peak (Hr)	Duration (Hr)
Rapid-Acting			
Humalog	0.25	1	3.5–4.5
Humulin R	0.5	2–4	6–8
NovoLog	0.25	0.75	3–5
Novolin R	0.5	2–5	8
Intermediate-Acting			
Humulin N	1–2	6–12	18–24
Novolin N	1.5	4–12	24
Humulin L (used less frequently)	1–3	6–12	18–24
Novolin L (used less frequently)	2.5	7–15	12
Long-Acting			
Humulin U	4–8	10–30	18–36
Lantus	1.1	none	24
Mixtures			
Humulin 50/50	0.5	3–5	24
Humulin 70/30	0.5–1	2–12	24
Novolin 70/30	0.5	2–12	24

When to Consult, Refer, Hospitalize
- Hospitalization is recommended for all newly diagnosed pediatric patients.
- Hospitalize adults and children with diabetic ketoacidosis (DKA) and severe infections.
- Co-management of pediatric type 1 DM patients with a pediatrician or pediatric endocrinologist.
- Refer unstable adult or geriatric patients; consider co-management of all type 1 DM patients.
- Refer all families to diabetic educator, registered dietitian.
- Ophthalmologist: Initial screening and annual exam for diabetic retinopathy and visual problems; all patients >9 years old who have diabetes for 3–5 years, and all patients >30 years old.
- Dentist: Routine check-ups and for dental complaints for all ages.
- Podiatrist: Routine foot care in elderly and foot problems as indicated.
- Consider psychological counseling if needed to address issues of altered body image and individual and family stressors related to disease and management.

Follow-Up
- Continue ongoing follow-up/consultation with endocrinologist and diabetic educator
- Routine diabetes visits: Daily for initiation of insulin or change in regimen, at least quarterly for patients not meeting their goals, and semiannually for other patients
- 24-hour urine collection or spot urine collection for microalbuminuria beginning at puberty and at 5 years' duration
- HbA1c every 3–6 months
- Glycosylated hemoglobin (HbA1c): Target goal 6%; normal range 4%–6%; each % correlates to 30 mg/dL FPG elevation; provides index of glycemic control for life of red blood cell, 8–12 weeks
- Serum fructosamine: Glycosylated protein (primarily albumin); normal value 1.5–2.4 mmol/L; provides index of glycemic control for preceding 2–3 weeks; low albumin levels will lower fructosamine levels; are useful when hemolytic states affect HbA1c measures
- Annual physical exam or routine well-child exam with primary care provider
- Thyroid function tests initially, then every 2–3 years for adults; annually for children
  - EXPECTED COURSE
    - Chronic, lifelong disease with no cure

  - COMPLICATIONS
    - Hypoglycemia signs/symptoms: Shakiness, weakness, sweating, headache, tachycardia, nervousness, dizziness, hunger, irritability, convulsions, coma
    - Somogyi effect: Early morning rebound hyperglycemia due to nocturnal hypoglycemia; around 3:00 a.m. serum glucose falls and patient is hypoglycemic; counterregulatory hormones compensate by mobilizing glucose stores; patient rebounds and becomes hyperglycemic by early morning; treated with reducing or eliminating p.m. or hs doses to eliminate nocturnal hypoglycemia
    - Dawn phenomenon: Hyperglycemia due to hepatic gluconeogenesis in early morning. Peripheral tissue insulin receptors become desensitized to insulin nocturnally, believed to be due to insulin receptor desensitizing property of growth hormone. Around 3:00 a.m. blood sugar measures either normal or high normal and gets progressively higher throughout the night, is elevated at 7 a.m. Treatment is to increase p.m. long-acting insulin or add an hs dose.

- Lipodystrophy (destruction of subcutaneous fat at injection sites): Seen less with use of synthetic human insulin rather than beef or pork insulin
- Retinopathy
- Nephropathy and renal failure
- Cardiovascular disease with lipid abnormalities; premature atherosclerosis
- Cerebrovascular disease
- Diabetic ketoacidosis
- Insulin resistance with long-term, high-dose therapy
- Peripheral neuropathy
- Autonomic nervous system problems, incontinence and erectile dysfunction
- Infections
- Foot and skin ulcerations
- Insulin allergy

Diabetes Mellitus Type 2

Description
- Metabolic disease causing hyperglycemia characterized by a relative insufficiency of insulin due to resistance to the action of insulin in target tissues, decrease in insulin receptors, and/or impairment of insulin secretion
- Formerly non–insulin-dependent diabetes mellitus (NIDDM), adult or maturity onset, type 2, nonketotic diabetes (because there is some endogenous insulin activity, usually diabetic ketoacidosis does not develop)

Etiology
- Genetically and clinically a heterogeneous disorder with familial pattern
- Influenced by environmental factors, lack of physical activity, diet high in refined carbohydrate and fat with low fiber
  - Two major types:
    - Obese type 2 diabetes: Most common type
      » Initial peripheral insulin receptor insensitivity, possibly due to cellular distention secondary to increased fat accumulation
      » Beta cell compensates by increasing insulin release; hyperglycemia does not occur
      » Eventually, beta cells may "burn out," insulin release falls, and hyperglycemia occurs as a result of the insulin receptor insensitivity
    - Non-obese type 2 diabetes
      » Initial problem may be blunted response of the beta cell to glucose
      » Glucose does not trigger adequate insulin release
      » Insulin resistance is not clinically significant
      » More common in certain Asian populations
- No human leukocyte antigen or islet cell antibodies
- Syndrome of hyperinsulinemia and insulin resistance resulting in hyperglycemia, hypertension, and hyperlipidemia to varying degrees in all patients

Incidence and Demographics
- Occurs predominately in obese adults >30 years but occasionally in adolescents with a genetic predisposition or obesity
- Incidence higher in females than males
- Accounts for nearly 90% of all diabetes mellitus cases in U.S.

Risk Factors
- Obesity/inactivity, >20% ideal body weight, or body mass index (BMI) >27 kg/m^2
- Family history of diabetes, mostly type 2
- Gestational diabetes increases risk for developing type 2 diabetes within 5–10 years post parturition
- Delivery of macrosomic infant, weight >9 lbs
- Previously impaired glucose tolerance
- Age >45
- African American, Asian American, Hispanic, Native American, or Pacific Islander
- Metabolic syndrome (syndrome X or insulin resistance syndrome): Cluster of disorders including hypertension, insulin resistance, truncal obesity, abnormal lipid levels, hyperinsulinism
- High-density lipoprotein (HDL) cholesterol <35 mg/dL and/or triglycerides >250 mg/dL

Prevention and Screening
- Adults >45 years screened every 3 years, and more often with FPG near 126 mg/dL
- Screening for gestational diabetes at 24–28 weeks gestation
- Secondary prevention of complications essential

Assessment
HISTORY
- More insidious onset, may not have classical signs of type 1 diabetes at early onset
- Obesity, blurred vision, chronic skin infections, polyuria, polydipsia, polyphagia, weight loss, fatigue, slow-healing wounds, recurrent infections (especially *Candida* and urinary tract infections), spontaneous abortion
- History related to type 2 diabetes: More prominent macrovascular changes than microvascular, such as vascular insufficiency, cardiovascular/cerebrovascular disease, and atherosclerosis
- History of HHNKS: Precipitating factors include treatment with calcium channel blockers, propranolol, corticosteroids, thiazides, phenytoin

PHYSICAL EXAM
- Usually discovered on routine exam with elevated glucose level
- Central obesity, hypertensive
- With more advanced stage:
  - Orthostatic blood pressure changes
  - Weight loss
  - Skin infections present
  - Visual and funduscopic changes: Microaneurysms with soft (cotton wool) and hard exudates, deep retinal hemorrhages, neovascularization, cataracts, glaucoma

– Oral *Candida* infections
– Peripheral vascular: Decreased circulation, cool extremities, decreased pulses, edema, capillary refill >3 seconds
– Neurologic: Decreased sensation of pain, proprioception, vibration, light touch, absent lower extremity reflexes, dysfunction in extraocular movements, weakness, ataxic gait

DIAGNOSTIC STUDIES
- Diagnosis confirmed with:
  – FPG) >126 mg/dL on two occasions OR
  – Random glucose level >200 mg/dL *plus* symptoms of polyuria, polydipsia and weight loss OR subsequent day FPG >126 mg/dL
  – OGTT no longer recommended for routine clinical use
- FPG >100 mg/dL and <126 mg/dL represents impaired fasting glucose (IFG)
- Urinalysis for protein, glucose, and ketones; microalbuminuria screening at initial diagnosis (ketonuria may occur but rare ketone accumulation in serum)
- BUN, urine and serum creatinine
- Fasting serum cholesterol and lipid profile
- Adult recommendations:
  – Glycemic control: Glycosylated hemoglobin A1c (HbA1c) <7.0%, preprandial capillary plasma glucose 90–130 mg/dL, peak postprandial capillary plasma glucose <180 mg/dL
  – Blood pressure 130/80 mmHg
  – Lipids: Low-density lipoproteins (LDL) <100 mg/dL, trigylcerides <150 mg/dL, high-density lipoprotiens (HDL) >40 mg/dL
- ECG and chest x-ray if clinically indicated for coronary and pulmonary pathology
- TSH
- Glycated serum protein: Index of glycemic control over past 1–2 weeks
- C peptide levels normal or above normal with type 2

Differential Diagnosis
- Diabetes mellitus type 1
- Diabetes insipidus
- Pancreatitis or pancreatic disease
- Pheochromocytoma
- Cushing syndrome
- Liver disease
- Glucosuria w/o hyperglycemia in renal tubular disease or benign renal glucosuria
- Secondary effects of oral contraceptives, corticosteroids, thiazides, phenytoin, nicotinic acid
- Severe stress from trauma, burns, or infection

Management

Common treatment plan with goal of FPG 80–100 mg/dL and HbA1c <7.0%

1. Diet and exercise
2. Oral monotherapy
3. Add a 2nd drug class
4. Add a 3rd drug class or add insulin

NONPHARMACOLOGIC TREATMENT

- Patient education: Basic pathophysiology, cause, general management and long-term complications of type 2 diabetes; oral glucose-lowering medications dosage, administration, and side effects
- Mainstay of treatment is correction of insulin resistance through diet, exercise, and weight loss; patients with FPG <250 mg/dL may be treated initially with medical nutritional therapy
    - Lifestyle modifications: diet, exercise, smoking cessation (if appropriate), avoid alcohol
    - Medical nutrition therapy prescribed by a registered dietician
    - Nutrition counseling following American Diabetes Association (ADA) guidelines; weight reduction of 5–10 lbs increases insulin sensitivity
    - General guidelines for adults and children: 10%–20% calories from protein, <10% from saturated fats, <10% from polyunsaturated fats, and 50%–70% from carbohydrates and monounsaturated fats
    - Moderate weight loss (10–20 lbs) and hypocaloric diets based on average daily intake can improve blood glucose levels
    - Daily exercise regimen for adults and physical activity for children reduces insulin resistance by increasing number of insulin receptors, increases glucose uptake for 48–72 hours, contributes to lipid control and weight loss
- SMBG when medications are initiated or altered—before each meal, at bedtime, and 2–4 in morning. for 3 days, then before breakfast and dinner for 7 days; once glucose is controlled, monitor daily at random times; maintan SMBG log
- Teach patient/parent how to modify therapy if they are ill; "sick day guidelines" for adults require continuing usual dose medication, frequent SMBG, increase intake of fluids; for pediatric patients, consult with pediatrician or pediatric endocrinologist
- Counsel regarding contraception and discuss importance of glucose control prior to and during pregnancy
- Perform stress test if >35 years with DM
- Referral to local support groups and American Diabetes Association
- MedicAlert or similar identification bracelet or necklace
- Foot care plan
- Annual influenza and pneumococcal vaccinations

PHARMACOLOGIC TREATMENT

- Step approach
- Treat to the target; start with 10 units insulin q hs and adjust weekly based on mean FBG on preceding 2 days:
  - >180, increase 8 units
  - 140–180, increase 6 units
  - 120–140, increase 4 units
  - 100–120, increase 2 units
- Goal of therapy: HbA1c control is looser than in type 1 DM; tight control is associated with fewer long-term microvascular complications but may increase the risk of severe hypoglycemia and weight gain
- If FPG >250 mg/dL and <400 mg/dL without symptoms of acidosis, dehydration, or ketosis, in addition to nutrition therapy and exercise begin monotherapy with oral antidiabetic agent (30%–40% patients may not respond)
- Antidiabetic agents listed in Table 17–2; select based on blood glucose level, age, and weight of the patient, taking into consideration precautions and contraindications specific to the classification of agent selected
- For obese patients: Begin metformin with a low dose, increase dosage every 1–2 weeks on basis of glycemic control; treatment should continue for 4 weeks prior to changing to another agent; then add insulin-release stimulator if control inadequate; then add thiazelolidinedione if first two agents do not provide adequate control; if no control, then stop oral insulin-release stimulator and add or switch to insulin
- For non-obese patients: Use insulin-release stimulator as initial agent; metformin if inadequate control with the first agent, thiazelolidinedione if the first two agents do not provide adequate control; then add insulin if needed, but do not discontinue the oral insulin-release stimulator
- Alpha-glucosidase inhibitors may also be added to the regimen to achieve better control in some patients
- If insulin is required, follow regimen of type 1 regarding insulin and SMBG
- If FPG >400 mg/dL or patient has signs of ketoacidosis, insulin therapy is required
- In metabolic syndrome (syndrome X or insulin resistance syndrome), it is theorized that the insulin receptors' insensitivity leads to hyperinsulinemia; this leads to increased hepatic very low density lipoprotein (VLDL) production, which leads to increased sodium retention; hyperinsulinemia also leads to endothelial proliferation, accelerating atherosclerosis with associated hypertension; these patients require treatment for hyperglycemia, hypertension, dyslipidemia, and weight loss

Table 17-2. Oral Antidiabetic Agents

Generic and Class	Brand Name	Action	Dosage Range	Usual Maximum Dosage	Comments and Major Side Effects
Sulfonylureas: Pancreatic islet beta cell insulin-release stimulator					
Chlorpropamide 1st generation	Diabinese	Long-acting	250–750 mg, single or divided	750 mg/day	Rarely used; hypoglycemia, disulfiram-like reaction with alcohol
Glimepiride	Amaryl	Intermediate-acting	1–4 mg daily	8 mg/day	Hypoglycemia
Glipizide 2nd generation	Glucotrol	Intermediate-acting	5–15 mg daily	15 mg/day or 40 mg divided	Hypoglycemia
	Glucotrol XL	Long-acting	5–40 mg/day, divided 5–10 mg daily	20 mg/day	Good in controlling postprandial hyperglycemia
Glyburide 2nd generation	DiaBeta Micronase	Intermediate-acting	1.25–20 mg, single or divided	20 mg/day	Hypoglycemia
Glyburide, micronized 2nd generation	Glynase Pres Tab	Intermediate-acting	0.75–12 mg, single or divided	12 mg/day divided	Hypoglycemia
Meglitinides: Pancreatic islet beta cell insulin-release stimulator					
Repaglinide	Prandin	Short-acting	0.5–4 mg within 30 min. of meals 2–4x/day	16 mg/day	Take with meals, quick onset; hypoglycemia; many drug interactions
Nateglinide	Starlix	Short-acting	60–120 mg tid within 30 min. before meals	120 mg tid	Quick onset, which may be useful in adolescents with irregular eating schedules; do not take if a meal is skipped; use with caution in severe renal disease; may be used as an adjunct with metformin

Table 17–2. Oral Antidiabetic Agents (cont.)

Generic and Class	Brand Name	Action	Dosage Range	Usual Maximum Dosage	Comments and Major Side Effects
Biguanides: Decrease hepatic glucose production; increase action on muscle glucose uptake					
Metformin	Glucophage	Intermediate-acting	500 mg–2.55 g divided into 2 or 3 doses	2.55 g/day	Contraindicated in renal dysfunction, chronic heart failure requiring treatment, use cautiously in many conditions that may predispose to lactic acidosis
Thiazolidinediones: Increase insulin action on muscle and fat glucose uptake					
Pioglitazone	Actos	Long-acting	15 or 30 mg daily	45 mg/day	Precautions with hepatic dysfunction, cardiac disease, anovulatory conditions
Rosiglitazone	Avandia	Long-acting	4–8 mg single or divided into 2 doses	8 mg/day	Precautions with hepatic dysfunction, cardiac disease, anovulatory conditions
Alpha-glucosidase inhibitors: Delay carbohydrate digestion and decrease postprandial glucose					
Acarbose	Precose	Short-acting	50–100 mg tid	<60 kg: 150 mg/day divided >60 kg: 300 mg/day divided	Take before meals Contraindicated in inflammatory bowel disease and other intestinal conditions; use glucose rather than sucrose for hypoglycemia
Miglitol	Glyset	Short-acting	50 mg tid	300 mg/day divided into 3 doses	Take before meals Contraindicated in inflammatory bowel disease and other intestinal conditions; use glucose rather than sucrose for hypoglycemia

Special Considerations
- Pregnancy:
  - Routine screening at 24–28 weeks gestation in all pregnant women with OGTT: Oral 50 g glucose (regardless of fasting) solution with a 1-hour blood glucose assay
  - Positive screening (>140 mg/dL) necessitates a standard glucose tolerance test prior to diagnosis
  - Criteria for diagnosis of gestational diabetes following 100 g oral glucose load: 1 hour—190 mg/dL, 2 hour—165 mg/dL, 3 hour—145 mg/dL
  - IFG refers to higher than normal serum glucose levels but not diagnostic of diabetes mellitus
  - Gestational diabetes is treated through a multidisciplinary approach, including nutrition therapy and insulin, if necessary
  - Pregnant patients with gestational diabetes requiring insulin management should be managed by an endocrinologist and perinatologist
  - Refer all gestational diabetic patients who require insulin therapy
- Elderly
- Frail or mentally disabled elderly are likely to have hypoglycemic events resulting from forgetting to take medication as prescribed; incidence of falls may increase

When to Consult, Refer, Hospitalize
- Endocrinologist referral for uncontrolled hyperglycemia
- Pediatric endocrinologist for pediatric DM type 2 patients until stabilized
- Hospitalize for severe infections, HHNKS, characterized by blood glucose >600 mg/dL, minimal ketosis, serum osmolality >340, and profound dehydration
- Diabetic educator for further teaching for all patients and for pregnancy/lactation
- Registered dietitian for further nutritional teaching
- Ophthalmologist: Initial screening and annual exam for diabetic retinopathy and visual problems; all patients >9 years who have diabetes for 3–5 years, and all patients >30 years
- Podiatrist for routine foot care in elderly and foot problems as indicated

Follow-Up
- When first diagnosed or when adjusting medications, see weekly, then biweekly, monthly; well-controlled diabetic patients, see every 6 months
- Annual urine protein, FPG, lipid profile, creatinine, ECG, full physical exam with funduscopic and neurologic exams, complete foot inspection
- If treated with medication, obtain HbA1c every 3–6 months; goal <7%
- Thyroid function tests as indicated
    - EXPECTED COURSE
        - Chronic, lifelong disease that requires long-term control to minimize complications

    - COMPLICATIONS
        - Hyperglycemic hyperosmolar nonketotic coma, Charcot foot secondary to neuropathy; also see type 1 DM complications

Hypoglycemia

Description
- Hypoglycemia is defined as plasma glucose concentration <50 mg/dL (value may vary by lab); may be asymptomatic; plasma glucose level of <30 mg/dL usually symptomatic.
- Can be classified as reactive (within 5 hours of eating), or fasting (occurs >5 hours after a meal).
- Reactive hypoglycemia is rare; more likely is pseudo hypoglycemia (symptoms without the drop in blood glucose; unclear cause).

Etiology
- Most commonly caused by excess exogenous insulin in diabetics but may result from use of some oral antihyperglycemic agents; precipitated by change in quantity and timing of activity and food.
- At the onset of hypoglycemia, the parasympathetic nervous system is activated causing hunger, which is followed by activation of the sympathetic nervous system (nervousness, sweating, tachycardia). Known as "Whipple's Triad," which consists of low plasma glucose, parasympathetic and sympathetic symptoms, and relief with ingestion of carbohydrates.
- Other causes: Benign functional disturbance of insulin secretion, pancreatic beta-cell tumor (insulinoma); autoimmune process (very rare); ethanol ingestion; glucocorticoid and growth hormone deficiencies; malnutrition; gastrointestinal surgery; chronic disease states (hepatic, renal, chronic heart failure [CHF]).
- In neonates, occurs due to erythroblastosis fetalis; insulinomas; B-cell nesidioblastosis; functional B-cell hyperplasia; Beckwith syndrome; panhypopituitarism; infants of mothers with DM and gestational DM; very ill or immature neonates; intrauterine malnutrition; metabolic defects.

Incidence and Demographics
- Most prevalent in diabetic patients on insulin and sulfonylureas
- Occurs in 1–3 per 1,000 live births, including approximately 5%–15% of infants with intrauterine growth retardation (IUGR)

Risk Factors
- Type 1 DM, type 2 DM on insulin or sulfonylureas
- Enzyme defects
- Liver disease, insulinoma
- Medication use such as disopyramide (Norpace), pentamidine, quinine
- Pregnancy, third trimester
- Pituitary or adrenal insufficiency
- Alcohol abuse
- Neonatal: Prematurity, hypoxia, hypothermia, IUGR, maternal DM, maternal glucose infusion during labor, small-for-gestational age (SGA)

Assessment
HISTORY
- Symptom history, especially if occurs postprandially or fasting; may be following excessive exercise
- Initial symptoms of headache, hunger, difficulty problem-solving; may be sweating, shakiness, tremor, anxiety, irritability, behavior change
- Progresses to coma and seizures without treatment
- Insulinoma: Morning headaches, morning confusion, nocturnal or early morning seizures
- Infants/children: SGA (highest risk), IUGR, prematurity
  - Hypothermia, hypoxia, or drug withdrawal at birth
  - Maternal DM, gestational DM history, or glucose infusion at birth
  - History of apnea of prematurity

PHYSICAL EXAM
- Altered mental status; tachycardia; hypotension; pale, cool, and clammy skin; coma; positive Babinski
- In neonates, onset may be a few hours to 1 week after birth: Jitteriness; convulsions; episodic cyanosis, apnea or tachycardia; lethargy and poor feeding; high-pitched cry; diaphoresis; pallor; hypothermia

DIAGNOSTIC STUDIES
- Adults: Serum glucose level <50 mg/dL indicates hypoglycemia (varies by laboratory)
- Consider drug testing for ethyl alcohol or sulfonylurea, liver function, BUN, creatinine, cortisol tests to identify associated factors in a diabetic patient
- In nondiabetic patient, also get C peptide levels, insulin, insulin antibodies, oral glucose tolerance test
- If cause not identified, additional testing after 72-hour fast may be done by specialist
- Neonates/children: Serum glucose level <35 mg/dL at 1–3 hours of age; <40 mg/dL at 3–24 hours of age; <45 mg/dL after 24 hours of age

Differential Diagnosis
- Pseudo hypoglycemia
- Anxiety and panic
- Pheochromocytoma
- Factitious hypoglycemia
- Other causes of coma
- See conditions listed under Etiology

Management
NONPHARMACOLOGIC TREATMENT
- Avoid fasting, alcohol use; snack before exercise
- Caffeine restriction (mimics symptoms)
- Avoid simple carbohydrates or beverages with large sugar content
- Diet: High protein with complex carbohydrates, frequent small meals approximately 6x/day

- Avoid causative agents
- Insulinomas and nesidioblastosis: Surgery
- In neonates: Oral or gavage feeding of high-risk, normoglycemic neonates and monitor for hypoglycemia

PHARMACOLOGIC TREATMENT
- If able to take oral substances, consume two glucose tablets or five Life Savers candies (equivalent to 10–15 g glucose) at onset of symptoms, followed by complex carbohydrates after the acute reaction is controlled
- If unconscious or unable to swallow, home or office management could include 1 mg glucagon IM or SC (adult and adolescent); 0.5–1 mg glucagon (5–10 years); 0.25–0.5 mg (<5 years), roll on side in case of vomiting; patient should be transported to an acute care facility for further monitoring and treatment
- If oral or gavage feedings are not tolerated in a normoglycemic, high-risk neonate, refer to neonatal specialist for further care

Special Considerations
- Some drugs, such as beta adrenergic antagonists, mask symptoms of hypoglycemia.
- Men can fast for 72 hours and maintain plasma glucose level above 50 mg/dL, while women exhibit progressive decrease in plasma glucose during prolonged fasting.
- Geriatric patients may have blunted autonomic response, present with confusion and impaired central nervous system (CNS) function.

When to Consult, Refer, Hospitalize
- Refer for suspected insulinoma and nesidioblastosis to adult or pediatric surgeon as appropriate
- Consult with physician or refer to endocrinologist for any unknown or uncontrollable cause
- Activate the emergency medical system for all unconscious patients

Follow-Up
- Educate patient and family about prevention, symptoms, and treatment of hypoglycemia
- Monitor insulin and sulfonylurea dosage carefully based on patient's diet and activity
- Monitor children with hypoglycemia for attainment of developmental milestones as intellect can be affected, especially in low birthweight infants and infants of diabetic mothers
  EXPECTED COURSE
  - Variable and dependent on etiology, but favorable prognosis with appropriate treatment

  COMPLICATIONS
  - Brain damage and tissue death from prolonged low glucose level

THYROID DISORDERS

Hyperthyroidism (Thyrotoxicosis)

Description
- Clinical condition caused by increased level of thyroid hormones T4 (thyroxine) and T3 (triiodothyronine)
- Manifestations include excessive metabolic activities

Etiology
- Excessive and uncontrolled secretion of thyroid hormone from a variety of causes:
  - Autoimmune Graves' disease (diffuse toxic goiter): Most common cause
  - Hyperfunctioning single nodular and multinodular goiter (toxic nodular goiter, Plummer's disease)
  - Solitary hyperfunctioning adenoma; transient subacute thyroiditis; postpartum
  - Drug-induced, such as iodide and iodide-containing drugs (amiodarone) and contrast media
  - Exogenous ingestion of thyroid hormone (factitia)
  - Rare causes include toxic thyroid carcinoma, HCG-secreting tumors (choriocarcinoma, hydatiform mole), TSH-secreting pituitary tumors, testicular embryonal carcinoma

Incidence and Demographics
- Graves' disease accounts for >85% of cases of hyperthyroid; autoantibodies against diffuse fractions of the gland catalyze accelerated hormone production and release
- Affects women > men, 8:1
- Typical age at onset in adulthood: Mid-20s through 30s but can occur in older adults
- Typical age at onset in childhood: 12–14 years, can occur at any age; less likely in neonates

Risk Factors
- Family history of thyroid disorders and autoimmune disorders
- Thyroid replacement hormone ingestion
- Other history of autoimmune disorder
- Mother with Graves' disease (neonates)

Prevention and Screening
- Monitor TSH and T4 for patients taking thyroid replacement hormones

Assessment
HISTORY
- Weight loss, increased appetite, nightmares, hypersensitivity to heat, fatigue, weakness, palpitations
- Mental: Insomnia, irritability, nervousness, anxiety, psychosis, in elderly severe depression
- GI: Increased frequency of bowel movements, diarrhea, pernicious vomiting
- Medication history, past medical history, and family history of autoimmune diseases

PHYSICAL EXAM
- Adrenergic: Nervousness, sweating, tachycardia, palpitations, tremor, lid lag, excitability
- Skin: Onycholysis, myxedema, hyperpigmentation, flushes, diaphoresis, thin/fine hair, spider angiomas
- Eyes (only Graves' disease): Periorbital edema, exophthalmos, chemosis, ophthalmoplegia, papilledema, blurred vision, photophobia, diplopia
- Neck: Goiter smooth or nodular, thyroid bruit or thrill
- Cardiac: Arrhythmia such as atrial fibrillation, sinus tachycardia, systolic flow murmurs, heart failure, widened pulse pressure
- Respiratory: Dyspnea on exertion, tachypnea
- Muscle: Proximal myopathy, periodic paralysis, progressive wasting of muscles
- Lymph nodes: Lymphadenopathy, splenomegaly
- Bone: Osteoporosis, hypercalcemia
- Reproductive: Abortion, infertility, abnormal menses, testicular atrophy, gynecomastia
- Neurologic: Hyperactive reflexes, tremors
- Thyroid storm (rare in children): Hyperpyrexia, tachyarrhythmia, encephalopathy, shock brought on by infection, trauma, noncompliance with antithyroid drugs, or other precipitating event

DIAGNOSTIC STUDIES
- TSH decreased or undetectable; free T4 (unbound thyroxine) usually elevated, if normal order T3 (5% hyperthyroid patients have normal T4); T3 elevated; hypercalcemia; elevated alkaline phosphatase; low hemoglobin/hematocrit; elevated serum antinuclear antibody; elevated TSH receptor antibody
- Urine pregnancy test in females if abnormal menses present
- CT scan for unilateral eye findings to rule out tumor; ECG in the elderly patient
- High radioactive iodine uptake scan for Graves' disease, goiter; low radioactive iodine uptake scan for thyroiditis
- Thyroid uptake scan or ultrasound for palpable nodules to rule out cold nodule (possibly cancer)
- Biospy

Differential Diagnosis
- Psychological disorders (e.g., anxiety, panic, psychosis)
- Pheochromocytoma
- Infection
- Thyrotoxic phase of Hashimoto's thyroiditis
- Hormone ingestion
- Plummer's disease
- Acromegaly
- Malignancy
- Chronic heart failure
- New onset or worsening angina
- Orbital tumors (cause exophthalmos)
- Myasthenia gravis (ophthalmoplegic changes)

Management

NONPHARMACOLOGIC TREATMENT
- Treatment may not be necessary in mild cases
- Surgery last option due to complications of hypoparathyroidism and vocal cord paralysis
- Educate parents about thyroid disease if appropriate

PHARMACOLOGIC TREATMENT
- Radioactive iodine (I_{131}) treatment choice for Graves' disease, symptomatic multinodular goiter, and single hyperfunctioning adenoma; treatment of choice in elderly
  - 1–2 doses orally; euthyroid in 2–6 months
  - Contraindicated in pregnancy and children
  - Hypothyroidism can occur
- Adjunctive therapy to control symptoms
  - Propranolol (Inderal) 10–60 mg q6h to abate catecholamine symptoms; children 1 mg/kg/day
  - Atenolol 50–100 mg qd; not recommended in children
- Antithyroid medication is often first-line therapy for children
  - Propylthiouracil (PTU) 100–150 mg q8h initially, then 50–100 mg bid maintenance dose
    · Neonates and children: 5–7 mg/kg/day in divided doses
    · 6 –12 weeks to reach euthyroid state
    · Relapses with PTU rarely occur except postpartum
  - Methimazole (Tapazole) 20–30 mg q 12 h initially, then 5–10 mg qd or bid maintenance
    · Children: 0.4 mg/kg/day in divided doses, then 0.2 mg/kg maintenance dose
    · 4–6 weeks to reach euthyroid state
  - Usually remain on drug for 1–2 years, then gradually withdrawn
  - Agranulocytosis: Rare side effect of drugs, order WBC before initiating antithyroid drugs
- Other medications as needed
  - Diltiazem (Cardizem) for patients unable to take betablockers
  - Gradually discontinue as euthyroid develops
  - Multivitamin, calcium replacement, and vitamin D rebuild bone density
  - Ophthalmopathy: Eye lubricants for mild cases

Special Considerations
- Elderly may develop arrhythmia (usually atrial fibrillation), CHF, and angina.
- Pregnancy: Thyroid autoantibodies, including TSH receptor antibody, may be ordered.
- Nonthyroidal illnesses such as active hepatitis, cirrhosis, nephrotic syndrome, infections, malnutrition, and severe acute illness can affect thyroid functioning serum tests.
- PTU at lowest doses during pregnancy, does not cross placenta.
- Spontaneous remission in 25% of children within 2 years, and in 50% of children within 4–5 years; relapse can occur in 30%–40% of cases.

When to Consult, Refer, Hospitalize
- Refer to endocrinologist for management of all patients; may co-manage after initial therapy
- Hospitalize for thyroid storm
- Pituitary tumor: Immediate referral to neurosurgeon
- Surgical referral for thyroidectomy
- Ophthalmologist for evaluation of eye pathology

Follow-Up
- Monitor free T4 and TSH every 4–8 weeks until patient becomes euthyroid or hypothyroid, then thyroid replacement therapy
- Maintenance visits every 3 months, then 6 months, then annually
- After radioactive iodine therapy order TSH every 6 weeks, 12 weeks, 6 months, then annually
- Baseline CBC, LFT every 3–6 months, ECG
  - EXPECTED COURSE
    - Usually requires long-term maintenance for replacement therapy, or follow-up for recurrence after remission

  - COMPLICATIONS
    - Thyroid storm
    - Hypothyroidism following surgery or radiation
    - Severe depression post treatment
    - Visual disturbance from ophthalmopathy
    - Hypoparathyroidism and vocal cord paralysis post surgery

Hypothyroidism

Description
- Decreased secretion of thyroid hormone due to dysfunction in thyroid gland or pituitary gland, occurring after the neonatal period
- Congenital hypothyroidism is present at birth

Etiology
- Primary: Inability of thyroid gland to produce TSH
  - Autoimmune thyroiditis (Hashimoto's) is the most common
  - Transient hypothyroidism in acute or subacute thyroiditis (viral etiology): Transient postpartum thyroiditis
  - Ablation of gland due to surgery, radiation, thioamide drugs, radioactive iodine
  - Congenital: Ectopic thyroid gland; aplasia of the thyroid gland; ineffective synthesis or utilization of thyroid hormones; transient hypothyroidism related to maternal antithyroid medications or fetal/neonatal exposure to high levels of thyroid hormone; congenital hypopituitarism
  - Iodine deficiency
- Secondary: Lesions in pituitary gland (less common)
  - Pituitary adenoma
  - Certain drugs such as lithium and para-aminosalicylic acid; previously treated hyperthyroidism, especially postpartum; coexisting autoimmune disorders (lupus, pernicious anemia, rheumatoid arthritis
- Tertiary: Thyrotropin-releasing hormone (TRH) deficiency from hypothalamus

Incidence and Demographics
- Predominant age >40; more frequent in women
- Hashimoto's thyroiditis can occur before age 3 years but usually after age 6 years, with an increasing incidence in adolescence
- Congenital hypothyroidism occurs in 1 in 3,700 live births in North America; more frequent in Far Eastern and Hispanic descent

Risk Factors
- Previous hyperthyroidism treatment
- Autoimmune diseases; presence of thyroid antibodies
- Family history of thyroid or autoimmune disorders
- Pituitary disease; hypothalamic disease
- Postpartum women, maternal TSH-binding antibodies
- Lithium treatment
- Diabetes mellitus type 1 (10% will develop hypothyroidism)
- Infertility problems, repeated spontaneous abortions
- Fetal or newborn exposure to antithyroid drugs or excessive amounts of iodine
- Children with Down, Turner, Klinefelter, or Noonan syndrome

Prevention and Screening
- No official screening guidelines; however, periodic TSH screening for patients treated for hyperthyroidism or those who are symptomatic; some clinicians screen adult women >45 or 50
- Mandatory newborn screening at 2–6 days (5%–10% false-negative rate); thyroid dysfunction must be confirmed with a venous sample
- Retest children with Down syndrome at age 3 months and periodically thereafter
- Screen those with autoimmune diseases

Assessment
HISTORY
- Adults: Anorexia, dry skin, coarse dry hair, alopecia, receding hairline, constipation, cold intolerance, lethargy, increase in weight, irregular or heavy menses, memory loss, depression, muscle aches, paresthesias, medication history (especially lithium)
- Neonates: Persistent jaundice, constipation, poor feeding, lethargy/somnolence, prolonged gestation, increased birthweight
- Children: Family history, poor growth, learning disabilities or poor school performance, fatigue, constipation, weight gain, cold intolerance

PHYSICAL EXAM
- Weight gain, short stature in pediatric patients, failure to grow, subnormal temperature, decreased level of consciousness
- Face: Dull, blank expression, swollen; eyes—periorbital edema; ears—decreased auditory acuity
- Skin: Dry skin, coarse dry hair, brittle nails, hair loss, temporal thinning of eye brows
- Mouth: Swollen tongue, slow speech, hoarseness; thyroid—enlarged gland or atrophy, tender, nodules

- Cardiac: Bradycardia, decrease heart tones, mild hypotension or diastolic hypertension, cardiomegaly
- Respiratory: Dyspnea, pleural effusion; breasts—galactorrhea; electrolytes—hyponatremia
- Abdominal: Hypoactive bowel sounds, ascites
- Extremities: Swollen hands/feet, leg edema
- Neurological: Dementia, paranoid ideation, slow/delayed reflexes, cerebellar ataxia, carpal tunnel syndrome
- Hematologic: Anemia; hyperlipidemia, hypercholesterolemia
- Neonates: Occasional large birthweight, jaundice, large fontanelles, respiratory distress, hoarse cry, large abdomen, umbilical hernia (possibly), hypothermia, cool/mottled extremities, bradycardia with murmurs and cardiomegaly, anemia

DIAGNOSTIC STUDIES
- TSH assay (use third-generation assay): Elevated in primary hypothyroidism; TSH will be low in cases due to pituitary insufficiency
- Order free T4 when TSH elevated; low free T4 confirms diagnosis of hypothyroidism
- Subclinical hypothyroidism—normal T4 and elevated TSH
- If secondary to pituitary or hypothalamic failure—normal TSH, low or mildly elevated T4
- Further tests when secondary hypothyroidism suspected, such as serum prolactin level, neuroradiologic studies, pituitary-adrenal and pituitary-gonadal function
- CBC, serum electrolytes, BUN, creatinine, glucose, calcium, phosphate, albumin levels, pregnancy test, urine protein, lipid studies as indicated
- Free thyroxine index (FTI) in most cases provides indirect estimate of T4
- Children: Bone age if short stature is suspected
- Neonates: Thyroid scan

Differential Diagnosis
- Depression
- Obesity
- Dementia
- Ischemic heart disease
- Chronic heart failure (CHF)
- Kidney failure
- Cirrhosis
- Nephrotic syndrome
- Chronic renal disease
- Coexisting secondary cause
- Congenital hypothyroidism
- Transient hypothyroidism
- Hypopituitarism
- Sick euthyroid
- Iodine ingestion
- Thyroid hormone resistance

Management

NONPHARMACOLOGIC TREATMENT

- Education, high-fiber diet for constipation, diet and exercise for weight loss if obese
- Avoid drug interactions: Cholestyramine; ferrous sulfate; aluminum hydroxide antacids; sucralfate; foods such as cabbage, turnips, kale, and soybeans that increase the loss of thyroid hormone as they may interfere with levothyroxine absorption, should be spaced 4 hours from these medications
- Take medication in the morning on an empty stomach to increase absorption
- For congenital hypothyroidism, monitor growth and development and be alert for signs of behavior changes

PHARMACOLOGIC TREATMENT

- Primary hypothyroidism: Correct hormone deficiency with thyroxine replacement
  - Levothyroxine (T4) first-line therapy for primary hypothyroidism
  - Adults: Starting dose: 50–100 mcg po qd, increase 25 mcg every 1–3 weeks based on clinical condition and laboratory results; average dose 125 mcg qd with maximum dose of 300 mcg
  - Elderly with coronary artery disease: Start levothyroxine at 25–50 mcg po qd with gradual increase every 4–6 weeks as tolerated, with maximum dose of 75–150 mcg
- Children: Congenital hypothyroidism is a true endocrine emergency; goal is to begin therapy by 14 days of life
  - Levothyroxine at 2–5 mcg/kg/day; recheck T4 and TSH at 1 month and titrate to maintain normal levels
- Subclinical hypothyroidism
  - Treat pharmacologically if TSH >10 mU/mL with presence of thyroid autoantibodies
  - Just monitor the elderly due to risk of coronary artery disease (CAD) with treatment
- Transient, subacute hypothyroidism
  - Self-limited with symptoms resolving after 2–3 months
  - No therapy for minimal symptoms
- Congenital hypothyroidism
  - Initially, levothyroxine 10–15 mcg/kg/day po; recheck thyroid function tests within 2–3 weeks (goal: raise T4 and decrease TSH; TSH may not decrease to normal levels for several months, despite normal T4)
  - Management is usually with a pediatric endocrinologist
  - May consider stopping levothyroxine at age 2–3 years in children with congenital hypothyroidism to reevaluate, if medication was started prior to a thyroid scan or if child had a normal gland on initial scan
  - Hashimoto's thyroiditis may be self-limited in older children, re-evaluate periodically throughout life

Special Considerations
- Adults/geriatric patients: Concomitant use of CNS depressants, digoxin, insulin may decrease efficacy of thyroid replacement dosage; elderly are at risk for angina as thyroid levels increase
- Pregnancy: If hypothyroidism is present during pregnancy, monitor TSH every trimester
- Children: T4 may be normally low and TSH high in premature infants; soy-based formula may interfere with absorption of levothyroxine; untreated hypothyroidism in children leads to facial edema, hirsute forehead, growth delays, and mental retardation

When to Consult, Refer, Hospitalize
- Refer developing myxedema coma, hypothermia, decreased mentation, respiratory acidosis, hypotension, hyponatremia, hypoglycemia, hypoventilation, significant cardiac disease, secondary hypothyroidism, or radically abnormal thyroid function tests to an endocrinologist
- Consult or refer for co-management of congenital hypothyroidism
- Refer pregnant and pediatric patients to an endocrinologist for ongoing management
- Hospitalization is not usually required

Follow-Up
- Adults: Measure TSH 4–6 weeks after initial dosage, then every 2 months until within normal limits, then every 6–12 months (TSH levels may remain elevated for several months despite effective treatment); if drug dosage changed, recheck TSH levels in 2–3 months
- Annual lipid levels
    EXPECTED COURSE
    - Improvement within 1 month of starting medication; symptoms resolve within 3–6 months
    - Treatment is usually lifelong; maintain medication at lowest dosage to maintain euthyroid state
    - Excellent prognosis with appropriate treatment

    COMPLICATIONS
    - Chronic heart failure
    - Depression, psychoses
    - Miscarriages during pregnancy
    - Thyrotoxicity, myxedema coma (rare)
    - Bone demineralization due to over-treatment
    - Mental retardation in children

Thyroid Nodule

Description
- Localized enlargements within thyroid gland; may function independently of hypothalamic/pituitary feedback
- Evaluation of thyroid nodule is important to detect thyroid cancer

Etiology
- Unknown etiology

- Autonomously functioning nodules (hot nodule on thyroid scan) are usually benign and may cause symptoms of hyperthyroidism
- Nonfunctioning nodule (cold nodule) may be malignant carcinoma

Incidence and Demographics
- Solitary nodules in 4%–7% of U.S. population
  - More common with age, women, exposure to ionizing radiation, living in areas with iodine deficiency
- <10% solitary nodules are malignant
- 10,000–20,000 new cases of thyroid cancer per year
- Papillary carcinoma 75% of thyroid cancers; follicular carcinoma (aggressive) < 10% of thyroid cancers
- Papillary nodules are twice as common in women than men, slow-growing
- Cysts comprise 15%–25% of thyroid nodules
- Uncommon in children; if they occur, usually asymptomatic and 25%–75% malignant

Risk Factors
- For thyroid nodule:
  - Female, increasing age, residing in area of endemic iodine deficiency
- For thyroid cancer:
  - Family history of thyroid cancer or multiple endocrine metaplastic type II carcinoma
  - Male gender, extremes in age (<15 and >70)
  - Exposure of head, neck or chest to radiation
  - Single nodule

Assessment
HISTORY
- Hoarseness, cough, dysphagia, obstruction, neck tenderness, neck swelling or enlargement
- History of hypo- or hyperthyroidism; external radiation to head, neck, chest; or nuclear fallout
- Family history of thyroid disease
- Medication history
- Pregnancy status
- Benign or malignant nodules often asymptomatic but may have symptoms of hypo- or hyperthyroidism

PHYSICAL EXAM
- Malignant: Hoarseness; enlarged cervical lymph nodes; dyspnea; tumor palpable as fixed, painless, hard, irregular-shaped mass; does not move with swallowing
- Benign: Multiple nodules palpable (nodular Hashimoto's thyroiditis or multinodular goiter)

DIAGNOSTIC STUDIES
- Fine-needle biopsy aspiration initial test with palpable nodules >1.5 cm
- Serum TSH; if low, order free T4
- Multinodular goiter is usually euthyroid

- Radionuclide scans to determine cytologic results; hot nodules are benign in 98% of cases; 5%–10% cold nodules are malignant (meaning decreased amount of radionuclide uptake)
- Ultrasound to determine if cystic
- Serum calcitonin with family history of medullary thyroid carcinoma
- Evaluate anithyroperoxidase antibodies and antithyroglobulin antibodies to rule out thyroiditis

Differential Diagnosis
- Malignant nodules versus benign nodules
- Cysts
- Thyroiditis

Management
NONPHARMACOLOGIC TREATMENT
- Adequate iodine intake
- Surgery for malignant or disfiguring tumors
- Carefully follow patients with benign nodules (see Follow-Up)
- Instruct patients to follow up for size changes, lymphadenopathy, dysphasia, hoarseness, new or worsening symptoms of hypo- or hyperthyroidism

PHARMACOLOGIC TREATMENT
- Treat abnormal thyroid hormone levels following guidelines for hypo/hyperthyroidism

Special Considerations
- Pregnancy and lactation: Avoid radionuclide scan

When to Consult, Refer, Hospitalize
- Refer all patients with thyroid nodules to endocrinologist for evaluation to rule out malignancy

Follow-Up
- Reevaluate euthyroid patients with benign nodules annually to check size and TSH
- Benign nodules with abnormal thyroid function require frequent monitoring according to hypothyroidism and hyperthyroidism guidelines
- Patients with malignancy must be followed up by an endocrinologist and possibly oncologist
  #### EXPECTED COURSE
  - Good survival rate with malignant nodules unless due to follicular carcinoma

  #### COMPLICATIONS
  - Tumor recurrence
  - Hypo- or hyperthyroidism

ADRENAL DISORDERS

Cushing Syndrome

Description
- Syndrome of clinical abnormalities resulting from exogenous glucocorticoid excess (mainly cortisol)
- Cushing syndrome is due to endogenous hypercorticosolism related to adrenal or pituitary dysfunction

Etiology
- Excess glucocorticoid production caused by adrenocorticotrophic hormone (ACTH)-secreting pituitary tumor (two-thirds of cases), or ectopic production by a nonpituitary tumor (small cell carcinoma of lung); or ACTH-independent adrenal tumor
- Prolonged use of glucocorticoids
- Serum concentration of glucocorticoids is regulated by the negative-feedback loop of the hypothalamic-pituitary-adrenal (HPA) system. Corticotropin-releasing hormone (CRH) stimulates the production and release of ACTH by the anterior pituitary, which stimulates the adrenal cortex to produce cortisol. Cortisol levels increase in response to increased ACTH levels and will decrease in response to decreasing ACTH levels.

Incidence and Demographics
- Cushing syndrome and primary adrenal tumors more common in women
- Pituitary tumors five times more frequent in women than men
- Age of onset 20–40 years
- Rare in childhood and infancy

Risk Factors
- Adrenal tumor
- Pituitary tumor
- Long-term or frequent high-dose corticosteroid use

Prevention and Screening
- Limit corticosteroid use
- Screen for unprescribed steroid use

Assessment
HISTORY
- Acne, back pain, headache, emotional lability, depression, mental changes, muscle weakness, fatigue, poor wound healing, thin skin, menstrual disorders/amenorrhea, hyperglycemia, susceptibility to infections, weight gain, easy bruising, decreased libido, insomnia
- Therapeutic or factitious use of corticosteroids

PHYSICAL EXAM
- High blood pressure
- Truncal obesity with thin extremities, dorsal fat pad "buffalo hump," moon face
- Skin: Thin, atrophic, acne, hirsutism, ecchymosis, hyperpigmentation; purple striae around breasts, abdomen, thighs

- Eyes: Increased intraocular pressure
- Musculoskeletal: Weakness, atrophy of muscles, thinning bones

DIAGNOSTIC STUDIES
- Glycosuria and elevated urine cortisol (24-hour urine for free cortisol)
- Plasma cortisol level elevated evenings (>5–7.5 mcg/dL)
- Serum glucose elevated, hypokalemia without hypernatremia
- Screening tests: Refer to endocrinologist
- Dexamethasone overnight suppression test: suppression cortisol level <5 mcg/dL normal result; if abnormal, more reliable suppression test performed by giving dexamethasone 0.5 mg po q6h for 2 days
- CT scans, chest and abdomen, for adrenal tumors and MRI for pituitary tumors

Differential Diagnosis
- Alcoholism
- Obesity
- Depression
- Familial cortisol resistance
- Hirsutism
- Anorexia nervosa
- Drugs such as phenytoin, phenobarbital, primidone accelerate dexamethasone metabolism, causing "false-positive" dexamethasone suppression test

Management
NONPHARMACOLOGIC TREATMENT
- High-protein diet
- Reduce pituitary ACTH by transsphenoidal resection or radiation
- Reduce adrenal cortisol secretion by bilateral adrenalectomy
- Ectopic ACTH-secreting tumors surgically removed

PHARMACOLOGIC TREATMENT
- Refer to endocrinologist for ongoing management
- Replacement glucocorticoid therapy up to 1 year post adrenal surgery and lifelong if bilateral adrenalectomy
- If patient is taken off glucocorticoid therapy, may need to restart if become ill

Special Considerations
- Pregnancy can exacerbate symptoms

When to Consult, Refer, Hospitalize
- Refer all cases to endocrinologist and coordinate their primary care
- Refer to surgeon and oncologist for adrenal or pituitary tumor

Follow-Up
- For recurrence symptoms, measure urine free cortisol
  ### EXPECTED COURSE
  - Posttreatment for pituitary adenoma: Normal ACTH suppressed and require 6–36 months to recover to normal function; hydrocortisone replacement therapy necessary

- Normal HPA function within 3–24 months after surgery if one adrenal gland left
- 10%–20% failure rate with transsphenoidal surgery; those with complete remission will have 15%–20% recurrence rate over next 10 years

COMPLICATIONS
- Hypertension, CAD
- Osteoporosis, compression fractures of spine, aseptic necrosis femur head
- Diabetes mellitus
- Overwhelming infection
- Nephrolithiasis
- Psychosis
- If untreated, morbidity and death

Adrenal Insufficiency/Addison's Disease

Description
- Primary adrenal insufficiency is a loss of all adrenal hormones, including mineralocorticoids, glucocorticoids, and adrenal androgens. It is an insidious, chronic disease of adrenal destruction, also known as Addison's disease or primary adrenal failure.
- Secondary adrenal insufficiency is a lack of glucocorticoids due to pituitary dysfunction; tertiary adrenal insufficiency is lack of glucocorticoids caused by hypothalamic failure.

Etiology
- Autoimmune destruction of the adrenal gland accounts for 80% of Addison's disease, followed by tuberculosis as second leading cause.
- Rarer causes include AIDS and other infections, genetic disorder, carcinoma, amyloid disease, hemochromatosis, antineoplastic chemotherapy, bilateral adrenal hemorrhage, or may be idiopathic.
- Secondary and tertiary adrenal insufficiency result from suppression of HPA axis through glucocorticoid replacement, adrenalectomy; pituitary tumor, trauma, surgery, infarction; or hypothalamic disease.

Incidence and Demographics
- Usually affects those ages 30–50, but may occur at any age; females > males
- Prevalence approximately 4:100,000

Risk Factors
- Autoimmune disease
- Family history of adrenal insufficiency
- Prolonged steroid use followed by infection, trauma, surgery
- Medications: Ketoconazole, Dilantin, rifampin, opiates

Assessment

HISTORY

- Progressive weakness, fatigue, weight loss, lightheadedness, anorexia, possible nausea and vomiting, diarrhea, cold intolerance, abdominal pain (like peptic ulcer disease), salt craving, emotional changes

PHYSICAL EXAM

- Postural hypotension
- 90% systolic blood pressure <110 mmHg and rarely >130 mmHg
- Skin: Hyperpigmentation (especially hand creases, knuckles, elbows, buccal mucosa) in Whites, multiple freckles, change in body hair distribution with scant axillary and pubic hair, areas of vitiligo
- Breasts: Dark nipples and areola
- Cardiac: Small heart
- Lymph: Hyperplasia, lymphadenopathy
- Acute adrenal insufficiency or Addisonian crisis may present with profound fatigue, dehydration, severe abdominal pain, nausea and vomiting, hypotension, hypoglycemia, and shock with vascular collapse and renal shutdown; is precipitated by surgery, infection, exacerbation of comorbid illness, sudden withdrawal of long-term glucocorticoid replacement

DIAGNOSTIC STUDIES

- Diagnostic: Low plasma cortisol <5 mcg/dL at 8 a.m.
- Sodium, chloride, glucose, and bicarbonate levels low with high potassium level
- BUN, plasma renin, ACTH, calcium all elevated
- CBC, decreased hemoglobin, neutrophils, and eosinophils
- Serum anti-adrenal antibodies in 50% cases of autoimmune Addison's disease
- ECG: Nonspecific changes
- EEG: Generalized slowing
- Abdominal CT scan: Small adrenals
- Chest x-ray: Small heart size and adrenal calcification

Differential Diagnosis

- Hyperparathyroidism
- Depression
- Mild thyrotoxicosis in elderly
- Gastrointestinal malignancy
- Chronic infection
- Heavy metal poisoning
- Hemochromatosis, anemia
- Salt-wasting nephritis
- Myopathies
- ACTH-secreting tumors

Management

NONPHARMACOLOGIC TREATMENT
- Monitor fluid and electrolytes
- Adequate dietary intake of sodium
- Treat all infections immediately and vigorously and raise cortisol dose

PHARMACOLOGIC TREATMENT
- Chronic phase: management initiated by endocrinologist—replace deficient hormones
- Cortisol 10–20 mg po every morning; 5–10 mg po at 4–6 p.m. (total of 15–25 mg of hydrocortisone daily in two divided doses with two-thirds morning and one-third afternoon) OR prednisone 3 mg po every morning, 2 mg po every evening
  - Dose will be increased in case of stress, trauma, surgery, stressful diagnostic procedures, postural hypotension, hyperkalemia, or weight loss
- Fludrocortisone acetate 0.05–0.3 mg po qd or qod for cases of primary adrenal insufficiency if insufficient sodium retention with cortisol alone
  - If edema, hypokalemia, or hypertensive crises occurs, lower dose
  - Salt additives for excess heat or humidity
- Acute adrenal insufficiency: Hospitalize for IV hydrocortisone, mineralocorticoid, normal saline

When to Consult, Refer, Hospitalize
- Refer all suspected cases to endocrinologist for management
- Hospitalization with acute crisis, dehydration, severe stress

Follow-Up
- Periodic evaluations of blood pressure, weight, electrolytes and other labs, muscle strength, appetite, cardiac status
- MedicAlert or similar identification bracelet or necklace

  EXPECTED COURSE
  - Excellent prognosis with lifelong steroid replacement therapy

  COMPLICATIONS
  - Acute adrenal crisis
  - Complications of steroid therapy: Osteoporosis, psychosis, hyperglycemia, Cushing syndrome

PITUITARY DISORDERS

Pituitary Adenoma

Description
- Pituitary tumors can manifest by disturbance of function (hyper or hyposecretion of trophic hormones), anatomic invasion into surrounding structures (enlargement of tumors), or combination.
- Microadenoma is <10 mm and macroadenoma is >10 mm in size.

Etiology
- Occasionally part of MEN1 (multiple endocrine neoplasia type 1) syndrome, autosomal dominant chromosomal mutation
- Etiology largely unknown
- If adenoma is secretory, usually only one hormone is secreted (frequently growth hormone, ACTH, or prolactin), causing characteristic symptoms. Secretion of prolactin (common) causes syndrome of hyperprolactinemia.

Incidence and Demographics
- More frequent in women
- Growth hormone secretion with gigantism almost always occurs in males
- Fairly common and may be asymptomatic; often found on autopsy

Assessment
HISTORY
- Headaches, visual field loss due to pituitary enlargement; rare loss of consciousness, seizures, mental state changes, brainstem dysfunction
- Amenorrhea, infertility, galactorrhea, impotence due to hyperprolactinemia
- Symptoms of Cushing syndrome with ACTH secretion (acne, weight gain, depression)
- Symptoms of acromegaly with growth hormone secretion (enlargement of head and face, feet and hands)

PHYSICAL EXAM
- Body habitus for signs of gigantism, acromegaly, Cushing syndrome
- Eyes: Ocular motor dysfunctions, pupillary dysfunction, limited visual fields
- Breast exam: Bilateral galactorrhea (milky discharge)

DIAGNOSTIC STUDIES
- Serum prolactin, growth hormone, adrenal steroids may be elevated
  - Prolactin should be considered for complaint of headache with visual changes, amenorrhea, or galactorrhea
- MRI of brain preferred over CT scan for pituitary imaging; angiography, visual field testing
  - Imaging indicated for men or women with serum prolactin >200 ng/mL

Differential Diagnosis
- Pituitary inflammation
- Other causes of headache
- Other causes of amenorrhea and galactorrhea
- Aneurysm
- Cushing syndrome

Management

NONPHARMACOLOGIC TREATMENT
- Transsphenoidal surgery or stereotactic radiosurgery to remove pituitary adenoma
- Radiation to pituitary

PHARMACOLOGIC TREATMENT
- Dopamine agonist bromocriptine (Parlodel) for hyperprolactinemia; may shrink tumors by 50% in 40% of patients within 3 months; treatment many be long-term. Withdrawal from drug may result in recurrent hyperprolactinemia
- Octreotide (Sandostatin), a somatotropin for treatment of acromegaly
- Postoperative substitution including adrenal steroids, thyroxin, and testosterone or estrogen may be given

Special Considerations
- Stop bromocriptine treatment with pregnancy/lactation

When to Consult, Refer, Hospitalize
- All suspected cases refer to endocrinologist, neurologist if surgery indicated

Follow-Up
- MRI scans at 6 months, 12 months, and annually for those treated with bromocriptine
- Growth of tumor indicates need for surgery or radiation therapy

EXPECTED COURSE
- Recurrence can occur within 5–10 years

COMPLICATIONS
- Hypopituitarism
- Pituitary hemorrhage, infarct
- Diabetes insipidus
- Surgical complications including menstruation ceases and infertility

Short Stature

Description
- Genetic: Height below the 3rd percentile (or 2.5 standard deviations below the norm) with no known etiology with appropriate growth in relation to parents' heights; normal growth rate and bone age
- Constitutional delay in growth also a normal variant of short stature. Well child who is short, takes longer to get to his/her eventual height (which is usually average height), with a biologically slower maturation and delay in puberty; delayed bone age by about 2 years; often progress to delayed puberty; parents' heights are normal; predicted final height is comparable to target height.
- Turner syndrome: Short stature in females due to an absence or abnormality of an X chromosome

Etiology
- Genetic: Usually, normal variant; possible genetic tendency toward growth hormone (GH) deficiency or GH receptor defect; possible inherited pathologic condition (e.g., hypochondroplasia)
- Constitutional delay in growth: Often no known cause; possible causes include decreased GH secretion, abnormal GH structure, GH receptor defect
- Turner syndrome: Absence or defect of an X chromosome, usually 45,X (monosomy) or 46,XX (mosaicism)

Incidence and Demographics
- Genetic: 3% of all normal children are below the 3rd–5th percentile in height; equal incidence in boys and girls
- Constitutional delay in growth: Increased incidence in boys
- Turner syndrome: Occurs in 1 in 2,000 live female births (no males)

Risk Factors
- Genetic: Parents who are below the 3rd–5th percentile in height or with a pathologic cause for short height (e.g., hypochondroplasia)
- Constitutional delay in growth: Usually, a positive family history of growth delay
- Turner syndrome: No known risk factors

Prevention and Screening
- No known prevention
- Assess parents' heights
- Fetal ultrasound may detect abnormality associated with Turner syndrome (no known prevention)
- Amniocentesis or chorionic villus sampling may detect Turner syndrome but also has the potential to over-diagnose an X chromosome abnormality

Assessment

HISTORY

- Genetic: Normal birth size; no intrauterine growth retardation; short parents below the 3rd–5th percentile with or without known pathologic reason
- Constitutional delay in growth: Normal birthweight and size; gradual decrease in rate of growth in the first 2 years of life; then maintains growth curve approximately 2 standard deviations (SDs) below normal
- Turner syndrome: No family history, slightly small birth size, puffy hands and feet in neonatal period; short stature with a marked deviation of a decreased height on the normal growth curve

PHYSICAL EXAM

- Genetic: Gradual decrease in growth rate within the first 2 years of life; normal growth rate after age 2 years; normal onset of puberty
- Constitutional delay: Aside from short stature, healthy; reduced growth rate until about age 2 years secondary to delayed bone age; in early adolescence, rate of growth decreases secondary to delayed puberty but then resumes after onset of puberty with some catch-up growth noted (see Table 17–3)
- Turner syndrome: Short stature, small jaw, short or webbed neck (20%–30% cases), high arched palate; absence or delayed puberty with ovarian failure; skeletal abnormalities; possible cardiovascular and renal abnormalities; recurrent otitis media, hearing loss, Hashimoto's thyroiditis, usually normal intelligence
- Height should be assessed on a carefully calibrated scale with a built-in level for children and on measuring boards for infants

DIAGNOSTIC STUDIES

- X-rays for bone age: Normal in genetic, delayed in constitutional delay
- Check for decreased serum GH and GH receptor defect
- Diagnostic tests for Turner syndrome should be directed by a pediatric endocrinologist and may include chromosomal karyotype, FSH and LH, thyroid function tests, glucose tolerance test, echocardiogram, renal and pelvic ultrasound

Table 17–3. Comparison of Normal Variants

	Familiar Short Stature	Constitutional Delay
Parents	Short (or family history)	Average height
Birth History and Early Years	Normal; often born at 25–75 percentile followed by a deceleration period until age 2, at which point they are in 3–5 percentile	Same growth shift as genetic short stature
Growth Velocity	Steady after age 2 to adulthood; parallels growth curve	Steady until puberty and because pubertal growth spurt is delayed, begins to fall away further from growth chart
Puberty Changes	Normal age	Males: failure to achieve Tanner genital 2 by age 13.8 years, or Tanner pubic 2 by 15.6 years: Females: failure to achieve Tanner breast 2 by age 13.3 years
Bone Age	Normal	Delayed (usually 2–4 years)
Ultimate Height	Short	Average (can be tall) Males >163 cm (64 inches) Females >150 cm (59 inches)
Diagnostic Studies	All normal	All normal except delayed bone age; A more extensive work-up likely will be done because of the delayed puberty
Treatment	Reassurance	None

Differential Diagnoses
- Constitutional short stature
- Familial short stature
- Malnutrition
- Chronic renal failure
- GI malabsorption
- Skeletal defects
- Pulmonary disease
- Cardiac disease
- Failure to thrive
- Metabolic diseases
- DM type 1
- Anemia
- Hypothyroidism
- GH deficiency
- Turner syndrome
- IUGR
- Chromosomal abnormalities

Management

NONPHARMACOLOGIC TREATMENT

- Genetic: No treatment is necessary as this is usually a normal variant; occasional uses of subcutaneous injections of GH have not proven to significantly increase final height
- Reassurance that child is healthy aside from short stature

PHARMACOLOGIC TREATMENT

- Constitutional delay: Treatment with injections of GH occasionally renders a brief increase in growth, but is unclear whether final height is truly affected; appropriate time to discontinue therapy is controversial
- Adolescents with constitutional delay may be treated with low doses of androgen
- Turner syndrome: Consists of hormone replacement at puberty, GH therapy, and anabolic steroid therapy managed by a pediatric endocrinologist

Special Considerations

- Educate families that growth hormone treatment will not make their child tall but will restore the normal growth pattern

When to Consult, Refer, or Hospitalize

- Consult with pediatrician or pediatric endocrinologist for evaluation and diagnosis; no further referral needed for genetic short stature
- Constitutional delay and Turner syndrome: Refer to pediatric endocrinologist for management

Follow-Up

- Continue to assess growth and development in routine physical exams
- Follow up with pediatric endocrinologist and other pediatric specialists as appropriate for clinical manifestations
- Periodic monitoring of thyroid function in all ages and lipid levels in adults is indicated at 6-month intervals for patients treated with GH who have constitutional delay
- Careful monitoring of bone maturation and serum glucose levels in patients with Turner syndrome

PUBERTAL DISORDERS

Normal onset of puberty is 8–13 years in girls and 9–14 years in boys; see Table 3–7 for classification of sexual maturity (Tanner staging).

Precocious Puberty

Description
- Early onset of pubertal changes (secondary sexual development) before age 6
  - Girls <6–8 years of age
  - Boys <9 years of age
- Normal development sequence is thelarche followed closely by pubarche and 2–3 years later menarche
- Normal variants of early onset puberty
  - Premature thelarche: Benign breast development (typically Tanner 2) usually in toddlers (see next section)
  - Premature adrenarche: Small amounts of pubic hair before age 8 in girls and before age 9 in boys (possibly axillary hair and body odor). No growth spurt, breast development, testicular enlargement (needs to be differentiated from true and pseudo precocious puberty)

Etiology
- True precocious puberty or central precocious puberty (CPP) results from premature activation of the hypothalamic-pituitary-gonadal axis; referred to as gonadotropin-releasing hormone–dependent. Hypothalamic-pituitary (CNS) stimulation of gonads produces estrogen and testosterone, which induces the pubertal changes. May be:
  - Idiopathic: No identifiable cause (system turns on spontaneously at an earlier than expected age); 75% of precocious puberty in females is idiopathic; approximately 33% in males
  - Neurogenic: Damage to areas of the CNS that affect the hypothalamic pituitary axis and may include CNS tumors, infections, trauma, radiation, cerebral malformations, hydrocephalus, seizure disorders, neurofibromatosis, and tuberous sclerosis
- Pseudo (or peripheral) precocious puberty:
  - Cause is from a source outside the central hypothalamic-pituitary system such as the ovaries or adrenals; the hypothalamic-pituitary system is not activated and does not mature
  - Results in the same secretion of pubertal amounts of estrogen and testosterone
  - Can occur from ovarian or testicular tumors, liver tumors (hepatomas), congenital adrenal hyperplasia, exposure to exogenous sex steroids from food (e.g., soybeans), drugs (e.g., oral contraceptives or estrogen-containing creams), or familial trait (e.g., familial testotoxicosis)

Incidence and Demographics
- More common in girls than in boys
- Usually idiopathic in girls
- In boys, approximately 50% related to a tumor, congenital adrenal hyperplasia, or familial testotoxicosis

Risk Factors
- CNS insult
- Family history

Prevention and Screening
- No known prevention

Assessment

HISTORY
- Pubertal changes: Age of onset, progression and specific symptoms (e.g., breast budding, hair, menses)
- Symptoms of possible underlying etiology such as headaches, weight loss, fatigue and constipation (hypothyroid)
- History of CNS insult (meningitis, radiation)
- Exogenous sources of hormones
- Family history of early-onset puberty

PHYSICAL EXAM
- Assess all pubertal changes: Breast development, testicular size, pubic hair staging, presence of adult body odor, acne, any growth spurt (plot on growth chart)
- Obtain blood pressure: Increased blood pressure may be consistent with increased intracranial pressure or congenital adrenal hyperplasia
- Thorough neurological exam including funduscopic exam (papilledema), visual acuity, and visual fields
- Palpate scrotum/testicles for any masses; the abdomen for possible hepatomegaly or enlarged ovary or uterus
- Assess skin for café-au-lait spots, myxedema
- Palpate the thyroid

DIAGNOSTIC STUDIES
- Results of tests will vary depending on the etiology.
- Levels of FSH and LH are usually in the prepubertal ranges with true precocious puberty; therefore, in order to document the premature activation of the hypothalamic-pituitary axis, a gonadotropin-stimulating test must be obtained. If premature activation has occurred, an increase in LH in response to a GnRH stimulation (i.e., serum concentration > 10 IU/L 30–40 minutes after administering GnRH SQ) will occur. A positive response indicates the presence of true precocious puberty (not the cause but the presence). If LH/FSH is high, follow with prolactin.
- In both true and pseudo precocious puberty, levels of testosterone or estradiol will be elevated. Levels are normal for normal variants such as premature adrenarche.
- Adrenal androgens, particularly dehydroepiandrosterone sulfate (DHEAS), are obtained to rule out congenital adrenal hyperplasia. Levels would be elevated.
- Thyroid function studies (free T4 and TSH) if hypothyroidism suspected.
- Bone age should be obtained on all patients to assist with determining etiology (i.e., advanced with true precocious puberty, normal with normal variants), height potential, and if treatment is warranted. May need to be repeated in the follow-up of patients.

- Pelvic and testicular ultrasounds may be obtained to rule out tumors.
- Cranial CT scan or MRI of the hypothalamic/pituitary regions can determine tumors or structural abnormalities.
- CT scan of the adrenals if adrenal tumor suspected.

Differential Diagnosis

- Premature thelarche
- Premature adrenarche
- Ovarian tumors
- Ovarian cysts
- Adrenal tumors
- McCune-Albright syndrome
- Exogenous sex steroids
- Congenital adrenal hyperplasia
- Familial testotoxicosis (Leydig cell tumors)
- Cerebral lesions

Management

NONPHARMACOLOGIC TREATMENT

- Treatment directed at underlying cause
- Reassurance if pubescent and postpubescent if evaluation negative and lack of pathology
- Referral to surgeon if fibrous tissue present causing breast enlargement, or breast mass present
- Weight reduction

PHARMACOLOGIC TREATMENT

- Antiestrogens (tamoxifen, clomiphene), dehydrotestosterone, diethylstilbestrol in elderly
- Eliminate or decrease any medication that may have a side effect of gynecomastia
- Treat specific hormone disorders

Special Considerations

- None

When to Consult, Refer, Hospitalize

- Refer to adult endocrinologist if diameter >4 cm or abnormalities persist >2 years, physical abnormalities in addition to gynecomastia, males >18 years, history and/or work-up compatible with pathologic origin
- Urologist if cryptorchidism, testicular neoplasm
- Surgeon for removal of mass if indicated

Follow-Up

- Pubescent males every 3–6 months
- Watch for signs of abnormal progression of puberty, chronic illness, or emotional/psychological disorders
- Perform/repeat diagnostic work up if clinical picture changes

EXPECTED COURSE
- Pubescent males should normalize within 2-year period
- Usually good prognosis

COMPLICATIONS
- Self-image problems
- Increased risk of breast cancer in patients with Klinefelter syndrome

Obesity

Description
- Condition involving accumulation of excess adipose tissue >20% over ideal body weight or body mass index (BMI) >30

Etiology
- May be secondary to diseases processes or a primary result of overeating and inadequate exercise
- Genetic predisposition; 60% risk of obesity if one parent obese, 90% risk if both
- Multifactorial, including environmental and psychological factors
- Abdominal fat (visceral fat) associated with metabolic disorders (diabetes mellitus, Cushing syndrome) and cardiovascular disease
- Hip and thigh fat (subcutaneous fat) more common in women and pose less medical risk than abdominal fat
- Waist measurements >35 inches in women and >40 inches in men pose significant health risk for cardiovascular disease; risk of death increases with BMI >30
- Secondary problems such as adrenal problems, hypothyroid, polycystic ovary disease cause <1% of cases
- Many medications cause increased appetite and weight gain, including steroids, antidepressants, hormones, mood stabilizers, antipsychotics

Incidence and Demographics
- Most prevalent chronic medical disorder in world
- Incidence and prevalence increasing in all genders and ages
- One-third of U.S. population is obese
- Prevalence rates higher in Hispanic and African-American women, Asian and Pacific Islanders, Native Americans, Native Hawaiians, and Alaskan Natives
- Among children and adolescents, prevalence is 13.7% and 11.5% respectively
- New onset in elderly is rare, requires investigation

Risk Factors
- Overeating or other poor dietary habits
- Sedentary lifestyle
- Genetic predisposition

Prevention and Screening
- Balanced dietary intake throughout life span
- Exercise regularly

Assessment

HISTORY

- Obtain weight history of life span
- Collect comprehensive diet history including food categories, amount of servings, number of meals per day, fluid intake, snacks
- Exercise history
- Motivation to lose weight and prior attempts to lose weight
- Smoking and alcohol intake
- Occupational history
- Past medical history of diabetes mellitus, thyroid disease, cardiovascular disease, cerebral vascular disease, hypertension, orthopedic problems
- Medication use, particular attention to laxatives, diuretics, hormones, nutritional supplements, OTC medications
- Family history of obesity, overeating, metabolic disorders, cardiovascular disease, cerebral vascular disease, hypertension, diabetes mellitus

PHYSICAL EXAM

- Height and weight; calculate BMI by using tables or formula (see Diagnostic Studies)
- Obtain waist and hip measurement; waist >35 inches in females and >40 inches in males is dangerous
- Children: weight exceeds 120% of that expected for their height (95th percentile on weight-for-height plot)
- Complete physical exam to assess for conditions associated with obesity
  - Skin: Assess for changes of Cushing syndrome or intertrigo caused by obese skin folds, striae, dermatitis, poor wound healing
  - Respiratory: Compromise due to restrictive lung disease, hypoventilation
  - Cardiovascular: Hypertension, coronary artery disease
  - Peripheral vascular: Venous insufficiency
  - Musculoskeletal: Arthritis

DIAGNOSTIC STUDIES

- Adults: Calculate BMI = weight in kg ÷ by height in meters squared
  - Pounds ÷ 2.2 = kg; inches x 0.0254 = meters
  - Also can be calculated by [weight in pounds ÷ height in inches ÷ height in inches] x 703
  - BMI between 18.5 and 25 is healthy normal weight
  - BMI 30–34.9 Class I obesity; 35–39.9 Class II obesity; >40 Class III obesity
- Waist–hip ratio: Estimate fat distribution using waist–hip ratio by measuring waist at navel and measure hips over buttocks, then divide waist measurement by hip measurement to get ratio
  - Men: Low risk <0.85, moderate risk 0.85–0.95, high risk >0.95
  - Women: Low risk <0.75, moderate risk 0.75–0.85, high risk >0.85
  - Upper body obesity has more significant health consequences than lower body obesity; therefore, large abdominal circumference or increased waist-to-hip ratio suggests increased risk of diabetes or vascular disease
- Calculate ideal body weight:
  - Men: Height (cm) = 64.19 – (0.04 x age) + (2.02 x knee height)
  - Women: Height (cm) = 84.88 – (0.24 x age) + (1.83 x knee height)
  - Rough estimate of ideal body weight can be obtained by starting with

100 lbs (women) or 106 lbs (men) and adding 5 lbs (women) or 6 lbs (men) for each inch over 5 feet
- Instruments to quantify body adipose tissue: hydrostatic densitometry (gold standard), skin-fold thickness measurement (simplest, most common), dual energy X-ray absorptiometry (DEXA) scan (most reliable and accurate, especially in elderly)
- Lipid profile, fasting blood glucose, metabolic and chemistry panel, thyroid function, consider urine free cortisol measures for work-up of secondary cause of obesity, or complication of obesity
  - Children: calculate BMI (interpretation depends on the child's age) and plot the BMI-for-age according to sex-specific charts through puberty
  - BMI = [weight in pounds ÷ height in inches ÷ height in inches] x 703
  - Fractions and ounces must be entered as decimal values
  - BMI-for-age <5th percentile = underweight
  - BMI-for-age >85th percentile = at risk of overweight
  - BMI-for-age >95th percentile = overweight

Differential Diagnosis
- Endocrine disorders presenting with obesity include hypothalamic disease, thyroid disease, pituitary dysfunction, Cushing syndrome, polycystic ovary disease

Management
NONPHARMACOLOGIC TREATMENT
- U.S. Preventive Services Task Force suggests a combination of diet, exercise, and behavioral modifications are essential to obtain and maintain weight reduction
- Children: develop an alliance with the family; treat parents also; use positive reinforcement; emphasize importance of family involvement in physical activity program
- Long-term lifestyle changes
- Comprehensive multidisciplinary approach to weight reduction includes dietary control, exercise, eating behavior modifications, psychosocial modification
- To lose 1 pound, 3,500 more calories must be expended than consumed (500 calories/day to lose 1 pound per week)
- Moderate calorie deficit or low-calorie diet for obese men and women attempting to lose weight—800–1,200 cals/day adult women; 800–1,500 cals/day adult men
- Follow U.S. Department of Agriculture (USDA) food pyramid; avoid controversial fad diets; high-fiber, low-fat diets have proven most successful
- Exercise: For energy expenditure, exercise 5–7 times a week for minimum of 30 minutes of moderate intensity activity (walking, jogging, cycling, ice/roller skating, swimming)
- May require cardiac stress test prior to initiating exercise plan
- Eating behavior modification: Emphasize planning and record-keeping
- Psychosocial modification: Support for losing weight essential, whether form of close friend, peer, therapist, or formal organization of people (such as Overeaters Anonymous, TOPS, Weight Watchers)
- Surgical approach with morbid obesity includes gastric operations, such as vertical-banded (Mason) gastroplasty and gastric bypass
- Pediatric obesity is best managed by increasing the child's activity level and improving nutrition; avoid medication or hypocaloric approaches

PHARMACOLOGIC TREATMENT
- Recommended for BMI >30 in conjunction with diet modification and exercise regimen or BMI >27–29 with at least one major comorbidity
- Appetite suppressant: sibutramine (Meridia) 5, 10, or 15 mg dosage qd; initial dosage usually 10 mg qd
    – Monitor blood pressure and CNS side effects
- Fat blocker: orlistat (Xenical) 120 mg tid with meals (no systemic absorption); discuss GI side effects; consider fat-soluble vitamin supplementation
- Over-the-counter products are not recommended

LENGTH OF TREATMENT
- Sibutramine is approved for 1 year; orlistat is approved for 1–2 years if no nutritional deficits result

Special Considerations
- Encourage patient to set goal of 10% weight loss for improved health and repeat as necessary

When to Consult, Refer, Hospitalize
- May consider registered dietitian when designing a low-calorie diet after determination of caloric requirements based on daily energy intake, expenditure, and average weight loss goal of 1 pound/week after the first month
- Counselor for behavior modification
- Refer adults and children with morbid obesity to specialists

Follow-Up
- Frequently, at least initially, to evaluate progress
- Monthly follow-up to monitor blood pressure if taking sibutramine
- Regular monitoring and reinforcement of progress until goal weight reached
    EXPECTED COURSE
    - Slow progress with expected loss from ½ lb to 2–3 lbs per week maximum
    - Continue to monitor for obesity complications
    - Many regain if do not maintain the lifestyle modifications

COMPLICATIONS
- Cardiovascular disease: Hypertension, coronary artery disease, varicose veins, CVA
- Metabolic disorders: Hyperinsulinemia, diabetes mellitus type 2, hyperlipidemia
- Pulmonary: Sleep apnea syndrome, chronic respiratory infections, hypo-ventilation
- Cholelithiasis; nephrotic syndrome
- Depression, loss self-esteem; psychosocial disability
- Degenerative joint disease, chronic orthopedic problems
- Structural disorders; skin disorders
- Cancers: Colon, rectum, prostate, uterine, biliary tract, breast, ovary
- Surgery increases perioperative morbidity and mortality

CASE STUDIES

Case 1. 52-year-old Hispanic female arrives at your clinic. She states she has been fatigued for 3 months, has gained weight since her last visit (6 months ago), and is urinating more frequently, but states that she is consuming more water and relates the urination to increased intake of fluids.
PMH: Hypertension and obesity; medications benazepril (Lotensin) 10 mg qd, and Prempro 0.625 mg/2.5 qd.

    1. What additional history would you ask?

Exam: Vital signs: BP 130/88, HR 72, RR 12, T 97.9°F, Wt 196 lbs, Ht 5' 4", BMI 33.7; general appearance is alert without distress. HEENT exam is normal, lungs clear and heart rate and rhythm regular without murmurs; abdomen is obese with waist circumference 39 inches, no masses or tenderness. Extremity pulses are normal; skin is warm and dry, sensation intact without lesions. Neuro exam is within normal limits.

    2. What diagnostic tests would you order?
    3. If your suspicions were correct, what actions would be required?
    4. What is your treatment plan and follow-up?

Case 2. A mother arrives at your clinic with her 7-year-old daughter, stating that she is developing breasts early and she has noticed hair under her arms.
PMH: Normal growth and development at well-child visits; current on immunizations

    1. What additional history would you ask?
Exam: Vital signs within normal limits, Height 95th percentile on the growth curve, Tanner stage III; the rest of the exam is normal.

    2. What diagnostic tests would you order?
    3. What is your next course of action?

Case 3. African-American parents bring their 11-year-old son to the community clinic stating he has lost 15 pounds in 3 weeks and is urinating frequently. He is also "drinking a lot."
PMH: Recent recovery from chicken pox (4 weeks); otherwise normal growth and development; immunizations up to date.

    1. What additional history would you ask?

Exam: Alert and oriented but appears ill, thin; fruity odor to breath, vital signs stable; mucous membranes slightly dry.

    2. What are your differential diagnoses?
    3. What diagnostic tests would you order?
    4. Your lab results return with a glucose of 420 mg/dL (fasting) and urine dip positive for ketones and glucose. What is your next course of action?

REFERENCES

American Association of Clinical Endocrinologists. (1998). AACE/ACE position statement on the prevention, diagnosis and treatment of obesity (1998 rev.). *Endocrine Practice, 4*(5), 297–350.

American Society of Plastic and Reconstructive Surgeons. (1996). Gynecomastia: Brief summary. *National Guideline Clearinghouse.* Retrieved February 1, 2008, from http://www.ngc.gov

Centers for Disease Control and Prevention. (2008). *Overweight and obesity.* Retrieved March 24, 2008, from http://www.cdc.gov/nccdphp/dnpa/obesity/

Dambro, M. R. (2007). *Griffith's five-minute clinical consult.* Philadelphia: Lippincott Williams & Wilkins.

Edmunds, M. W., & Mayhew, M. S. (2004). *Pharmacology for primary care providers* (2nd ed.). St Louis, MO: Mosby.

Goroll, A. H., & Mulley, A. G. (2006). *Primary care medicine* (4th ed.). Philadelphia: Lippincott Williams & Wilkins.

Hay, W., Hayward, A. R., Levin, M J., & Sondheimer, J. M. (2006). *Current pediatric diagnosis and treatment.* New York: Lange Medical Book/McGraw Hill.

Kleigman, R. M., Marcdante, K J., Jensen, H. B. & Behrman, R. E. (2006). *Nelson essentials of pediatrics* (5th ed.) Philadelphia: Elsevier Saunders.

McPhee, S. J., Papadakis, M. A., & Tierney, L. M. (2008). *Current medical diagnosis & treatment* (44th ed.). Norwalk, CT: Appleton and Lange.

National Center for Chronic Disease Prevention and Health Promotion. (2007). *Body mass index-for-age: BMI is used differently with children than it is with adults.* Retrieved February 1, 2008, from www.cdc.gov/nccdphp

National Guideline Clearinghouse. (2003). *American Association of Clinical Endocrinologists medical guidelines for clinical practice for growth hormone use in adults and children—2003 update.* Retrieved February 1, 2008, from http://www.guideline.gov/summary/summary.aspx?doc_id=37 26&nbr=002952&string=Gynecomastia

National Guideline Clearinghouse. (2004). Standards of medical care for patients with diabetes mellitus. *Diabetes Care, 27,* S15-S35. Retrieved February 1, 2008, from http://www.guidelines. gov/summary/summary.aspx?ss=15&doc_id=10400&nbr=005446&string=diabetes

Riddle, M. C., Rosenstock, J., & Gerich, J. (2003). Treat to the target trial: Randomized addition of glargine or human NPH insulin to oral therapy of type 2 diabetic patients. *Diabetes Care, 26*(11), 3080–3086.

Schwartz, M. W. (2008). *The 5 minute pediatric consult.* Philadelphia: Lippincott Williams & Wilkins.

Sinclair, A. J., Conroy, S. P., & Bayer, A. J. (2008). Impact of diabetes on physical function in older people. *Diabetes Care, 31*(2), 233–235.

Taylor, R. (2007). *Manual of family medicine* (2nd ed.). Philadelphia: Lippincott Williams & Wilkins.

Weinzimer, S. A., Ternand, C., Howard, C., Chang, C. T., Becker, D. J., & Laffel, L. M. (2008). A randomized trial comparing continuous subcutaneous insulin infusion of insulin aspart versus insulin lispro in children and adolescents with type 1 diabetes. *Diabetes Care, 31*(2), 210–215.

Psychiatric–Mental Health Disorders

Mary-Ann Krisman-Scott, RN, PhD, FNP-BC

GENERAL APPROACH

- Mental illnesses are common, serious brain disorders that affect thinking, motivation, emotions, and social interactions.
- Untreated mental illness contributes adversely to other physiological illnesses.
- Obtain a complete history, including mental status exam.
- Distinguish between a mental disorder and a medical condition or substance abuse.
- Concomitant disorders are common.
- Most mild mental disorders can be effectively treated in a primary care setting.
- Consider a child's developmental level. The clinician should consider a psychiatric disorder with the presence of a developmental delay.
- Approximately 20%–25% of children visiting pediatric outpatient settings have psychiatric disorders, either diagnosed or undiagnosed.

Red Flags
- Individuals with mental illness often self-medicate with alcohol or other substances.
- Consult, refer, or hospitalize when presenting symptoms are severe, chronic, or unresponsive.
- Suicidal ideation and attempt are always psychiatric emergencies.
- Individuals who represent a clear and present danger to themselves or others should never be left alone and should be immediately hospitalized even when it is contrary to their wishes.

ANXIETY DISORDERS

Description
- Acute or chronic fearful emotion with associated physical symptoms. Subtypes include:
  - Panic disorder:
    - Episodes of recurrent and intense fear or feeling of impending doom that occur without apparent warning
    - Physical symptoms include palpitations, shortness of breath, tachycardia, sweating, abdominal distress, dizziness, tightness in chest, fear of dying, "losing one's mind," "going crazy," or a sense of unreality
    - May be accompanied by agoraphobia in which patients rigidly avoid situations in which it would be difficult to get help; they prefer to be accompanied by a friend of family member in tunnels, elevators, crowded streets, subways, airplanes, etc.; some patients may refuse to leave their homes
  - Obsessive-compulsive disorder (OCD):
    - Recurrent, repetitive, and intrusive thoughts and/or behaviors that are extremely difficult or impossible to control, unreasonable, excessive, and that interfere significantly with a person's ability to function
  - Posttraumatic stress disorder (PTSD):
    - Exposure to an extreme traumatic stressor such as rape, sexual or physical abuse, natural disasters, war, or other perceived or actual threat to a person's physical being or self-concept
    - Results in persistent symptoms including nightmares, flashbacks, numbing of emotion, dissociative episodes, or inability to recall specific events
    - Acute form identified as lasting less than 3 months; chronic form lasting 3 months or longer
  - Acute stress disorder (ASD):
    - Exposure to a traumatic event that involved actual or threatened death or serious injury
    - Response to the event is intense fear, helplessness, or horror
    - Results in the same symptoms as PTSD but these symptoms occur within 4 weeks of the event
    - Lasts for a minimum of 2 days and a maximum of 4 weeks
  - Phobias:
    - Social phobia:
      - Severe, persistent fear of social or performance situations provoking an immediate and intense anxiety response; extreme, irrational fear leads to avoidance of people or social situations
    - Specific phobia:
      - Extreme, irrational fear of specific objects such as elevators, snakes, or insects that leads to avoidant behavior of that particular object
  - Generalized anxiety disorder (GAD):
    - Excessive worry, feelings of apprehension, panic, or dread accompanied by symptoms of physiological arousal (palpitations, muscle tension and restlessness, fatigue, sweating, difficulty concentrating); anxiety may seem groundless, or may appear disproportionate to the issue
    - Symptoms present at least 6 months, occurring more days than not, with the individual reporting little or no control, along with significant distress and impairment in social, occupational, and interpersonal areas

Etiology
- Psychodynamic theory:
  - Severe conflict between the id and superego
  - Irrational guilt and shame
- Behavioral theory:
  - Conditioned behavioral response to earlier interpersonal or social experiences
- Biologic theory:
  - Genetic predisposition
  - Overstimulated autonomic nervous system, stress response
  - Abnormalities of neurotransmitter receptors in the central nervous system (CNS), specifically GABA receptors
- Existential theory:
  - Response to an awareness of a vast void in existence and meaning

Incidence and Demographics
- Anxiety disorders are one of the most common mental illnesses in the U.S.
- 19 million people are affected each year; 60% of cases are women; onset 25–30 years.
- Anxiety disorders account for 15% of the population seen in general practice settings.
- Panic disorders occur more frequently in women than men.
- Anxiety is a common concomitant disorder in patients with a history of early traumatic experiences such as abuse, separation, loss of a parent.
- Separation anxiety and overanxious disorders are syndromes unique to pediatric patients.
- Phobias affect children and adults with a lifetime prevalence of 10%.
- Adult onset of obsessive-compulsive disorder affects men and women equally; childhood onset is more common in boys.
- Generally onset of anxiety is prior to early adult years. If first episode after this age consider other non-psychological source.

Risk Factors
- Family history; genetic predisposition
- Exposure to traumatic events

Prevention and Screening
- Public and patient education and awareness
- Reduced exposure to real or potential trauma
- Strong social support systems and strategies to develop personal resilience

Assessment
HISTORY
- Determine onset, frequency, and duration of symptoms
- Determine degree of distress and symptom interference with daily function
- Elicit predisposing factors or stressors such as divorce, financial difficulties, job loss, victimization
- Obtain complete medical history, medications, over-the-counter drugs (OTCs), and supplements taken
- Obtain history and current patterns of use of caffeine, alcohol, nicotine, and other substances
- Feelings of loss of control, panic, impending doom or dread, depersonalization, difficulty concentrating

- Excessive worry, irrational fear, concern over "losing one's mind" or death, memory changes
- Difficulty concentrating, making decisions, irritable, agitated mood, motor restlessness
- Sleep disturbances (insomnia, frequent awakenings), fatigue, irritable, agitated mood
- Nausea, diarrhea, vomiting, frequent urination
- Feeling of lump in the throat, difficulty swallowing, dry mouth
- Obsessive-compulsive disorder:
  - Either recurrent and persistent unwanted thoughts that are difficult or impossible to control, and/or
  - Repetitive, uncontrollable behaviors such as excessive handwashing, counting
  - Present most days for >2 weeks
- Posttraumatic stress disorder:
  - Recurring dreams or nightmares of a previously experienced traumatic event or intrusive recollections of the event
  - Hyperarousal
  - Avoidance of stimuli associated with the event
  - Intense psychological distress at exposure to reminders of the original event
- Phobias:
  - Excessive, persistent fear and avoidance of specific objects or situations
  - Avoidance of school and impaired social, family, and academic functioning in children
  - Avoidance of work, social activities in adults
- General anxiety and panic attacks:
  - Palpitations, tachycardia, tightness in chest or chest pain
  - Difficulty breathing, tachypnea, hyperventilation
  - Light-headed, dizziness, diaphoresis
  - Tingling, numbness in extremities
  - Fear of losing control or going crazy
  - Fear of dying

PHYSICAL EXAM
- Perform general exam to rule out serious central nervous system, cardiopulmonary, or endocrine disorder
- Focus on vital signs, cardiac and pulmonary exam

DIAGNOSTIC STUDIES
- Diagnostic labs such as ECG, TSH, CBC, chemistry panel to rule out medical conditions
- Minnesota Multiphasic Inventory (MMPI-II), Hamilton Anxiety Scale may be done

Differential Diagnosis
- Any medical condition with central nervous system involvement
- Substance abuse, including acute withdrawal or intoxication
- Metabolic disorders

- Seizure disorders
- Mood disorders
- Caffeine, nicotine
- Delirium, especially in older adults

Cardiac disorders
- Arrhythmias
- Myocardial infarction (MI)
- Cardiovascular disease
- Chronic heart failure (CHF)

Endocrine disorders
- Cushing syndrome
- Hyperthyroidism
- Hypothyroidism
- Hypoglycemia

Pulmonary disorders
- Chronic obstructive pulmonary disease (COPD)
- Asthma
- Pulmonary embolism
- Pneumothorax

Medications that may produce anxiety as a side effect
- Anticholinergics
- Antihistamines
- Corticosteroids
- Antihypertensives
- Antipsychotics
- Antidepressants
- Bronchodilators
- Amphetamines
- Anesthetics

Management
- Mild cases of anxiety disorders and GAD are responsive to treatment in general practice.
- Refer primary anxiety disorders that meet DSM IV criteria to a mental health provider.
- Patient education to ensure compliance and effective treatment.
     NONPHARMACOLOGIC TREATMENT
     - Cognitive-behavioral therapy; supportive psychotherapy, insight-oriented psychotherapy, group therapy (especially for PTSD)
     - Stress management education, courses, workshops; behavioral conditioning, biofeedback
     - Community self-help and support groups
     - Education of patient and family about the disorder and treatment

PHARMACOLOGIC TREATMENT
- Benzodiazepines are effective in the short-term management of some anxiety disorders (Table 18–1)
    - Significant potential for dependence and abuse; limit use to 1 month
    - Rapid onset of action with quick symptom relief
    - Alprazolam (Xanax) and clonazepam (Klonopin) are frequently used to treat panic disorders
    - Patients with substance abuse histories are at risk for abuse
- Other anti-anxiety medications:
    - Buspirone (Buspar): 7.5 mg bid up to 20–30 mg a day
    - Slower onset of action may take up to 4 weeks for anti-anxiety effects
    - Maximum therapeutic effect may not be reached for 4–8 weeks

Table 18-1. Benzodiazepine Therapy for Anxiety Disorders

Benzodiazepines	Initial Dose	Therapeutic Dose
Alprazolam (Xanax)	0.25–0.5 mg tid	0.5–6 mg/day
Clonazepam (Klonopin)	0.25–1 mg bid	1–4 mg/day
Lorazepam (Ativan)	1–1.5 mg bid	1–3 mg/day
Diazepam (Valium)	2–10 mg bid	4–40 mg/day

- Antidepressants are commonly the first-line drug of choice for anxiety disorders (Table 18–2)
    - Potential for substance abuse and dependence is significantly less than with benzodiazepines
    - Main therapeutic effect may take 2–4 weeks
    - Patient education of time required to reach main effect of the drug is essential for compliance

Table 18-2. SSRI/SNRI Therapy in Anxiety Disorders

SSRI/SNRI Medications	Initial Dose	Therapeutic Dose
Fluoxetine (Prozac)	20 mg qd	20–60 mg/day
Paroxetine (Paxil)	20 mg qd	20–50 mg/day
Sertraline (Zoloft)	25 mg qd	25–200 mg/day
Fluvoxamine (Luvox)	50 mg qd at hs	100–300 mg/day
Venlafaxine (Effexor)	12.5–25 mg bid	150–375 mg/day
Escitalopram (Lexapro)	10 mg qd	20 mg/day

Note. SSRI = selective serotonin reuptake inhibitor; SNRI = serotonin-norepinephrine reuptake inhibitor

LENGTH OF TREATMENT
- Length varies according to individual response and symptom management
- Mild and situational anxiety usually resolves within 2 months
- Long-term use of antidepressants often is required
- Chronic, disabling anxiety requires a psychiatric consultation and referral

Special Considerations
- It is common for anxiety disorders to occur concomitantly with other disorders such as depression, eating disorders, and substance abuse; or with ADHD, depression, OCD, and Tourette syndrome in children.
- Anxiety disorders are commonly seen with medical disorders. Always rule out underlying medical causes and ensure appropriate treatment of any concomitant disorders.
- Patients with anxiety disorders need reassurance that their disorder can be effectively treated.
- The establishment of a trusting, safe, therapeutic relationship with the primary practitioner is essential for compliance and effective treatment.

When to Consult, Refer, Hospitalize
- Severe panic attacks, intense PTSD, and disabling OCD always require a psychiatric consult or referral and usually require a combination of pharmacotherapy and cognitive-behavioral therapy.
- There have been few studies documenting the results of treatment of anxiety in children and adolescents and few anti-anxiety agents are approved in children. Referral to a psychiatrist is indicated for anxiety in children.

Follow-Up
- Patients should be seen weekly during the acute phase of treatment.
- Medications need to be monitored for effectiveness, appropriate dose, and potential abuse.

    COMPLICATIONS
    - Drug abuse or dependence, dysfunctional social or occupational performance
    - Treatment resistance or undertreatment, side effects from medications

MOOD DISORDERS

Grief/Bereavement

Description
- A normal emotional and physiological reaction to loss.
- Uncomplicated grief presents as depressed mood that is situational and time-limited.
  - May cause varying degrees of symptoms such as feeling of profound sadness, crying spells, insomnia, loss of appetite, survivor guilt

Risk Factors
- All persons are at risk for uncomplicated grief.
- Risk of developing more complicated mood disorders: Poor coping skills, lack of support, history of previous mood disorder, alcohol or substance abuse.

Assessment
    HISTORY
    - Feelings of sadness and profound loss, crying spells
    - Insomnia, loss of appetite, and weight loss
    - Survivor guilt

PHYSICAL EXAM
- May be no objective findings

DIAGNOSTIC STUDIES
- Depression screening if grief extends beyond 8 weeks

Differential Diagnosis
- Major depressive illness
- Mood disorder

Management

NONPHARMACOLOGIC TREATMENT
- Encourage the expression of grief and mourning over loss
- Offer reassurance that grief is a normal, nonpathologic reaction to loss and is self-limited
- Encourage participation in support groups

PHARMACOLOGIC TREATMENT
- Mild anti-anxiety agents in lowest effective dose may be used to treat symptoms but do not treat symptoms of major depression

When to Consult, Refer, Hospitalize
- Grief that lasts longer than 2 months should be evaluated for mood disorders; assess suicide ideation and refer to mental health specialist.

Follow-Up
- The duration of normal grief reaction varies among different cultures, but usually begins to show marked improvement within 8 weeks. The diagnosis of major depressive disorder is not given unless symptoms are still present after 2 months and represent a significant change in function and impairment.
- The elderly and patients without adequate social/familial support are at high risk for developing major depression and suicidal ideation.
- Children may harbor feelings of guilt and responsibility and may require referral to psychiatrist or mental health specialist.

Depression

Description
- Major depression is a complex mood disorder lasting at least 2 weeks, with sad, blue mood that may or may not be accompanied by the loss of interest or pleasure in nearly all activities, every day.
- In children the mood may be irritable rather than sad.
- Depression is associated with abnormalities in neurotransmission, neurophysiology, and neuroendocrine function.
- Clinical manifestations of childhood depression vary according to the child's developmental age.

- Subtypes of depression include:
  - Adjustment disorder with depressed mood
- Depressive disorders:
  - Major depressive disorder: Single or recurrent episodes of depression associated with other symptoms lasting at least 2 weeks but without mood elevation, elation, or mania
  - Dysthymic disorder: Chronic, sustained depressed mood ongoing for a minimum of 2 years, more days than not, symptoms less severe than depressive disorder
  - Premenstrual dysphoric disorder
- Mood disorders due to illness and drugs
- Bipolar disorder (mania, cyclothymic disorder): Recurrent episodes of depression with episodes of mania characterized by lack of impulse control, excessive energy, grandiose or delusional thinking, elated mood, inappropriate behaviors, hyperactivity, pressured speech, and decreased need for sleep
- Atypical depression: Characterized by hypersomnia, fatigue, rejection sensitivity, overeating
- Melancholic depression: Characterized by insomnia, early morning or frequent awakenings, anxiety, loss of appetite, difficulty concentrating, fatigue
- Postpartum: Symptom onset within 2 weeks to 6 months postpartum

Etiology

- Genetic predisposition
- Biological dysregulation of the hypopituitary axis (stress response). The core symptoms of depression—such as sleep, appetite, and mood disturbances—are related to the functions of the hypothalamus and the pituitary glands and associated hormones such as cortisol, leptin, and corticotropin-releasing hormone (CRH).
- Abnormalities in neurotransmitters in the brain associated with serotonin, acetylcholine, dopamine, norepinephrine, epinephrine, and GABA; possible structural changes in the brain
- Additional environmental factors and learned behaviors may influence neurotransmitter function or exert independent influence

Incidence and Demographics

- Depression is the most common mental illness seen in primary care practices.
- Lifetime prevalence for the U.S. population is 7% for women and 3% for men.
- 15% of the individuals diagnosed with severe major depression die of suicide.
- Patients with depression have 2–3 times the normal death rate at any age (independent of suicide) and are more likely to incur long-term medical consequences such as premature osteoporosis, coronary artery disease, dysfunction of inflammatory mediators and the immune system, and increased insulin resistance.
- Bipolar disorder has a mean age of 30 and ranges from age 5 to 50.
- Mean age for onset of major depressive disorder is 40.
- Dysthymic disorder occurs up to 7x more often in women than in men.
- Suicide rates are highest in the elderly.

Risk Factors
- Recent stressful life events are the most powerful predictors of onset of a depressive disorder
- Prior episodes of depression
- Persons without close interpersonal relationships
- Losing a parent prior to age 11
- Family history, especially having a first-degree relative who is diagnosed
- Alcohol and substance abuse
- Postpartum period
- Significant psychosocial stressors such as divorce, finances, job loss, trauma, or abuse
- Chronic medical illness
- Risk factors for suicide:
  - Personal or family history of one or more mental or substance abuse disorders
  - Severe psychosocial stressors: Divorce, unemployment, legal problems, perception of poor health
  - Anxiety
  - Depression in childhood or adolescence
  - Prior suicide attempt(s)
  - Family or domestic violence, including physical or sexual abuse
  - Firearms in the home
  - Specific plan
  - Family history of suicide

Prevention and Screening
- Patient education/public awareness of the signs, symptoms, and treatment modalities available
- Early recognition, intervention, and initiation of treatment

Assessment
HISTORY
- Establish frequency, type, and duration of symptoms
- Degree of disruption or impairment in daily activities
- Prior personal psychiatric history
- Family psychiatric/psychosocial history
- Identify acute and chronic stressors
- Ask about suicidal thoughts, impulses, and history of prior attempts or current plans
- According to the DSM-IV-TR (*Diagnostic and Statistical Manual of Mental Disorders,* Fourth Edition, Text Revision), sad, blue, or depressed mood and/or absence of pleasure plus four or more of listed symptoms must be present for a minimum of 2 weeks and represent a change from previous function in order to diagnose major depression. Classic symptoms of major depression (DSM-IV-TR):
  - Depressed mood most of the day, nearly every day; in children can be irritable mood
  - Significant weight loss when not dieting, or weight gain, or an increase or decrease in appetite
  - Markedly diminished interest or pleasure in all or almost all activities
  - Psychomotor agitation or retardation

- Alcohol and substance abuse
- Mononucleosis

Endocrine disorders
- Hypothyroidism
- Hyperthyroidism
- Cushing syndrome
- Addison's disease
- Diabetes

Neurological disorders
- Neoplasms
- Stroke
- Severe trauma
- Head injury
- Multiple sclerosis
- Seizure disorders
- Parkinson's disease
- Dementia
- Chronic pain

Cardiac disorders
- Arrhythmia
- CHF
- MI
- Hypertension

Medications that can induce depression
- Opioids
- Steroids
- Estrogen
- Antihypertensive agents
- Digoxin
- Anti-Parkinson drugs
- NSAIDs
- Beta blockers
- Sedatives and hypnotics
- Antibacterial/antifungals
- Antineoplastic drugs
- Psychotropic drugs
- Analgesics
- Anti-inflammatories

Management
- Mild depression or hypomania may be safely managed by a primary practitioner with frequent evaluation.
- Frequent follow-up necessary to educate patient regarding the illness and to adequately treat.

- Tricyclic antidepressants and SSRIs may precipitate a manic episode in those patients prone to manic depressive or bipolar illness.
- Patient education concerning the nature of the illness, course of treatment, and expected outcome is essential.
- A complete diagnostic evaluation is essential with evaluation of suicide risk.

NONPHARMACOLOGIC TREATMENT

- Pharmacologic treatment should always be accompanied by some form of psychotherapy
- Cognitive-behavioral therapy with a focus on cognitive distortions and behaviors that exacerbate depressive illness
- Psychoanalysis or psychotherapy with a focus on interpersonal skills
- Suicidal ideation or behavior should always be evaluated further and treated by a mental health practitioner
- Electroconvulsive therapy: Indicated for severely depressed or suicidal patients who don't respond to pharmacological agents; main side effect is temporary memory impairment that may last up to 2 weeks
- Provide community resources, hotlines, and list of local support groups

PHARMACOLOGIC TREATMENT

- SSRIs (Table 18–3) are the first-line drug of choice due to their effectiveness and safety record in adults; Fluoxetine is the SSRI with a pediatric indication; use of other SSRIs in children is an off-label use; dosing information is not based on FDA recommendations, but on other literature
- Fluoxetine is now available as a generic product. As a brand-name product it is available as a once-a-week sustained release product
- Information from an increasing number of studies indicates an increase in suicidal and homicidal behavior with SSRI use in some children; an FDA advisory panel has recently recommended warnings on all antidepressants indicating that suicide risk may be increased in children taking these products, therefore they should be seen once a week when initiating treatment or when changing dosages until stable
- Other cautions include abrupt withdrawal of SSRIs may cause unpleasant somatic complaints (fatigue and irritability) so SSRIs should be tapered; during treatment children may experience "behavior activation" (the underactive child may become agitated and impulsive)

Table 18-3. Common SSRI and SNRI Therapy for Treatment of Adult Depression

Medication	Initial Dose	Target Dose
Fluoxetine (Prozac)	20 mg qd in a.m.	20–80 mg qd
Sertraline (Zoloft)	50 mg qd	50–200 mg qd
Paroxetine (Paxil)	20 mg qd in a.m.	20–50 mg qd
Citalopram (Celexa)	20 mg qd	40–60 mg qd
Escitalopram (Lexapro)	10 mg qd	10–20 mg qd
Duloxetine (Cymbalta)	40 mg qd	40–60 mg qd in divided dose

- Tricyclic antidepressants (Table 18–4) are also effective but are associated with greater incidence of side effects
- Tricyclics block cholinergic muscarinic receptors, resulting in possible constipation, dry mouth, urinary retention, blurred vision, and sinus tachycardia; other side effects include sedation, postural hypotension, weight gain, potentiation of CNS medications, dizziness
- Tricyclics are contraindicated in patients with cardiac conduction disorders, narrow angle glaucoma, and prostatic hypertrophy
- Tricyclics cause weight gain; monitor weight and BMI

Table 18-4. Common Tricyclic Antidepressants

Medication	Initial Dose	Target Dose
Amitriptyline (Elavil)	25 mg q hs	50–150 mg divided
Desipramine (Norpramin)	25 mg qd	75–300 mg qd
Imipramine (Tofranil)	25 mg q hs	75–300 mg q hs
Nortriptyline (Pamelor)	10–25 mg hs	75–150 mg qd or divided

- Monoamine oxidase inhibitors (MAOIs), such as phenelzine (Nardil) and tranylcypromine (Parnate), are used in the treatment of refractory or treatment-resistant depression; potentially serious and lethal side effects, such as hypertensive crisis, may occur; these drugs should be ordered by psychiatrist
- Other antidepressants used in adults are listed in Table 18–5; dose should be increased weekly until therapeutic dose is reached

Table 18-5. Other Antidepressants Commonly Used in Treating Adults and Children

Medication	Initial Dose	Target Dose
Bupropion (Wellbutrin)	75 mg bid; avoid bedtime dosing	300–400 mg/day divided 3–4x daily
Mirtazapine (Remeron)	15 mg q hs	15–45 mg q hs
Venlafaxine (Effexor)	25–50 mg qd with food in 2–3 doses	75–375 mg qd divided

LENGTH OF TREATMENT

- Duration and course of treatment is individualized, depends upon severity of illness and response to treatment
- If the patient is nonresponsive to medication, increase to maximum dose slowly, then if no response, change within class (one SSRI to another) or to another antidepressant (Wellbutrin, Effexor, Remeron); next to second-line tricyclics; and finally, refer out for MAOIs
- Depression is a chronic illness with frequent episodes of recurrence
- Antidepressants are most effective when taken for at least 1 year after remission of symptoms
- If patient has had two or more episodes, should consider remaining on antidepressants

Special Considerations
- Patients treated for major depression in a general practice setting have more pain and physical illness, social and interpersonal impairment than other patient populations.
- Sustained release (SR) or extended release (XR) are more easily tolerated.
- Tricyclic medications have a high potential for lethality in overdose.
- Depression in the elderly may be difficult to diagnose due to the greater incidence of dementia and number and types of medications taken for other medical conditions.
- Elderly patients require smaller starting doses but may require same therapeutic dosage as younger adults and frequently require closer medical management.

When to Consult, Refer, Hospitalize
- All patients who present with suicidal ideation, prior attempt, or plan should immediately be referred to an emergency room or psychiatrist for further evaluation and treatment.
- All patients should be referred to the appropriate mental health practitioner for therapy.
- Consult for all women who are pregnant or plan on becoming pregnant prior to the initiation of medication.
- Patients who are severely impaired by their symptomology or present with comorbid disorders such as obsessive-compulsive disorder, substance abuse, eating disorders, or no social support should be referred to a psychiatrist or other mental health specialist.
- Patients who represent a clear and present danger to themselves or others should be immediately hospitalized.
- Children should be referred to a child and adolescent psychiatrist and at minimum be consulted.
- Antidepressant medication in children should be managed by a mental health professional.

Follow-Up
- Patients should initially be seen weekly to titrate dosage, monitor symptom management and compliance.
- Medication compliance is a serious issue with patients often discontinuing treatment before medication has time to work and symptoms subside.
- Educate patients concerning risks, benefits, and possible side effects of medications.
    - EXPECTED COURSE
        - Most patients respond to antidepressants within 2–3 weeks of treatment but should be educated that drug therapy may take months to reach full effect
        - Risk factors for recurrence are several prior episodes and early discontinuance of medication
        - To ensure the most effective response, antidepressants need to be taken at least 1 year after remission of symptoms as depression is a chronic disease with frequent episodes of recurrence

    - COMPLICATIONS
        - Social isolation, impairment of vocation and interpersonal relationships, suicide

SUBSTANCE USE DISORDERS

Tobacco Use and Smoking Cessation

Description
- Nicotine addiction is the number-one health problem in the nation

Incidence and Demographics
- An estimated 45.3 million Americans smoke
- Greater incidence of smoking in men than women
- An estimated 4,000 youths under age 18 begin smoking each day

Risks of Tobacco Use
- 430,000 individuals die each year of tobacco-related illnesses.
- Deaths from cancer are 2x greater for smokers than nonsmokers.
- Direct and indirect health costs each year are estimated at over $100 billion.
- >40% of U.S. children are exposed to environmental tobacco smoke in their own homes.
- 23% of high school students currently use some form of tobacco, most commonly cigarettes. Teenage smokers experience decreased physical fitness, lung function; later in life, increased risk lung cancer, heart disease.

Prevention and Screening
- Discuss the effects of tobacco use at all healthcare visits with children and adolescents and smoking adults.
- Screen individuals for exposure to second-hand smoke.
- Inquire at adolescent health visits if the teen's friends are smokers. If a teen's friends smoke, the teen is more likely to smoke.
- Take a complete smoking history at all healthcare visits and encourage attempts to quit.

Assessment
- Evaluate smoker's readiness to quit

Management
Smoking Cessation
- Combination of education, support, behavioral strategies, bupropion, and nicotine replacement therapies are more effective than any method alone. Encourage patient to quit and offer therapy at every visit.
- Nicotine replacement therapy and bupropion double the probability of success.
- Nicotine replacement product adverse reactions include local irritation of skin or mucous membranes, withdrawal symptoms, GI upset, tachycardia, spontaneous abortion. Avoid use immediate post-MI, accelerated hypertension, severe angina, chronic nasal disorders (spray), hepatic and renal dysfunction, hyperthyroidism, and other disorders.
- Encourage cessation of smoking first without pharmacologic interventions; if unsuccessful, may educate regarding products available for assistance (see Table 18–6). They should not be used by adolescents with heart disease, especially arrhythmias, or during pregnancy (unless under supervision). Efficacy in teens has not been proven.

Follow-Up
- Patient must stop smoking before nicotine preparation is used.
- Pregnant women should be encouraged to stop smoking without pharmacologic support.

- Relapse is common and frequently occurs within the first 1–2 weeks during withdrawal.
- Provide weekly visits during attempts to quit.
- Long-term success is greater with multiple attempts.

Table 18–6. Pharmacologic Preparations to Assist in Smoking Cessation

Pharma-cotherapy	Precautions/ Contraindications	Side Effects	Dosage	Duration	Availability
Bupropion SR	History of seizure History of eating disorders Do not use in patients younger than 18	Insomnia, Dry mouth	150 mg every morning for 3 days then 150 mg twice daily (Begin treatment 1–2 weeks pre-quit)	7–12 weeks maintenance up to 6 months	Zyban (prescription only)
Varenicline	Caution with hx psychiatric illness (suicidality, depression) or impaired renal function. Do not use in patients younger than 18	Nausea/ vomiting, insomnia, constipation, diarrhea, fatigue	0.5 mg daily for 3 days, then 0.5 mg bid for 4 days, then 1 mg po daily for 11 weeks	12 weeks May continue an additional 12 weeks if treatment successful	Chantix (prescription only)
Nicotine Gum		Mouth soreness, dyspepsia	If smoked 1–24 cigs/day: 2 mg gum (up to 24 pcs/day) If smoked 25+ cigs/day: 4 mg gum (up to 24 pcs/day)	Up to 12 weeks	Nicorette, Nicorette Mint, Nicorette Orange (OTC only)
Nicotine Inhaler		Local irritation of mouth, throat	6–16 cartridges/ day	Up to 6 months	Nicotrol Inhaler (prescription only)
Nicotine Nasal Spray		Nasal irritation	8–40 doses/day	3–6 months	Nicotrol NS (prescription only)
Nicotine Patch		Local skin reaction, insomnia	21 mg/24 hours 14 mg/24 hours 7 mg/24 hours 15 mg/16 hours	4 weeks then 2 weeks then 2 weeks 8 weeks	Nicoderm CQ, (OTC only), Generic patches (prescription and OTC) Nicotrol (OTC only)

From *Treating tobacco use and dependence: PHS clinical practice guideline* by the U.S. Department of Health and Human Services, 2001, Washington, DC: Author. Available from www.surgeongeneral. gov/tobacco/clinicaluse.htm.

Alcoholism

Description
- The physiological dependence on alcohol as indicated by evidence of tolerance, symptoms of withdrawal, and impairment of function in social, interpersonal, and occupational areas of one's personal life.
- Alcoholism is often characterized by a preoccupation with the substance, loss of control over the amount and frequency of use, physical and psychological dependence and tolerance.

Etiology
- Alcohol is absorbed rapidly from the gastrointestinal tract and acts as a CNS depressant.
- Excessive quantity will cause stupor, coma, and death (from respiratory depression or toxicity to neurons).
- Physical and psychological dependence vary; there may be genetic predisposition to alcoholism as well as social and cultural conditioning to its use.

Incidence and Demographics
- Alcohol dependence and abuse are prevalent worldwide.
- First episode of alcohol intoxication is likely to occur in adolescence.
- Alcohol is the most frequently used depressant in the world.
- Alcoholism is more common in men than women.
- Alcoholism rates are highest in African-American and Hispanic males.
- Alcoholism is present cross-culturally and in all socioeconomic classes.
- Estimated that more than 50% of violent crimes committed occur under the influence of alcohol.

Risk Factors
- Family history; 40% of Japanese have aldehyde dehydrogenase deficiency, which increases susceptibility to alcoholism; Native Americans
- Abuse of other substances; presence of a psychiatric disorder
- Cultural conditioning, college students
- Domestic violence or abuse

Prevention and Screening
- Routinely ask questions to assess problem with alcohol (e.g., CAGE [Table 18–7])
- Early public education as to the nature, course, and consequences of alcohol
- Primary intervention programs in the community and schools
- Increased social and public awareness through educational mass media campaigns
- Community groups such as MADD (Mothers Against Drunk Drivers)

Table 18-7. CAGE Questionnaire

Memory Clue	Question to Ask
C	Have you ever felt you ought to **C**ut down on your drinking?
A	Have people **A**nnoyed you by criticizing your drinking?
G	Have you ever felt bad or **G**uilty about your drinking?
E	Have you ever had a drink the first thing in the morning (**E**ye-opener) to steady your nerves or get rid of a hangover?

Scoring and interpretation: Person receives one point for each positive answer. One "yes" answer indicates hazardous drinking. Two or more "yes" answers indicate alcohol abuse or dependence.

Adapted from "Screening for alcohol abuse using the CAGE questionnaire" by B. Bush, S. Shaw, P. Cleary, T. L. Delbanco, & M. D. Aronson, 1987, *American Journal of Medicine, 82*, 231–235.

Assessment

HISTORY
- Inquire about patterns of use; however, denial is a common coping mechanism
- History of prior substance abuse treatment
- Psychiatric history and mental status exam
- Current use of prescribed and OTC medications

PHYSICAL EXAM
- Clinical manifestations of alcoholism and alcohol abuse include:
    - Withdrawal symptoms such as tremors, confusion, hallucinations, disorientation, seizures
    - Neurological: Memory impairment, forgetfulness, loss of time or blackouts, hyperreflexia, ataxia, confabulation
    - Cardiovascular: Cardiomyopathy, hypertension, and arrhythmias
    - Compromised immune system, frequent infections
    - Gastrointestinal: Peptic ulcer; diarrhea; nausea; gastric distention; ascites; enlarged liver; hepatitis; cirrhosis; pancreatitis; malnutrition; thiamin, folic acid, and vitamin B deficiency
    - Musculoskeletal: Muscle wasting, frequent fractures
    - Generally unkempt appearance, poor personal hygiene
    - Integumentary: Cushingoid appearance, flushed face, spider nevi, ecchymosis
    - HEENT: Nystagmus, angiomas, smell of alcohol on breath, blurred vision
    - Impotence, sexual dysfunction
    - Generalized edema
    - Higher incidence of STDs, HIV infections
- Acute intoxication: Ataxia, drowsiness, disinhibition, delayed responses, nystagmus, psychomotor dysfunction
- Overdosing: Coma, respiratory depression, seizures, stupor
- Chronic indicators of alcoholism: Flushed face, frequent accidents, positive response to CAGE questionnaire, scleral injection, unexplained work/school absences

DIAGNOSTIC STUDIES
- Blood alcohol levels; CBC: Decreased WBC, platelets, hematocrit; increased MCV
- Chemistry profile for liver function studies (AST, ALT, GGT, LDH, alkaline phosphatase, total bilirubin), cholesterol, triglycerides, uric acid, amylase all increased (AST > ALT by factor of 2)
- Consider HIV, thyroid function tests, glucose, electrolytes to clarify the diagnosis
- Prothrombin time, PTT if liver disease suspected
- Urinalysis, ECG, chest x-ray to fully evaluate health

Differential Diagnosis
- Major depressive mood disorders
- Anxiety disorders
- Bipolar disorder
- Personality disorders
- Polysubstance abuse disorder
- Endocrine disorders such as Cushing syndrome
- Neurological disorders, seizure disorders
- Cardiovascular disease

Management
NONPHARMACOLOGIC TREATMENT
- Substance abuse counseling; treatment program such as Alcoholics Anonymous, employee assistance programs
- Cognitive-behavioral therapy, psychoanalysis

PHARMACOLOGIC TREATMENT
- Detoxification for symptoms of withdrawal; commonly used agents include the benzodiazepines lorazepam (Ativan), chlordiazepoxide (Librium), oxazepam (Serax); use of atenolol (Tenormin) to reduce need for benzodiazepines; clonidine, carbamazepine when benzodiazepines not good choice
- Maintenance therapy includes disulfiram (Antabuse), naltrexone (ReVia), thiamine, folic acid, and B complex
- Pharmacologic and medical management of underlying medical disorders as appropriate

LENGTH OF TREATMENT
- Physical withdrawal can be treated in 1 week; however, psychological dependence is long-term

Special Considerations
- Alcohol abuse during pregnancy can lead to severe birth defects, fetal alcohol syndrome.
- Alcoholism and alcohol abuse have long-term medical, social, and legal consequences.
- Severe intoxication is a medical emergency and may lead to coma, respiratory depression, aspiration, and death.

When to Consult, Refer, Hospitalize
- Refer patients diagnosed or suspected of alcoholism to a substance abuse specialist.
- Hospitalize for acute intoxication and withdrawal.
- Refer social issues to a mental health specialist for long-term management.
- Refer all legal issues to the appropriate legal authority.

Follow-Up
EXPECTED COURSE
- Treatment and outcome are variable for each individual with recovery as a lifelong commitment

COMPLICATIONS
- Peak at 65–74 years of age depending on length of exposure, frequency, and quantity of consumption
- See Assessment for list of medical complications; fetal alcohol syndrome

Illicit Substance Use and Dependence

Description
- A maladaptive pattern of substance use manifested by recurrent and significant adverse medical, psychosocial, and legal consequences related to the repeated use of the substance
- Drug dependence manifests as substance-seeking behaviors, physical dependence, tolerance, and withdrawal

Etiology
- Acquired brain disease, not well understood
- Neurons in the locus caeruleus are thought to adapt to chronic opiate exposure and fire at a higher than normal rate when withdrawal occurs, and are responsible for producing the physical symptoms of withdrawal
- Contributing factors to individual vulnerability:
  - Genetic predisposition
  - Neurotransmitter abnormalities
  - Environmental stressors
  - Psychodynamic factors such as unstable childhood, impaired developmental stages, personality disorders
  - Social-cultural factors such as increased availability and prevalence, cultural acceptance and peer pressure, impaired family and peer relations, stress, lack of valued alternatives

Incidence and Demographics
- Abuse and dependence are more common in men than in women.
- The average onset age of substance use is 12–14 years of age.
- There is a link between substance use and suicide in adolescents.
- Usage crosses all cultural and socioeconomic barriers.
- Marijuana is the most commonly used substance, excluding alcohol and tobacco.
- Strong links occur among alcohol, substances, and nicotine abuse.
- Highest prevalence of abuse occurs during ages 18–25.

- 70% of all admissions to treatment programs are men, 30% are women.
- 76% of men and 65% of women with a diagnosis of substance abuse have psychiatric disorders.

Risk Factors
- Genetic vulnerability
- Personal or family history
- Social, cultural, peer acceptance, and frequent use
- Psychiatric diagnosis, history of previous addiction
- Chronic pain

Prevention and Screening
- National and local public education and awareness through mass media educational campaigns
- Early prevention and education programs in school systems
- Cognitive-behavioral therapy to enhance coping skills

Assessment

HISTORY
- Personal, family history of abuse
- Patterns of use, substances of choice
- History of accidents, traumas, overdoses; legal difficulties
- Effects can be found in Table 18–8

PHYSICAL EXAM
- Stimulants:
  - Anxiety, agitation, panic, restlessness, irritability, aggression
  - Mood swings, grandiose, elated mood, hallucinations
  - Tachycardia, arrhythmias, chest pain, hypertension; hypothermia, hyperthermia
  - Abdominal pain, nausea, vomiting, insomnia, mydriasis
  - Hypersexuality, frequent urination
- Depressants:
  - Dysphoria, depressed affect, apathy, psychomotor retardation, slurred speech, drowsiness
  - Diaphoresis, hypotension, miosis, rhinorrhea, sneezing, headache, nausea, vomiting
  - Myalgia, muscle pain, ataxia, tremors, impaired coordination, impotence
  - Mood swings, aggression, combativeness, lack of impulse control, disinhibition
  - Impaired attention, memory and judgment, hallucinations, paranoia
- Hallucinogens:
  - Mydriasis, nystagmus, tachycardia, hypertension, ataxia, tremors
  - Severe anxiety, panic, mood swings, aggression, hallucinations, paranoia, flashbacks
  - Impaired concentration, memory, judgment, ability to make decisions
- Cannabis:
  - Paranoia, confusion, hallucinations, distortion of time and spatial orientation

• Inhalants/solvents:
  – Odor on breath, ataxia, slurred speech, euphoria, agitation, tachycardia, arrhythmias
  – Delirium, confusion, stupor, hallucinations, organic brain damage

Table 18–8. Effects of Drugs Abuse

Name of Drug	Effect	Method of Use	Characteristics	Effects on User
Tobacco	No alterations in mood or effect	Smoked, chewed	Addicting	Frequent respiratory symptoms, infections. Lowered HDL cholesterol, increased heart disease; smokeless tobacco increases incidence of oral cancer, periodontal disease
Alcohol	Initial euphoria, impaired judgment Long-term depressant effects	Swallowed	Withdrawal symptoms with frequent, prolonged use	Gastritis, vomiting, anorexia; blackouts with heavy use
Marijuana	Relaxation, depressant; may have mild hallucinogenic effects	Smoked, swallowed	Referred to as "gateway" drug, may lead to use of other products; tolerance with regular use	Chronic users develop apathy, decreased motivation, flat affect, global cognitive impairment (memory, problem-solving), chronic cough
Cocaine	Stimulant, produces euphoria, increased physical activity, may lead to aggression, paranoia	Smoked, snorted, sniffed	Highly addictive, tolerance develops	Hypertensive crisis, coronary artery vasospasm, arrhythmias may occur
Methamphetamine	Stimulant, similar to cocaine	Snorted, smoked, ingested	Withdrawal symptoms with cessation	Similar to cocaine, tachycardia
Hallucinogens (LSD, PCP, MDMA "Ecstasy")	Visual, auditory hallucinations, altered mood and dream-like state	Ingested	Ecstasy often called a "date rape" drug	Hallucinations may occur weeks after use; renal damage may occur with ecstasy

Table 18-8. Effects of Drugs Abuse (cont.)

Name of Drug	Effect	Method of Use	Characteristics	Effects on User
Inhalants (glue, paint thinner, gasoline, freon)	Euphoria, dream-like state, often with hallucinations; some products may have aphrodisiac properties	Directly inhaled or inhaled by huffing (putting a substance-soaked cloth in a bag and inhaling)	Commonly used by younger teens because of easy access	Most are CNS toxins, possible permanent sequelae such as peripheral neuropathy, ataxia, cognitive loss, language difficulty, loss of coordination; lung, kidney damage may occur
Heroin	Sedation, soothing and numbing effect with euphoria	Snorted, sniffed, subcutaneous (skin popping) and IV use	Sniffing most common method of use with adolescents	Chronic symptoms include constipation, chronic pruritus, bronchospasm

DIAGNOSTIC STUDIES
- Urine and serum toxicology screens
- CBC, chemistry profiles, liver, kidney, cardiac, thyroid functions to rule out other disorders
- VDRL, HIV because of high rate of STDs and bloodborne disease in this population
- CT, MRI scans, x-rays as indicated by history and physical to rule out other conditions

Differential Diagnosis
- Polysubstance abuse
- Psychiatric disorders
- Hypothyroidism, hyperthyroidism
- Hypoglycemia, hyperglycemia
- Head trauma
- Stroke, dementia, delirium, seizure disorder

Management
- Treatment and management depends on patient motivation, characteristics, and ability to engage in a therapeutic relationship. Nonjudgmental support by provider facilitates recovery.
- Before treatment, identify type and amount of substance ingested and route taken.
- Minimization and denial are hallmark characteristics and interfere with recovery.
    NONPHARMACOLOGIC TREATMENT
    - Multiple treatment modalities and interventions
    - Behavioral therapy
    - Narcotics Anonymous, Cocaine Anonymous, Marijuana Anonymous
    - Long-term residential treatment programs

PHARMACOLOGIC TREATMENT
- Methadone hydrochloride, levo-alpha-cetyl methanol (LAAM) used in treatment of heroin addiction, to block effects of heroin and yield stable, noneuphoric state free from drug craving
- Buprenorphine (Buprenex), a controlled narcotic similar to morphine with longer duration of action and no physical dependence upon withdrawal
- Stimulant abuse:
    - Diazepam (Valium) 5–10 mg q3h; drug of choice for cocaine toxicity
    - Monitor cardiac rate and rhythm
- Depressant abuse:
    - Phenobarbital for withdrawal
    - Haloperidol (Haldol) is commonly used to treat assaultive and psychotic behaviors

LENGTH OF TREATMENT
- Varies according to individual response
- Substance abuse commonly occurs with psychiatric disorders, requiring treatment of other disorder
- Prognosis and recovery are highly dependent on personal motivation and social support
- Residential treatment needs to exceed 90 days to be effective
- Methadone maintenance is 12 months minimum
- Opiate treatment is a minimum of 2 years

Special Considerations
- Legal issues are common with substance abuse disorders.
- Abuse of substances during pregnancy increases the risk of spontaneous abortion, premature birth, preeclampsia and eclampsia, low birthweight, and birth defects.
- DSM-IV-TR criteria applies to adult population and may not be applicable to adolescents and children.

When to Consult, Refer, Hospitalize
- Role of the primary provider is diagnosis, referral to substance abuse specialist, and co-management of medical consequences.
- Hospitalize for severe intoxication and medical compromise.

Follow-Up
- Frequency of follow-up dictated by substance abuse specialist.
    EXPECTED COURSE
    - Substance abuse is a chronic disorder characterized by periods of relapse and remission
    - Outcomes are contingent on adequate length of time in treatment, support systems

COMPLICATIONS
- Long-term use results in significant changes in brain function as well as severe impairment in social, vocational, and interpersonal relations
- High-risk behavior places substance abusers at risk for infections such as HIV, STDs, hepatitis
- Poor nutritional status, dental problems, poor personal hygiene

DOMESTIC VIOLENCE AND ABUSE

Domestic Violence

Description
- Physical, emotional, economic, or sexual pain and injury inflicted deliberately upon a partner or family member with the express goal of controlling, manipulating, or intimidating that individual within the relationship

Etiology
- Genetic predisposition toward aggression
- Personality disorders (antisocial disorder, narcissistic disorder, borderline personality disorder)
- Environmental stressors; comorbid medical disease (depression, mania, schizophrenia)
- Low self-esteem; exposure to violence at an early developmental age

Incidence and Demographics
- Domestic violence is the leading cause of injury to women ages 15–44.
- 1 in 4 pregnant women have a history of domestic violence.
- 22%–35% of all women seen in emergency rooms suffer injuries as a result of domestic violence.
- 50% of homeless women are victims of domestic violence.
- Women who leave are at 75% greater risk of being murdered than those who stay.
- Profile of known, reported abusers: Male under age 25, lower socioeconomic status, inner city resident; male victims are under-reported.

Risk Factors
- Female gender
- Physical, emotional, financial dependence
- Poverty, housing problems, lack of education, lack of vocational skills
- Divorced and single-parent families
- Psychiatric diagnosis
- Alcohol and substance abuse
- Pregnancy or other physical and emotional disabilities
- Family or personal history of physical or sexual abuse; long-term exposure to violence
- Social isolation, lack of support systems

Prevention and Screening
- Public education and awareness campaigns
- Educated primary providers

- Provide community resources, support
- Community emergency shelters, hotlines, and safe houses
- Organizations such as the National Coalition Against Domestic Violence

Assessment
HISTORY
- **Interview individuals alone**
- Inclusion of questions concerning domestic violence in medical history
- Appropriate documentation
- Trouble expressing anger
- Passive role in the relationship

PHYSICAL EXAM
- Withdrawn, fearful, evasive
- Poor personal hygiene, neglect; bruises, burns, fractures, injuries to abdomen, breasts, torso, pelvic region; injuries inconsistent with explanation offered
- Significant delay between time of injury and treatment
- Substance abuse; depression, anxiety; suicidal or homicidal ideation; somatization of symptoms

DIAGNOSTIC STUDIES
- As injuries warrant:
  - X-ray
  - CT, MRI
  - CBC, chemistry profiles, electrolytes, STD testing, VDRL, HIV

Differential Diagnosis
- Accidental injuries
- Depression or anxiety
- Hypochondriasis
- Substance abuse
- Borderline personality disorder

Management
NONPHARMACOLOGIC TREATMENT
- Establishment of safe, supportive environment
- Development of plan of action regarding safety and escape
- Provide community resources, shelters, and hotlines
- Cognitive-behavioral therapy

PHARMACOLOGIC TREATMENT
- Varies according to individual injuries
- Antidepressants
- Anti-anxiety agents

Special Considerations
- Individuals who are victims of domestic violence have greater incidence of substance abuse.
- Individuals with a history of being a victim of domestic violence are more likely to commit violent acts.
- Individuals who are feeling trapped or hopeless have a greater incidence of suicidal ideation and depression.
- It is mandatory by law to report all acts of violence or abuse against children or the elderly; check state laws for reporting domestic violence.

When to Consult, Refer, Hospitalize
- Refer all cases to mental health specialist for counseling.
- Refer those with injuries to an Emergency Department.

Follow-Up
- Long-term follow-up with mental health specialist is often needed, or return to therapy at later time.

Elder and Disabled Adult Abuse and Neglect

Description
- Emotional or physical injury deliberately inflicted upon an elderly partner or family member with the goal of control and intimidation by a person who has control or a position of trust. Goal is manipulation, intimidation, or control of the dependent individual.

Etiology
- Physical, emotional, sexual, and financial dependency due to disability or age; unreasonable physical restraint; deprivation of food, water, shelter, or medical treatment; and physical abandonment
- Limited economic and financial resources

Incidence and Demographics
- More than 2 million adults >60 years of age are abused annually.
- Individuals >84 are more likely to be abused.
- Women are more likely to be victimized than men.
- Greater incidence of abuse by family members than paid providers.
- More than 50% of victims are cognitively impaired.

Risk Factors
- Over age 84
- Social isolation, lack of support
- Cognitively impaired
- Physical, financial dependency

Prevention and Screening
- Public education and awareness
- Social programs such as Adult Protective Services
- Caregiver support/respite
- Assess caregivers for depression

Assessment
HISTORY
- Interview patient alone
- Mental status exam
- Determine primary caregivers, living arrangements, legal custodian, and power of attorney
- History of medical treatment, accidents, fractures, physical injuries, traumas, overdose of medications
- Determine environmental, psychosocial, and financial stressors

PHYSICAL EXAM
- Monitor nutritional status for dehydration, malnutrition
- Lacerations, bruises, wounds, burns, fractures
- Poor skin and personal hygiene
- Fearful, evasive, guarded, depressed

Other
- Unusual or inappropriate activity in bank accounts
- Numerous unpaid bills
- Lack of amenities
- Missing belongings
- Missed medical appointments

DIAGNOSTIC STUDIES
- Specific to presenting symptomology
- Signs of poor nutritional status

Differential Diagnosis
- Accidental injury
- Depression
- Self-neglect due to cognitive status or physical impairment

Management
NONPHARMACOLOGIC TREATMENT
- Goal is to maintain independence of the patient and caregiver; if patient needs care beyond the ability of caregiver, consider institutionalization, home care services, respite for caregiver, adult day care program, etc.
- Potential removal from the home for care and safety
- Monitor nutritional status and vital signs, cognitive status, medical status as symptomology presents
- Counseling for the perpetrator and the abused may be indicated; consider need for psychiatric or alcohol abuse treatment

PHARMACOLOGIC TREATMENT
- Antidepressants may be indicated

Special Considerations
- It is mandatory by law to report all elder and disabled adult abuse and neglect to Adult Protective Services.

When to Consult, Refer, Hospitalize
- Hospitalization or institutionalization when in the best interest of the individual

Follow-Up
- Routine medical follow-up for signs of further abuse

COMPLICATIONS
- Wide variety of medical and emotional consequences are possible

Child Abuse and Neglect

Description
- Physical or emotional pain and injury inflicted deliberately upon a child or failure to provide a child with adequate food, clothing, shelter, supervision, or care
- Includes physical abuse; sexual assault; unreasonable physical restraint; deprivation of food, water, shelter or medical treatment; emotional deprivation; and physical abandonment

Etiology
- No single set of factors produce abusive and/or neglectful individuals
- Often the abuser was a victim of abuse

Incidence and Demographics
- 2.5 million cases are reported each year in the U.S.

Risk Factors
- History of abuse in family is common
- Non-biologic primary caregiver, live-in girlfriend/boyfriend of child's parent
- Increased family stress and social isolation are linked to abuse
- Low socioeconomic level and financial stress are correlated with increased rates of neglect and abuse
- Some psychiatric conditions in parents or guardians are associated with abuse and neglect
- Alcohol and drug abuse are related to high rates of neglect and abuse
- Characteristics of the child, including dependency, being a fussy baby, slow growth, developmental delay, disability, and male gender increase rates of abuse and neglect

Prevention and Screening
- Public education and awareness
- Government social programs such as Child Protective Services

Assessment
HISTORY
- Interview child and parents separately
- If physical injury present, ask specific questions eliciting detailed answers including when and how it occurred
- Inconsistencies, contradictions, and failure to adequately explain should arouse suspicion of abuse

- Take complete social history including information about parents, caretakers, and family functioning and determine environmental, psychosocial, or financial stressors
- Explore child's past and present history of medical treatment including accidents, fractures, physical injuries, traumas, ingestions, illnesses
- Explore child's developmental and behavioral history including the perinatal period, labor and delivery, neonatal period, feeding difficulties, sleeping problems, toilet training, encopresis or enuresis

PHYSICAL EXAM

- Measure height and weight, utilizing growth chart and comparing findings to norms and child's own growth curve, note nutritional status and hydration
- Findings on physical exam suggestive of abuse include:
  - Bruising: In unexpected areas (abdomen, lower back, inner thighs, neck, around the mouth, pinna, inner aspects of arms—as child raises arms to protect face), in infants <6 months of age, and multiple bruises in various stages
  - Marks with characteristic shapes: Belt buckles, looped cords, palm of hand, human bite marks, marks around the wrists or ankles may indicate tying the child down
  - Burns: Cigarette marks, specific objects (curling iron), immersion burn into a hot bathtub (discrete water level marks are around buttocks and feet and hands); scalds from tap water are the most common type of intentional burn
  - Hair: Patchy areas of alopecia from pulling out hair
  - Mouth: Torn frenula, petechial lesions, lacerations or bruising to the palate
  - Neurological signs (signs of increased intracranial pressure [ICP] from bleeding into the head)—bulging anterior fontanelle, palpable split in suture lines, increasing head circumference, papilledema, behavior changes and/or decreased level of consciousness, vomiting; most subdural hematomas are due to abuse; head trauma accounts for approximately 50% of deaths due to physical abuse
  - Eyes (fundus): Retinal hemorrhages (from shaking), papilledema (from increased ICP)
  - Abdomen: Vomiting, abdominal distention, tenderness, decreased or absent bowel sounds may indicate trauma; bruising on the abdomen may not always be present; abdominal trauma is the second leading cause of death from physical abuse
  - Genitalia and buttocks: Most sexual abuse leaves no visible scars and injuries that occur heal quickly; in girls, possible findings include unusually enlarged hymenal opening (requires expert evaluation because of wide range of normal in sizes and shapes), extensive vaginal adhesions, purulent vaginal discharge. In boys, penile and/or scrotal injuries are uncommon; most findings are in the rectal area and may include abrasions, perirectal skin tags outside the midline (develop as small areas of bleeding that heal), hemorrhoids (normally very uncommon in children), poor rectal tone (dilation >15 mm), penile erection during entire exam in prepubertal boys (may be a normal variant). In both sexes any sexually transmitted skin lesions such as warts are highly suggestive of abuse.

DIAGNOSTIC STUDIES
- Bony injuries are most common in children <3 years
- Fractures highly suggestive of abuse include metaphyseal (or buckle handle fracture), rib, scapular, vertebral, spiral fractures of the humerus or femur in the young infant and/or fractures of the hands or feet in children <2 years of age
- Metaphyseal injuries are fractures through newly forming bone that occur when limbs are forcefully moved (usually rotated), such as commonly seen in the distal humerus and femur or proximal tibia; they are highly suggestive of abuse; changes may not be seen on x-ray for days to weeks
- Skull fractures suggestive of abuse are wide fractures (>3 mm), complex fractures (branching, involvement of suture lines), occurring outside the parietal area, and/ or multiple skull fractures; simple skull fractures may or may not be associated with abuse; falls less than 2½ feet do not usually result in a skull fracture
- Multiple fractures in various stages of healing is almost pathognomic of abuse once osteogenesis imperfecta is ruled out
- Fractures not highly suggestive of abuse are fractures of the distal radius and ulna (from falling on outstretched hands), simple linear fracture of a long bone, mid-clavicular fractures, and nondisplaced spiral fracture of the tibia in a toddler
- Blunt trauma to a bone can cause subperiosteal hemorrhage with subsequent periosteal thickening and elevation visible on x-ray
- Full skeletal surveys are recommended in children <3 years of age who are suspected of being abused
- New, nondisplaced fractures may not be evident on x-ray for 1–2 weeks and a repeat x-ray or a bone scan is recommended
- Sexual abuse requires a specialized exam and collection of laboratory and forensic evidence

Differential Diagnosis
- Unintended injury
- Poverty resulting in poor hygiene, poor clothing, or poor nutrition
- Osteogenesis imperfecta

Management
- Suspicion of neglect or abuse mandates reporting to local (or state, depending on region) child protection authority. Consider reporting to local law enforcement authority.
- Inform parent/guardian that you are required by law to report.

Special Considerations
- The child protection agency is responsible for investigating the case and assisting the family and child to access support services.
- Documentation is critical and should be done carefully as it may be part of a court case.

When to Consult, Refer, Hospitalize
- If injuries are severe or involve suspected sexual abuse, child should be referred to the hospital for evaluation and treatment with child abuse team.

Follow-Up
- The FNP has the responsibility to follow up closely and advocate for safety and medical well-being of the child.
  - COMPLICATIONS
    - Victims are at risk for depression; other psychological, educational, and behavioral problems; and repeating the cycle of violence

Sexual Assault and Abuse

Description
- Any sexual act or penetration committed through coercion or physical force including rape, incest, sodomy, oral and anal acts, or use of a foreign object

Etiology
- Character disorders
- Behavioral: Act of violence is reinforcing; once done, likely to do again
- Social: Exposure to violence in culture, media, and home

Incidence and Demographics
- Women have a greater incidence of being assaulted; men are more frequently perpetrators.
- Most common form of abuse is by fathers, stepfathers, uncles, older siblings, and dates.
- Incestuous behavior is reported more frequently among families of low socioeconomic status.
- Alcohol involved in 34% of all rapes.
- Only 1 out of 4 rapes is reported.

Risk Factors
- OF THE ABUSER
  - Substance abuse disorders, psychiatric disorders
  - Divorce, pregnancy
  - Family or personal history of physical or sexual abuse
  - Long-term exposure to violence
  - Lower socioeconomic status
  - Social isolation, lack of support systems
  - Factors such as unemployment, financial difficulty, housing problems, overcrowding

- OF THE ABUSED
  - Vulnerable, dependent, young
  - Opportunity for abuser to be alone with them

Prevention and Screening
- Public education and awareness campaigns
- Provide community resources, support
- Community emergency shelters, hotlines, and safe houses
- Organizations such as the National Coalition Against Domestic Violence
- Assertiveness and self-defense training

Assessment

- FNP is required to know and follow specific rape evaluation protocols regarding history, physical, and collection of specimens or information/findings may not be admissible in court.
- If FNP not educated in rape evaluation, refer to a specially trained provider.

  HISTORY
  - Social history, living environment, relationships
  - Inclusion of questions concerning domestic violence in medical history
  - Interview individuals alone when possible

  PHYSICAL EXAM
  - Withdrawn, frightened appearance, depressive symptoms
  - Dislocations and fractures
  - Unexplained bruises, abrasions, cuts, laceration, burns, soft tissue swellings, hematomas
  - Sexually transmitted diseases, genital rash, discharge
  - Rectal tissue swelling, discharge

  DIAGNOSTIC STUDIES
  - Forensic specimens and extensive STD testing per protocol, including HIV screening
  - Pregnancy test now and at later time
  - X-rays, CT scans, MRI as indicated

Differential Diagnosis

- Consenting sex among adults
- Accidental injury to pelvic and groin area
- Posttraumatic stress syndrome

Management

- Ensure safety, well-being, confidentiality
- Accurate documentation
- Be aware of depressive symptoms and potential for suicide

  NONPHARMACOLOGIC TREATMENT
  - Cognitive-behavioral therapy
  - Psychoanalysis
  - Support groups and community resources
  - Legal intervention

  PHARMACOLOGIC TREATMENT
  - Emergency contraception (rule out pregnancy with urine or serum HCG first)
    - Emergency contraceptive tablet or
    - Norgestrel 0.3 mg and ethinyl estradiol 0.03 mg (Lo/Ovral) or other 30 mcg pill: 4 tablets within 72 hours of incident with 4 tablets 12 hours later
    - Levonorgestrel 0.25 mg and ethinyl estradiol 0.05 mg (Preven) 2 tablets within 72 hours of incident then 2 tablets 12 hours later
    - Antiemetic may be necessary with emergency contraception

  LENGTH OF TREATMENT
  - Varies with individual medical and emotional needs

Special Considerations
- Individuals with other mental disorders at higher risk of abusing others
- Nature of relationship between abuser and the individual affects recovery
- Individuals with developmental delays are at risk of being abused

When to Consult, Refer, Hospitalize
- All injuries and all cases of recent rape should be referred to Emergency Department (with rape protocol).
- Refer all those with recent or past sexual abuse to mental health professional with experience in sexual abuse for treatment of psychosocial issues and possible post-traumatic stress syndrome.

Follow-Up
- Depends on individual coping strategies and support system

> COMPLICATIONS
> - Posttraumatic stress disorder, injuries to external genitalia, STDs

EATING DISORDERS

Disorders that are characterized by severe disturbances in eating behavior. The two major types are anorexia nervosa and bulimia nervosa. Binge eating also is a disorder that exists by itself.

Anorexia Nervosa

Description
- Eating behavior characterized by an individual's refusal to maintain a normal body weight (and body weight is <85% of expected), severe restriction of caloric intake, intense fear of gaining weight and a severely distorted perception of one's body, and absence of menses; weight loss to >15% below expected weight for height
- Types: restricting, binge eating and purging

Etiology
- Biological:
  - Genetic vulnerability and predisposition, neurotransmitter abnormalities
- Psychodynamic:
  - Reaction to the demand of adolescence; perfectionist personality with obsessive, rigid characteristics
  - Lacking self-confidence; close, troubled relations with parents; influence of family dynamics; parents may be overbearing/demanding; father may be distant while mother is overprotective and intrusive
- Social/cultural:
  - Peer pressure to be thin; media and cultural emphasis on thinness, youth, body image
- Pathophysiology of starvation:
  - Lack of energy and nutrients causes fat and protein store breakdown.

Incidence and Demographics
- Approximately 90% of patients are female
- 85% of cases have onset usually at 14–18 years of age
- Maximum frequency of occurrence is age 17–18
- Mortality rates are 5%–18%, making it the psychiatric disorder with the highest rate of fatalities
- Associated with depression in 65% of cases, social phobia in 34%, obsessive-compulsive disorder in 26%

Risk Factors
- Family histories of mood disorders, alcoholism, or eating disorders
- Perfectionistic, compulsive, high expectations of self
- White, middle-class females; adolescence
- Dancers, athletes, gymnasts

Prevention and Screening
- Public education and awareness
- Early intervention

Assessment
HISTORY
- Weight history, onset of weight loss
- Symptoms such as constipation, cold hands and feet, fatigue
- Dietary habits, patterns of eating, food rituals, weight loss, binge eating or purging
- Menstrual history: Amenorrhea
- Perception of body weight and shape, fears of gaining weight
- Exercise history, frequency and duration—may be excessive
- Use of medication for weight control
- Psychiatric history including comorbidity and previous eating disorders
- Family history of eating or psychiatric disorders
- Previous psychiatric treatments

PHYSICAL EXAM
- Weigh patient without clothes.; weight is often 15% below ideal body weight with significantly low BMI
- Amenorrhea, lanugo, delayed growth, sexual maturation
- Altered vital signs: Hypothermia, hypotension, bradycardia
- Muscular atrophy, ridges in fingernails, erosion of enamel of teeth from stomach acid

DIAGNOSTIC STUDIES
- A multitude of endocrine and medical problems can occur secondary to the starvation that occurs with this disorder; there are no definite laboratory tests used to diagnosis anorexia
- ECG (look for flattening or inversion of T waves, ST segment depression, lengthening of QT interval), CBC (anemia, leukopenia), chemistry panel with electrolytes (low potassium level), LH and FSH diminished, TSH, T3, T4, glucose levels

Differential Diagnosis
- Bulimia nervosa
- Mood disorders
- Medical disorders such as cancer, diabetes mellitus, Crohn's disease, endocrine disorders
- Substance abuse

Management
- First consideration in treatment is to restore the individual's nutritional state.
  ### NONPHARMACOLOGIC TREATMENT
  - Nutritional and medical management
    - Establish appropriate eating habits
    - Rehydrate and correct electrolyte balance
    - Restore weight; stop exercising
  - Psychotherapy
    - Cognitive–behavioral therapy is the treatment of choice
    - Individual and family therapy
    - Nutritional and dietary education and weekly monitoring

  ### PHARMACOLOGIC TREATMENT
  - SSRI antidepressants are most commonly used and may or may not be helpful in treating anorexia, but may be used in prevention of relapse of symptoms after weight is restored
  - Other antidepressants such as TCAs or amitriptyline (Elavil), antipsychotics (olanzapine—Zyprexa), mood stabilizers, and appetite stimulants (cyproheptadine—Periactin) have also been tried

  ### LENGTH OF TREATMENT
  - Varies according to individual characteristics, severity of symptoms and motivation
  - Inpatient stays may last 4–8 weeks, followed by day treatment program of 4–6 weeks

Special Considerations
- Denial is a classic characteristic of this disorder
- Individuals resist medical treatment
- Symptoms of bulimia occur in 30%–50% of anorexic individuals
- Poor nutritional status may endanger fetus and status of the pregnancy

When to Consult, Refer, Hospitalize
- A psychiatric consult should always be obtained.
- Mandatory hospitalization should occur when the risk of death from complications of malnutrition is likely.
  - Required when total body weight is 30% below expected

Follow-Up
- The role of the primary care provider is to monitor the medical component, including weekly weight and nutritional status, periodic lab tests, and collaboration with involved professionals.

EXPECTED COURSE
- The course of anorexia nervosa varies widely
- 10-year outcome: ½ markedly improved, ¼ recovered completely
- Short-term response to hospitalization is good, but relapse is common
- Food rituals, low self-esteem, and distorted body image commonly persist after treatment
- Indicators of a favorable outcome are decreased denial; admission of hunger; improved self-esteem and perceptions of body image and self

COMPLICATIONS
- Cardiac arrhythmias if purging, heart failure, convulsions, osteoporosis, infertility

Bulimia Nervosa

Description
- Recurrent episodes of overeating followed by purging behavior (episodes occur at least twice a week for 3 months). Feeling of self-worth unduly influenced by weight.
  - Eating a larger amount of food than most in a discrete time period
  - Sense of lack of control over eating during episode
- Recurrent compensatory behavior to prevent weight gain with use of laxative, diuretic, enema, induced vomiting (purging type); or fasting or excessive exercise (nonpurging type).

Etiology
- Neurotransmitter abnormalities: Poor serotonergic function; depression
- Poor impulse control disorder as high prevalence of alcoholism and drug abuse in this population
- Genetic predisposition
- Social, cultural, and peer pressure to be thin
- Demands of adolescence
- Family dynamics, particularly family disorganization and lack of interest

Incidence and Demographics
- More common in females than in males
- More common than anorexia but may occur together
- Occurs in late adolescence

Risk Factors
- Approximately 90%–95% of individuals are female; adolescence and young adults; family history of obesity, family conflict
- Poor impulse control, low self-esteem; high expectations of self performance
- Normal weight or overweight; history of dieting, obesity, fluctuating weight
- Substance abuse, mood disorders

Prevention and Screening
- Public education and awareness
- Early intervention

Assessment

HISTORY
- Onset of symptoms such as constipation, muscle cramps; menstrual history
- Dietary habits, patterns of eating, food rituals, and purging behaviors
- Use of medication especially for weight control, use of laxatives
- Weight history, exercise history
- Psychiatric history, body perception

PHYSICAL EXAM
- Complete physical exam to rule out medical causes
- Weight measurement without clothes (weight fluctuations—typically remains within 20% normal)
- Dental carries, dental erosions, gum disease, parotid swelling
- Abdominal distress (from putting pressure on the abdomen to vomit), esophagitis, irritation of the pharynx
- Ridges in fingernails, calluses or abrasions on knuckles (Russell's sign)

DIAGNOSTIC STUDIES
- CBC, chemistry panel with electrolytes (low potassium), ECG, TSH, T3, T4
- Amylase levels will be elevated with vomiting and return to normal in 72 hours after vomiting stops

Differential Diagnosis
- Anorexia nervosa
- Gastrointestinal disorders
- Endocrine disorders
- Neurological disorders
- Mood disorders
- Anxiety disorders
- Personality disorders

Management

NONPHARMACOLOGIC TREATMENT
- Cognitive-behavioral therapy including individual and family therapy
- Nutrition counseling: Goal to restore appropriate eating patterns
- Community support groups and resources

PHARMACOLOGIC TREATMENT
- Antidepressant medications, SSRIs and TCAs, are considered effective in reducing binge eating and purging behaviors. Use doses given in the treatment of depressive disorders
- Avoid MAO inhibitors due to potential for severe food interactions and hypertensive crisis
- Medication is used as adjunct therapy, combined with psychological and nutritional counseling

LENGTH OF TREATMENT
- Duration of treatment varies: Often months to years

Special Considerations

- Patients will try to hide behaviors associated with the disorder; family may see patient make frequent trips to bathroom after eating, excessive exercise, up during night binging.

When to Consult, Refer, Hospitalize

- Refer all cases to mental health professional who is an eating disorder specialist.
- Treatment may be managed on an outpatient basis in consultation with a nutritionist and psychotherapist.
- Hospitalization indicated when outpatient treatment is unsuccessful, or if cardiac complications, hemodynamic instability, or hypovolemia present.

Follow-Up

- Role of primary care provider is to monitor medical aspects, including nutritional status (weekly weight), periodic lab testing, and coordinate care with other involved professionals.

  #### EXPECTED COURSE
  - Frequent relapses
  - Better prognosis than anorexia
  - Prognosis depends on severity, electrolyte imbalances, and other medical complications

  #### COMPLICATIONS
  - Chronic induced emesis results in volume depletion, renal compensation, cardiac arrhythmia, esophagitis, dental decay

OTHER DISORDERS

Attention-Deficit Hyperactivity Disorder (ADHD)

Description

- ADHD is a neurobiological disorder affecting attention, impulse control, and level of activity.
- One of the most common psychiatric disorders of childhood and adolescence; also recognized in adults.
- Main behavioral aspects of ADHD: Inattentiveness, impulsivity, and hyperactivity, more frequent and severe than what would be expected for child's developmental level. Symptoms vary from individual to individual and may include:
  - Easily distracted
  - Daydreams
  - Appears to be in another world
  - Fidgety, restless
  - Inappropriate or excessive activity
  - May seem to be "driven by a motor," always on the go
  - Talks constantly
  - Interrupts others
  - May have difficulty getting along with others
  - Forgetfulness: Fails to turn in work or complete assignments ("forgets")

- Poor sustained attention
- Poor self-esteem
- Symptoms may vary with the type of setting. Often minimized in highly supervised situations, one-on-one encounters, and/or when an activity is new or enjoyable. Symptoms may worsen when the activity is non-preferred, difficult, or unstructured.
- Age of onset of symptoms is usually prior to age 7 (diagnosis may be made later).
- Subtypes (DSM-IV-TR)
  - Attention-Deficit Hyperactivity Disorder, Combined Type
  - Attention-Deficit Hyperactivity Disorder, Predominantly Inattentive Type
  - Attention-Deficit Hyperactivity Disorder, Predominantly Hyperactive-Impulsive Type

Etiology
- No single known cause for ADHD, may be multiple etiologies. Possible causes of ADHD:
  - Genetic factors: Up to 50% of children may have inherited this disorder
  - Adoption: Adopted children five times more likely to have ADHD than nonadopted children; may be related to poor prenatal care, malnutrition, or lack of stimulation
  - Neurochemical differences: Possible dopamine or norepinephrine deficiencies
  - Brain structure differences: Possible frontal lobe and striatum alterations
  - Pregnancy and delivery complication
  - Prenatal substance abuse
  - Low birthweight
  - Traumatic brain injury

Incidence and Demographics
- Approximately 3%–7% of all school-age children have ADHD.
- Ratio of boys to girls with ADHD approximately 3:1; however, girls may be under-diagnosed because although they are inattentive, their behavior tends to be less aggressive than boys.
- ADHD is the most common psychiatric disorder in school-age children; less recognized in adults.
- ADHD is one of the most common referrals for mental healthcare providers.

Risk Factors
- See Etiology

Prevention and Screening
- Public education and awareness
- Early screening and evaluation
- Patient and family education

Assessment
HISTORY
- Specific symptoms, age of onset (<7 years), duration of symptoms (>6 months), presence in more than one setting
- Has a negative impact on child's quality of life
- Central nervous system insult/injury such as fetal alcohol syndrome, prematurity, CNS infection/injury, lead poisoning, neurodegenerative disorders and seizures

- Family/child history of medical conditions such as anemia, thyroid dysfunction, fragile X syndrome
- Interpersonal dynamics: Interactions between the child and each family member and peer relationships
- Past or present stressors such as divorce or loss of a parent
- School history: Grades (past and present), school problems, absenteeism
- Family history of psychiatric illnesses, ADHD, or "school problems" (diagnosed or undiagnosed)
- History should be obtained from multiple sources including parents, child, teachers, or other individuals involved with the child such as mental health care providers

PHYSICAL EXAM
- Usually no findings on physical exam; there may be an increased incidence of neurological "soft signs," which can aid with diagnosis
- A complete physical exam to rule-out possible medical etiologies
- Obtain vision and hearing tests

DIAGNOSTIC STUDIES
- No laboratory tests diagnose ADHD
- Parent and teacher rating scales, such as Connor's, Vanderbilt, Achenbach, and Barkley's, should be used in addition to the clinical history
- Psychological, educational, and language evaluations may be performed if learning disabilities are suspected; psychoeducational testing may be obtained through the child's school or a psychologist
- If indicated obtain a CBC, lead level, and/or thyroid studies
- EEGs may be obtained to rule out seizure disorders; MRIs are only indicated for children with neurological findings

Differential Diagnosis
- Anxiety
- Depression
- Learning disabilities
- Pervasive developmental disorder
- Substance abuse
- Medical disorders—absence seizures, hypothyroidism, anemia, lead poisoning
- Hearing and vision impairment
- Disorganized and chaotic family

Possible comorbid or co-existing conditions
- Depression
- Dysthymia
- Learning disabilities
- Oppositional defiant disorder
- Conduct disorder
- Bipolar disorder
- Tourette syndrome
- Drug or alcohol abuse
- Adjustment disorder
- Post traumatic stress disorder

Management
NONPHARMACOLOGIC TREATMENT
Education of Child and Family
- Assess their understanding of ADHD and provide information as needed
- Discuss the treatment plan with the child and family, including behavioral and educational plans and medication use
- Often find that one of the parents has symptoms and may need to provide support and assistance for them; adults often have history of problems in school, jobs, and require assistance with organization, social skills

Social Skills Training
- Children with ADHD often have problems with peer relationships due to their inability to read social cues and impulsive, hyperactive or aggressive behaviors; tend to be immature
- Training facilitates the child in recognizing problem areas in relationships and teaches strategies to help improve social skills

Psychotherapy
- Often helpful in understanding ADHD and its impact on the child and family
- May include cognitive-behavioral therapy (CBT) for the child and family, and group therapy
- Behavioral and educational interventions (Table 18–9)

PHARMACOLOGIC TREATMENT
- Approximately 80% of children with ADHD respond positively to medication; adults may also respond (see Table 18–10)
- Some positive effects of medication include improvement in attention, concentration and academic achievement; decrease in hyperactive behaviors, disruptive and aggressive behaviors, and emotional lability (emotional ups and downs)
- Psychostimulants are the first-line choice for the treatment of ADHD

Table 18–9. Selected Behavioral and Educational Interventions for Children With ADHD

Behavioral Interventions at Home	Accommodative Interventions at School
Establish a list of appropriate behaviors (a targeted small number but consistently reinforced)	Assess for possible learning disorders
Provide a structured environment (predictable routines)	Tutoring
	Untimed testing
	Preferential seating in the classroom
Give only 1–3 shortly stated instructions at a time	Note-taking services
Use chart for reminders	Modified textbooks
Use timers or bells for transitions	Tailoring of homework assignments
Reward positive behaviors	Organizational aids
Ignore minor misbehaviors or give nonverbal cues	Use visual cues
Consistently discipline targeted behaviors	Use peer helper

Table 18-10. Pharmacologic Management of ADHD

Medication	Daily Dose Range	Maximum Dose
Methylphenidate HCl		
(Ritalin, Ritalin LA, Ritalin SR)	5–60 mg	60 mg
(Metadate CD, Metadate ER)	10–60 mg	60 mg
(Concerta)	18–54 mg	54 mg
Dextroamphetamine Sulfate (Dexedrine, Dexedrine Spansule)	5–30 mg	40 mg
Dextroamphetamine/amphetamine (Adderall, Adderall XR)	5–30 mg	40 mg / 30 mg (XR)
Dexmethylphenidate HCl (Focalin)	2.5–10 mg	20 mg
Atomoxetine HCl (Strattera)	10–60 mg	100 mg
Pemoline (Cylert)*	18.75–75 mg	112.5 mg

*Not used as first-line therapy due to liver toxicity

- Side effects of the psychostimulants include:
  - Decreased appetite, insomnia, headache, stomachache, irritability, dysphoria
  - Rebound effect (increased hyperactive or impulsive behavior or marked irritability as medication wears off)
  - Most side effects dissipate after several days; however, if they persist, medication change should be considered
  - Less common side effects seen particularly with methylphenidate are tics in susceptible children (5%–10%) and possible growth suppression at high doses
  - Nonstimulant medication may be used to treat ADHD if the child does not respond or tolerate stimulants; these may include clonidine (Catapres), imipramine (Tofranil), venlafaxine (Effexor), and/or bupropion (Wellbutrin)
  - Unlike psychostimulants, nonstimulants may not treat all behaviors associated with ADHD; a combination of stimulants and nonstimulants may be needed

LENGTH OF TREATMENT
- The child may continue on medication throughout adulthood; however, as the child matures, he or she may learn compensatory mechanisms, therefore decreasing the need for medication

Special Considerations
- The diagnosis of ADHD prior to the age of 4 years should be done cautiously.
- Females may often be under-diagnosed, particularly if child is inattentive but does not exhibit impulsive or hyperactive behavior.
- Adolescents typically are not hyperactive but restless.
- Hyperactive children often exhibit quiet behavior while in an office setting.
- If hyperactive behavior appears suddenly, this is often due to a stressor in the child's life, not ADHD.

- Inattention or lack of motivation may be easily confused with ADHD and need to be examined further.
- Children with ADHD are at an increased risk for developing other conditions such as substance abuse, depression, conduct and anxiety disorders and driving violations.

When to Consult, Refer, Hospitalize
- If the child has an atypical ADHD presentation or has a complicated comorbid condition
- When the child does not respond to treatment
- If the child exhibits severe antisocial or aggressive behavior
- If the child is threatening or attempting suicide

Follow-Up
- Medications should be monitored closely to determine effectiveness and possible side effects.
- Behavioral rating scales are useful to establish the effectiveness of medication during school.
- Initially frequent telephone follow-up with an office visit 1 month after starting medication.
- Frequent follow-up when titrating medication dosage and every 3–6 months when stabilized.
- Monitor height, weight, and blood pressure at every visit.
- Provide close monitoring of the child's functioning in school and at home, and make appropriate adjustments and recommendations as needed.

Conduct Disorder

Description
- Persistent antisocial behavior, violating another's rights and inconsistent with societal norms. Conduct disordered individuals exhibit at least one of the symptom clusters below:
    - Aggressive, bullying behavior toward people or animals,
    - Vandalism, fire-setting, and property destruction
    - Lying, "conning," or theft
    - Serious violation of rules (truancy) or running away from home overnight
- No sign of remorse for misconduct.

Etiology
- No single known etiology. Multiple genetic and environmental factors suspected to play a role.
    - Parental inconsistency, chaotic home environment, harsh and punitive parenting
    - Parental depression, parental antisocial personality disorder
    - Children who lack permanent family or absent father
    - Children with ADHD and oppositional defiance disorder
- New evidence suggests neurotransmitters such as serotonin and abnormalities in catecholaminergic and peptidergic systems are linked to aggressive conduct disorder.

Incidence and Demographics
- Occurs in 1%–10% of children, more common in boys.
- As much as 50% of patients <18 years seen in outpatient psychiatric care have a conduct disorder.
- Prevalence in U.S. is increasing. Boys <18 years have 6%–16% prevalence. Girls have a 2%–9% prevalence.

Risk Factors
- Dysfunctional family
- Socioeconomically deprived
- Family history of antisocial personality
- Substance abuse
- Learning disorders or ADHD

Prevention and Screening
- Early management of associated disorders decreases the likelihood that antisocial behaviors will develop
- Parent education about child development and parenting techniques
- Social skills training

Assessment
HISTORY
- Specific behaviors of the individual and effects on self and others
- Comorbid conditions such as depression, anxiety, substance abuse, learning disabilities, ADHD
- Academic history, past and present
- Family history of sociopathic and/or psychiatric illnesses
- Family functioning
- CNS insults/injuries, disorders, or symptoms

PHYSICAL EXAM
- Evaluate for trauma or abuse
- Evaluate for medical causes (uncommon)

DIAGNOSTIC STUDIES
- Neuropsychiatric assessment
- Psychoeducational testing to rule out learning disabilities

Differential Diagnosis
- Oppositional defiant disorder
- Depression
- ADHD
- Specific developmental disorders
- Substance abuse
- Bipolar disorder
- Psychotic disorders
- Dissociative disorder
- Posttraumatic stress disorder

Management
NONPHARMACOLOGIC TREATMENT
- Psychotherapy and anger management; individual and family therapy
- Parent training
- Treat comorbid conditions if present (depression, personality disorders, anxiety)

PHARMACOLOGIC TREATMENT
- Medications helpful for management of aggressive and antisocial behavior include lithium, risparidone (Risperdal), olanzapine (Zyprexa); atypical antipsychotics (diminish aggression); stimulants (with co-existing ADHD); clonidine (Catapres), and SSRIs (with coexisting depression or anxiety)

LENGTH OF TREATMENT
- Variable

Special Considerations
- Early age of onset and higher number of behaviors correlate with poorer prognosis
- Medication and patient management should be by a psychiatrist who specializes in this area

When to Consult, Refer, or Hospitalize
- All cases should be referred to mental health professional
- Emergency referral or hospitalization for aggressive, threatening behavior that jeopardizes safety of others or patient; homicidal or suicidal ideation

Follow-Up
- Close monitoring of medications and support to child and family as needed
  EXPECTED COURSE
  - Course is variable and dependent on multiple factors including patient's receptivity to treatment, stability of family, and access to resources; early intervention has a more favorable outcome

  COMPLICATIONS
  - Treatment failure may result in criminalization and placement in a correctional facility

Insomnia

Description
- Chronic insomnia:
  - Difficulty initiating or maintaining sleep of a restorative nature that lasts for at least 1 month and causes significant distress or social, educational, or occupational impairment
- Transient insomnia:
  - Lasts only a few days and is induced by substances, medications, jet lag, medical illness, stressful events

Etiology
- Normal sleep has two basic phases: REM (time of physical and mental activation) and NREM (deep rest), which cycle in 90 minutes and repeat 4–5 times a night; with insomnia, the typical pattern is lost due to:
  - Substance or medication effects
  - Situational stressors
  - Medical disorders

– Sleep apnea conditions
– Disturbance in circadian rhythms from jet lag, shift work
– Psychiatric disorders such as anxiety, major depressive disorders
– Primary sleep disorders with unknown etiology

Incidence and Demographics

- It is estimated that close to 60% of the population has suffered from insomnia at any given time
- Most common and widely recognized sleep disorder
- More prevalent with increasing age
- More common in women than men

Risk Factors

- Elderly individuals
- Individuals under severe situational stress such as divorce, job loss, financial distress
- Occupations that require shift work, frequent travel through time zones
- Alcohol and substance abuse

Prevention and Screening

- Regular bedtime routines
- Normalized work hours
- Reduced daily stress, avoid stimulants late in the day

Assessment

HISTORY
- Inquire about onset, frequency, and duration of insomnia
- Elicit present and past history of sleep patterns, routines, and naps
- Inquire about patterns of use of caffeine, nicotine, alcohol, or substances
- Review current medications, including OTC and herbal products
- Obtain psychiatric and medical history

PHYSICAL EXAM
- Physical exam should be tailored to the presenting symptomology, as primary insomnia is an illness of exclusion of other underlying medical conditions

DIAGNOSTIC STUDIES
- CBC, chemistry profile, electrolytes, ECG
- EEG if warranted by abnormal exam or associated symptoms

Differential Diagnosis

- Alcohol or substance abuse
- Medication side effects
- Acute reaction to stressful life events
  PSYCHIATRIC DISORDERS SUCH AS
  - Anxiety disorder
  - Major depressive disorder
  - Grief reactions
  - Bipolar disorder

MEDICAL CONDITIONS SUCH AS
- Cardiac disease
- Gastrointestinal disease
- Respiratory problems
- COPD
- Sleep apnea
- CNS lesions
- Endocrine disorders

Management

NONPHARMACOLOGIC TREATMENT
- Primary treatment consists of treating underlying cause
- Eliminate or restrict use of caffeine, nicotine, and other CNS stimulants; alcohol may cause rebound stimulation
  - Establish routine
  - Consistent bed time
  - Only go to bed when tired
  - Do not use the bedroom for any activity other than sleeping and sexual activity
  - Rise from bed at the same time every day regardless of hours slept
  - Do not nap during the day
  - Provide individual with literature and community resources

PHARMACOLOGIC TREATMENT
- Medications commonly prescribed for the treatment of insomnia include benzodiazepines, zolpidem (Ambien) and trazodone (Desyrel); most medications (Table 18–11) have some adverse effects such as hangover, loss of effectiveness (tolerance), dependence, constipation; Trazodone has TCA adverse reactions; Benzodiazepines are addictive; zolpidem may cause psychological dependence
- Melatonin is not FDA-approved but has shown some effectiveness in self-treatment of insomnia

Table 18-11. Insomnia Medications

Medication	Dose
Non-Benzodiazepines	
Zolpidem (Ambien)	10 mg hs
Zaleplon (Sonata)	10–20 mg hs
Trazodone (Desyrel)	25–100 mg hs
Ramelteon (Rozerem)	8 mg hs
Benzodiazepines	
Triazolam (Halcion)	0.125–0.25 mg hs
Temazepam (Restoril)	15–30 mg hs
Flurazepam (Dalmane)	15–30 mg hs
Estazolam (ProSom)	1–2 mg hs
Quazepam (Doral)	15–30 mg hs

LENGTH OF TREATMENT
- Non-Benzodiazepines: Prescribe for short term (1 month), except Rozerem—can be used long term
- Benzodiazepines: Prescribe for 7–10 days
- Use lowest effective dose and discontinue gradually
- Rebound insomnia may occur when medications discontinued
- Be aware of potential for drug tolerance, dependence, and withdrawal with benzodiazepines

Special Considerations
- Do not prescribe for pregnant or lactating women or persons with sleep apnea, renal or hepatic disease
- Dose in the elderly is usually lower and short-acting agents generally are safer
- Benzodiazepines have a potential for abuse; do not prescribe if history of substance abuse or mental illness

When to Consult, Refer, Hospitalize
- Refer to mental health specialist when symptoms are secondary to anxiety disorder or mood disorder
- When symptoms continue for longer than 1 month, refer to a sleep disorder specialist, neurologist, psychiatrist, or other qualified mental health practitioner

Follow-Up
- Weekly monitoring of effectiveness of treatment, compliance, and potential abuse
  EXPECTED COURSE
    - Most cases of primary insomnia will resolve with short-term management

  COMPLICATIONS
    - Medication dependence

CASE STUDIES

Case 1. A 7-year-old male child is brought in by his mother because he is having difficulty in school. The mother has brought a note from the school nurse and teacher. The child makes careless mistakes in schoolwork, is unable to sustain attention to tasks, does not listen, does not follow through on assignments, or finish schoolwork. This 7-year-old boy is constantly on the move, interrupts, cannot wait his turn, blurts out answers, and talks in class. He has lost his backpack twice and has difficulty remaining in his seat on the school bus.
PMH: Fracture left tibia at age 5 years due to bike accident, 7 stitches for laceration to forehead due to a fall from tree-climbing at age 6 years. No serious illnesses, no hospitalizations.

    1. What additional history would you ask?
    2. What do you think is happening?
    3. What diagnostic tests would you offer?
    4. What is your treatment plan?

Case 2. An 18-year-old female, on break from her first semester at college, presents to you with her mother. The chief complaint is amenorrhea, fatigue, and weight loss. The mother blames the weight loss and fatigue on the poor quality of college food, dorm life, and being away from home.
HPI: It is revealed that the patient is a dance major with daily dance classes at the university and evening dance classes at a private studio. She has always been a competitive student and graduated from high school with a grade point average of 4.0. During her senior year she was the school social activities director, participated in extracurricular activities and volunteer work. Although the patient is new to college life, she already is involved in dance performances, volunteer work, has joined the poetry club, and is co-editor of their publication.

    1. What additional history would you ask?

Exam: BP is 110/70, respiratory rate 18 and regular, heart rate 80 and regular, skin is dry, weight just at the 30th percentile with low BMI, negative for syncope or orthostatic hypotension, negative for parotid enlargement, negative for oral lesions or dental caries, alert with intact cranial nerves, good muscle strength and coordination. Normal pubic hair development and small breasts. Fingernails dry and brittle, no ridges, skin over knuckles intact and normal.

    2. What do you think is happening?
    3. What diagnostic tests would you offer?
    4. What is your treatment plan?

Case 3. A 70-year-old male presents to you reporting several incidents of shortness of breath and a choking sensation, accompanied by dizziness, diaphoresis, feelings of doom and loss of control. These "spells" have occurred four times in the past 4 weeks and start without warning. He denies seizure disorder and has not experienced loss of consciousness. Two days ago he went to the hospital emergency room because he thought he was having a heart attack. He was told it was not a heart attack and to see his regular provider.

    1. What additional history would you ask?

Exam: Patient appears calm, alert, oriented and concerned. Physical exam is unremarkable with normal vital signs.

2. What do you think is happening?
3. What diagnostic tests would you offer?
4. What is your treatment plan?

REFERENCES

Adesman, A. (2003). A diagnosis of ADHD? Don't overlook the probability of comorbidity! *Contemporary Pediatrics, 20*(12), 91–106.

American Academy of Pediatrics. (2007). *What do I need to know about child abuse?* Retrieved April 2, 2008, from http://www.aap.org/publiced/BK0_ChildAbuse.htm

American Psychiatric Association. (2000). *Diagnostic and statistical manual of mental disorders* (4th ed., text rev.). Washington, DC: Author.

Barrickman, L. (2003). Disruptive behavioral disorders. *Pediatric Clinics of North America, 50*(2), 1005–1017.

Brickner, M. (2007). Elder abuse detection and intervention: A collaborative approach. *Care Management Journals 8*(4), 219–223.

Bush, B., Shaw, S., Cleary, P., Delbanco, T. L., & Aronson, M. D. (1987). Screening for alcohol abuse using the CAGE questionnaire. *American Journal of Medicine, 82*, 231–235.

Centers for Disease Control and Prevention. (2007). Cigarette smoking among adults in the United States, 2006. *MMWR: Morbidity and Mortality Weekly Report, 44*, 1157–1161.

Edmunds, M. W., & Mayhew, M. S. (2004). *Pharmacology for the primary care provider* (2nd ed.). St. Louis, MO: Mosby.

Eisendrath, S. J., & Lichtmacher, J. E. (2008). Psychiatric disorders. In L. M. Tierney, S. J. McPhee, & A. Papadakis (Eds), *Current medical diagnosis and treatment* (47th ed., pp. 847–948). New York: Lange Medical Books/McGraw Hill.

Gephart, H. R. (2003). Where we are, and how well we can succeed, at treating ADHD. *Contemporary Pediatrics, 20*(12), 77–87.

Goroll, A. H., May, L. A., & Mulley, A. G. (Eds.). (2006). *Primary care medicine: Office evaluation and management of the adult patient.* Philadelphia: Lippincott Williams & Wilkins.

Griffith, H. W., & Dambro, M. R. (2008). *The 5 minute consult.* Malvern, PA: Lea & Febinger.

Institute for Clinical Systems Improvement (ICSI). (2004). *Tobacco use prevention and cessation for adults and mature adolescents.* Bloomington, MN: Author. Retrieved March 5, 2008, from http://www.guidelines.gov/summary/summary.aspx?doc_id=5454&nbr=003731&string=%22Tobacco+use+prevention%22+and+cessation

Kase, L., & Ledley, D. R. (2007). *Anxiety disorders.* Hoboken, NJ: John Wiley & Sons, Inc.

Levenkron, S. (2001). *Anatomy of anorexia.* New York: W. W. Norton & Company.

Liu, Y. H., & Leslie, L. K. (2003). Diagnosing ADHD: Putting AAP guidelines to the test—and into practice. *Contemporary Pediatrics, 20*(12), 51–73.

McPhee, S. J., Papadakis, A., & Tierney, L. M. (Eds.) (2008). *Current medical diagnosis and treatment 2008* (47th ed.). New York: Lange Medical Books/McGraw Hill.

Pritts, S. D., & Susman, J. (2003). Diagnosis of eating disorders in primary care. *American Family Physician, 67*(2), 297–304.

Reece, R. M., & Christian, C. (2008). *Child abuse: Diagnosis and treatment* (3rd ed.). Elk Grove, IL: American Academy of Pediatrics.

Rhodes, K. V., & Levinson, W. (2003). Interventions for intimate partner violence against women: Clinical applications. *Journal of the American Medical Association, 289*, 601–605.

Sadock, B. J., & Sadock, V. A. (2003). *Kaplan and Sadock's synopsis of psychiatry: Behavioral sciences/clinical psychiatry* (9th ed.). Philadelphia: Lippincott Williams & Wilkins.

Sharp, L. K., & Lipsky, M. S. (2002). Screening for depression across the lifespan: A review of measures for use in primary care settings. *American Family Physician, 66*(6), 1001–1014.

Silver, L. B. (1999). *Attention-deficit hyperactivity disorder.* Washington, DC: American Psychiatric Press, Inc.

Stahl, S. M. (2000). *Essential psychopharmacology: Neuroscientific basis and practical applications* (2nd ed.). New York: Cambridge University Press.

Stahl, S. M. (2006). *Essential psychopharmacology: The prescriber's guide.* New York: Cambridge University Press.

Stein, M. T., & Perrin, J. M. (2003). Diagnosis and treatment of ADHD in school-age children in primary care settings: A synopsis of the AAP practice guidelines. *Pediatrics in Review, 24*(3), 92–98.

U.S. Department of Health and Human Services. (2008). *Treating tobacco use and dependence: 2008 Update: PHS clinical practice guideline.* Retrieved March 1, 2008, from http://www.ncbi.nlm.nih.gov/books/bv.fcgi?rid=hstat2.chapter.28163

Walsh, K. H. (2002). Welcome advances in treating youth anxiety disorders. *Contemporary Pediatrics, 19*(9), 66–82.

Web sites with important information:
Centers for Disease Control and Prevention: http://www.cdc.gov
National Institutes of Health: http://www.nih.gov
National Institutes of Mental Health: http://www.nimh.nih.gov

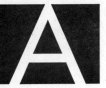

Case Studies and Discussion

CHAPTER 2

Case 1. Joan graduated from a family nurse practitioner program 5 years ago and has worked part-time in a college health center since graduation. She is now accepting a job as an FNP in a family practice setting and was asked to cover the prenatal clinic 1 day a week, in addition to providing regular family practice care. The collaborating physician assures her that he will provide her with direct supervision during the first 6 to 8 weeks of her experience and that he will be present in the clinic while she is seeing patients.

1. Is Joan legally authorized to provide care to prenatal women? To children?
   If her certification has been maintained as a family nurse practitioner, then she is legally authorized.
2. Should she accept this assignment? Why or why not?
   She is legally authorized and she can accept this assignment because adequate supervision will be provided to her during this training period.
3. What standards of care should she follow in providing care to prenatal patients?
   Standards of care are developed by professional organizations such as the American Nurses Association, which has created the Standards for Advanced Practice Nursing. Practice standards that guide safe and appropriate care for prenatal patients may be developed by the NP as protocols or guidelines for practice may be already published.

Case 2. Lee Ann is a 14-year-old who presents in the clinic for a physical exam and immunizations. She is alone and reports that her mother is working and does not know that she has come to the clinic. Lee Ann reports that she must have the exam and immunizations for school. The school has advised you in writing that Lee Ann's immunizations are not up-to-date, and she cannot return to school until a record is provided to validate her updated immunization history.

    1. What are the legal issues presented in this case?
       The main legal issue is the provision of care to minors without the consent of parent or legal guardian. Informed consent is necessary to provide care.
    2. What ethical principles will guide you in making a decision regarding this case?
       You will involve Lee Ann in the decision-making process by asking whether she would like to call her mother and making a new appointment with her mother present. In this way, you are using the principle of beneficence-duty to help others, as well as compassion and caring. You also can speak with the mother and call the school nurse to clarify the need for Lee Ann's absence from school.

Case 3. Alice is a 49-year-old African-American mother and grandmother. She has three children living at home and the oldest daughter, in high school, now has a baby. Alice reports that she is very angry with her teenage daughter, who does not want to help out around the house or care for her baby. Alice feels like there is chaos all the time and she complains of having frequent stress-related headaches.

    1. What theoretical model will assist you in planning an intervention for Alice?
       The developmental model proposes that families progress through developmental processes and that they are predictable. Since this is a non-traditional family, Alice may be experiencing some disappointment that she cannot enjoy just being mother in the launching phase of family life, but instead must also assume the role as grandmother and caretaker for her daughter's child. In addition, the daughter's developmental stage of adolescent carries with it several developmental tasks that are not being met when caring for a child. Alice's daughter may be exhibiting conflict over not being able to finish high school and the need to care for her child rather than spend time with her peers. Conflict over development processes is apparent.
    2. What additional information would you like to obtain?
       What coping mechanisms and support systems does Alice have for handling stress? Who else would be considered part of the family—does Alice have a partner? What about the baby's father? What roles do other members of the family assume? What are the financial resources? What are the strengths of the family? Are there any safety issues for the baby, Alice, or her daughter?
    3. How can you best help her today?
       Acknowledge the stress in Alice's life and treat her headaches. Ask about her willingness to engage a counselor for additional help for both her and her daughter, either alone or in family therapy. Identify and strengthen Alice's coping skills. Encourage Alice to see that she, her daughter, and the baby maintain regular health promotion visits. Consult with social services for a referral to a program for teenage mothers.

CHAPTER 3

Case 1. Emily, 2 months old, is coming to the clinic for her well-baby exam. Her birth history is unremarkable, with a birthweight of 7 pounds, 8 ounces (16.5 kg) and length of 20.5 inches. She is breastfed on demand, about every 3–4 hours. She has not had any immunizations.

1. What vaccines will Emily need today?
   DTaP, IPV, HBV, HIB, PCV
2. What developmental milestones will you assess for in a 2-month-old?
   Regards faces, eyes follow to midline, smiles, laughs, squeals, vocalizes, lifts head to 45° when prone, responds to bell, equal movements
3. There is no fluoride in the tap water; when should you start Emily on fluoride? How much will you give her per day?
   Begin at 6 months with 0.25 mg per day.
4. Emily's mother is thinking about discontinuing breastfeeding and starting infant formula. What information should you provide to her that might encourage her to continue to breastfeed?
   Breast milk is nutritionally balanced, contains antibodies and macrophages, and is free of bacteria. Allergic reactions are rare. Breastfeeding saves time and money.

Case 2. Travis, a 4½-year-old, comes to the clinic for a school physical. His last check-up was at 3 years of age. He is 40 pounds and 39 inches. His immunization records indicate he has had 4 DtaP, 3 IPV, 1 MMR, 2 hepatitis B, and 3 Hib vaccine shots.

1. What vaccines will he need today?
   DtaP, IPV, MMR, Hepatitis B, and Varicella
2. What safety issues will you discuss with Travis and his parents?
   Recreational sports protection gear (helmets, pads); swimming safety; automobile (street safety, seatbelts); knows his address and phone number, and how to call 911; Ipecac on hand for accidental poisoning; smoke alarms in the house; guns in the home

Josh, Travis's 14-year-old brother, needs a pre-participation sports physical. Josh weighs 225 pounds and is 5 feet, 8 inches tall.

3. What will your assessment examination focus on?
   History, immunization status, vital signs, pubertal development, musculoskeletal and cardiopulmonary systems
4. What counseling does Josh need?
   Weight management (his BMI is 34.2), safety (seatbelts, recreational protective gear)
5. What immunizations might Josh need?
   Hepatitis B (check that all 3 were given), Varicella (if no history of vaccine or disease), tetanus-diphtheria (due 6–10 years after last DTP), MMR (second shot, if not given previously)

Case 3. You have been asked to set up a health fair for a large computer company. The company would like to focus on the employees, their families, and the retired workers. You research the company and find out that there are equal numbers of employees with young children, single employees, and retired employees planning to attend the health fair.

1. What primary prevention topics will you address for parents of young children?
   Nutrition, iron intake, fluoride, safety (car seats, falls, poisonings, drowning), immunizations, sunscreen
2. What secondary prevention topics will you address for adults ages 18–50?
   Clinical breast exam, pap smears, serum cholesterol
3. What secondary prevention topics will you address for adults 50 and older?
   Clinical breast exam, mammography, pap smears, serum cholesterol, testicular exam, digital rectal exam, PSA, fecal occult blood, flexible sigmoidoscopy, dental/oral screening, blood pressure
4. How would you educate the participants about stress management?
   Large amounts of stress can lead to disease. Discuss stress management techniques (relaxation, imager, time management). Seek out support. Recognize sources of stress for the geriatric clients (e.g., loss).

CHAPTER 4

Case 1. 18-year-old male freshman complains of losing weight and fatigue x 1 month. He states he is chronically tired, can't get enough sleep, and feels feverish, but he doesn't have a thermometer in his dorm room. He has occasional aching joints. Of note is a cold a few weeks ago with a sore throat. He went to the university clinic at that time, had a rapid strep test done, and was told it was negative. He is concerned because he has missed more than 8 classes this month.
PMH: Usually healthy. Few occasional colds. Was told he had a heart murmur but not sure if he still does. Chickenpox at age 8. No past surgeries or hospitalizations; not sure of his immunizations status. No current medications, NKDA.

1. Should you be concerned about measles, mumps, rubella, polio, diphtheria, and pertussis since he does not know if his immunizations are up-to-date?
   No, it is unlikely that he has missed these immunizations because they would have been required on entrance to college.
2. What other history is needed?
   Health of his roommates, dormmates and friends; any rash, specific joint pain, or swelling; how much weight has he lost; whether he had any night sweats or cough; tick bite or outdoor exposure; and what is his sexual preference and partner history (how many, use of STD protection, any symptoms of STDs in partners), history and symptoms of STDs, any swollen glands, other associated symptoms.

Exam: No lymphadenopathy, pharynx pink without exudate, systolic murmur best heard over the 2nd ICS, no joint swelling or tenderness, no rash or skin lesions

3. What is your differential diagnosis?

   Rheumatic fever, mononucleosis (unlikely with no lymphadenopathy), Lyme disease (dependent on history of exposure), HIV primary infection (unlikely without additional symptoms), viral illness (unusual to last this long and be unaccompanied by rash)

4. What initial diagnostic and management plan is appropriate?

   Aortic murmur is significant and rheumatic fever should be highly suspected. Immediate referral to cardiologist is essential with initiation of penicillin treatment. Initial diagnostic testing would include CBC, ESR, C-reactive protein, streptococcal antibody titre, and ECG.

Case 2. 6-year-old male with both parents who are quite worried because his "hands are swollen and his eyes are red." Has had a low-grade fever for over 1 week; highest 101°F. Also had runny nose so mother thought he had a cold. Yesterday, his eyes were red, but didn't notice anything about the hands. Today, eyes are very red, lips are red and swollen, and hands are swollen and beginning to peel.

PMH: No childhood illnesses; occasional colds; 1 or 2 ear infections as a baby. Bilateral hernia repair at age 9 months. Immunizations up to date.

1. What are you looking for on physical exam?

   Fever, cervical lymphadenopathy, rash, skin desquamation in groin; eye, ear, nose, throat exam for signs of local infection; cardiac exam for signs of pericarditis, myocarditis; neurologic exam for signs of meningitis; abdominal exam for hepatosplenomegaly; musculoskeletal exam for arthritis

2. What do you suspect from this child's presentation?

   Kawasaki disease

3. What is your management plan?

   Immediate referral to pediatric cardiologist

Case 3. 14-month-old female with father who states, "She had a high fever a few days ago. Now she has a rash."

HPI: Visited 4 days ago for persistent fever of 2-day history. Fever as high as 104°F. Diagnosed with viral syndrome and sent home with instructions for fever management and to push fluids. Now returns, afebrile today, but has a light red rash on chest and back. Appetite poor, drinking liquids. Her face was flushed when she had the fever, but now face is pale.

PMH: History of recurrent otitis media, 4 episodes in 9 months. Immunizations up to date. No current medications.

1. What other history is needed?

   Her contact to other children and whether any of them have been ill; whether she seems to have a sore throat; how she is eating and sleeping; her activity level

2. What screening tests need to be done?

   If sore throat is present, a throat swab and a CBC with differential will rule out group A B-hemolytic streptococcal infection

3. What is the likely diagnosis and what management is appropriate?

   Given the history of high fevers that relented on the onset of rash on Day 4, this is likely to be roseola. Expected PE findings would be a blanching erythematous maculopapular rash and may have adenopathy. Rule out otitis media. Continue supportive management.

CHAPTER 5

Case 1. A 6-year-old male child presents to your clinic after playing outside all week while parents worked to clear a vacant adjacent lot. Within 2 days, the mother noticed the child to be scratching at legs. Upon close examination, an erythematous linear rash was noted on both lower extremities.
PMH: Asthma
Medications: Montelukast 5 mg po q pm and Albuterol inhaler PRN

1. What pertinent history is it important to ask?
   Any fever, systemic symptoms, any bites or other forms of exposure? Is there a history of allergies, irritant dermatitis, or other rashes?
2. What is the most likely diagnosis based on this history?
   Contact dermatitis, due to a plant such as poison ivy
3. What would you expect to find on PE?
   Eruptions along areas of skin exposure on arms and legs. Papules, dry scaling and erythema. May see scratch marks. Later will see weeping and excoriation.
4. Is he contagious?
   No, contact dermatitis is not contagious unless clothing or other items are contaminated with the oil from the plant.
5. How would you treat this patient?
   Identification and removal of offending agent; relief of symptoms with colloidal oatmeal, astringent, topical corticosteroids (do not use over large areas or if infected), antihistamines, antibiotics (only if infected).

Case 2. A 26-year-old White male comes in with a complaint of a "funny rash" on his back and across his shoulders that has resulted in "brown and white patches." He reports to you that he has had this rash for 6 months; however, his girlfriend noticed that the rash was spreading.
Social history: Works in an automobile factory and enjoys playing volleyball in his off time. Recently joined a church volleyball league.
PMH: Healthy, does not smoke, drinks 2–3 nights per week with friends

1. What pertinent history is it important to ask?
   Has he used any new products? Allergies? Medications? Previous episodes of same? Any itching, scaling, flaking? Any associated symptoms of disease?
2. You note discrete, scattered, or confluent patches. Wood's lamp exam reveals faint yellow-green scales. What is the most likely diagnosis?
   Tinea versicolor
3. What laboratory tests would you order to confirm the diagnosis?
   KOH and microscope visualization
4. How would you treat this patient?
   Topical selenium sulfide 2.5% shampoo to skin for 30 minutes the wash off for tinea versicolor; repeat 2 weeks later

Case 3. A 5-year-old girl presents to the clinic with skin lesions that the mother reports were at first vesicular by description and have now become honey-crusted. They are in various stages of healing on her face, arms, and legs. Nothing itches at all. Has had no fever. Attends day care.
PMH: No hospitalizations, 2–3 bouts of otitis media per year

1. What pertinent history is it important to ask?

   How long have the lesions been there? Fever? Remedies tried so far? Crowded living conditions? In day care? Any contacts with similar? Vaccines current?

2. What is the most likely diagnosis given this presentation?

   Impetigo

3. What would you look for on PE?

   Possible poor hygiene evident in child's grooming; breakdown and secondary infection (impetiginizing) of neglected skin lesions; honey-colored fluid oozing from open lesions and others with crusted covering; may see bullous (large vesicle or bullae containing clear yellow fluid on erythematous base); ecthyma (ulceration with thick adherent crust); possible tenderness; possible regional lymphadenopathy

4. Is she contagious?

   Yes

5. What laboratory tests would you order?

   Diagnosis is primarily clinical; cultures may be warranted if diagnosis is in doubt or if the lesions fail to respond to an appropriate course of antibiotics; possible gram stain; cultures demonstrate S. aureus, group A streptococci, possible methicillin resistant S. aureus; if recurrent, serology for anti-DNAse beta to look for prior strep infection.

6. How would you treat this patient?

   Wash area with soap to remove crusts prior to applying topical antibiotic penicillin for streptococci, Dicloxacillin for staphylococcus; erythromycin may be used if allergic to penicillin; topical mupirocin for small lesions.

CHAPTER 6

Case 1. A 16-year-old female presents with a "severe cold" x 4–5 days

HPI: Was previously well. Until last week, she had a cold, which is persisting without much improvement. Patient's mother very concerned that she needs antibiotics; claims they are always used to treat her daughter's head colds by previous providers. Feels feverish, has dry cough, runny nose, mostly clear drainage with some yellow mucus in the mornings, scratchy sore throat, and ears "popping." Tried Advil cold and sinus product with benefit.

PMH: Is in general good health, single, and sexually active with boyfriend x 2 months. Denies food, drug, or environmental allergies, smokes 5 cigarettes per day.

Medications: Oral contraceptive, took amoxicillin 500 mg bid yesterday—left over from prescription she was given 2 months ago for "sinusitis."

1. What additional history do you need?

   Details on history of frequent head colds (review the symptoms and signs, number of episodes in past few years, how treated, whether the episodes resolved). Any change in environment (dusty or damp, pets)? Has she ever had allergy tests or radiographic sinus imaging or endoscopy? Does she have asthma or allergic symptoms? Any symptoms/signs of systemic disease (diabetes)? Any intranasal (or other) drug use? ETOH? OTC nasal decongestants? Does she use condoms? Assess her STD risk.

2. What are the risk factors for possible diagnoses?

Cigarettes predispose to allergic rhinitis and sinusitis. Allergic rhinitis predisposes to sinusitis. Oral contraceptives may cause vasomotor rhinitis. Oral sex and new partner may cause gonococcal pharyngitis, risk for HIV, and immunosuppression

Exam: Temp is 99.0°F, thin-appearing White female, NAD, looks mildly ill. Voice quality "nasal." Posterior oropharynx has mild erythema, no lesions or exudate, tonsils not enlarged, neck supple with no lymphadenopathy, ear canals and TMs clear bilaterally. Nasal turbinates mildly erythematous and edematous, watery discharge. Heart: RRR at 88 BPM, lungs clear.

3. What diagnostic tests would you order?

Probably none at this time unless the history and physical exam suggests HIV risk or other systemic disease (diabetes, anemia)

4. What is your differential diagnosis?

Infectious rhinitis, probably viral; allergic rhinitis; acute bacterial sinusitis; vasomotor rhinitis

5. What treatment plan will you carry out?

Patient/family education on various types of rhinitis/sinusitis and what treatment is appropriate in this case versus indiscriminate use of antibiotics; also prevention measures and maintenance care. Suggest saline lavage qid, intranasal corticosteroid steroid spray, non-sedating antihistamine, OTC oral decongestants, infection prevention, allergy control in her environment

Case 2. 22-year-old female college student presents with sore throat and ear ache.

HPI: Sore throat began 3 days ago, was seen at student health center 2 days ago and treated with Pen V K 250 mg qid. Sore throat worse last night and especially c/o severe right ear pain. Notes fever and chills, but did not take temperature; and overall feels very tired and achy. Hurts to swallow, only drinking liquids. Lives in the dormitory. Denies problems with SOB, chest pain, rash, joint pains, nausea, vomiting, or diarrhea.

PMH: Healthy, denies any preexisting medical problems.

Medications: Pen V K, Advil prn for fever and pain x 3 days, last dose 4 hours ago

Exam: Young Asian female, looks ill. Temp 102.3°F, sinuses nontender, nasal mucosa clear. Ear canals and TMs negative. Throat 4+ erythema on posterior wall, white-yellow purulent exudate on right tonsillar area. Positive trismus, palatal bulge on the right. Neck positive for anterior cervical lymphadenopathy, tender, soft, and mobile. Chest clear. Heart RRR at 110 BPM.

1. What are the most likely possibilities for a differential diagnosis?

Peritonsillar abscess, streptococcal tonsillitis, infectious mononucleosis, antibiotic noncompliance, acute otitis media, antibiotic resistant infection

2. What information in the history is the most significant?

Failure to improve on antibiotics; symptoms worse with ear pain, which may be referred from pharynx

3. What physical examination components are especially useful for this presentation?

Fever, erythematous posterior pharynx with exudative tonsil, trismus, palatal bulge, tender lymphadenopathy, negative ear findings

4. Are the findings from the history and physical adequate to make the diagnosis and what diagnostic studies will rule in or out any of the possibilities?
   The history and physical are very revealing for peritonsillar abscess; however, CBC with differential, mono screen test, quick streptococcal screen, throat culture, and possibly blood cultures will help define her diagnosis.
5. What treatment plan will you carry out?
   Start parenteral antibiotics (ceftriaxone is a good choice) and consult with ENT specialist for urgent evaluation and possible admission. If urgent referral to ENT is not possible, make arrangements for her to be evaluated at the nearest emergency department for evaluation and treatment.

Case 3. A 6-year-old boy presents with severe right ear pain.
HPI: Child was well until this morning, when he awoke at 6 crying with right ear pain. Mother noted that he felt very hot, did not take temp. Gave Children's Tylenol and he slept a little. Mother later noted drainage from the ear on his pillow.
PMH: Frequent otitis media as an infant/toddler, which he seemed to "grow out of"; never required long-term antibiotics or ventilation tubes; last otitis media was about 2 years ago.
Exam: Young African-American male, looks moderately ill. Temp 101.2°F orally, right ear canal has whitish crust and is moist, no erythema or edema, tragus nontender with manipulation. TM red and bulging, small perforation present. Oropharynx clear, nose clear, neck supple, no lymphadenopathy, heart RRR 110, respirations 32, lungs clear.

1. What additional history is important?
   Any recent URI? Cigarette smoke exposure? Is the child in day care? Any siblings? Recent swimming? Has he ever had otitis externa or TM rupture?
2. What is the differential diagnosis?
   Acute otitis media with perforation, acute otitis externa, foreign body
3. What historical and physical exam features support the differential?
   The external auditory canal is without erythema or edema, no tragal tenderness, so otitis externa is ruled out; the red, bulging TM with a perforation and acute illness supports acute otitis media; the whitish crust in the ear canal is from the perforation of the tympanic membrane with extrusion of exudate.
4. What are the risk factors for otitis media?
   Male, day care, eustachian tube dysfunction, secondhand cigarette smoke exposure
5. How will you treat this child?
   Amoxicillin 40 mg/kg/day given tid; or ofloxacin (Floxin) otic 5 gtts bid; acetaminophen or ibuprofen for pain and fever; follow up in 2 weeks but instructed to return if not improving in 48–72 hours

CHAPTER 7

Case 1. A 15-month-old female is brought in by her mother with a cough, runny nose, and low-grade fever. Her mother states she seems to have a cold all the time.

HPI: This current episode started 2 days ago and the mother is concerned about the frequency of colds. The rhinorrhea is yellow-green, appetite decreased, no symptoms of otitis media but she does have a history.

1. What additional history would you like?

   Frequency of the colds (a child normally will have 7–9 colds a year, particularly if he or she attends day care or has older siblings), onset, description of cough; sleep, activity, appetite, vomiting, change in stools; immunization status, particularly for Haemophilus and pneumococcal; history of respiratory disease, GERD, feeding problems; family history of asthma, allergies, cystic fibrosis; social factors such as siblings, day care, smokers in the home, foreign-born

Exam: Temp 100.6°F, pulse 110, resp 32. Alert and quiet in mother's lap. Nose has moderate amount of thick yellow discharge; cough is wet, deep, and seems barky. Lungs with scattered wheezing and rhonchi in all fields, mild intercostal retractions, no nasal flaring. Rest of exam normal.

2. What are the possible diagnoses?

   Bronchiolitis because of low grade fever, URI symptoms, tachypnea, retractions, wheezing, rhonchi; croup because of barky cough, concurrent URI; viral pneumonia because of fever, cough, URI symptoms; cystic fibrosis because of frequent recurrence, cough, would have foul smelling stools

3. What diagnostic tests would you initially order?

   Pulse oximetry to help determine degree of respiratory distress; CXR to determine infection, congenital anomaly; CBC with differential to determine infection; sweat test to rule out cystic fibrosis

4. Your working diagnosis is bronchiolitis. What is your treatment plan?

   Encourage parent to offer lots of clear liquids; acetaminophen as needed for fever; educate parents on signs and symptoms of respiratory distress and to return immediately or go to ER if present. Trial of bronchodilator in office, if significant reduction is wheezing, give Rx to use at home: albuterol 5mg/ml 0.1–0.15mg/kg in 2cc of saline q4–6 hr if no nebulizer available for home use, oral Alupent 2mg/5ml 0.1mg-0.15mg/kg q 4-6 hr. Follow up the next day.

5. On follow-up your patient is doing much better, but the results of the sweat test have returned positive. What is your course of action now?

   The child most likely has cystic fibrosis. Referral to a specialist is indicated.

Case 2. A 76-year-old male resident of an assisted living facility presents to your office complaining of recent weight loss (10–15 pounds in the last 2 months) and shortness of breath on exertion. Denies any fevers, diaphoresis, chest pain. Has had a nagging cough for the last 3 months, mostly nonproductive.

PMH: Hypertension, hypercholesterolemia.

Medications: Cardizem 180 mg qd, atorvastatin (Lipitor) 20 mg qd. Former smoker, 1 ppd x 30 years

1. What additional history would you like to obtain?

   Living situation; any known exposures to others with pneumonia, flu, TB? Any recent travel? Does cough get worse at night or with exercise? Any history of asthma, wheezing? When the cough is productive, what does it look like—color, consistency, any blood? Any URI symptoms? Any symptoms of indigestion? Hx of allergies, clear nasal discharge, postnasal drip? Any night sweats?

Exam: Temp 97.4°F, pulse 80, resp 20, BP 150/90; alert, cooperative male in no apparent distress. Nose: mild edema; chest: slight increase in AP diameter, no retractions, hyperresonance on percussion, no abnormal breath sounds.

2. What are the most likely differential diagnoses?

   Postnasal drip, most common cause of chronic cough; COPD; lung cancer; TB; CHF; aginal equivalent; GERD; psychogenic cause (recent loss of wife)

3. What diagnostic tests would you order?

   CXR—rule out COPD, lung cancer, TB; CBC—infection, cancer; PPD—TB; pulmonary function tests—COPD; upper GI if above negative—rule out GERD; bronchoscopy, based on results of other tests

4. If the PPD is negative, would you do anything further?

   Consider repeating the PPD in 1 week because of booster effect

5. What would you do for this patient on this visit?

   Discuss possibility of grief reaction to loss of wife, depression; assess eating habits, humidification, cough suppressant at night; consider nasal antihistamines or nasal steroids; would avoid decongestants due to slight elevation in BP and potential for urinary retention in a man this age; update immunizations, pneumovax, flu (depending on season) and tetanus

Case 3. A 35-year-old married Hispanic female presents with a chief complaint of cough for 7 days. She is the mother of three and works in a hardware store. The cough is productive of yellow phlegm and gets worse at night. She also notes some shortness of breath on exertion. She has felt warm off and on for the last 2 days, has had some yellowish rhinorrhea, denies earaches, sore throat.

PMH: Nonsmoker. No past history of asthma, bronchitis, pneumonia. Her children have had colds but currently well. She moved to the U.S. about 6 months ago from Guatemala. No other significant PMH.

Medications: Has tried OTC cold preparations with some relief

Exam: Temp 100°F, pulse 82, resp 18, BP 128/86. Nose: erythema and edema; throat mild erythema; neck: shotty anterior cervical nodes; lungs: scattered adventitious breath sounds with partial clearing post cough; rest of PE normal.

1. What are your working differential diagnoses?

   URI, bronchitis, viral pneumonia, TB, occupational exposure

2. What diagnostic tests would you order?

   PPD because of immigrant status, cough, low grade fever. Other diagnostic tests are not indicated at this time. This patient has no signs of respiratory distress, bacterial pneumonia, or sinusitis.

3. What would you do for this patient at this visit?

Nonpharmacological: Increase fluids, rest, humidification, avoidance of secondhand smoke

Pharmacological: Antipyretic as needed, cough suppressant at night if having difficulty sleeping due to cough, bronchodilator inhaler

Follow-up: 48–72 hr to read PPD and see if symptoms have improved

4. On return visit, the PPD is positive at 10 mm. She tells you her symptoms are not improved and her fever has been 101°F, but responds well to Tylenol. What is your differential diagnosis now?

TB; bronchitis with secondary bacterial infection

5. What diagnostic tests would you order?

CXR; CBC with differential

6. What would you do regarding the other family members?

Have all family members get a PPD; discuss communicability of illness

7. The CBC with differential results are WBC 12,000, segmented 50%, lymphs 48%; CXR shows increased hilar markings. Would you order an antibiotic? If so, which and why?

Yes. Because this is a previously healthy patient with no recent antibiotic use, you would select a broad spectrum antibiotic that would cover for most of the causative organisms of secondary bacterial infection, which are S. pneumoniae, Haemophilus, Chlamydia, Mycoplasma and Moraxella. You would choose a macrolide (Azithromycin, Clarithromycin, Erythromycin) or Doxycycline. Alternatively, you could also use a beta-lactam such as Augmentin, Ceftin or Vantin. Although the CXR was suggestive of pneumonia and not TB, her positive PPD warrants prophylaxis with INH as well. She will require baseline ALT and AST and benefit from some pyridoxine (vitamin B6) to prevent neuropathy.

CHAPTER 8

Case 1. Lori is a 44-year-old White female who presents to the clinic for a well-woman exam. She works as a telephone operator in a busy law firm office. Lori voices no complaints today. Diet recall indicates high-fat meals, including junk foods. She states she loves cheese.

PMH: Smokes 2 packs per day for 15 years; past medical history significant for hypertension; drinks 3 beers daily

Medications: Hydrochlorothiazide 50 mg qd

1. What additional history would you ask regarding her cardiovascular status?

Personal and family history of CHD, DM, hyperlipidemia; any previous lipid evaluation; history of activity/exercise; comprehensive health maintenance history; previous attempt of smoking/alcohol cessation; history of psychosocial stressors; any comorbid disease; abdominal pain; rheumatic disorders; medication history, including OTCs

Exam: Vital signs: BP 128/84; Wt: 133 lbs, Ht: 64 inches, eyes: yellow-orange raised lesions on eyelids; remainder of exam is unremarkable.

2. Would you order any diagnostic test on this patient?

Baseline EKG; fasting lipid profile (total cholesterol, triglycerides, HDL, LDL, VLDL, risk ratio); apolipoprotein b; comprehensive metabolic panel, U/A, TSH, freeT4; mammogram; possibly CXR

3. If your suspicions are correct, what actions would be required?

Step 2 diet and exercise program; referral to nutritionist for diet counseling; tobacco and alcohol cessation program; counseling for stress reduction

4. When Lori returns to the clinic 6 months later with total cholesterol 252, HDL 30, and LDL 170, how will you intervene?
   Reinforce Step 2 diet and exercise. Start on a statin such as atorvastatin (Lipitor) 10mg/day; plan on monitoring hepatic function panel every 4–6 weeks after starting therapy for 3 months and again with any dose increases.
5. What complications can occur with this problem and the treatment regimens?
   Hyperlipidemia—CAD progression, stroke, peripheral vascular disease. Drug treatment—pancreatitis, rhabdomyolysis, hepatic dysfunction

Case 2. Baby Joe is 1 month old and presents to the clinic because he is not feeding well and his mother states he is losing weight. Baby Joe was delivered vaginally at 36 weeks gestation. His birthweight was 4 lbs 9 oz. The baby is taking 2 oz of formula over a 55-minute period
Medications: None

1. Are there any other history questions you would like to ask?
   Weight history since birth; prenatal/delivery history; voiding/stooling history in past 24 hrs; 24 hr intake history; feeding behavior

Exam: Vital signs: Temp: 98.0°F/ear, Resp: 60, HR: 180, Wt: 5 lbs 2 oz. Crying and irritable, sweating; systolic thrill, II/VI continuous murmur at the upper LSB, rate 180; respiratory rate 60 with bilateral crackles; hepatomegaly noted.

2. What are your differential diagnoses?
   Patent ductus arteriosus, atriovenous malformations, venous hum, ventricular septal defect with aortic regurgitation, pulmonary atresia, persistent truncus arteriosus, aortopulmonary septal defect, peripheral pulmonary stenosis, total anomalous venous connection, CoA, tetralogy of Fallot
3. What is your management plan?
   Refer child to emergency room for admission and evaluation with cardiologist.

Case 3. Mr. Jones is 56 years old and presents to the clinic complaining of decreased appetite, shortness of breath, and swelling in his feet. He is unable to perform normal activities without becoming winded and has a productive cough.
PMH: 6 lb weight gain in the past 7 days. Past medical history significant for hypertension, hyperlipidemia, and MI.
Medications: Lipitor 20 mg/day, Monopril 40 mg/day

1. What additional history would you ask?
   Characteristics of cough and sputum; need for additional pillows to sleep—orthopnea; fever; detailed history on comorbid diseases

Exam: Vital signs: BP 90/40; Pulse 120; Resp 24; Skin: cyanotic; CV: S3 gallop, jugular distention; Lungs: basilar rales and wheezing; Abdomen: hepatomegaly, ascites; Extremities: 3+ pedal edema bilaterally

2. What diagnostic studies would you order?
   CXR, EKG, echocardiogram, electrolytes, U/A, pulse oximetry, arterial blood gases

3. What is your differential diagnosis?

CHF, renal disease, COPD, nephrotic syndrome, cirrhosis, pulmonary emboli, MI, pneumonia, asthma, chronic venous insufficiency

4. What is your management plan?

Give oxygen and consult with physician to plan hospital admission to stabilize; identify and treat underlying disease. At follow-up, educate about sodium and fluid restriction, control leg edema with elastic pressure stockings and elevation of legs, record daily weights; multiple medications needed to treat—diuretics, ACE, beta-blocker, glycoside, vasodilators, and anticoagulants.

CHAPTER 9

Case 1. A 6-week-old infant presents to the clinic for a well-baby exam. The mother tells you about how much the baby is spitting up with every feeding. She has decreased the amount per feeding and increased the frequency but still the child spits up a large portion of the feeding. He is on Isomil and Mom is feeding 1–2 oz q 1–2 h around the clock. There is no weight loss; he has gained 6 oz since his 2-week visit. Denies projectile vomiting.

PMH: He is the product of an uncomplicated pregnancy and full-term birth. Currently on no medications.

1. What other history would you ask?

Any choking during feeding (congenital anomalies), any bile or blood in regurgitation (obstruction), fevers URI sx (infection), other illnesses. Appropriate developmental milestones (smiling, lifting head when prone), neurological disorders, stooling pattern, irritability, consolability (intussusception, Hirschsprung's disease), any projectile vomiting (pyloric stenosis), feeding position and postfeeding position. Family history of food allergies (food intolerances or allergies).

Exam: Vital signs, growth parameters stable. HEENT: normal, Lungs: clear, Heart: RRR, no murmur, Abdomen: normal bowel sounds, soft, no masses or organomegaly

2. What laboratory tests would you order?

CBC to look for infection, anemia; electrolytes to evaluate hydration status; U/A to look for UTI, hydration status

3. What other studies would you order

CXR to look for congenital anomalies, lung status, cardiac enlargement

4. What is the most probable diagnosis and what treatment would you provide?

If all studies are normal, consider change in formula to Nutramigen for possible allergy. Upright with feeding and postfeeding. Review burping techniques and frequency during feedings. Close follow-up and, if not resolved, referral to pediatric gastroenterologist.

Case 2. An 18-year-old female presents with abdominal pain. She has had some vague lower abdominal cramping off and on for the last 2 months, but today the pain intensified and she was unable to attend school. She has had episodes of loose stools and that has seemed to ease the pain until today; otherwise, her bowel habits have been normal.

1. What other history questions would you ask this patient?

   Stool pattern >3/day or <3/week, straining or feeling of incomplete evacuation, mucus in stools, feeling abdominal distention (IBS), any blood in stools, nocturnal diarrhea (UC), fever, anorexia, weight loss (UC), LMP, birth control, hx of STDs (PID, ectopic pregnancy), any association with certain foods (lactose intolerance), UTI sx, family hx of bowel disease, nausea, vomiting, low fiber diet (diverticulosis)

Exam: Alert and oriented female lying in a fetal position. Vital signs stable, Abdomen—increased bowel sounds, softly distended, no masses or organomegaly, diffuse tenderness in R & LLQ, no rebound or guarding. Rectal—no masses or tenderness, hemoccult—negative, pelvic—normal.

2. What laboratory tests would you order?

   CBC—infection, anemia, blood loss; ESR—inflammatory process; HCG—pregnancy; stool for WBCs, culture, O&P—infectious etiology; albumin—malabsorption, chronic disease

3. What other studies would you consider?

   Abdominal US—ectopic, ovarian abscess; sigmoidoscopy–UC; colonoscopy–Crohn's disease

4. What is the likely diagnosis if laboratory tests are normal and what treatment would you provide?

   If all laboratory tests are normal, the most likely diagnosis is IBS. Have patient keep a diary of food intake and symptoms, avoid foods that increase symptoms, trial for 2 weeks of a lactose-free diet, increase fiber. Antidiarrheal or anticholinergic as needed. Close follow-up; if unresponsive, refer for further evaluation.

Case 3. A family of three presents to you complaining of vomiting and diarrhea times 2 days. It started with the 3-year-old son and then the mother and now the father. They are most concerned about their son because he has not eaten or drank anything since yesterday and has had a fever of 101°F. He is otherwise healthy and has had no past medical illness other than an occasional cold.

1. What other questions would you ask this family?

   Frequency of vomiting, color of vomitus, waking at night to vomit; frequency of diarrhea, description of stools, blood, mucus; fever, lethargy, urine output, crying with tears; recent travel, camping, day care; any common food source that all members have eaten

Exam: 3-year-old Black male appears lethargic. Temp: 101.4°F, Pulse: 120, Resp: 22
HEENT: normal, Heart: RRR, no murmur, Lungs: clear
Abdomen: Increased bowel sounds; soft; no masses, tenderness, or organomegaly

2. What laboratory tests would you order?

   CBC with diff—infection, parasites; U/A—hydration status; stool for WBCs, culture, O&P

3. Are any other diagnostic studies warranted at this time?

   No

4. What is the likely diagnosis and treatment would you provide?

Acute gastroenteritis. While awaiting lab results, maintain and improve hydration status. Give ORT at 50 ml/kg over a 4-hour period, start with sips and gradually increase, if no vomiting occurs; if vomiting occurs, either wait 1 hour and retry or give an antiemetic, then try to rehydrate again with ORT. Once child is rehydrated (crying with tears, alert, good urine output, thirsty), resume regular diet

CHAPTER 10

Case 1. A 49-year-old woman with a history of hypothyroidism complains of mid-back pain for 2 days. This is pain that she has never experienced in the past. She also complains of urinary frequency, dysuria, and intermittent nausea.

PMH: Gravida 2 Para 2. Multiple UTIs during early reproductive years. Medications include Synthroid 100 mcg, Prempro. She has a 15 pack-year smoking history.

1. What additional history will you need?

Characteristics and duration of pain, presence of abdominal or chest pain, other gastrointestinal symptoms, fever, gross hematuria, current symptoms of UTI; PMH of kidney stones or urologic structural abnormalities, any new sexual partners.

Exam: Vital signs stable, afebrile, appears in moderate distress, positive left-sided CVA tenderness.

2. What are the differential diagnoses?

Pyelonephritis, back strain, urolithiasis, MI, gallbladder disease, other gastrointestinal problem because of the patient's history of frequent UTIs during her reproductive years. Current dysuria and urinary frequency, plus the CVA tenderness on exam. Pyelonephritis is first in the differential.

3. What diagnostic studies will you consider?

Urinalysis, CBC with differential; BUN, creatinine, KUB

Results: Urinalysis shows 2+ hematuria with 1+ proteinuria, negative leukocytes, negative nitrates. A KUB was then ordered and demonstrated a small stone in distal ureter, 4 mm.

4. What treatment will you consider?

Strain urine; save any retrieved stones for laboratory analysis. Increase fluid intake to maintain urinary output at 2–3 L/day, increase fiber in diet; decrease animal fat in diet. Pain management with NSAIDS and opioids as required; antiemetics as needed. Return if inadequate pain relief from NSAIDs, severity of pain increases, urine output decreases despite increasing fluids, unable to keep fluids down. Because patient was afebrile and urinalysis was negative for infection, pyelonephritis became the top differential, confirmed by KUB. The size and location of the stone indicate she will pass this spontaneously with conservative measures. Further work-up will be required only if she does not improve or she has a recurrent symptoms.

Case 2. A 25-year-old female, recently married, comes in complaining of painful urination for 2 days. She has no fever. She uses a diaphragm for birth control.

HPI: No medications. Reports burning, frequency, hematuria, urgency. PMH significant for one urinary tract infection at age 19. Otherwise in good health.

    1. What are the differential diagnoses?
      Cystitis, vaginitis, female urethral syndrome, meatal stenosis

Exam: Vital signs are stable, afebrile, mild suprapubic tenderness. Normal pelvic exam.

    2. What diagnostic studies will you order?
      Urinalysis; urine culture not necessary because she is afebrile and it is not a recurrent infection. Physical exam confirmed cystitis as the top differential.
    3. What risk factors can you identify?
      Female, diaphragm use, recently married
    4. What treatment measures will you prescribe?
      Hygiene measures, hydration, voiding after coitus. Trimethoprim/sulfamethoxazole (Bactrim) DS bid, or ciprofloxacin (Cipro) 500 bid for 3 days. Phenazopyridine (Pyridium), 200 mg tid for no more than 2 days for pain relief.
    5. What follow-up is necessary?
      No follow-up necessary. Expect resolution of symptoms in 72 hours.
    6. What will you do if this patient follows up 2 weeks later with another UTI?
      Obtain culture and sensitivity and retreat as indicated. Trial of cranberry juice or tablets. Review hygiene, use of diaphragm, and voiding after coitus. Consider postcoital antibiotic prophylaxis or alternate method of birth control.

Case 3. A 10-year-old boy comes in with his parents to discuss bedwetting. He has daytime continence but has always had nocturnal enuresis once or twice a week. He has been diagnosed with attention-deficit disorder, but is not receiving any drug treatment; however, he has recently been placed in a special education class in school. Episodes of enuresis are now occurring almost nightly.

HPI: Normal gestation, normal labor and delivery. No serious childhood illnesses. No history of UTI. No medications, no allergies

    1. What additional history would you like?
      What the family thinks about his bedwetting, what he thinks about it, family history of bedwetting

Exam: Physical exam and neurological exam are normal (i.e., no anatomic abnormalities, normal gait, reflexes).

    2. What are the differential diagnoses?
      Primary nocturnal enuresis (PNE), UTI, diabetes
    3. What diagnostic studies will you order?
      Urinalysis

4. What treatment would you consider?

Discuss with patient and parents the causes of PNE (i.e., primarily an arousal disorder). Reinforce to the family that bedwetting is nobody's fault, is a common problem, and over time generally resolves on its own. However, he has had some changes in his daily routine that may be also causing him to wet the bed more frequently. Describe motivational and conditioning exercises as well as use of alarms and pharmacologic agents. Start by having parents restrict fluids 2 hours before bedtime and begin bladder exercises. Keep a motivational chart that has rewards for every morning his bed is dry. Have patient return in 2 weeks for follow-up. Consider addition of either DDVAP or an alarm at that time.

CHAPTER 11

Case 1. A 39-year-old sexually active woman presents with a 3-week history of white vaginal discharge, no itching, but notices a fishy odor.

HPI: Denies abdominal pain, nausea and vomiting, fever, genital lesions, lymphadenopathy, dysuria. Patient is in a monogamous relationship with same partner for 6 years.

1. What additional history would you obtain?

LMP, current method of contraception, use of tampons or douching, symptoms noted in partner

Exam: Thin, white-gray vaginal discharge coating vaginal walls, cervix without inflammation or discharge, no cervical motion tenderness on bimanual examination.

2. What might you find on examination of vaginal fluid if this woman has bacterial vaginosis?

Thin, homogenous, white-gray discharge; pH >4.5; clue cells visible on microscopic exam; positive KOH whiff test

3. Should her partner be evaluated and treated?

No, treatment of men has not shown to alter relapse/reinfection rate in female partners.

4. What is the standard treatment for nonpregnant women?

Metronidazole 500 mg bid for 7 days or metronidazole gel 0.75% intravaginally bid for 5 days

5. What does the patient need to know regarding use of this medication?

Patient is to avoid alcohol for 48 hours prior to initiating medication treatment, while taking the medication, and for 48 hours after taking the last dose due to the antibuse effect of this drug.

Case 2. Jane S. comes to your office for her first prenatal visit. She has had a positive home pregnancy test. This is her third pregnancy. She reports that she has made frequent attempts to stop smoking without success.

1. What further history do you need from Jane?

Age, LMP, menstrual history, gynecologic history, obstetric history, PMH, medications, social history

2. What will you include in her physical assessment?

Height, weight, blood pressure, complete physical exam, pelvic exam including bimanual exam for fundal height

3. What screening tests will you order?

Urine screen for protein and glucose followed by urinalysis and urine culture; CBC, blood type, Rh and antibody screen; RPR; rubella titre; hepatitis screen; Pap smear; STI screening if indicated

4. What prenatal education will she need?

Include plan for smoking cessation. Nutrition, exercise, changes during pregnancy, prenatal vitamin and folic acid supplementation, smoking cessation through behavior modification techniques.

Case 3. A 52-year-old woman presents with complaints of hot flashes and no menstrual period for 4–5 months. She asks if there is a blood test to determine if she has gone through menopause and would like your advice on hormone replacement therapy.

HPI: LMP 4–5 months, two periods prior to that were late and scantier than usual. Hot flashes occur daily with profuse sweating, but denies mood change or vaginal dryness. Has tried an herbal over-the-counter product without relief.

1. What additional history would you like before advising her on treatment?

Obstetric and gynecologic history; complete medical history for history of breast cancer or breast mass, thromboembolic disease, gallbladder disease, hypertension, cardiovascular disease, hyperlipidemia, liver tumor, migraines; osteoporosis risk factors; method of contraception, chance of pregnancy

2. What laboratory tests will you do to confirm menopause?

No tests are essential; by history she is perimenopausal. TSH not necessary unless having additional symptoms of hyperthyroidism; LH, FSH, and estradiol will fluctuate. Significant FSH and LH elevations may not be seen until 1 year after cessation of menses.

3. What information will you review about hormonal treatment in menopause?

Hormone replacement now reserved for short-term use in patients with severe symptoms. Long-term use is not cardioprotective and may increase risk for stroke, MI, breast cancer and perhaps dementia. Advise herbal preparations or symptomatic treatment rather than HRT at this time.

4. What other recommendations should the FNP provide?

Calcium intake of 1200–1500 mg per day; vitamin D 400–800 IU per day; exercise and weight management; vaginal lubrication for intercourse if dryness occurs, Kegel exercises to prevent urinary incontinence, check active ingredient and dosage of herbal product to determine its value (black cohosh, soy in large amount, flaxseeds may be helpful).

CHAPTER 12

Case 1. A 17-year-old male is brought to your office by his mother complaining of several days of unilateral testicular pain and swelling thought to be caused by injury while wrestling with a friend. The patient is reluctant to give more information.

1. How can you elicit more information from this patient?

Ask his mother to step out of the room during the examination and continue to question him in a matter-of-fact, nonjudgmental manner. Tell him you review this information with all adolescents and adults. Tell him what the differential diagnosis is because it is important to treat the right cause. Assure him that confidentiality is always respected in adolescents seeking treatment for STIs.

2. What additional information would you like?
   Other symptoms such as fever, urinary complaints, urethral discharge; history of STIs and current sexual practices; description of the injury

Exam: Edematous, tender hemi-scrotum with indistinguishable, tender epididymis; positive Prehn's sign; positive cremasteric reflex; no urethral discharge; temp 101°F.

3. Can testicular torsion be ruled out?
   Yes, by positive Prehn's sign, no nausea or vomiting.
4. What is the most likely diagnosis?
   Epididymitis
5. Is diagnostic testing necessary to initiate treatment?
   No. Test for gonorrhea and Chlamydia, but empirically initiate treatment with ceftriaxone and doxycycline. Also consider testing for syphilis and HIV.
6. What additional intervention is needed?
   Advise bedrest and scrotal elevation until fever and pain subside. Avoid sexual activity and pelvic strain until infection completely resolved. Refer if no improvement in 3 days. Teach safe sex practices, use of condoms, notify partners within past 30 days, and advise need for STI evaluation and treatment prior to resuming intercourse.

Case 2. Parents bring in their 1-week-old, full-term male infant, reporting that his penis is red and swollen. He has been crying continuously since his bath several hours ago. Previously, the baby had been healthy; nursing well, gaining weight.
HPI: Previously healthy baby has been crying for several hours.

1. What additional history would you like?
   Has the baby been circumcised? How have the parents been caring for the uncircumcised penis? Was the foreskin retracted?

Exam: The exam is unremarkable except for moderately edematous and reddened glans penis with retracted prepuce.

2. What is the differential diagnosis?
   Balanitis, phimosis
3. How would you treat this patient?
   Replace foreskin to non-retracted position if possible. If unable, obtain emergency urologic consult.
4. What follow up is necessary?
   Attention to penis during well-child visits.
5. What infant care teaching do parents need?
   Care of uncircumcised penis

Case 3. A 67-year-old retired postal worker presents with a 3-month history of difficulty urinating. He denies urinary burning, hematuria, foul-smelling urine, and abdominal pain. He does complain of hesitancy, dribbling, and retention.
PMH: No history of UTIs, prostate trouble, or renal disease. Worked as mail carrier for 30 years. Has been sedentary since retirement 5 years ago. HTN identified 3 years ago, treated until about 1 year ago when he felt better so did not return for follow-up. Does not smoke, drinks 3–4 beers several days a week.

1. What additional history would you like?

   Any irritative symptoms; sexual activity; medications, including over-the-counter antihistamines and decongestants, saw palmetto, or other herbal products; family history of prostate cancer; last complete physical exam, DRE, and PSA.

Exam: BP 168/102, pulse 72 regular, afebrile. Abdomen nontender with no bladder distension, no CVA tenderness. DRE: Good sphincter tone, prostate smooth, firm, nontender with obliteration of median sulcus.

2. What diagnostic tests would you perform?

   Urinalysis, serum creatinine, PSA

3. What does the clinician need to know regarding the indicated diagnostic test necessary for this patient?

   The PSA needs to be drawn prior to the digital rectal exam (DRE) being performed.

4. Can you make a diagnosis?

   Diagnosis of BPH based on clinical findings can be made and treatment could be instituted with medications. Refer if AUA score >8, unresponsive to medication, suspicious for malignancy, or complications with medications.

5. What is your treatment plan?

   Treat with an alpha-adrenergic blocker (terazosin or doxazosin) for both BPH and HTN. Increase dose gradually over 1 month and monitor BP until therapeutic effect is reached in 4–6 weeks. Avoid bladder irritants, decrease fluid in the evening. Once medication therapy is initiated, encourage patient to keep a log noting urinary symptoms in relation to medication dosage, and bring log to each follow-up visit for evaluation.

6. What follow up and screening recommendations would you give this patient?

   DRE and PSA annually; baseline ECG, serum cholesterol, annual fecal occult blood testing and sigmoidoscopy every 3–5 years (see Chapter 3, Adult Screening Guidelines); BP check-ups every 3–6 months when stable (see Hypertension, Chapter 8).

CHAPTER 13

Case 1. A 23-year-old sexually active male presents with a 4–5 day history of dysuria he feels is caused by a urinary tract infection.

HPI: Denies frequency, fever, flank pain, hematuria, history of urinary tract infections.

1. What additional information will help you evaluate this patient?

   Presence and characteristics of penile discharge, number of sexual partners, history of STIs

Exam: Mucopurulent urethral discharge, no inguinal adenopathy, no genital lesions.

2. What is the differential diagnosis?

   Gonococcal urethritis, NGU

3. Should any diagnostic tests be done?

   Tests for gonorrhea and Chlamydia using one of the following: Gram stain (gonorrhea only), culture using special media for each, DNA probe, nucleic acid amplification test on first void urine

4. What are your treatment considerations?

Consider empiric therapy for both gonorrhea and chlamydia, notify partner(s) of need for evaluation and treatment, abstain from intercourse until treatment complete (7 days), report to public health department after confirmation of gonorrhea or Chlamydia. No follow-up necessary if resolves. Refer for persistent or recurrent urethritis.

Case 2. A 17-year-old female comes to the family planning clinic for routine pelvic exam and contraception. She has had 4 sexual partners in the past year and only occasionally uses condoms. She requests an HIV test because one of her recent partners is an IV drug user. *PMH:* History of 2 pregnancies with 2 abortions, no major illnesses, does not smoke, drinks 2–3 beers on the weekend, lives with mother and grandmother, in 11th grade, failing some classes.

1. What additional information should you obtain?

History of STIs, current symptoms of STIs, signs and symptoms of primary HIV infection (fever, adenopathy, pharyngitis, rash, myalgias, diarrhea, headache, nausea and vomiting, thrush)

Exam: Complete physical exam with no significant findings except flat-topped, fleshy colored lesions on labia minora and thin yellow vaginal discharge.

2. What screening tests should be done?

Pap smear; gonorrhea and chlamydia tests; vaginal microscopy for trichomoniasis, bacterial vaginosis, and candidiasis; syphilis serology; HIV testing; pregnancy test

3. What treatment should be considered today?

Rule out pregnancy before treatment of HPV and other infections.

4. What education and prevention topics should be discussed with this patient?

HIV risk factors; perinatal transmission of HIV; how to change unsafe sexual behavior; additional birth control measures; annual screening for cervical cancer, gonorrhea, chlamydia; use of condoms to prevent transmission of HPV to partner

CHAPTER 14

Case 1. 13-year-old White male presents with pain in right hip that has worsened over the past 2 weeks.

HPI: Prefers to play video games, does not play sports, denies trauma
PMH: PETs at age 5, >100% for weight on growth chart

1. What other history would you like?

Recent illness, description of pain, associated symptoms?

2. What type of examination should be done?

Observe gait, assess for muscle atrophy and tenderness, assess for limited ROM.

Exam: Patient has local tenderness over hip with decreased flexion, abduction, and internal rotation.

3. What diagnostic tests should be ordered?

AP and lateral of hip/frog-leg X-ray

4. What is the diagnosis and plan for management?

Slipped capital femoral epiphysis; refer to orthopedic surgeon immediately for evaluation.

Case 2. 34-year-old man with complaint of left elbow pain for the last 2 weeks.
HPI: Played in two golf tournaments 2 weeks ago. Denies trauma. C/o dull ache in elbow joint that radiates down forearm. Denies numbness or tingling.
PMH: Overweight, history of "borderline hypertension"

1. What other history would you like?
   Any fever or other recent illnesses
2. What should be done on physical exam?
   Inspect for edema, redness, palpate joint for crepitus, fluctuancy. Assess for muscle atrophy and limited ROM.

Exam: Medial epicondyle is tender to palpation, + pain with pronation, flexing wrist against resistance, or squeezing hard rubber ball

3. What diagnostic tests should be ordered?
   None indicated
4. What is the diagnosis and plan for management?
   Epicondylitis nonpharmacologic Treatment will consist of RICE protocol. Avoid aggravating activities and oral NSAIDs. Symptoms should resolve in 3 months with conservative treatment.

Case 3. A 15-year-old girl presents with complaint of right knee pain during and after exercise.
HPI: Pain in anterior right knee area, just below knee joint during and after exercise. Denies trauma, plays basketball on her high school team, currently practicing nightly for an upcoming tournament
PMH: Well, no history of serious illness, accidents, or medical problems

1. What other history would you like?
   Precipitating factors, description of pain, any redness or swelling, associated symptoms, alleviating factors
2. What type of examination should be done?
   Vital signs, inspection for redness and swelling; palpation for warmth, tenderness, effusion; swelling at tibial tubercle, ROM, ligament stability

Exam: No fever; no redness, edema, warmth, or effusion; ROM/ligaments all intact; bony tenderness, slight swelling at tibial tubercle on right

3. What diagnostic tests should be ordered?
   None indicated unless symptoms do not improve
4. What is the diagnosis and plan for management?
   Osgood Schlatter's disease. Avoid activities that cause pain; ice for 20 minutes after exercise; quad strengthening exercises; NSAIDs if necessary.

- Difficulty concentrating or making decisions
- Change in sleep patterns (insomnia or hypersomnia)
- Low self-esteem; feelings of worthlessness or excessive, inappropriate guilt,
- Recurrent thoughts of death, suicidal ideation with or without a specific plan, prior suicide attempt
- Decreased energy and fatigue; increased somatic complaints such as headache
- Feelings of hopelessness
- Adjustment disorder:
  - A less severe form of depression in which symptoms occur within 3 months of identifiable stressor, mild sadness, inability to concentrate, excess worry, somatic complaints
- Bipolar disorder:
  - Extreme swings in mood, hyperactivity, flight of ideas, decreased need for sleep, grandiosity, impaired judgment, depression, aggressive behavior, sexual acting out, delusions, or ideation
- Depression in children:
  - Sadness, crying, withdrawal, fatigue, anger, irritability or agitation, somatic complaints, separation anxiety, difficulty concentrating, feelings of guilt or worthlessness, weight change, change in sleep patterns, increased social isolation, substance abuse, or suicidal ideation
- Dysthymic disorder:
  - Depressed mood most of the day, present almost continuously, patient complains he/she has always been depressed

PHYSICAL EXAM
- Complete physical exam with a mental status exam to rule out any underlying medical conditions
- Observe personal appearance, grooming, hygiene, affect

DIAGNOSTIC STUDIES
- Primarily a clinical diagnosis; tests (CBC, TSH, sedimentation rate, chemistry profile, B12 and folate, VDRL, CT scan) are used to rule out suspected underlying medical causes
- ECG prior to initiation of tricyclic antidepressants (TCA)
- Cortisol levels, EEG may be done by specialist
- Psychometric tests include Minnesota Multi Personality Index (MMPI-2)
- Self-report scales commonly used are the Beck Depression Inventory, Hamilton Rating Scale for Depression, Zung Self-Rating Depression Scale, and Geriatric Depression Scale

Differential Diagnosis
- Electrolyte imbalances
- Chronic fatigue syndrome
- COPD
- Bereavement or grief reaction over recent loss
- Bipolar disorders
- Psychotic disorders, schizophrenia

CHAPTER 15

Case 1. 49-year-old African-American female presents with new onset headache over the last 2 months.

HPI: She states that prior to these episodes, she never thought of herself as a "headachey" person. She relates that the headaches are "nearly always" occipital, and are often accompanied by pain so severe that it feels like the top of her head will come off. When questioned, it is clear that she is both photo- and phonophobic and also experiences lightheadedness associated with the headache.

PMH: Healthy female; perimenopausal.

Medications: Monthly Advil for menstrual cramps. Has tried Excedrin migraine with these headaches to no avail.

1. What other history is needed?

   Family history of headache, including migraine. Are patient's symptoms becoming progressive? History of head injury? Does she have headache with exertion, staining, sexual activity, or coughing? Any change in mental state, focal neurologic deficits, or fever?

2. What type of physical exam would you do?

   Screening neurological exam including funduscopic, cranial nerves, motor exam, gait and coordination, reflexes (would be normal in primary headache syndrome). Focused general exam to include vital signs, HEENT, and other systems as the history suggests to rule out secondary headache. Heart and lung exam routine for woman this age.

3. What screening tests would you do?

   CBC if chronic anemia or infection is suspected. Consider CT due to new onset headache lasting more than a few weeks. Do immediate CT if headache with exertion, straining, sexual activity, or coughing; or on exam there is change in mental state, focal neurologic deficits, or fever. Other diagnostic testing as directed by history and physical exam to rule out infectious, metabolic or autoimmune process

4. What is the most likely diagnosis?

   Migraine headache

5. How would you manage this patient?

   The patient has started with analgesics, Excedrin, which did not work. Can try NSAID, but avoid opioids to prevent rebound headache. Move on to 5-HT agonists if non-narcotic analgesics ineffective. Sumatriptan (Imitrex): oral: 25 mg taken as soon as possible at onset, 25–100 mg every 2 hours up to 300 mg in 24 hours. Injection: 6 mg SC adults. Perform first injection in office. Intranasal: Single dose of 5, 10, or 20 mg administered in one nostril, may repeat once after 2 hours, not to exceed 40 mg in 24 hours. See her at weekly to monthly intervals until headaches under control. Consider prophylactic treatment for attacks occurring more then twice a month, or impairing daily function, or medications contraindicated due to hypertension or cardiovascular disease

Case 2. A 3-year-old Asian male comes in for follow-up after management in the emergency department for multiple febrile seizures.

PMH: No prior history of virus-induced high fevers associated with seizing. No medications except over-the-counter acetaminophen liquid for fevers.

1. What other history do you want to obtain?

   How long has he been febrile? (Febrile seizure usually occurs within the first 24 hours of fever.) Any symptoms of URI, otitis, tonsillitis? Is there a family history of febrile seizures? Other risk factors for febrile seizures, such as neonatal discharge > or equal to 28 days; delayed development; day care attendance; very high fever? Complete description of the seizure, duration, recovery, motor involvement, etc. Any history of recent illness or exposure to illness, onset of headaches, vomiting, or unusual symptoms? Recent trauma; lead, toxin, or medication exposure? Prenatal/perinatal history, including developmental history.

2. What physical examination would you perform?

   Complete physical exam. Identify underlying illness requiring treatment; look for signs of physical abuse. Complete neurological exam, including level of consciousness, presence of meningismus, or a tense bulging fontanel; obtain head circumference. Look for neurocutaneous skin lesions.

3. What further diagnostic tests would you want to order?

   Probably none; lumbar puncture would have been done in ER if any clinical suspicion of meningitis or for children under age 18 months with first seizure; MRI would be done for child with focal seizures. Consider serum lead and routine lab studies only if no source of fever can be elicited on physical examination.

4. How will you initially manage this patient?

   Because febrile seizures are very frightening to the parents, parental reassurance and education are vitally important, as is an active search for the underlying cause of the fever and appropriate treatment with each incidence. Vigorous control of fevers by antipyretics and sponging with tepid water. Acetaminophen 10–15 mg/kg per dose either orally or per rectum. Ibuprofen 10 mg/kg per dose orally.

Case 3. A 78-year-old male presents with his wife and daughter complaining of an episode over the weekend of sudden-onset right-sided weakness that completely resolved in about 2 hours. He did not seek medical attention at the time because it resolved.

PMH: Smoker, 64 pack-year history. Mild hypertension diagnosed in 1985. Was told he had elevated lipids "a few years back" but refused to take medication or change his lifestyle at that time. Has not been back to see a provider since.

Medication: Hydrochlorothiazide 50 mg/day "for a year or so," 1985–1986. Occasional acetaminophen.

1. What other history is important?

   Onset, duration, and progression of symptoms most important in determining etiology and management. Resolution of symptoms in minutes to hours is suggestive of a TIA. Detailed description of symptoms or deficits including visual changes, aphasia, motor weakness, paresthesias may give clue to location of lesion. Review of systems for associated seizure, loss of consciousness, syncope, vertigo, vomiting, chest pain. Past medical history: Cardiac disease; peripheral vascular disease; diabetes; IV drug abuse; and previous neurologic conditions such as seizure, head trauma, dementia, brain tumors. Review all medications, including home remedies and supplements, particularly those which can alter level of consciousness or cause bleeding.

2. What systems will you examine?
Complete neurologic exam for any neurologic deficits (no lasting deficits with TIA).
Cardiovascular exam for hypertension, atrial fibrillation, heart murmurs, carotid bruits,
abdominal bruits.

3. What is the most likely diagnosis?
TIA; also has significant risk factors for cardiovascular and cerebrovascular disease.

4. What is your plan?
Consult with primary care physician or refer to neurologist immediately for work-up that will
include CT scan; consider obtaining CBC, ESR, baseline coagulation studies, chemistry
panel, lipid profile, RPR, ECG, and chest x-ray in meantime. Provide initial education
to patient and family about need for immediate response for subsequent episodes which
could be stroke. Also provide initial education about risk factors—smoking, hypertension,
hyperlipidemia—that will need to be modified. Prescribe aspirin 325 mg daily to be started
immediately, until more definitive management is begun.

CHAPTER 16

Case 1. L.O. is a 9-month-old Hispanic male brought to the clinic by his mother for a routine
well-child check-up. His mother states all is going well. L.O. lives at home with his mother,
father, and his maternal grandmother, who cares for him while his parents are at work. He is
eating table food and drinking cow's milk.
PMH: UTD on immunizations; no illnesses requiring antibiotics.
Current medications: None
Exam: This is a very plump male infant who is interactive with his mother and the examiner.
His vital signs are WNL. His weight is in the 95th percentile for his age whereas his height is in
the 50th percentile. In your office setting you perform a Hgb, which is 9g.

1. What additional history would you like?
Diet recall, any pica, family history of anemia, any gastrointestinal ailments

2. What type of anemia is most likely in this case?
Iron deficiency anemia

3. What is the most likely cause of L.O.'s anemia?
Inadequate dietary intake of iron due to intake of cow's milk before 12 months of age and
onset of rapid growth

4. What corrective actions might you recommend at this time?
Parental education about appropriate diet for age, referral to nutritional assistance program
if needed, consider vitamin with iron supplement, follow up in 1 month and then monitor at
well-child exams

Case 2. B.C. is a 48-year-old White female who presents to your clinic complaining of feeling
tired all the time. She works full time and cares for her elderly mother in the home. B.C. reports
"getting plenty of sleep and eating well." She finds little time for exercise and "doesn't have the
energy to even go for a walk." ROS: Pertinent only for heavy bleeding during her periods which
she states began about 8 months ago. B.C. reports having to stay close to home and using a
hand towel to supplement peri-pads.
PMH: Denies any hospitalizations or surgeries. Anemia during pregnancy. LMP: 1 week prior to
clinic visit. Otherwise healthy; does not smoke or drink alcohol

1. What type of physical exam would you do?
   General appearance, presence of cyanosis or pallor, vital signs, thyroid exam, neurological exam, breath sounds, cardiac auscultation, abdominal exam, pelvic exam, rectal exam for occult blood.
2. At this point, what might you include in your differential diagnosis?
   Anemia due to blood loss, hypothyroidism, fatigue due to depression (related to caregiver burden)
3. What diagnostic studies would you order?
   CBC, TSH, chemistry panel; consider lipid panel, ECG

Test Results: Hgb: 10g; RBC: 3.6; MCV: 72; TSH: 1.56 (normal)

4. What would your recommendations be for B.C. at this point?
   Iron supplementation to treat iron deficiency anemia due to heavy periods. Consider additional laboratory studies such as serum iron, ferritin, TIBC. Work-up or referral for menorrhagia. Offer support for caregiver burden. Follow up monthly until corrected.

Case 3. B.W., an 85-year-old African-American male, is brought to the clinic by his daughter for evaluation of possible dementia. She is worried that he cannot care for himself as evidenced by the fact that he forgets his car at church some Sundays and walks home, and by his apparent weight loss. She is concerned that he cannot prepare his own meals anymore.
PMH: Hypertension—controlled; bladder irritability responsive to medication. NKDA; currently taking Vasotec 5 mg qd, Ditropan 5 mg qd
SH: B.W. lives alone in his own home one block from his church. There is a gentleman who lives on his block who assists him with paying his bills, going for doctor's appointments, and getting medication refills. B.W. reports being able to fix his own meals and denies feeling hungry.
ROS: Denies SOB, CP, anorexia, but admits he has lost some weight. Denies bowel changes. Does have some trouble remembering things but has always been able to find his car because the only place he drives is to church.

1. What would you include in your differential diagnosis at this time?
   Dementia due to Alzheimer's disease or multi-infarct dementia; reversible causes of dementia such as vitamin B12 deficiency; depression; occult malignancy; sensory deficits

Exam: Alert, well-dressed 85-year-old African-American male who looks younger than his stated age. His vital signs are WNL. He scores 27 on the MMSE. CN II–XII are intact. He is able to ambulate without assistance. Romberg's intact, no evidence of ataxia. No lymphadenopathy. Lungs are clear without adventitious breath sounds. Heart: Regular rate and rhythm without murmur or gallop. Abd: no distention, bowel sounds positive. No palpable masses. No hepatosplenomegaly or CVAT. Genital exam WNL. Rectal *exam:* Normal size prostate, enlarged without nodules. Stool is brown and heme negative.

2. What diagnostic studies would you order at this time?
   CBC, chemistry panel, TSH, B12, and folate levels, RPR and PSA, fecal occult blood tests (FOBT) x 3

3. B.W. comes to see you 1 week later and has the following laboratory results: Hgb: 9 g; Hct: 27.2%; MCV=72; reported as hypochromic; all other parameters are WNL. He has lost two more pounds, despite the fact that his daughter has been cooking for him and encouraging him to eat. His FOBT are all positive. What type of anemia does this man most likely have and what would be the next step in your diagnostic work-up of this gentleman?

Iron deficiency anemia, probably due to blood loss. You urgently refer him to a surgeon or gastrointestinal specialist for colonoscopy, and order iron replacement therapy. You caution him to gradually increase the iron pills to three a day between meals and increase fluids and fiber to prevent constipation.

CHAPTER 17

Case 1. 52-year-old Hispanic female arrives at your clinic. She states she has been fatigued for 3 months, has gained weight since her last visit (6 months ago), and is urinating more frequently, but states that she is consuming more water and relates the urination to increased intake of fluids.

PMH: Hypertension and obesity; medications benazepril (Lotensin) 10 mg qd, and Prempro 0.625 mg/2.5 qd.

1. What additional history would you ask?

   Allergies, sleeping pattern, appetite/weight change, level of activity/exercise, 24-hour diet recall, social history including ETOH and cigarette use, family history of DM, thyroid disorders, hypertension, cardiovascular disease. ROS questions should include statement on how the patient feels in general; changes in skin integrity, nails, or hair; visual changes; problems with breathing; chest pain/palpitations; urinary symptoms such as incontinence, urgency, or burning; vaginal dryness; frequent yeast infections; bowel habit changes such as constipation, diarrhea, bloating; frequent hunger or thirst.

Exam: Vital signs: BP 130/88, HR 72, RR 12, T 97.9°F, Wt 196 lbs, Ht 5' 4", BMI 33.7; general appearance is alert without distress. HEENT exam is normal, lungs clear and heart rate and rhythm regular without murmurs; abdomen is obese with waist circumference 39 inches, no masses or tenderness. Extremities' pulses are normal; skin is warm and dry, sensation intact without lesions. Neuro exam is within normal limits.

2. What diagnostic tests would you order?

   Complete metabolic panel to check glucose level, renal and hepatic function due to the history of hypertension and exam findings; complete blood count to rule out anemia or other blood dyscrasias due to complaint of fatigue; thyroid panel to rule out hypothyroidism due to increased risk of age and gender and the complaint of fatigue and weight increase; lipid profile for risk of lipid abnormalities with the history of hypertension, obesity and age; urinalysis to rule out infection as a result of the history of frequency; may consider EKG and CXR as baseline studies.

3. If your suspicions were correct, what actions would be required?

   Order fasting blood glucose on a separate day to confirm the diagnosis

4. What is your treatment plan and follow-up?

Blood glucose between 250 mg/dl and 400 mg/dl would require immediate treatment with oral medications. If her blood glucose was <250 mg/dl, diet and exercise would be the initial therapy. Nonpharmacologic therapy to include patient education: basic pathophysiology, cause, general management, and long-term complications of Type 2 diabetes, lifestyle modifications including diet and exercise counseling and plan, foot care, medic alert bracelet, self-glucose monitoring and log. Pharmacotherapy would include initial monotherapy. The medication will be adjusted based upon home glucose monitoring in 1 week. Referral to a diabetes educator and dietician should be considered.

Case 2. A mother arrives at your clinic with her 7-year-old daughter, stating that she is developing breasts early and she has noticed hair under her arms.
PMH: Normal growth and development at well-child visits; current on immunizations

    1. What additional history would you ask?
    Family history, medication use or medications in the home, history of chronic disease, onset of menses, recent increase in rate of growth, changes in behavior or mood, illness, or head trauma

Exam: Vital signs within normal limits, Height 95th percentile on the growth curve, Tanner stage III; the rest of the exam is normal

    2. What diagnostic tests would you order?
    Consider hormone and GnRH testing, thyroid function test. May consider bone age, MRI of pituitary gland and CT of adrenal glands
    3. What is your next course of action?
    Refer to a pediatric endocrinologist for management if precocity is confirmed.

Case 3. African-American parents bring their 11-year-old son to the community clinic stating he has lost 15 pounds in 3 weeks and is urinating frequently. He is also "drinking a lot."
PMH: Recent recovery from chickenpox (4 weeks); otherwise normal growth and development; immunizations up to date.

    1. What additional history would you ask?
    Incidence of fatigue, abdominal pain, nausea, vomiting or diarrhea, headaches, medication use or drug ingestion; changes in behavior of school performance

Exam: Alert and oriented but appears ill, thin; fruity odor to breath, vital signs stable; mucous membranes slightly dry

    2. What are your differential diagnoses?
    DM Type 1, urinary tract infection, hypercalcemia, sepsis, acute abdomen, salicylate intoxication
    3. What diagnostic tests would you order?
    Blood glucose (by monitor) and urine dip for glucose, ketones, and signs of infection; urgent comprehensive metabolic panel
    4. Your lab results return with a glucose of 420 mg/dl (fasting) and urine dip positive for ketones and glucose. What is your next course of action?
    Consult with pediatrician or endocrinologist for hospitalization and management; educate parents on cause/course of illness and need for hospitalization.

CHAPTER 18

Case 1. A 7-year-old male child is brought in by his mother because he is having difficulty in school. The mother has brought a note from the school nurse and teacher. The child makes careless mistakes in schoolwork, is unable to sustain attention to tasks, does not listen, does not follow through on assignments, or finish schoolwork. This 7-year-old boy is constantly on the move, interrupts, cannot wait his turn, blurts out answers, and talks in class. He has lost his backpack twice and has difficulty remaining in his seat on the school bus.

PMH: Fracture left tibia at age 5 years due to bike accident, 7 stitches for laceration to forehead due to a fall from tree-climbing at age 6 years. No serious illnesses, no hospitalizations.

1. What additional history would you ask?

   Family history, prenatal history, developmental history, history of neurologic compromise or head trauma, behavioral history, academic history, history of ear infections, vision or hearing problems, any comorbid conditions like depression or anxiety. Any siblings or family members with ADHD, learning disabilities, or attending/attended special education programs. Onset of symptoms, duration, environmental influences or changes, stressors or precipitators. Ask about symptoms to determine inattentive, hyperactive, impulsivity per DSM-IV criteria. Explore parenting skills, discipline techniques, possibility of abuse or neglect.

2. What do you think is happening?

   Probable attention-deficit / hyperactivity disorder

3. What diagnostic tests would you offer?

   Blood tests are not routinely done. Sometimes a CBC, TSH, or serum lead may be done if there is anything in the history or physical to suggest these. ADHD rating scales may be used by the teacher and parents. Vision and hearing screening should be done to rule out deficits in these areas. ADHD is a clinical diagnosis made by history, clinical observation, and neuropsychological testing.

4. What is your treatment plan?

   Refer to a pediatric neurologist or psychiatrist for pharmacologic management. Psychostimulant medication has been helpful and the medication most frequently used is methylphenidate (Ritalin). Offer information, counseling, resources, and support to parents. Behavior modification programs and social skills training are frequently helpful. With parental consent, communicate with school officials and advocate for child's appropriate educational placement and accommodations as needed.

Case 2. An 18-year-old female, on break from her first semester at college, presents to you with her mother. The chief complaint is amenorrhea, fatigue, and weight loss. The mother blames the weight loss and fatigue on the poor quality of college food, dorm life, and being away from home. HPI: It is revealed that the patient is a dance major with daily dance classes at the university and evening dance classes at a private studio. She has always been a competitive student and graduated from high school with a grade point average of 4.0. During her senior year, she was the school social activities director, and participated in extracurricular activities and volunteer work. Although the patient is new to college life, she is already involved in dance performances, volunteer work, has joined the poetry club, and is co-editor of their publication.

1. What additional history would you ask?

   Onset of symptoms, weight history, dietary history with patterns of eating and caloric intake, identify any food rituals, binging, or purging. Menstrual history, age of menarche, and date of LMP, sexual history, exercise history, psychiatric history including history of eating disorders and previous treatments, family history of psychiatric or eating disorders, use of medication for weight control, history of substance abuse, history of abuse or neglect, perception of body. Identify presence of other physical symptoms such as bowel habits, cold hands or feet, fatigue, signs of sexual maturation, patterns of hair growth, skin changes or acne, temperature tolerance, ridges in fingernails, parotid hypertrophy, calluses on fingers, dental erosion. Determine medical history and recent illnesses.

Exam: BP is 110/70, respiratory rate 18 and regular, heart rate 80 and regular, skin is dry, weight just at the 30th percentile with low BMI, negative for syncope or orthostatic hypotension, negative for parotid enlargement, negative for oral lesions or dental caries, alert with intact cranial nerves, good muscle strength and coordination. Normal pubic hair development and small breasts. Fingernails dry and brittle, no ridges, skin over knuckles intact and normal.

2. What do you think is happening?

   Possible eating disorder—anorexia nervosa, restrictive type. Rule out medical disorders such as thyroid disease, diabetes, pregnancy, CNS lesion or malignancy, or a communicable disease such as acquired immunodeficiency.

3. What diagnostic tests would you offer?

   Start with CBC, chemistry panel with electrolytes and FBS, LH, FSH, HCG, thyroid panel (TSH, T3, T4), electrocardiogram. Other tests based on history and physical findings.

4. What is your treatment plan?

   Psychiatric referral or consultation with a specialist in eating disorders. Make sure patient is hydrated and in stable condition. Primary care provider may monitor medical status in collaboration with specialist.

Case 3. A 70-year-old male presents to you reporting several incidents of shortness of breath and a choking sensation, accompanied by dizziness, diaphoresis, feelings of doom and loss of control. These "spells" have occurred 4 times in the past 4 weeks and start without warning. He denies seizure disorder and has not experienced loss of consciousness. Two days ago he went to the hospital emergency room because he thought he was having a heart attack. He was told it was not a heart attack and to see his regular provider.

1. What additional history would you ask?

   Ask about onset, duration, and severity of symptoms and to what extent daily functioning is impaired. Identify any precipitating events or recent life changes. Obtain complete medication history, caffeine intake, alcohol or drug use, prescription, OTC medication, and alternative medication or treatments, including herbal supplements. Obtain complete past medical history, any current medical problems, psychiatric history, social history, and family medical and psychiatric history.

Exam: Patient appears calm, alert, oriented and concerned. Physical exam is unremarkable with normal vital signs.

2. What do you think is happening?
   Panic attacks.
3. What diagnostic tests would you offer?
   Diagnostic labs depend on physical findings. Consider chest x-ray and electrocardiogram due to symptoms and age; consider chemistry panel, TSH, and CBC to rule out other medical conditions; Hamilton Anxiety Scale, or similar rating tool.
4. What is your treatment plan?
   Referral for cognitive behavioral therapy. Pharmacologic treatment with SSRI. With the elderly, dose is half the usual starting dose and increased slowly.

Review Questions

1. A 6-month-old infant is brought to the clinic for a well-child visit. The developmental assessment should include evaluation of the infant's ability to:
   a. Pick up small objects with the thumb and forefinger
   b. Say "no-no" and "bye-bye"
   c. Sit up, with and without support
   d. Pull-up to a standing position

2. A 17-year-old male comes in for routine treatment of acne vulgaris. He has been using benzoyl peroxide facial scrubs with no improvement. Numerous open and closed comedones are seen on exam, as well as numerous papules and a few pustules. No cysts or scarring are noted. The preferred treatment regimen would be:
   a. Isotretinoin (Accutane) in the morning and minocycline hydrochloride (Minocin) 100 mg bid
   b. Erythromycin 1% gel (E-Mycin) gel in the morning and 0.025% tretinoin (Retin-A) cream at bedtime
   c. Tretinoin (Retin-A) 1% cream at bedtime
   d. Oral erythromycin 250 mg tid

3. A 21-year-old female is having a very severe asthma exacerbation. Which of these physical findings may be absent during an asthma attack?
   a. Tachypnea
   b. Wheezing
   c. Prolonged expiration
   d. Tachycardia

4. The differential diagnosis of gastroesophageal reflux (GERD) in an infant (>2 months old) would include all of the following except:
   a. Overfeeding
   b. Hirschsprung's disease
   c. Urinary tract infection
   d. Gastroenteritis

5. A 62-year-old nulliparous diabetic female presents with complaint of watery vaginal discharge without itching or irritation. You notice no discharge, erythema, or lesions on pelvic exam. Your initial work-up should include all except
   a. Microscopy with KOH for fungal elements and spores
   b. CA 125
   c. Pap smear and transvaginal ultrasound
   d. Microscopy for clue cells

6. You suspect that a 27-year-old woman with profuse, yellow vaginal discharge has trichomoniasis. Besides characteristic trichomonads on microscopy, what other findings would support your diagnosis?
   a. Clue cells and fishy odor
   b. Hyphae
   c. Pruritus and cervical motion tenderness
   d. Vaginal pH >4.5

7. An older patient is taking carbidopa-levodopa (Sinemet) for Parkinson's disease. He develops depression. Which of the following medications to treat depression would be contraindicated for this patient?
   a. Monoamine oxidase inhibitor (MAOI)
   b. Serotonin selective reuptake inhibitor (SSRI)
   c. Tricyclic antidepressant
   d. Lithium

8. The preferred medication regimen for treating newly diagnosed hypothyroidism in older clients who have heart disease is:
   a. 100 mg of propylthiouracil, followed by an increase in dosage every 2–3 weeks
   b. 150 mg of propylthiouracil, followed by an increase in dosage every 4–6 weeks
   c. 0.025 to 0.05 mg of levothyroxine sodium (Synthroid), followed by an increase in dosage every 4–6 weeks
   d. 0.1 mg of levothyroxine sodium (Synthroid), followed by an increase in dosage every 4–6 weeks

9. Joanne is planning to go for an interview for a job with a physician practice that has not hired NPs previously. Joanne is asked, "How can we bill for the services you provide?" Joanne should explain:
   a. In most states NPs can be primary care providers under managed care plans, so she will be reimbursed by managed care plans
   b. Medicaid is the only insurance plan that does not reimburse FNPs
   c. Medicare will reimburse for Joan's services at 85% of the customary physician rate
   d. Reimbursement is available from Medicare at the full physician rate even if the MD is not in the office

10. A mother brings her 2-year-old child in for a sick visit. The child's face looks as though it has been slapped. What is the most likely cause?
    a. High fever
    b. Varicella
    c. Fifth's disease
    d. Roseola

11. A 10-year-old boy complains of a sore throat, fever, and fatigue for 2 days. Findings include pharyngitis, anterior cervical adenopathy, and an oral temperature of 101.6° F (38.6° C). Which of the following tests should be ordered at this time?
    a. Antistreptolysin O titer
    b. Cytomegalovirus titer
    c. Culture for streptococcal infection
    d. Monospot and complete blood count

12. A client who is starting warfarin sodium (Coumadin) therapy should be counseled to avoid:
    a. Alcohol, salicylates, and large amounts of green leafy vegetables
    b. Alcohol, antacids, and large amounts of yellow vegetables
    c. Anything containing acetaminophen
    d. Participation in contact sports

13. Initial symptoms of acute glomerulonephritis most commonly seen by the clinician include:
    a. Generalized edema and anorexia
    b. Periorbital edema and hematuria
    c. Fever and hypotension
    d. Flank pain and pyuria

14. A 22-year-old male with history of undescended testicles presents for his first adult health maintenance examination. You will make all of these recommendations except:
    a. Self-testicular exam and annual clinical exam to detect testicular cancer
    b. DRE and PSA level every 3–5 years for early detection of prostate cancer
    c. Use of condoms if sexually active to prevent unintended pregnancy and infection with a sexually transmitted infection
    d. BP check every 2 years to detect hypertension

15. An overweight adolescent boy complains of pain in his hip that radiates to the medial aspect of his knee He denies trauma and has not had a fever. You note upon exam that he is walking with a limp. The most likely diagnosis is:
    a. Transient toxic synovitis
    b. Slipped capital femoral epiphysis
    c. Avulsion fracture of the tibial tuberosity
    d. Legg-Calve Perthes

16. Factors that may precipitate sickle cell crisis include which of the following?
    a. Increased environmental humidity
    b. Overhydration
    c. Exposure to extreme cold or heat
    d. Lack of activity and exertion

17. In addition to features of depression, bipolar disorder is characterized by:
    a. Excessive worry and feelings of apprehension
    b. Refusal to maintain normal body weight due to intense fear of gaining weight
    c. Grandiose or delusional thinking
    d. Increased sleep

18. In what Tanners stage is a 10-year-old female with pubic hair mainly around the labia and breast budding?
    a. Stage 1
    b. Stage 2
    c. Stage 3
    d. Stage 4

19. A mother reports that her 14-year-old child has developed generalized itching and hives after being stung by a bee. Further assessment for more serious signs indicating the need for emergency intervention would be:
    a. Fluid oozing from lesions
    b. Pain, erythema, and honey-colored crusting of lesions
    c. Angioedema, shortness of breath, and wheezing
    d. Tachycardia

20. A 68-year-old man with chronic obstructive pulmonary disease (COPD) has continuous symptoms. Which medications should be considered for initial treatment?
    a. Steroids
    b. Theophylline
    c. Antibiotics
    d. An anticholinergic

21. A 1-year-old presents for a well-child exam and you notice that the child has fallen off the growth curve for height and weight; otherwise, the P.E. is normal. You begin a work-up for FTT. What diagnostic tests would you initially order?
    a. CBC, CT of abdomen
    b. CBC, U/A, electrolytes
    c. CBC, TSH, abdominal flat plate
    d. CBC, HIV, U/A

22. Latoya, 22, presents for her annual Pap smear and mentions that she has had a yellowish, irritating vaginal discharge with dysuria and dyspareunia for 7–10 days. If she is a reliable patient, what is generally recommended in regards to her Pap smear when an infection is present?
    a. Perform the Pap smear today knowing that you will be able to diagnose the vaginal problem and obtain accurate cervical cytology at the same time
    b. Assess for and treat likely infectious process and defer Pap smear for 3–6 months
    c. Obtain Thin Prep sample instead of conventional Pap smear
    d. Obtain Pap smear and cultures for sexually transmitted infections

23. A patient with a positive DNA probe test for chlamydia has no medication allergies, is on no medications, and had an LMP 3 weeks ago. You will treat her with:
    a. Azithromycin 1 g po in a single dose
    b. Bactrim DS bid for 14 days
    c. Defer treatment until pregnancy can be ruled out
    d. Metronidazole gel 0.75% intravaginally bid for 5 days

24. How often should blood levels of anticonvulsant medications be routinely checked on a patient with a clinically controlled seizure disorder?
    a. Every 3 months
    b. Annually
    c. When adjusting dosage and when there has been a change in seizure frequency
    d. If neurological sequelae appear, such as intention, facial tics, or slurred speech

25. Which of the following statements indicates a client's understanding of what should be done to care for the client's diabetes mellitus when he or she is ill?
    a. "I should take my usual dose of insulin."
    b. "I should avoid eating sweets, especially when I'm sick."
    c. "I should check for ketones if my blood sugar is over 150."
    d. "I should alter my regular insulin but take my usual NPH insulin."

26. Which of the following statements about Duvall's theory of the stages in family development is true?
    a. The stages cannot overlap.
    b. The stages are based on the age and school placement of the firstborn child.
    c. There are four stages.
    d. Marriage is strongest during the fourth stage.

27. The nurse practitioner has just diagnosed a 27-year-old with Lyme disease. What is the appropriate management?
    a. Bactrim 400 mg bid for 14–21 days
    b. Amoxicillin 100 mg tid for 10 days
    c. Doxycycline 100 mg bid for 14–21 days
    d. Keflex 500 mg qid for 14 days

28. Acute otitis media can be distinguished from otitis media with effusion by:
    a. Hearing loss with ear popping and crackling
    b. Otalgia and decreased mobility of tympanic membrane
    c. Temporomandibular joint pain
    d. Eustachian tube obstruction

29. A new 58-year-old patient has a blood pressure reading of 162/90 mm Hg. The nurse practitioner should:
    a. Tell the patient she has hypertension and begin treatment today
    b. Have the client return for a total of three successive blood pressure checks and discuss therapeutic lifestyle changes.
    c. Initiate treatment with 25 mg of hydrochlorothiazide daily
    d. Plan to recheck the client in 3 months.

30. A patient complains of burning sensation during urination. The patient's history reveals that she has recently become sexually active and is on oral contraceptives. A urine dipstick reveals leukocyte esterase and nitrite. The best course of action would be to:
    a. Place the client on amoxicillin 250 mg 4 times a day for 14 days.
    b. Place the client on nitrofurantoin (Macrodantin) 100 mg 4 times a day for 5 days
    c. Perform a pelvic exam and obtain cultures to rule out vaginitis and cervicitis; then place the client on trimethoprim-sulfamethoxazole (Bactrim DS) 160/800 mg every 12 hours for 3 days
    d. Obtain a urine culture result prior to placing on antibiotic therapy

31. Your evaluation of a 6-year-old male with an asymptomatic, firm, pear-shaped sac behind the testicle would include:
    a. Fluid aspiration for culture and sensitivity
    b. Transillumination
    c. Doppler ultrasound
    d. If on right side, immediate referral

32. You examine a patient you suspect has a meniscus injury. To assess for this injury, you examine the patient supine and the knee fully flexed. The tibia is externally rotated and mild varus or valgus stress is placed on the knee. This test is called:
    a. Lachman's test
    b. McMurray's
    c. Anterior drawer
    d. Thompson test

33. P.I. presents to clinic requesting a pregnancy test. The test is positive. Besides referral for obstetrical care, what dietary supplements might you recommend at this time?
    a. None, the patient is healthy and does not need supplements
    b. Prenatal vitamin with folic acid
    c. Vitamin C
    d. Vitamin E

34. A 12-year-old boy is brought in by his parents for increasing behavior problems in school and in the neighborhood. Which of the following descriptions would prompt your referral for a possible conduct disorder?
    a. Disregards the rights of others
    b. Shows remorse for misconduct
    c. Easily distracted, forgetful, does not complete tasks
    d. Mood swings, agitation, restlessness

35. A 22-year-old female presents to your office with a complaint of sudden onset of shortness of breath. Her history reveals she is sexually active and takes oral contraceptives. She has just returned from a trip to Australia and tells you she slept and watched movies for the whole 22-hour flight. You are immediately concerned that this patient may have:
    a. Hepatitis
    b. Pulmonry embolis
    c. Migrane headaches
    d. Urinary tract infection

36. You diagnosed pityriasis rosea in a 28-year-old male who came to you presenting with a maculopapular scaling rash for 2 days. Upon history, he revealed that he had a large single bright red patch that preceded this rash eruption by about 2 weeks. Where would the location of the current rash most likely present and what is the origin?
    a. Across the entire body; is metabolic in origin
    b. Over the cheeks and chin; most likely contact in origin
    c. Across the trunk; most likely infectious in origin
    d. Across the entire body; most likely infectious in origin

37. You order a PPD on a 7-year-old who has a parent with suspected TB. The PPD result is 7 mm in duration. Your treatment plan is:
    a. Counsel family about TB and repeat PPD in 3 months
    b. Order a chest x-ray (CXR) and begin medication if CXR is suggestive of pulmonary disease
    c. Order a chest x-ray (CXR) and refer patient to begin treatment with INH
    d. Begin INH

38. A 70-year-old man presents with anemia, recent weight loss, and heme positive stools. He has no GI complaints. The diagnosis until proven otherwise is:
    a. Ulcerative colitis
    b. Peptic ulcer disease
    c. Hemorrhoids
    d. Colon cancer

39. All of the following are symptoms of premenstrual syndrome EXCEPT:
    a. Difficulty concentrating
    b. Psychotic episodes
    c. Fatigue, lethargic
    d. Irritability

40. You are working in a college health clinic that offers free HIV testing. A student has had unprotected intercourse with a new partner. You advise:
    a. Chlamydia screening, gonorrhea testing, and syphilis prophylaxis
    b. Review history, chlamydia screening, HIV testing, provide hepatitis B vaccination
    c. Use of condoms for 3 months, then HIV testing
    d. Qualitative viral RNA level to assess for HIV

41. A 12-year-old male with a recent history of otitis media presents with 1 day of acute right facial weakness, including flattening of the forehead furrows, inability to completely close the ipsilateral eye, flattening of the nasolabial fold, and drooping of the mouth. What is the most likely diagnosis?
    a. Bell's palsy
    b. Acoustic neuroma
    c. Recurrence of otitis
    d. Trigeminal palsy

42. The family nurse practitioner sees an active 11-year-old girl who has type I diabetes. The child plays softball and basketball, and swims on the school team. The nurse practitioner tells the child and her mother that:
    a. Insulin dosing and eating patterns should not be changed during periods of frequent exercise
    b. Nocturnal hypoglycemia may occur on significantly active
    c. Type I diabetic patients should avoid strenuous physical activity
    d. Nocturnal hyperglycemia may occur on weekends

43. The nurse practitioner should:
    a. Rely on tradition, intuition, and personal preference to deal with clinical problems
    b. Accept and use clinical practice guidelines regardless of the source of the recommendations
    c. Understand that cultural influences rarely influence health behaviors
    d. Use evidence-based practices and critically evaluate and participate in outcome studies

44. A 34-year-old male presents for your care with what appears to be obvious oral candidiasis. You treat him with nystatin oral suspension 500,000 units swish and swallow 3–5 times/day for 10 days. His infection clears, but he returns with the same symptoms in 1 month. Which of the following would NOT be part of your evaluation for this patient?
    a. Diabetes mellitus
    b. HIV infection
    c. Malnutrition or substance abuse
    d. Multiple sclerosis

45. Which of the following helps you differentiate croup from bronchiolitis?
    a. Age
    b. Presence of fever
    c. Tachypnea
    d. Wheezing

46. During a clinic visit, a woman known to rely on advertising claims for a wide variety of alternative therapies tells the nurse practitioner that her husband is limiting his daily fluid intake to one glass of liquid in order to keep him from passing blood in his urine. Which of the following responses by the nurse practitioner would be most appropriate?
    a. "Your husband can become dehydrated with small amounts of fluid."
    b. "Your husband needs to be seen for a kidney evaluation as soon as possible."
    c. "Tell me how you think this is helping your husband."
    d. No response is necessary as the nurse practitioner does not see the woman's husband

47. Initial treatment for lateral epicondylitis includes all of the following except:
    a. NSAIDs
    b. Tennis elbow band
    c. Cortisone injection
    d. Physical therapy

48. In a female with vitamin B12 deficiency, you would expect which laboratory profile?
    a. Hgb <36, MCV < 80
    b. Hgb <36, MCV >100
    c. CBC normal between episodes of hemolysis
    d. Decreased hgb and hct, normal MCV

49. A sexually active patient with multiple partners presents with fever, adenopathy, rash, myalgias, headache, pharyngitis, and hepatosplenomegaly. You suspect:
    a. Syphilis
    b. Primary herpes simplex, type 1 infection
    c. Disseminated gonorrhea
    d. Primary HIV infection

50. A G1 P1 mother of a 7-day-old presents with right breast pain and fever since yesterday night. She is breastfeeding but uses 2–3 ounces of formula at one to two nighttime feedings. On exam you note that her nipples have a small central fissures and the right breast has some redness in the lower outer quadrant. She has no allergies and her temperature is 100.5° F. The infant is gaining adequate weight. Which of the following statements is false?
    a. When indicated, one possible antibiotic choice is dicloxacillin (Dycill 500 mg po qid) for at least 10 days.
    b. Breastfeeding should be continued and encouraged more frequently and exclusively irrespective of the usual antibiotic therapy
    c. Using formula to replace a feeding is a possible etiology of mastitis
    d. Sore nipples with skin breakdown are normal and no improvement of the latch is necessary

Answers to the Review Questions

1. A 6-month-old infant is brought to the clinic for a well-child visit. The developmental assessment should include evaluation of the infant's ability to:
   a. Incorrect. Pincer grasp occurs at about 9 months
   b. Incorrect. Occurs between 9 and 12 months
   c. Correct. Sit up, with and without support
   d. Incorrect. Occurs between 8 and 12 months

2. A 17-year-old male comes in for routine treatment of acne vulgaris. He has been using benzoyl peroxide facial scrubs with no improvement. Numerous open and closed comedones are seen on exam, as well as numerous papules and a few pustules. No cysts or scarring are noted. The preferred treatment regimen would be:
   a. Incorrect. Accutane is used for cystic acne only
   b. Correct. Use of topical antibiotic due to pustules and tretinoin as an effective comedolytic
   c. Incorrect. This dose of tretinoin is too high; and topical antibiotic also should be tried, due to pustules.
   d. Incorrect. Topical agents should be tried first.

3. A 21-year-old female is having a very severe asthma exacerbation. Which of these physical findings may be absent during an asthma attack?
   a. Incorrect. Tachypnea is always present in severe asthma
   b. Correct. Wheezing absent when there is severe constriction of the bronchial tree
   c. Incorrect. Prolonged expiration is always present
   d. Incorrect. Tachycardia always present

4. The differential diagnosis of gastroesophageal reflux (GERD) in an infant (>2 months old) would include all of the following except:
   a. Incorrect. Can present similar to GERD in infants
   b. Correct. Hirschsprung's disease presents with constipation and abdominal distention rather than vomiting or spitting up
   c. Incorrect. Can present similar to GERD in infants
   d. Incorrect. Can present similar to GERD in infants

5. A 62-year-old nulliparous diabetic female presents with complaint of watery vaginal discharge without itching or irritation. You notice no discharge, erythema, or lesions on pelvic exam. Your initial work-up should include all except
   a. Incorrect. Although this may be part of the work-up, the patient does not have classic signs of yeast infection; greater importance should be placed on ruling out endometrial cancer.
   b. Incorrect. This is a marker for ovarian cancer, which does not present with watery vaginal discharge.
   c. Correct. Pap smear may show AGCUS and ultrasound may show increased endometrial stripe, requiring referral for further endometrial cancer work-up.
   d. Incorrect. Although this may be part of total work-up, bacterial vaginosis does not need to be treated unless symptomatic; greater importance should be placed on ruling out endometrial cancer.

6. You suspect that a 27-year-old woman with profuse, yellow vaginal discharge has trichomoniasis. Besides characteristic trichomonads on microscopy, what other findings would support your diagnosis?
   a. Incorrect. These are characteristic of bacterial vaginosis.
   b. Incorrect. These are found on microscopy in candidiasis.
   c. Incorrect. Pruritus may be present, but cervical motion tenderness is significant for PID.
   d. Correct.

7. An older patient is taking carbidopa-levodopa (Sinemet) for Parkinson's disease. He develops depression. Which of the following medications to treat depression would be contraindicated for this patient?
   a. Correct. Nonspecific MAO inhibitors are contraindicated in combination with levodopa (this does not include selegiline).
   b. Incorrect. This would be a good choice for treatment.
   c. Incorrect. These are not contraindicated with levodopa.
   d. Incorrect. This is not contraindicated with levodopa and would only be used to treat bipolar depression.

8. The preferred medication regimen for treating newly diagnosed hypothyroidism in older clients who have heart disease is:
   a. Incorrect. Propylthiouracil is used in the treatment of hyperthyroidism.
   b. Incorrect. Propylthiouracil is used in the treatment of hyperthyroidism.
   c. Correct. Lower starting dosage to avoid adverse effect of angina in a patient who has preexisting CAD.
   d. Incorrect. Elderly patients with CAD require lower starting dosage.

9. Joanne is planning to go for an interview for a job with a physician practice that has not hired NPs previously. Joanne is asked, "How can we bill for the services you provide?" Joanne should explain:
   a. Incorrect. This is not the case in most states, and is one of the issues of great concern to FNPs.
   b. Incorrect. Medicaid does reimburse FNPs, however, it is dependent on state interpretation.
   c. **Correct. This is true provided that the FNP has her own Medicare provider number.**
   d. Incorrect. If the physician is not in the office, the NP must bill under her own provider number at 85% of the physician rate.

10. A mother brings her 2-year-old child in for a sick visit. The child's face looks as though it has been slapped. What is the most likely cause?
   a. Incorrect. It is possible, but not characteristic and taking the child's temperature can quickly rule it out.
   b. Incorrect. Does not cause rash to the cheeks.
   c. **Correct. Slapped cheek appearance with a sick appearing child is likely to be Fifth's disease.**
   d. Incorrect. Rash is generalized, not characteristic of cheeks.

11. A 10-year-old boy complains of a sore throat, fever, and fatigue for 2 days. Findings include pharyngitis, anterior cervical adenopathy, and an oral temperature of 101.6° F (38.6° C). Which of the following tests should be ordered at this time?
   a. Incorrect. Used to determine previous Streptococcal infection.
   b. Incorrect. Pharyngitis is not prominent feature of CMV.
   c. **Correct. Used instead of or in combination with quick strep test.**
   d. Incorrect. Mononucleosis is less likely in a 10-year-old.

12. A client who is starting warfarin sodium (Coumadin) therapy should be counseled to avoid:
   a. **Correct. Due to increased risk of GI bleed and the large amounts of Vitamin K in the food.**
   b. Incorrect. Although antacids decrease INR, they do not need to be avoided, but INR needs to be monitored.
   c. Incorrect. Acetaminophen is potentiated by protein bound drugs.
   d. Incorrect. Not contraindicated in the controlled patient.

13. Initial symptoms of acute glomerulonephritis most commonly seen by the clinician include:
   a. Incorrect. These are symptoms of chronic renal failure.
   b. **Correct. Edema and gross hematuria are the major symptoms of post-streptococcal glomerulonephritis.**
   c. Incorrect. These are symptoms of sepsis.
   d. Incorrect. These are symptoms of pyelonephritis.

14. A 22-year-old male with history of undescended testicles presents for his first adult health maintenance examination. You will make all of these recommendations except:
    a. Incorrect. This is the recommended screening, especially in male with history of undescended testicle (see Testicular Cancer, Prevention and Screening).
    b. **Correct. This is not recommended at age 22 (see Prostate Cancer, Prevention and Screening).**
    c. Incorrect. This would be recommended since cryptorchid male may still be fertile and capable of contracting STD (see Cryptorchidism).
    d. Incorrect. This is appropriate screening (see Chapter 3, Adult Screening Recommendations).

15. An overweight adolescent boy complains of pain in his hip that radiates to the medial aspect of his knee. He denies trauma and has not had a fever. You note upon exam that he is walking with a limp. The most likely diagnosis is:
    a. Incorrect. Transient toxic synovitis occurs most commonly in children under 10 and presents with hip pain.
    b. **Correct. Slipped capital femoral epiphysis is most common in adolescents who are obese. It usually presents with a limp and knee pain referred from the hip.**
    c. Incorrect. Avulsion of the tibial tubercle, or Osgood Schlatter disease, occurs commonly in adolescents who are physically active. Pain occurs below the knee at the tibial tubercle.
    d. Incorrect. Leg-Calve Perthes disease usually occurs in younger children and is not associated with obesity. It does present with a limp and can present with referred knee pain.

16. Factors that may precipitate sickle cell crisis include which of the following?
    a. Incorrect. Humidity has no effect.
    b. Incorrect. Dehydration may cause crisis.
    c. **Correct. This is a risk factor for crisis.**
    d. Incorrect. Overexertion may cause crisis.

17. In addition to features of depression, bipolar disorder is characterized by:
    a. Incorrect. These are features of anxiety disorder.
    b. Incorrect. This is characteristic of anorexia nervosa.
    c. **Correct. This is part of the diagnostic description for bipolar disorder.**
    d. Incorrect. Bipolar disorder is characterized by decreased need for sleep.

18. In what Tanners stage is a 10-year-old female with pubic hair mainly around the labia and breast budding?
    a. Incorrect. There are no puberty changes during stage 1.
    b. **Correct.**
    c. Incorrect. This stage involves darker, curlier hair with breast and areola enlargement.
    d. Incorrect. This stage involves adult-like pubic hair with areola and papilla form second breast mound.

19. A mother reports that her 14-year-old child has developed generalized itching and hives after being stung by a bee. Further assessment for more serious signs indicating the need for emergency intervention would be:

    a. Incorrect. Fluid oozing is a nonspecific sign.

    b. Incorrect. Describes infection

    c. Correct. These are signs of anaphylaxis.

    d. Incorrect. Tachycardia is nonspecific, could be from previous exercise or anxiety.

20. A 68-year-old man with chronic obstructive pulmonary disease (COPD) has continuous symptoms. Which medications should be considered for initial treatment?

    a. Incorrect. Used after all other drugs have failed.

    b. Incorrect. Used after anticholinergic and beta 2 agonist have failed.

    c. Incorrect. Only used in acute exacerbation.

    d. Correct. This drug is in line with national guidelines.

21. A 1-year-old presents for a well-child exam and you notice that the child has fallen off the growth curve for height and weight; otherwise, the P.E. is normal. You begin a work-up for FTT. What diagnostic tests would you initially order?

    a. Incorrect. Would only be done if history and physical exam revealed abnormality.

    b. Correct.

    c. Incorrect. Would be done if history and physical exam revealed abnormalities.

    d. Incorrect. HIV test done only if history and physical exam raise suspicion for HIV disease.

22. Latoya, 22, presents for her annual Pap smear and mentions that she has had a yellowish, irritating vaginal discharge with dysuria and dyspareunia for 7–10 days. If she is a reliable patient, what is generally recommended in regards to her Pap smear when an infection is present?

    a. Incorrect. Pap smear may be false positive due to infectious processes; also does not accurately diagnose all possible infections.

    b. Correct. Pap smear more likely to be accurate after inflammatory process has cleared.

    c. Incorrect. Inflammatory changes of cells caused by infectious process may still cause false positive Pap smear.

    d. Incorrect. It is not cost effective since the Pap smear will have to be repeated in 3–6 months.

23. A patient with a positive DNA probe test for chlamydia has no medication allergies, is on no medications, and her had an LMP 3 weeks ago. You will treat her with:

    a. Correct. This is first line treatment and ensures compliance.

    b. Incorrect. Drug choice and dose for chlamydia

    c. Incorrect. It is not necessary to defer treatment, since some drugs are safe in pregnancy.

    d. Incorrect. This is treatment for bacterial vaginosis.

24. How often should blood levels of anticonvulsant medications be routinely checked on a patient with a clinically controlled seizure disorder?
   a. Incorrect. Anticonvulsant level unnecessary if clinically controlled, although primary care visit and LFT levels (if on valproic acid) may be indicated.
   b. Incorrect. There is not set interval for anticonvulsant levels in clinically controlled seizure disorder; may want to try to discontinue medication if seizure-free for 2 years.
   c. Correct.
   d. Incorrect. These are not signs of medication problems or increased seizures.

25. Which of the following statements indicates a client's understanding of what should be done to care for the client's diabetes mellitus when the he or she is ill?
   a. Correct.
   b. Incorrect. Diabetics should always limit the sweets they are eating.
   c. Incorrect. Ketones should be checked if the blood sugar is over 300.
   d. Incorrect. Insulin should be taken regularly when ill, alterations are based upon self glucose monitoring.

26. Which of the following statements about Duvall's theory of the stages in family development is true?
   a. Incorrect. They can overlap.
   b. Correct.
   c. Incorrect. There are eight stages.
   d. Incorrect. The theory does not explain this.

27. The nurse practitioner has just diagnosed a 27-year-old with Lyme disease. What is the appropriate management?
   a. Incorrect. Not the drug of choice
   b. Incorrect. Dosage and length of treatment inappropriate
   c. Correct.
   d. Incorrect. Not the drug of choice

28. Acute otitis media can be distinguished from otitis media with effusion by:
   a. Incorrect. Occurs with otitis media with effusion, not acute otitis media.
   b. Correct.
   c. Incorrect. Not a prominent feature of either.
   d. Incorrect. Occurs with otitis media with effusion, not acute otitis media.

29. A new 58-year-old patient has a blood pressure reading of 162/90 mm Hg. The nurse practitioner should:
   a. Incorrect. Need three elevated B/P readings at separate visits to confirm hypertension.
   b. Correct. Exercise and reducing sodium and changing diet may help lower the blood pressure.
   c. Incorrect. This would be a good first choice after you have taken the 3 B/Ps and they are all elevated.
   d. Incorrect. This is too long to wait to reassess.

30. A patient complains of burning sensation during urination. The patient's history reveals that she has recently become sexually active and is on oral contraceptives. A urine dipstick reveals leukocyte esterase and nitrite. The best course of action would be to:
    a. Incorrect. The beta lactam class of medication is not as effective as other antibiotics for UTI; length of treatment is longer than needed.
    b. Incorrect. This does not offer the patient the most effective therapy for the shortest period.
    c. **Correct. Genital infection may present with dysuria, so needs to be ruled out in newly sexually active client. Short course therapy with the above antibiotic or a fluoroquinolone has been shown to be safe and effective against the organisms most often responsible for uncomplicated UTI (e.g., E. coli.)**
    d. Incorrect. History and symptom complex indicate high likelihood of UTI. No need to obtain culture before you begin treatment.

31. Your evaluation of a 6-year-old male with an asymptomatic, firm, pear-shaped sac behind the testicle would include:
    a. Incorrect. Not necessary if infection is not suspected
    b. **Correct. Should be red glow if hydrocele with shadow of testicle; smaller mass if spermatocele**
    c. Incorrect. Not done unless diagnosis is in question
    d. Incorrect. Varicocele requires referral if on right side because it is associated with right spermatic vein obstruction and retroperitoneal neoplasm

32. You examine a patient you suspect has a meniscus injury. To assess for this injury, you examine the patient supine and the knee fully flexed. The tibia is externally rotated and mild varus or valgus stress is placed on the knee. This test is called:
    a. Incorrect. The Lachman test is used to check for injury to the anterior cruciate ligament.
    b. **Correct. The McMurray test is used to check for injury to the meniscus. The exam is as described.**
    c. Incorrect. The anterior drawer test checks for injury to the anterior cruciate ligament.
    d. Incorrect. The Thompson test is assess for Achilles tendon injury or rupture.

33. P.I. presents to clinic requesting a pregnancy test. The test is positive. Besides referral for obstetrical care, what dietary supplements might you recommend at this time?
    a. Incorrect. Should begin vitamin supplementation as early in pregnancy as possible, even during period of time while trying to conceive.
    b. **Correct. Begin as early as possible during pregnancy; must have minimum of 400 mg of folic acid to help prevent neural tube defects.**
    c. Incorrect. Not a necessary supplement, probably sufficient intake in diet.
    d. Incorrect. Not a necessary supplement, probably sufficient intake in diet.

34. A 12-year-old boy is brought in by his parents for increasing behavior problems in school and in the neighborhood. Which of the following descriptions would prompt your referral for a possible conduct disorder?
    a. **Correct. This is a characteristic of conduct disorder.**
    b. Incorrect. Lack of remorse is a characteristic of conduct disorder.
    c. Incorrect. These are characteristics of ADHD.
    d. Incorrect. These may be seen with substance abuse.

35. A 22-year-old female presents to your office with a complaint of sudden onset of shortness of breath. Her history reveals she is sexually active and takes oral contraceptives. She has just returned from a trip to Australia and tells you she slept and watched movies for the whole 22-hour flight. You are immediately concerned that this patient may have:
    a. Incorrect. There are no data suggesting this.
    b. Correct. Patients on oral contraceptives with long periods of sitting such as airplane trips are at high risk for DVT and pulmonary embolism.
    c. Incorrect. There is no indication of migraine in the history.
    d. Incorrect. There is no indication of urinary symptoms or fever.

36. You diagnosed pityriasis rosea in a 28-year-old male who came to you presenting with a maculopapular scaling rash for 2 days. Upon history, he revealed that he had a large single bright red patch that preceded this rash eruption by about 2 weeks. Where would the location of the current rash most likely present and what is the origin?
    a. Incorrect. Neither option is correct.
    b. Incorrect. Usually across trunk; it is not contact in origin.
    c. Correct. Pityriasis rosea is defined as a maculopapular scaling condition across the trunk that is most likely infectious in origin. Unknown etiology, but suspected viral infectious agent.
    d. Incorrect. It is not across the entire body.

37. You order a PPD on a 7-year-old who has a parent with suspected TB. The PPD result is 7 mm in duration. Your treatment plan is:
    a. Incorrect. The PPD is considered positive in this high risk situation, so treatment is indicated.
    a. Incorrect. Preventative medication would be necessary even if the chest x-ray did not show active disease.
    b. Correct. Since child is a close contact of someone who may have TB, induration >5 is considered positive PPD.
    c. Incorrect. Chest x-ray is also indicated.

38. A 70-year-old man presents with anemia, recent weight loss, and heme positive stools. He has no GI complaints. The diagnosis until proven otherwise is:
    a. Incorrect. Would present with more complaints such as abdominal pain and bloody diarrhea.
    b. Incorrect. Would present with epigastric pain.
    c. Incorrect. Usually presents with rectal pain or palpable mass.
    d. Correct. Often presents in elderly in late stage with only anemia, bowel changes, heme positive stools, and possible weight loss.

39. All of the following are symptoms of premenstrual syndrome EXCEPT:
    a. Incorrect. This is a symptom of PMS.
    b. Correct. Psychotic episodes are not part of PMS.
    c. Incorrect. This is a symptom of PMS.
    d. Incorrect. This is a symptom of PMS.

40. You are working in a college health clinic that offers free HIV testing. A student has had unprotected intercourse with a new partner. You advise:
   a. Incorrect. See General Approach section.
   b. Correct. This woman is considered high risk because of new partner.
   c. Incorrect. Earlier HIV testing should be done and other STIs should be ruled out.
   d. Incorrect. See HIV Diagnostic Studies section.

41. A 12-year-old male with a recent history of otitis media presents with 1 day of acute right facial weakness, including flattening of the forehead furrows, inability to completely close the ipsilateral eye, flattening of the nasolabial fold, and drooping of the mouth. What is the most likely diagnosis?
   a. Correct. Bell's palsy affects the motor branch of the facial nerve, altering facial movements.
   b. Incorrect. Acoustic neuroma is a tumor of the 8th cranial nerve, the acoustic nerve.
   c. Incorrect. Otitis media does not affect the cranial nerves.
   d. Incorrect. Trigeminal palsy would affect temporal and masseter muscle function (i.e., jaw clenching and lateral movement of the jaw).

42. The family nurse practitioner sees an active 11-year-old girl who has type I diabetes. The child plays softball and basketball, and swims on the school team. The nurse practitioner tells the child and her mother that:
   a. Incorrect. Exercise requires additional energy; diet and insulin doses should be adjusted accordingly.
   b. Correct.
   c. Incorrect. Exercise is healthy and insulin doses should be adjusted appropriately.
   d. Incorrect. Nocturnal hypoglycemia may occur on days the patient is very active.

43. The nurse practitioner should:
   a. Incorrect. The NP should use scientific resources.
   b. Incorrect. The NP should use reliable sources for guidelines.
   c. Incorrect. Culture influences health behaviors.
   d. Correct.

44. A 34-year-old male presents for your care with what appears to be obvious oral candidiasis. You treat him with nystatin oral suspension 500,000 units swish and swallow 3–5 times/day for 10 days. His infection clears, but he returns with the same symptoms in 1 month. Which of the following would NOT be part of your evaluation for this patient?
   a. Incorrect. Diabetes is a risk factor for recurrent oral candidiasis.
   b. Incorrect. HIV infection is a risk factor for recurrent oral candidiasis.
   c. Incorrect. Poor nutrition or substance abuse can lead to decreased immunity and oral candidiasis.
   d. Correct. Multiple sclerosis is not a risk factor for oral candidiasis.

45. Which of the following helps you differentiate croup from bronchiolitis?
   a. **Correct. Croup affects children 3 months to 5 years; bronchiolitis is a disease of infants under 2 years, with peak incidence at 3–6 months.**
   b. Incorrect. Both have little or no fever.
   c. Incorrect. Both cause tachypnea.
   d. Incorrect. Both cause wheezing.

46. During a clinic visit, a woman known to rely on advertising claims for a wide variety of alternative therapies tells the nurse practitioner that her husband is limiting his daily fluid intake to one glass of liquid in order to keep him from passing blood in his urine. Which of the following responses by the nurse practitioner would be most appropriate?
   a. Incorrect. This approach may not be effective because it may be perceived as attacking the woman's beliefs.
   b. Incorrect. This approach may not be effective because it may be perceived as attacking the woman's beliefs.
   c. **Correct. Validates that you understand what she believes but need to understand more why this makes sense to her. Opens communication that may lead to a therapeutic intervention.**
   d. Incorrect. Does not allow for any intervention for a potentially serious problem and does not address concerns about the woman's healthcare decisions.

47. Initial treatment for lateral epicondylitis includes all of the following except:
   a. Incorrect. The initial treatment includes using NSAIDS to reduce the pain and inflammation.
   b. Incorrect. The initial treatment includes the use of a tennis elbow band to decrease the traction at the insertion of the tendon into the epicondyle.
   c. **Correct. The initial treatment does not include using a cortisone injection in the area. This is considered a second line treatment.**
   d. Incorrect. The initial treatment for epicondylitis may include physical therapy.

48. In a female with vitamin B12 deficiency, you would expect which laboratory profile?
   a. Incorrect. This is a microcytic anemia, such as thalassemia.
   b. **Correct. This is a macrocytic anemia, as in B12 deficiency.**
   c. Incorrect. This is true with G6PD deficiency.
   d. Incorrect. This is a normocytic anemia, as in anemia of chronic disease.

49. A sexually active patient with multiple partners presents with fever, adenopathy, rash, myalgias, headache, pharyngitis, and hepatosplenomegaly. You suspect:
   a. Incorrect. Hepatosplenomegaly and pharyngitis are not seen in syphilis.
   b. Incorrect. Hepatosplenomegaly is not seen in HSV infection.
   c. Incorrect. Hepatosplenomegaly is not seen in gonorrhea.
   d. **Correct. See HIV section.**

50. A G1 P1 mother of a 7-day-old presents with right breast pain and fever since yesterday night. She is breastfeeding but uses 2–3 ounces of formula at one to two nighttime feedings. On exam you note that her nipples have a small central fissures and the right breast has some redness in the lower outer quadrant. She has no allergies and her temperature is 100.5° F. The infant is gaining adequate weight. Which of the following statements is false?

   a. Incorrect. This antibiotic regimen is used only when mother is toxic.

   b. Correct. Breastfeeding helps increase antibiotic dissemination.

   c. Incorrect. No relationship.

   d. Incorrect. This is not normal.

Index

About the Authors

Elizabeth Blunt, PhD, MSN, FNP-BC, is the Coordinator of Nurse Practitioner programs at Villanova University. She is certified as both a Family Nurse Practitioner and an Adult Nurse Practitioner. Her practice is primarily emergency and trauma care, and she has held positions as a staff nurse, trauma program administrator, nurse manager, and director of nursing. She is active in both community and professional groups, and has multiple publications to her credit.

Shirlee Drayton-Brooks, PhD, FNP-BC, APRN-BC, is currently an Associate Professor of Nursing and the Director of the Family Nurse Practitioner Program at Widener University, School of Nursing. She received her BSN in 1977 from Temple University, MSN in 1983 in Adult Health from the University of Pennsylvania, and PhD in 1993 in organization change, group dynamics, and curriculum design from Temple University. In 1997, Dr. Drayton-Brooks received a post-master's certificate as a family nurse practitioner from Widener University. Dr. Drayton-Brooks has over 30 years' experience in nursing practice leadership and education. In addition to her Widener University duties, Dr. Drayton-Brooks serves as a part-time family–board certified family nurse practitioner at the Health Annex in Philadelphia, a Federally Qualified Health Center. She is involved in research on the health-promoting behaviors and metabolic syndrome. She is most proud of her recent appointment by Secretary Levitt to the National Advisory Council on Nursing Education and Practice (NACNEP) and as President-Elect of the National Organization of Nurse Practitioner Faculties (NONPF).

Deborah Gilbert-Palmer, EdD, FNP-BC, received her associate degree in nursing in 1985 from the University of West Virginia. Her nursing career includes pediatric oncology nursing for 10 years at St. Jude Children's Research Hospital and Emergency Medicine. In 1993, she completed her bachelor's degree in nursing at the University of Tennessee-Memphis, and went on to complete a master's degree in nursing in the Family Nurse Practitioner Program at the University of Tennessee in 1995. She was credentialed as a Family Nurse Practitioner by the

American Nurses Credentialing Center in 1995. She has practiced in primary care settings in rural Missouri and Arkansas for the past 13 years. In 2000, she joined the faculty at Arkansas State University and now, as an associate professor, coordinates the FNP program. In 2005, she completed her doctorate in educational leadership.

Mary Ann Krisman-Scott, RN, PhD, FNP-BC, is a certified Family Nurse Practitioner. Her research interests are nursing history, particularly care of the dying, and hospice. Mary Ann received her BSN from Catholic University and her MSN and PhD from the University of Pennsylvania. She has 23 years of experience as a family nurse practitioner and 20 years of teaching experience in both the university setting and in staff education. She is a recipient of the Provost's Award for Teaching at the University of Pennsylvania. She, along with her two co-authors, received the American College of Nurse Midwives Book of the Year Award for their textbook *Educating Advance Practice Nurses and Midwives: From Practice to Teaching*. She is a frequent presenter at professional meetings and has a number of peer-reviewed publications. Dr. Krisman-Scott is a veteran of Vietnam and is represented on a mural in Philadelphia saluting nurses in the United States. She has had significant involvement in international nursing and has been a consultant to a number of Eastern European nursing organizations, hospitals, and ministries of health.

Lisa Neri, MSN, CRNP, has practiced as a family nurse practitioner in Chester Springs, Pennsylvania, since 1999. Prior to 1999, Neri worked in critical care and emergency nursing. She has served as a preceptor for nurse practitioner students from Widener University and is active in the ChesMont chapter of the Pennsylvania Coalition of Nurse Practitioners (PCNP), where she served as president from 2001 to 2006. Neri continues to serve as their educational coordinator and representative to the executive board of PCNP.

Elizabeth Petit de Mange, PhD, MSN, BSN, NP-C, RN, is an Assistant Professor at Villanova University College of Nursing. She earned her PhD in nursing from the University of Colorado in 2002. She earned an associate degree in Nursing from Gloucester County College in 1980, a BSN from Thomas Jefferson University in 1986, an MSN in nursing administration from Widener University in 1989, and a post-master's Family Nurse Practitioner Certificate from Wilmington College in 2007. Dr. Petit de Mange has taught at the undergraduate and graduate levels in nursing since 1989 in classroom and virtual settings. Her clinical practice has included the care of children and adults in rural and urban healthcare settings. Dr. Petit de Mange's primary interests include an examination of health disparities among ethnic minorities and the healthcare needs of homeless populations. Dr. Petit de Mange also is interested in the interconnectedness between cultural beliefs and practices on health outcomes, particularly among Native American populations.

Barbara Rideout, MSN, APRN-BC, currently works as the nurse practitioner in Student Health at Drexel University. Student Health is operated by the Division of Family Medicine in the College of Medicine. She participates in precepting medical students, family medicine and pediatric residents, and nurse practitioner students who rotate through Student Health. Her previous experience includes teaching in associate degree, BSN, RN-BSN, and MSN (adult NP and FNP) programs. The focus of her teaching at the undergraduate level was fundamentals of nursing and medical-surgical nursing. She taught all of the GI and GU content across the curriculum. Rideout was assistant director of nursing for continuing education and quality assurance for 7 years before returning to teaching in 1988. She spent 20 years as clinical nurse specialist in ostomy and wound care, was a founding member of what is now the National Nursing Centers Consortium, and was clinical director of nurse-managed health centers for Temple University and Drexel University. Her degrees include BSN (as RN-BSN) from the University of Delaware, 1980; MSN (nursing education) from Villanova University, 1986; post-master's in adult primary care from Temple University, 1997; and post-master's family nurse practitioner, Drexel University, 2000.

Barbara Siebert, MSN, CRNP, FNP-BC, is a clinical assistant professor at Drexel University College of Nursing & Health Professions, Philadelphia, where she is the track coordinator for the Women's Health Nurse Practitioner Program and the Women's Health Nurse Practitioner MSN Completion Program. From 1993–2006, Siebert was the Associate Director of Planned Parenthood Federation of America's Women's Health Nurse Practitioner Program. In 1979, she received her diploma in nursing from Holy Name Hospital School of Nursing, in Teaneck, NJ, and her BSN from Dominican College of Blauvelt (NY) in 1981. She received her MSN as a family nurse practitioner from the Medical College of Virginia/Virginia Commonwealth University School of Nursing in 1986. In 1995, Siebert received a post-master's in graduate nursing education from the University of Pennsylvania's School of Nursing. As an FNP, she has extensive clinical experience providing comprehensive medical and family planning/gynecological health care to adolescents and primary health care to adults across the life span. She maintains a clinical practice at the Adolescent Health Department of St. Christopher's Hospital for Children in Philadelphia. In addition to her clinical and teaching responsibilities at Drexel University College of Nursing & Health Professions, Siebert lectures on anatomy and physiology of the male and female reproductive systems and conducts workshops for clinicians teaching comprehensive and gender-sensitive male and female genital examinations throughout the country.

NOTES